Seventh Edition

OUR GLOBAL ENVIRONMENT

A Health Perspective

Anne Nadakavukaren

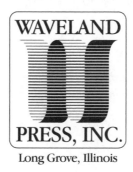

WAVELAND
PRESS, INC.

Long Grove, Illinois

For information about this book, contact:
    Waveland Press, Inc.
    4180 IL Route 83, Suite 101
    Long Grove, IL 60047-9580
    (847) 634-0081
    info@waveland.com
    www.waveland.com

Photo credits: Part 1 (page 1), Lynn Betts, Natural Resources Conservation Service; Part 2 (page 123), AP Photo; Part 3 (page 277), Tom Curtin.

10-digit ISBN 1-57766-686-0
13-digit ISBN 978-1-57766-686-8

Printed in the United States of America

7   6   5   4   3

OUR GLOBAL ENVIRONMENT

Contents

• • • • • • • • • • • • • • • •

Part 3
Environmental Degradation:
How We Foul Our Own Nest   277

• • • • • • • • • • • • • • • •

Preface

*O*ur Global Environment: A Health Perspective is intended as a text for introductory level courses in environmental health or human ecology, presenting a broad survey of the major environmental issues facing society early in the 21st century. The book combines an overall ecological concern with specific elements related to personal and community health, emphasizing the interrelatedness of the two and conveying to students an awareness of how current environmental issues directly affect their own lives.

Commencing with a rudimentary discussion of general ecological principles, the text focuses primarily on our present population-resources-pollution crisis and explains why human health and welfare depend on successful resolution of these challenges. Intended for a one-semester course, the text consists of 17 chapters and is divided into three main sections, each with its own introduction. Discussion within each chapter covers general aspects of the subject in question, while specific illustrative examples are treated in box inserts. The seventh edition features a new chapter on clean energy alternatives as well as extensive revisions and updates to material covered in previous editions.

In order to give students a perspective on the kinds of actions being taken to deal with identified problems, a brief description of federal statutes dealing with particular environmental issues is included wherever appropriate. Moreover, the text reviews the latest developments in international efforts to negotiate binding treaties on issues of global concern, such as climate change, ozone-layer depletion, and tobacco use, and incorporates numerous examples of environmental problems and solutions from other nations. Appendices at the end of the book describe the various federal agencies dealing with environmental and health issues and provide names and Web addresses of major non-governmental environmental organizations for the benefit of those students who wish to obtain further information or to become actively affiliated with such groups. The ability of citizens to influence public policy is stressed throughout the book, a basic purpose of the text being to provide students with sufficient information and insight into environmental problems to enable them to understand and participate in the public decision-making processes that will profoundly influence health and environmental quality in the decades ahead.

I would like to express my sincere gratitude to J. Randy Winter, Associate Director of the Center for Renewable Energy at Illinois State University, who reviewed the new chapter on clean energy alternatives and provided very useful comments and suggestions. I would also like to acknowledge the following: Heinz Russelmann, former Director of the Environmental Health Program at Illinois State University, whose encouragement, suggestions, and review of earlier editions of this text have been of invaluable assistance; Dr. Kenneth Jesse, Professor of Physics (retired) at Illinois State University, for his thoughtful review and valuable suggestions on matters pertaining to ionizing radiation and noise pollution; Dr. Anthony Otsuka, Professor in the Biological Sciences Department at Illinois State University, for his insightful comments on the sections dealing with mutations and cancer; former colleague Phil Kneller, now at Western Carolina University, and Tom Anderson of the McLean County Health Department for their suggestions and review of material on foodborne disease; Dr. Gregory Crouch, Associate Director of the Department of Environmental Health and Safety at Indiana University, for his valuable input on risk assessment and related topics; Laurie Prossnitz, Waveland Press, whose friendly cooperation and painstaking editorial efforts have been sincerely appreciated; Neil Rowe, publisher of Waveland Press, for his cooperation and help; and especially my husband and daughters for their loving support and understanding during the course of this project.

Anne Nadakavukaren

In nature there are neither rewards nor
punishments—there are consequences.
—R. G. Ingersoll

········ Part 1 ········

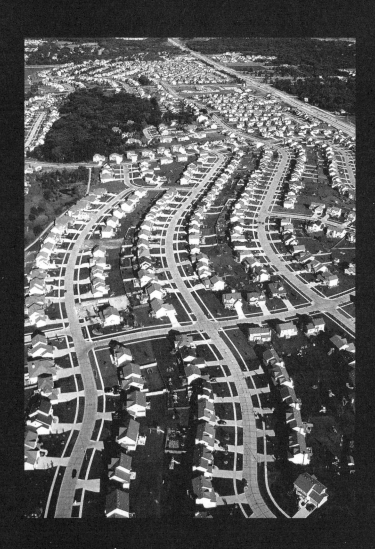

People, Progress,
and Nature

Is Conflict Inevitable?

Human beings, as a species, are unquestionably the dominant form of life on earth today. Inhabiting every continent, roaming the seas, exploring space, creating glittering cities and festering slums, taming rivers, bringing water to the desert, harnessing the atom, tinkering with the gene—people often deceive themselves into believing they are all-powerful creatures, apart from the rest of nature. Yet a half-million years of cultural evolution cannot alter the fact that humans, like all other living organisms, are inextricably bound up in the web of interdependency and interrelationships that characterize life on this planet. Human health, well-being, and indeed survival are ultimately dependent on the health and integrity of the whole environment in which we live. Today, the natural world that we share with all other forms of life on this planet is under unprecedented attack, not by outside forces of evil, as in a science fiction movie, but rather by a wide range of human activities and the sheer pressure of human numbers. Sometimes unwittingly, sometimes with full awareness of the consequences of our actions, we are rapidly altering the basic foundations of the environment that sustains us.

Although the destructive impact of human activities on the natural environment is nothing new—as the extinction of woolly mammoths by Prehistoric hunters or the deforestation of ancient Greece bears witness—the "human footprint" has expanded exponentially during the past two centuries, particularly in the years since World War II. What were once local or regional problems have now become issues of global concern, demanding unprecedented international cooperation if they are ever to be resolved. Achieving such cooperation and commitment requires a fundamental understanding of the nature of the problems facing society and a realization by policy makers and the public of the consequences of inaction.

In the United States, attitudes regarding humanity's relationship to the natural world have changed radically during the past 100 years. Reflecting prevailing beliefs in the "Old World" countries from which they came, most pre-20th century American immigrants considered themselves "above" nature and viewed the seemingly infinite resources of a sparsely populated continent simply as "things" to be exploited for human benefit. Though a few early American writers like Thoreau extolled the value of unspoiled surroundings, most of his contemporaries viewed wilderness as an enemy to be conquered and proceeded to do so. After the Civil War, destruction of America's natural heritage accelerated, as railroads connected the far-flung regions of a vast continent and millions of settlers streamed westward. By the end of the 1800s, the "frontier" was no more; most of the virgin forests east of the Mississippi had been felled, the enormous herds of bison that once blanketed the Great Plains had been reduced to a pitiful remnant, and the passenger pigeon was about to become extinct.

At the dawn of the 20th century, attitudes toward the natural world slowly began to change. At first, concerns focused on the rate at which Americans were depleting what had once seemed an inexhaustible supply of natural resources. The so-called Progressive Conservation Movement was led not by citizen activists but by scientific professionals—experts in forestry, botany, geology, hydrology—and championed by a young, intelligent, and energetic president, Theodore Roosevelt. Influenced by his conservationist friend, John Muir, Roosevelt set aside land for

2

national forest reserves and national monuments. By the time he left office in 1909, national forest acreage had nearly tripled to 100 million acres. Early 20th-century conservationists like Roosevelt, Muir, and forestry expert Gifford Pinchot bore little resemblance to present-day environmentalists, however; most were wealthy sportsmen, primarily interested in saving resources for use by future generations. The integrity of ecosystems or the human health impact of pollutants had not yet entered the consciousness of those who called themselves "conservationists." Nevertheless, our modern concern for wilderness, biodiversity, and natural beauty was born from the collective thinking of these pioneers of the movement.

Following Teddy Roosevelt, a succession of presidents, both uninformed and uninterested in the conservation issues so enthusiastically addressed by their predecessor, largely ignored such matters. Not until the Dust Bowl days of the 1930s was the conservation theme revived by President Franklin Roosevelt, whose administration first tackled the all-too-obvious problem of soil erosion by creating the Soil Conservation Service.

World War II brought an end to the Great Depression and spawned momentous new forces that radically altered life on this planet, greatly accelerating the pace and expanding the scope of environmentally destructive forces. WW II marked an epochal environmental turning point in numerous ways. Exposure to ionizing radiation in the form of fallout from nuclear bomb testing made the post-war generation of children the first to grow up with strontium-90 in their bones. The fruits of wartime research on DDT ushered in a new "Age of Chemicals" that promised to end the scourge of insect-borne disease and famine but subsequently proved to have a darker side as well. In the immediate post-war years, wartime austerity receded into memory, succeeded by a period of booming prosperity and reckless optimism regarding the benefits of growth. Industrial and agricultural production soared and Americans rushed forward in a feverish quest for the "good life" through rampant consumerism. While a few scientists fretted that the environmental life-support systems undergirding national prosperity were being undermined, most citizens believed that no price was too great to pay for economic growth.

The public's comfortable assumption that everything was rosy was irreversibly shattered in 1962 by an unassuming middle-aged woman, Rachel Carson, whose best-selling book, *Silent Spring*, constituted a scathing indictment of humanity's war against nature, especially the indiscriminate use of chemical pesticides. It's difficult for young people today to comprehend the impact *Silent Spring* had in 1962. To a large extent, the book's publication marked the opening salvo of the environmental revolution (in fact, Carson was the first to popularize the word "environment") because *Silent Spring* succeeded in

opening the public's eyes to the full extent of a problem they had hitherto ignored. *Silent Spring* expanded the earlier elitist focus on wilderness preservation and resource conservation to include toxics issues and human health—concerns to which the vast middle class of Americans could whole-heartedly relate. During the 1960s, "ecology" became a household word, introduced by career biologists who, having identified environmental abuses, raised the alarm at what they saw. By the late 1960s the public, too, had become aware of what was happening, reacting with dismay to pollution-choked rivers and smoggy skies, and demanding the policy actions that characterized the following decades.

The fledgling environmental movement gained momentum in 1969 due to a series of eco-disasters that convinced ordinary citizens "enough is enough!" Key events that year included an offshore oil rig blowout at Santa Barbara that fouled scenic California beaches with sticky crude and dying seabirds (an event that provoked as much public outrage and media attention as the notorious BP oil spill in the Gulf of Mexico in 2010); a spectacular fire raging across the surface of Cleveland's grossly polluted Cuyahoga River; and an application by giant oil companies for permission to build an oil pipeline across Alaska.

These and other mounting environmental insults prompted Wisconsin Senator Gaylord Nelson to suggest the nation hold an "Environmental Teach-In," an idea that quickly caught on and culminated in a coast-to-coast public relations event held on April 22, 1970—the first national celebration of Earth Day. Acclaimed as the "largest one-day outpouring of public support for any social cause in American history," Earth Day 1970 attracted participants from all walks of life—biologists, bureaucrats, homemakers, farmers, economists, educators, and millions of students. Older Americans protesting the gradual uglification of "America the Beautiful" also offered strong support, as did many existing national environmental organizations such as the Sierra Club, National Wildlife Federation, Audubon Society, and others. Not surprisingly, the burgeoning environmental movement had opponents as well, particularly among those who viewed activists' demands as a threat to corporate profits. Many observers at the time downplayed the significance of environmentalism, assuming it was simply the latest fad among white, liberal "flower children." But they were wrong. Environmentalism didn't fade away after April 1970 but rather was institutionalized in the form of an impressive array of far-reaching new laws enacted by Congress during the 1970s. These laws today constitute the legal framework for America's war against pollution and ecological degradation. Earth Day made environmentalism a permanent issue in U.S. political dialogue.

Over the years since the first Earth Day, the U.S. has devoted an enormous amount of time, money, and people power to solving the environmental problems highlighted by that event. Many of those efforts are still ongoing and some have met with a considerable degree of success—certainly the air Americans breathe today and the waterways in which they recreate are far cleaner than they were in the late 1960s and early 1970s. However, as in so many aspects of life, it seems that no sooner do we solve one problem than several more emerge to take its place. As U.S. air quality, water quality, and the management of solid and hazardous wastes gradually improved, concerns regarding global-scale challenges such as ozone-layer depletion, desertification, loss of biodiversity, and climate change took center stage—

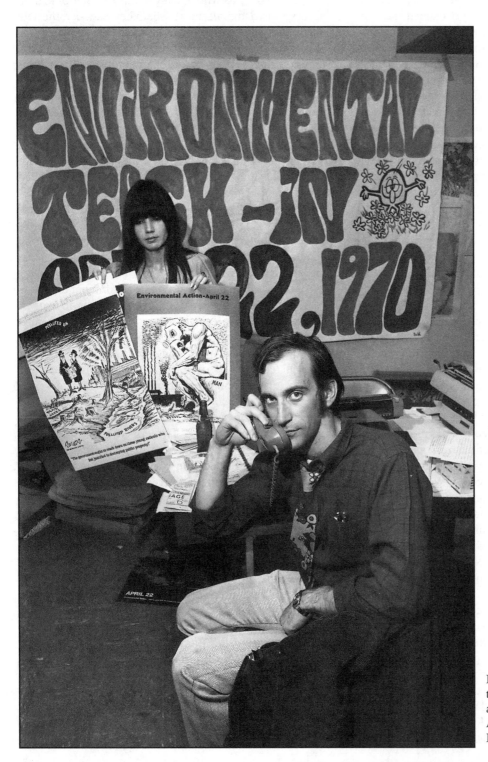

Denis Hayes, head of Environmental Teach-In, Inc., coordinated the activities for the first Earth Day on April 22, 1970, from his Washington, DC office. [*AP Photo*]

but have proven much more difficult to resolve. Solutions to these problems require far more than a quick technological "fix" like installing scrubbers on polluting power plants. Instead, success ultimately depends on halting population growth, devising new energy and transportation strategies, making fundamental changes in how the world's agricultural and forest lands are managed, and so forth.

The contrast between the public's response to the relatively straightforward environmental problems of the early 1970s and those confronting society today has been aptly described by Gus Speth, founder of the World Resources Institute and author of the thought-provoking book *Red Sky at Morning* (2004). Whereas the pollution/toxics problems evoking protests in the 1970s were close to home and easy to understand (what's confusing about a toxic waste dump in your backyard?!), those now on the global agenda are scientifically complex and still subject to a degree of uncertainty. The earlier problems were highly visible and immediate—robins dying of pesticide poisoning—but climatologists' warnings of the dire consequences associated with global warming a century hence strike many people as too theoretical and too far in the future to worry about today, even though scientists insist that meaningful action must be taken within the next few years in order to avert irreversible eco-catastrophe. Similarly, since the major impacts of climate change, tropical deforestation, and species loss will be on people and places far away rather than on our own communities, we're less motivated to take potentially painful policy actions than was the case four decades ago. All of these factors have diluted the once-emphatic demand that government "do something right now!" to address these issues.

Organized political opposition from vested interests who feel threatened by specific policies or actions proposed to address global environmental challenges have also increasingly blocked adoption of major new initiatives. Political leadership at the highest levels of government, such as that exemplified by Teddy Roosevelt over a century ago, had largely been lacking in the U.S. until the election of President Barack Obama in 2008 inspired new hope among American environmentalists. Though once the undisputed leader in cutting-edge environmental initiatives, during the Bush years the U.S. was widely criticized for obstructing international efforts to deal meaningfully with a wide array of global environmental problems, most notably that of climate change. As a result, the nations of Western Europe, largely indifferent to such issues until the mid-1980s, took over as the leading environmental actors on the world stage, moving ahead to forge an international climate change treaty, beginning to "green" their economies, and surpassing the United States in clean energy initiatives. However, in spite of laudable gains on the European front, it was obvious to all that without the active cooperation and engage-

ment of the world's largest economy and third most populous nation (i.e., the U.S.), future progress in resolving global environmental issues would be limited at best.

The election of President Obama marked a radical shift in U.S. environmental policy, though securing congressional approval for desired policy objectives has proven to be challenging. The Obama administration fully supports the prevailing scientific consensus on the urgent need to mitigate climate change by reducing carbon emissions and transitioning to a clean energy economy. Its commitment to fight climate change and strengthen environmental protection across the board is reflected in the appointments the president has made to key government agencies dealing with health and environmental issues and by efforts to engage other major powers—and major polluters—like China and India to take action as well. The challenges ahead are immense, but a new commitment on the part of the U.S. government to become actively involved in seeking solutions is a welcome change in direction, albeit one that needs to be followed up by legislative action.

The responsibility for protecting and preserving our global environment, however, rests with individuals as well as with their governments. Fortunately, one of the most hopeful trends for reversing the current downward spiral of environmental degradation is the worldwide proliferation of small grassroots organizations made up of committed citizens, working independently on their own local problems in the recognition that we don't have to sit back as passive spectators to the despoliation of our environment. They realize that much can be done to limit the impact of advanced technology on the natural world and to incorporate environmental considerations into national policy making. These activists, ordinary people from all walks of life, have an important message for the rest of us: to a great extent the technical know-how to prevent further deterioration exists—what is needed most is a societal commitment to get the job done.

The most important decisions being made in the environmental health arena today are political decisions, balancing ecological concerns with economic and social considerations. Individuals wishing to become involved in protecting and enhancing environmental quality will find their efforts most effective when directed toward influencing environmental policy-making bodies at every level of government. To be a successful eco-advocate, however, requires a thorough understanding of the nature of our environmental crisis, how the present situation developed, what the human impact of these threats may be, and what actions have already been taken in an attempt to restore and maintain a quality environment. These are the issues this book will attempt to address in the belief that a well-informed, politically active citizenry is an essential ingredient for staving off eco-catastrophe and embracing programs of sustainable development.

Hurt not the earth, neither the sea, nor the trees.
—Bible, Revelations 7:3

Introduction to Ecological Principles

In July of 1969, when astronauts Neil Armstrong and "Buzz" Aldrin became the first humans to land on the moon and gazed back at their home planet more than 200,000 miles away, they were filled with a sense of wonder at the beauty and uniqueness of Earth. Of all the heavenly bodies of which we are aware, our planet is neither the largest nor the smallest, the hottest nor the coldest, yet it *is* extraordinary in one vital respect—in all the universe Earth is the only planet known to support life. Within the narrow film of air, soil, and water that envelops the surface of the globe, extending vertically from the deepest ocean trenches more than 36,000 feet below sea level to about 30,000 or more feet above sea level, exists what ecologists call the **biosphere**—that portion of Earth where life occurs.

The known limits of the biosphere have been steadily expanding as scientific discoveries over the past several decades have revealed an astonishing array of species thriving in habitats once regarded as too extreme to support life. Such surprises include heat-loving bacteria living near deep-sea hydrothermal vents where water temperatures may reach 250°F (121°C) and microbes feasting on sulfur compounds in oil deposits more than 5,000 feet below the earth's surface (Smil, 2002; Kashefi and Lovely, 2003). Nevertheless, even though a number of bizarre aquatic species inhabit the ocean depths and bioaerosols such as microbial spores and pollen grains may be found

floating in the upper reaches of the atmosphere, by far the greatest number of living things are found in the region extending from the permanent snow line of tropical and subtropical mountain ranges (about 20,000 feet above sea level) to the limit of light penetration in the clearest oceans (about 600 feet deep). Here a vast assemblage of plant, animal, and microbial life can be found—approximately 1.8 million named species and millions more assumed to be awaiting discovery. These species interact both with each other and with their physical environment; over very long periods of time they become modified in response to environmental pressures and, in turn, they themselves modify their physical surroundings.

The first living organisms on Earth (probably forms similar to bacteria) are now thought to have arisen more than 3.5 billion years ago on a planet whose environment was considerably different from that of the present-day world. The life activities of those early organisms, feeding upon and reacting with the chemical compounds in the waters where they first arose, were responsible for the creation of the modern atmosphere, which made possible the emergence of higher forms of life. The first primitive organisms evolved in a world devoid of atmospheric oxygen but rich in carbon dioxide. This carbon dioxide in turn provided a carbon source for the evolutionarily more advanced photosynthetic organisms that could produce their own food by utilizing the sun's energy to convert carbon dioxide and water into carbohydrates, releasing oxygen as a waste product. It was through the action of such photosynthetic organisms that Earth's atmosphere gradually became an oxygen-rich one, permitting the development of the types of life with which we are familiar today. In this way, the life activities of one group of organisms profoundly altered the environment and created conditions that facilitated the emergence of other forms of life. The ability of living things to modify their surroundings and the tendency of other organisms to respond positively or negatively to such changes have been constant features of evolutionary progression throughout the ages and remain so today.

ECOSYSTEMS

The concept of nature as divided into basic functional units called **ecosystems** reflects scientists' recognition of the complex manner in which living organisms interact with each other and with the nonliving (or abiotic) components of their environment to process energy and cycle nutrients. The concept is admittedly imprecise, since few ecosystems have definitive spatial boundaries or exist in splendid isolation. Adjacent ecosystems commonly influence each other, as when a pond ecosystem is altered by materials washing into it from surrounding terrestrial ecosystems, and certain components (e.g., water birds, insects) may be moving in and out on a regular basis (Smith, 1986). Similarly, the concept of ecosystems is a broad one, its main usefulness being to emphasize the interdependence of the biotic and abiotic components of an area. An ecosystem has no defining size limitations: an abandoned tire casing containing trapped rainwater, microorganisms, and swarms of mosquito larvae can be regarded as an ecosystem; so can a family-room aquarium, a city park, a cornfield, a tide pool, a cow pasture, or, indeed, the entire planet Earth. Any of these widely diverse situations can be considered an ecosystem so long as living and nonliving elements are present and interacting to process energy and cycle materials (Stiling, 1992).

BIOTIC COMMUNITY

The most familiar classification system used for grouping plants and animals is one based upon presumed

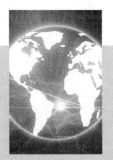

· · · · · · · 1~1 · · · · · · · ·

Western Forests Under Siege

For in nature nothing takes place in isolation. Everything affects every other thing . . .
Frederick Engels, *Dialectics of Nature,* 1895

An ecological tragedy has been unfolding over the past decade in the forests of the western United States and Canada. The complex cast of characters includes several species of pine, a tiny native beetle, a blue-stained fungus, drought, wildfires, grizzly bears, and climate change. Dramatizing the truism that "all components of nature are interrelated and interconnected," the cascading ecological repercussions of an unprecedented outbreak of the mountain pine beetle *(Dendroctonus ponderosae)* are devastating millions of acres of forest and wreaking long-term havoc on wildlife populations and on the physical environment.

The mountain pine beetle, a small (5–7.5 mm long) black insect native to western North America, lays its eggs in a vertical gallery under the bark of various pine tree species—lodgepole pine, whitebark pine, and ponderosa pine among its favorites. They also introduce a fungus that compounds beetle damage by staining the sapwood a telltale bluish-gray. Newly hatched larvae feed on the phloem layer within the tree, blocking the flow of sap that might otherwise drown the immature insects. In most cases, infested trees die within a month of being attacked, turning affected forests from a healthy green to a rusty red color. In the past, healthy pines usually managed to fend off their attackers by secreting copious amounts of resin to expel invading beetles. For a variety of reasons, however, pine trees across the West today are severely stressed and thus less able to protect themselves.

The origins of the current onslaught may extend back to the beginning of the 20th century, when fires and heavy logging cleared large areas of all trees. When the forest subsequently regenerated, all the trees were of approximately the same age and often of the same species, unlike the original forest cover that was less dense and more biologically diverse. Since mountain pine beetles typically target larger-diameter trees—particularly those 80 years of age or older—by the early 21st century these densely planted, old-growth forests were made-to-order for a beetle invasion.

Other factors have further contributed to the pines' vulnerability. Years of drought in the West have weakened the trees and undermined their natural defenses, as has forest overcrowding due to many decades of fire suppression. Among whitebark pines, an infestation of blister rust, an alien invasive fungal disease, has rendered the trees more susceptible to beetle attack. Most insidious of all has been the impact of climate change; over the past 40 years, temperatures in the United States have risen by about 0.4°C per decade, slightly more at higher elevations in the western states where these forests predominate (van Mantgem et al., 2009). While a warmer climate limits the range of certain pine species that are adapted to life in cool mountain areas, it facilitates spread of the mountain pine beetle to areas formerly too cold for the insect to survive over winter. Only with a return to former wintertime low temperatures of -30°F and below is the expansion in the mountain pine beetle's range likely to be checked—and, given climate change trends, that's not going to happen any time soon.

All these factors have combined to produce the most extensive insect infestation ever recorded in North America; by late 2008 British Columbia, the most severely affected area, had lost 33 million acres of lodgepole pine forest. In Colorado, Forest Service officials fear that every lodgepole pine over 5 inches in diameter will be dead within a few years and report that the beetles are now moving into lower-altitude ponderosa pine forests adjacent to residential areas. In Yellowstone National Park the whitebark pine forest could be functionally extinct before 2020; and, thanks to a freak windstorm in 2008 that blew mountain pine beetles over the continental divide from British Columbia into Alberta, experts warn that the insects could spread all the way to the Great Lakes (Robbins, 2008).

The ecological ramifications of western forest loss are devastating. In Yellowstone the demise of the whitebark pine, first to blister rust and now to the mountain pine beetle, threatens the survival of grizzly bears, for which whitebark pine nuts are a dietary staple. Red squirrels, Clark's nutcrackers, and black bears likewise are nourished by pine nuts, while deer, elk, and grouse are also dependent on the pine-dominated ecosystem for their survival (NRDC, 2009). Canadian forestry professionals worry that flash-flooding following tree loss will adversely affect salmon habitat due to increased siltation of streams—though they concede that woodpeckers and other insect-eaters stand to benefit from a bountiful food supply!

Proliferation of wildfires constitutes one of the most dangerous consequences of dying forests. Many western communities, like Colorado's Vail and Steamboat Springs, are now surrounded on all sides by dead trees. During the first few years following tree death, while the trunks are still standing, crown fires represent the greatest risk; after 4–5 years, however, trees begin to topple and the accumulated timber on the forest floor is a major hazard for catastrophic fires that can damage soil, inhibit regrowth of forest vegetation, cause mud slides during subsequent rain events, and result in siltation of natural waterways and reservoirs.

Beyond their obvious risk as a fire hazard, dead trees pose a safety threat as well. Park officials and ski resort owners are now busy removing dead trees, fearful that they could topple over and injure visitors; a number of campgrounds have been closed for that very reason. The Forest Service faces the monumental task of removing dead trees near highways before they fall onto roadways and block traffic. Finding a way to dispose of so much dead wood poses problems as well; there simply aren't enough sawmills still operating to process all of the dead timber from such a vast area. Innovative approaches to shred fallen trees for use in biomass boilers or process them into fuel pellets for wood-burning stoves or convert them into newsprint scarcely make a dent in the huge piles of dead wood. The economic implications of massive tree loss are of great concern to those in the commercial timber industry, dependent on high-quality lodgepole and ponderosa pine for a substantial share of their business. Even when beetle-infested timber can be salvaged, it typically sells for less than half the price of uninfested wood because of the blue stain left by the fungus. The tourist industry is worried as well, wondering how many visitors will want to vacation amidst desolate vistas of dead trees (Robbins, 2008).

There is as yet no conclusion to this story; government officials, business interests, conservation groups, and ordinary citizens continue to wrestle with the problem, searching for an effective response. In the meantime, the mountain pine beetle continues its inexorable spread, profoundly altering long-established biotic communities in western forests.

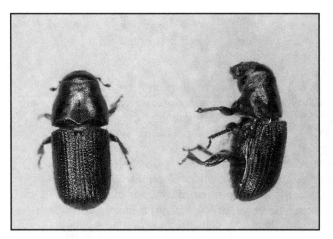

The diminutive mountain pine beetle is responsible for the most extensive insect infestation ever recorded in North America. [*USDA, Forest Service*]

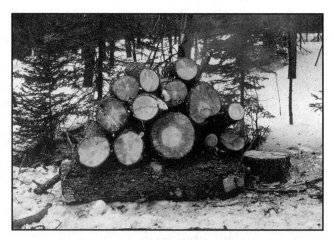

Beetle-infested trees are cut, piled, and ready to be burned. [*USDA, Forest Service*]

evolutionary relationships—lions, tigers, and leopards being grouped in the cat family; wheat, corn, and rice in the grass family; and so forth. However, ecologists tend to arrange species on the basis of their functional association with each other. A natural grouping of different kinds of plants and animals within any given habitat is termed by ecologists a **biotic community.**

Biotic community, like ecosystem, is a broad term that can be used to describe natural groupings of widely differing sizes, from the various microscopic diatoms and zooplankton swimming in a drop of pond water to the hundreds of species of trees, wildflowers, ferns, insects, birds, mammals, and so forth, found in an Appalachian forest. Biotic communities have characteristic trophic structures and energy flow patterns and also have a certain taxonomic unity, in the sense that certain species tend to exist together.

Individuals of the same species living together within a given area are collectively referred to as a **population.** Such populations constitute groups more or less isolated from other populations of the same species. A population within the biotic community of a region is not a static entity but is continually changing in size and reshuffling its hereditary characteristics in response to environmental changes and to fluctuations in the populations of other members of the community.

The community concept is one of the most important ecological principles because (1) it emphasizes the fact that different organisms are not arbitrarily scattered around the earth with no particular reason as to why they live where they do, but rather that they dwell together in an orderly manner; and (2) by illuminating the importance of the community as a whole to any of its individual parts, the community concept can be used by humans to manage a particular organism, in the sense of increasing or decreasing its numbers. Emphasizing biotic communi-

ties as a whole, rather than focusing on their constituent species, is helpful also in demonstrating why removing one species from a community (or, conversely, introducing a nonnative species into a community) can often have unintended—and sometimes disastrous—consequences.

European settlement of the sparsely populated North American continent launched a gigantic experiment in human interference with natural ecosystems. The sad tale of beaver exploitation provides one dramatic example of how a stable biotic community can unravel simply by eliminating one of its members. In the late 17th century, French traders began trapping these once-abundant mammals, shipping enormous numbers of valuable pelts back to Europe to accommodate the insatiable demands of the hat-making industry. So extensively and heavily were they hunted that within 150 years beavers faced extinction from the Great Lakes region all the way to Oregon and California. Only as their numbers plummeted did the beavers' role within their biotic community become apparent. With the demise of their architects, beaver dams were no longer maintained and eventually washed away. As a result, rates of stream flow sharply accelerated, destroying the spawning beds of fish species that relied on the quiet waters behind the dams for breeding. Marshy areas created by the dams were either drained or flooded, depending on location, and waterfowl populations declined as nesting sites were lost. Flooding increased in frequency and intensity, streamside erosion worsened, and siltation of river channels accelerated. Disappearance of the beaver, perceived by the trappers as a creature that was "going to waste" in the wilderness, thus led to surprisingly far-reaching effects (Ashworth, 1986). Some of these effects are now being reversed, thanks to an amazing comeback of beavers in North America. Since 1900, when beaver populations on the continent numbered but 100,000—almost exclusively in Canada—the regrowth of forests on abandoned farmland (and the fact that beaver hats are no longer fashionable!) has fostered a population explosion of these industrious mammals. Today there are an estimated 10–15 million beavers in the northern U.S. and Canada and their propensity for felling trees and damming streams in urbanized areas has caused some to regard them as unwanted pests. Nevertheless, they show no intention of retreating a second time and have brought many environmental benefits in the form of new wildlife habitat to the areas they have recently colonized (Dean, 2009).

Introducing a nonnative species (i.e., an exotic) into an established biotic community can be every bit as destabilizing as removing a component species. Time and again, accidentally or deliberately, humans have released plants or animals into a new environment only to see them quickly attain major pest status, usually due to the absence of natural predators that could keep their numbers under control. In the United States, West Nile encephalitis virus, zebra mussels, emerald ash borers, and northern snakeheads (the "pit bull" of fish) are but the most recent in a host of unwanted aliens to invade our shores—gypsy moths, European starlings, Asian carp, kudzu, purple loosestrife, water hyacinths, sea lampreys, Formosan termites—to mention but a few of the most notorious. Elsewhere in the world, exotic species have been equally disruptive; in the Netherlands, six North American muskrats brought to that country in 1906 have, in the absence of natural enemies, multiplied into the millions. Spreading throughout the country via the hundreds of thousands of miles of canals that characterize Holland, the muskrats have become major pests by burrowing into and weakening the vital dikes that protect the low-lying country from devastating floods. Along the Mediterra-

nean coast, a Pacific seaweed, *Caulerpa taxifolia*, accidentally released from aquarium tanks at Monaco's Oceanographic Museum, has proliferated from the French Riviera to the shores of Croatia. Wherever it goes, *Caulerpa* crowds out native plant and animal species, producing a monoculture that threatens to destroy the entire Mediterranean ecosystem. Another uninvited migrant native to the east coast of North America, Leidy's comb jelly, was discharged with ships' ballast water into the Black Sea where it has multiplied so rapidly since the late 1980s that a single cubic meter of seawater now contains as many as 500 of the tiny animals. Because the jellyfish out-competes native fish for the zooplankton both eat, populations of indigenous fish species have plummeted and the entire Black Sea ecosystem is now on the verge of collapse (Baskin, 2002; Bright, 1998).

In our attempts to "control" nature we must never forget that the intricate interdependencies that have evolved over the millennia among the biotic communities of the earth cannot be altered without provoking a corresponding change somewhere else in the ecosystem.

ECOLOGICAL DOMINANTS

Although all members of a biotic community have a role to play in the life of that community, it is obvious that certain plants or animals exert more of an influence on the ecosystem as a whole than do others. As George Orwell might have put it, "All animals are equal, but some animals are more equal than others." Those organisms which exert a major modifying influence on the community are known as **ecological dominants.** Such dominants generally comprise those species that control the flow of energy through the community; if they were removed from the community, much greater changes in the ecosystem would result than if a nondominant species were removed. For example, when farmers chop down the dominant hardwood trees in an eastern forest to clear the land for cultivation, the changes produced by this removal (i.e., loss of animal species that depend on the trees for food and shelter, loss of shade-loving plants that proliferate under the canopy, change in soil microbiota, raising of soil temperature, increase in soil erosion, and so forth) are much more pronounced than would be the changes brought about when the farmers' children wander into the forest and pick all of the trilliums and lady slippers they find growing there. In either case, the stability of the ecosystem is upset, but the loss of several species of spring wildflowers, while unfortunate, has much less effect on the forest community as a whole than does the loss of the dominant oaks, maples, and beeches.

In most terrestrial biotic communities certain plants comprise the dominant species because they not only provide food and shelter for other organisms, but also

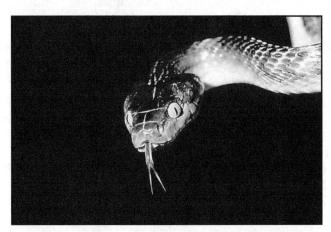

The brown tree snake, native to Australia, Papua New Guinea, and the Solomon Islands, is notorious for having nearly wiped out the native forest birds of Guam, where it appeared in the late 1940s or early 1950s, most likely having hitchhiked aboard military aircraft. [*USGS photo by G. Rodda*]

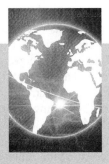

······· 1-2 ·······

Of Pythons and Porch Vines

Thoughtless actions often lead to unintended consequences. The growing popularity of exotic pets has given rise to a booming—and largely unregulated—trade in "unusual" animal companions from far-flung corners of the globe. Every year, according to the Union of Concerned Scientists, hundreds of millions of cute "pocket pets" such as pygmy hedgehogs, African dormice, fat-tailed gerbils, ferrets, and bush babies enter the United States from abroad, along with less-cuddly reptiles, tropical fish, and birds. Although generally beloved by their owners, these animals pose a potential threat to human health, as several past outbreaks of infectious diseases such as salmonellosis and monkeypox have been linked to the commercial trade in imported reptiles and Gambian rats, respectively. Equally problematic—and more dramatic—is the environmental havoc caused when some exotic species escape or are deliberately released by owners who have tired of caring for them. Not uncommonly, these freed pets become invasive in their new surroundings, preying on and out-competing native species and threatening the integrity of local ecosystems.

A prime example of the environmental harm that can result is the recent population explosion of Burmese pythons in the Florida Everglades. Purchased as cute (to some people!) little hatchlings at prices as low as $20 each, pythons can grow more than 20 feet long and weigh up to 200 pounds. Apparently a number of snake owners, unable or unwilling to care for their now-gigantic pets, have decided to release them into nearby forests or wetlands and let them fend for themselves. This might not be a major problem in places like northern Minnesota, but when it occurs in a semi-tropical setting like southern Florida, the reptiles thrive and multiply. Sightings of Burmese pythons are now being reported regularly in the Everglades, in mangrove swamps along the Florida coast, as well as in other wetland areas in the state. Everglades Park biologists estimate there are now tens of thousands of pythons slithering through state-managed lands around the Everglades. In 2006 several clutches of python eggs were discovered, evidence that the snakes are now breeding in the park and making eradication virtually impossible. In their new habitat pythons have found a bountiful food supply of small rodents, water birds, deer, even the occasional alligator! U.S. Fish and Wildlife Service personnel fear they may be competing for prey and living space with alligators and with the threatened eastern indigo snake; they are concerned about human safety as well.

Owners of exotic pets aren't the only group whose interests or hobbies unintentionally undermine ecological stability. For centuries, gardeners have carried plant species from one region of the world to another, often across ocean barriers that in earlier times protected established biotic communities from outside invaders. Most of these deliberately introduced crop plants, trees, and ornamentals have brought substantial benefits and few problems to their new environments, but a minority have become notorious invaders, outcompeting and overgrowing the native flora and posing an enormous economic burden in terms of lost production and eradication efforts. Among the more problematic species introduced by gardeners are dandelions, garlic mustard, water hyacinth, Cogon grass, English ivy, Japanese honeysuckle, barberry, mimosa, purple loosestrife, and multiflora rose. Most notorious, however, is kudzu *(Pueraria montana* var. lobata), originally known as "porch vine" for its decorative value around the verandas of southern homes.

Like so many introduced ornamental plants that subsequently became major pests, kudzu's spread was facilitated by human actions every step of the way. Native to China and Japan where it has numerous natural enemies that keep it under control, kudzu made its American debut in 1876 at Philadelphia's Centennial Exposition, where it was displayed among other horticultural plant varieties in the Japanese pavilion. The attractive vine captured the fancy of American gardeners and from 1876 until the early 1900s, the "porch vine" remained docile and well-behaved, used almost exclusively in residential settings. In 1902, however, the U.S. Department of Agriculture (USDA) saw kudzu as a potentially valuable plant for producing livestock fodder on degraded lands in the South and re-introduced it from Japan for that purpose. It was first planted commercially in 1910 in Florida and by the 1920s was being actively promoted as a forage crop by Florida nursery owners who did a brisk business selling kudzu plants by mail order. During the 1930s the

Soil Conservation Service began aggressively pushing kudzu for erosion control. The government was so convinced of kudzu's benefits for stabilizing soils that during the 1940s it distributed 85 million kudzu cuttings to farmers and paid them up to $8/acre to plant fields of it.

Unfortunately, kudzu soon proved itself to be a scourge; by 1953 it was removed from USDA's list of acceptable cover crops and attempts at eradication were launched. In 1972 USDA designated kudzu a "weed," meaning that it could no longer be used under the Agricultural Conservation Program; in 1998 it was given official status as a federally-listed "noxious weed." By then, however, it was far too late. In summertime, kudzu vines can grow up to a foot per day, 60 feet in a year. They climb up anything they come into contact with—trees, telephone poles, fences, abandoned buildings. By overgrowing trees and blocking their access to sunlight, kudzu infestations are destroying valuable southern forests and endangering the rich biodiversity they harbor. Southerners wryly joke that they "close their windows at night to keep the kudzu out." Today kudzu covers over 7 million acres in the southeastern United States, its northward spread limited primarily by the plant's intolerance of freezing weather. Kudzu is highly resistant to herbicide treatment and efforts to find a natural enemy to keep the vine under control have thus far been unsuccessful (some researchers believe that constant grazing can eliminate the vine and are experimenting with raising goats on wastelands overgrown with kudzu). As with python-infested wetlands, it looks as though southerners will have to accept kudzu as a landscape feature that's here to stay (Baskin, 2002; Winberry and Jones, n.d.).

Considering the immense adverse ecological and economic impacts of pythons, porch vines, and numerous other exotic species, little has been done to prevent future invasions, either in terms of public education efforts or through legislation. In regard to exotic pets, only a few governments, notably Australia, New Zealand, and Israel, require proactive screening to regulate the trade. In the United States, three states—California, Hawaii, and Florida—prohibit the sale of animals, especially small predators, that might become invasive if they were to escape into the wild. Elsewhere, unless an exotic animal eats plants or is on the list of endangered species banned from international trade, its entry as an article of commerce most likely will go unchallenged. Similarly, prior to importing new plant varieties into the U.S., neither horticulturalists nor the USDA's Agricultural Research Service routinely investigate their potential for becoming troublesome weeds. Even where regulations exist, Internet sales and transactions conducted at large garden shows and pet fairs make enforcement easy to circumvent. Legislation requiring that animal species be screened for their invasive potential prior to importation has been introduced in Congress almost every year since 2000 and is strongly supported by conservation groups; however, Congress has failed to act on the matter. In the meantime, the burden for preventing yet more harmful invasions will rest, by default, on individual pet owners and gardeners. Common sense can deter an invasion before the fact, but once an invader is well-established, solving the problem is nigh impossible.

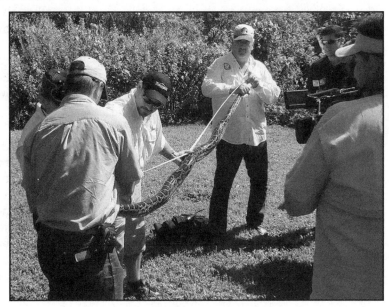

Burmese pythons have been found throughout Everglades National Park and adjacent areas. Here, Florida officials measure and photograph a 9-foot, 8-inch specimen in July 2009. [*Courtesy of Florida Fish and Wildlife Conservation Commission*]

directly affect and modify their physical environment. That is, they contribute to a build-up of topsoil, moderate fluctuations of temperature, improve moisture retention, affect the pH of the soil, and so on. As a general rule, the number of dominant species within a community becomes progressively fewer as one moves toward the poles and greater the closer the community is to the tropics. While a northern coniferous forest may consist of only spruces or firs, a jungle in Sumatra may have a dozen or more tree species that could be considered dominants. In addition to the effects of latitude, one can also generalize that dominant species are fewer in regions where climatic conditions are extreme, like tundra and deserts (Odum, 1959).

Among animal species in a biotic community, certain **keystone predators** help maintain greater biotic diversity than would exist in their absence. Keystone, or dominant, predators moderate competition among the species upon which they prey, reducing the density of strong competitors and thereby allowing less aggressive competitors to maintain their populations within the community. Sea otters along Alaska's Pacific coast represent a prime example of the importance of keystone predators. The stability of kelp "forests" in Alaskan coastal waters had long been maintained by sea otters that preyed heavily on kelp-eating sea urchins. With urchin populations held at tolerable levels, a food supply for other herbivores in that biotic community was maintained and a diverse range of species flourished. When otter numbers suddenly plummeted in the 1990s due to killer whale attacks, the population of sea urchins exploded, overwhelming their competitors and resulting in a sharp decline in the biodiversity of the kelp forest community (Estes et al., 1998).

BIOMES

The species composition of any particular biotic community is profoundly affected by the physical characteristics of the environment, particularly temperature and rainfall. The kinds of plants and animals one would see while touring Yellowstone National Park would differ significantly from those found on a trek through the Amazon. Ecologists have divided the terrestrial communities of the world into general groupings called **biomes,** areas that can be recognized by the distinctive life forms of their dominant species. In most cases, the key characteristic of a biome is its dominant type of vegetation. We might define a biome as a complex of communities characteristic of a regional climatic zone. Each biome has its own pattern of rainfall, its own seasons, its own maximum and minimum temperatures, and its own changes of day length, all of which combine to support a certain kind of vegetation. Since climatic zones change in a relatively uniform pattern as one moves from the poles toward the equator, the earth's biomes form more or less continuous latitudinal bands around the globe. Starting at the polar regions, let's take a brief look at the major biomes of the earth (note: ecologists list numerous subdivisions of the biomes described here, but for our purposes these general groupings will suffice).

Tundra

The northernmost of the world's land masses, tundra is characterized by permanently frozen subsoil called **permafrost.** In this biome rainfall is quite low, about 8 inches annually, but because the permafrost doesn't allow moisture to penetrate beyond the upper few inches of soil, the tundra in summer is dotted with numerous lakes and bogs—and probably the world's most voracious mosquitoes! The tundra is windy, with only a few stunted trees. The dominant vegetation here consists of moss, lichens, grass, and some small perennials. Animal life is limited in the number of species but very abundant in the number of individuals. These include caribou or reindeer, birds, insects, polar bears, lemmings, foxes, rabbits, and fish. Reptiles and amphibians are absent. The tundra is basically a very fragile environment. Because of the slow rates at which tundra plants grow and decompose (due to the low temperatures and the characteristics of permafrost), the thick, spongy matting of lichens, grasses, and sedges that typify tundra is especially slow to recover from disturbance. Tracks of vehicles or animals can remain visible for decades. Great care must be taken in building on tundra because heat from structures will melt the permafrost and cause uneven settling, which often badly distorts the buildings. Until the 1960s the tundra was relatively unexploited, but with the construction of the Alaska oil pipeline and similar kinds of mineral development in Canada and Siberia, that situation has changed. Impending climate change represents an even greater threat to tundra ecosystems, as rising temperatures result in widespread melting of permafrost—a process now well underway throughout the far North.

Taiga

A Russian word for "swamp forest," the taiga is sometimes called the **boreal forest.** This biome covers much of Canada, Scandinavia, and Russia. The Canadian taiga alone constitutes fully 10% of all forests worldwide and 25% of intact virgin forests. Here the dominant vegetation consists of conifer trees—mainly spruces, firs, and pines—that have needlelike leaves that stay on the trees for three to five years. Some deciduous trees such as aspens, alders, and larches are also prominent. In general, the trees are much less diverse in number of species than those in the deciduous forests farther south and the soils have a different kind of humus and are more acid. Precipitation in the taiga is only moderate but, because drainage is poor, lakes, ponds, and bogs are common here. Animals of the taiga include bears, moose, lynxes, weasels, wolverines, and 186 species of land birds; indeed, 30% of all land birds in Canada and the United States nest and raise their young in the boreal forest, though most migrate south as winter approaches (Blancher, 2002). Because of the huge stands of just one or two species of conifers, the taiga provides an opportunity for periodic outbreaks of pests like the spruce budworm, which can defoliate huge areas of forest. Perhaps because of the lack of diversity of species, taiga populations tend to undergo "boom or bust" cycles fairly regularly.

Temperate Deciduous Forest

This biome occurs in a belt south of the taiga where climate is milder and where rainfall is abundant relative to the amount of evaporation. This is the biome familiar to most of us because it is the one in which Western, as well as Chinese and Japanese, civilization developed. Soil types and elevations vary widely within this biome. Maples, beech, oaks, and hickories are common trees; many species of ferns and flowering herbaceous plants are also found. The deciduous forest has a great variety of mammals, birds, and insects, as well as a modest number of reptiles and amphibians. Because of the annual leaf drop, deciduous forests generate soils rich in nutrients, which in turn support a multitude of soil microbes. When such forests are cleared, the richness of the soils can be maintained if great care is taken to see that their supplies of nutrients and decaying organic matter are preserved (in a sense, raising crops or grazing animals is akin to mining the soil, since the nutrients leave along with the crops, meat, wool, or whatever is removed). All too often, however, short-term careless exploiters have allowed soils to deteriorate or have ignored opportunities to improve them. Unfortunately, economic considerations often lead individuals who are exploiting an ecosystem to use short-term strategies that are disastrous for humanity in the long run.

Table 1-1   100 of the World's Worst Invasive Alien Species

Micro-organisms	Land Plants *(cont'd.)*	Aquatic Invertebrates *(cont'd.)*	Fish *(cont'd.)*
avian malaria	kudzu	Mediterranean mussel	Mozambique tilapia
banana bunchy top virus	lantana	Northern Pacific seastar	Nile perch
rinderpest virus (cattle plague)	leafy spurge	rosy wolfsnail	rainbow trout
	leucaena	zebra mussel	walking catfish
Macrofungi	melaleuca		Western mosquito fish
chestnut blight	mesquite	**Land Invertebrates**	
crayfish plague	miconia	Argentine ant	**Birds**
Dutch elm disease	mile-a-minute weed	Asian longhorned beetle	Indian myna bird
chytrid frog fungi	mimosa	Asian tiger mosquito	red-vented bulbul
cinnamon fungus	privet	big-headed ant	starling
	pumpwood	common malaria mosquito	
Aquatic Plants	purple loosestrife	common wasp	**Reptiles**
caulerpa seaweed	quinine tree	crazy ant	brown tree snake
wakame seaweed	shoebutton ardisia	cypress aphid	red-eared slider
water hyacinth	Siam weed	Formosan subterranean termite	
	strawberry guava	gypsy moth	**Mammals**
Land Plants	tamarisk	khapra beetle	brushtail possum
African tulip tree	wedelia	little fire ant	feral cat
Australian acacia	yellow Himalayan raspberry	red imported fire ant	field mouse
Australian prickly pear		sweet potato whitefly	goat
Brazilian pepper tree	**Aquatic Invertebrates**		grey squirrel
cluster pine	Chinese mitten crab	**Amphibians**	long-tailed macaque
cogon grass	comb jelly fish	bullfrog	nutria
common cord-grass	fishhook waterflea	cane toad	pig
fire tree	flatworm	Caribbean tree frog	rabbit
giant reed	giant African snail		red deer
gorse	golden apple snail	**Fish**	red fox
hiptage	green crab	brown trout	ship rat
Japanese knotweed	marine clam	carp	short-tailed weasel
Kahili ginger		large-mouth bass	small Indian mongoose
Koster's curse			

Source: Courtesy of the Invasive Species Specialist Group, www.issg.org/database.

Grasslands

In regions where annual rainfall is not sufficient to sustain the growth of trees and evaporation rates are high, we find the grasslands of the world. These may be called by different names in various countries: prairie, veldt, savannah, steppe, pampas, llanos. All are characterized by the dominance of grasses and herds of grazing animals. Carnivores also abound, such as coyotes and lions, as do rodents and many species of reptiles. The grassland biome has a higher concentration of organic matter in its soil than does any other biome, the amount of humus in grassland soil being about 12 times greater than that in forest soils. The extraordinary richness of grassland soil has led to the establishment of extremely successful agricultural ecosystems in the grassland areas. These systems can break down rapidly, however, if careful soil conservation is not practiced. The interlaced roots and creeping underground stems of grasses form a turf that prevents erosion of the soil. When the turf is broken with a plow or overgrazed, the soil is exposed to the erosive influences of wind and water, resulting in such calamities as the "Dust Bowl" of the Great Plains in the 1930s. In temperate regions the widespread conversion of natural grasslands to cropland has greatly reduced the geographical extent of this biome. In the tropics, however, grasslands have expanded considerably as a result of deforestation; today tropical grasslands constitute the world's most extensive ecosystem (Smil, 2002).

Desert

Areas receiving less than 10 inches annual precipitation and featuring high daytime temperatures are classified as deserts. These areas are concentrated in the vicinity of 30° north and 30° south latitude. Lack of moisture is the essential factor shaping the desert biome. Most deserts are quite hot in the daytime and, because of the sparse vegetation and resultant rapid reradiation of heat, quite cold at night. Desert plants and animals are characterized by species that can withstand prolonged drought. Among plants such adaptations include waxy cuticle on stems or leaves, reduction in leaf size, and spiny growths to repel moisture-seeking animals. Plants may appear to be widely spaced, but if their roots were visible, the ground between them would be seen to be laced with a shallow root system to take maximum advantage of any rain that does fall. Proportionately more annual plants are found in the desert biome than in any other; because their seeds often require abrasion or a rain heavy enough to leach out inhibiting chemicals, the desert appears to bloom almost overnight after a heavy rain. For the most part, desert animals are active at night, remaining under cover during the heat of the day. Desert soils contain little organic matter and must ordinarily be supplied with both water and nitrogen fertilizer if they are to be cultivated. Human activities have already produced a great increase in the amount of desert and wasteland, removing many once-productive acres from cultivation. Occasional years of good rainfall cause people to forget that the desert is inherently a very fragile environment.

Tropical Rain Forest

This biome is found in Central and South America, central Africa, and South and Southeast Asia. It is characterized by high temperatures and high annual rainfall; 100 inches or more of annual precipitation is common in this biome. Year-round temperature variation is slight. Tropical rain forests are characterized by a great diversity of plant and animal species and by four distinct layers of plant growth—the top canopy of trees reaching 200 feet or more, a lower canopy of densely intertwined treetops at about 100 feet, a sparse understory, and only a very few plants growing at ground level. A wide variety of epiphytic plants can be found. Both plant and animal species exist in greater diversity in the tropical rain forest than anywhere else in the world, though numbers of individuals of a particular species are usually limited. To most people, the luxuriant growth of a tropical jungle implies a rich soil, and one hears many glowing promises of the agricultural riches to be reaped by turning the Amazon or Congo River basins into farmland. The truth of the situation is far different, however. Tropical forest soils in general are exceedingly thin and nutrient-poor. They cannot maintain large reserves of minerals needed for plant growth, primarily because heavy rainfall and a high rate of water flow through the ground to the water table leach them from the soil. The leaching process leaves large residues of insoluble iron and aluminum oxides in the upper levels of tropical forest soils, a process termed "laterization." With the exception of certain fertile river valleys, primitive slash-and-burn agriculture is the only type suitable to most areas of the tropical rain forest. Unfortunately, this fragile ecosystem is being destroyed more rapidly than any other biome due to human population growth and in some cases, such as in Brazil, as a direct consequence of governmental actions.

It should be noted that in areas where there are substantial variations in altitude, the biomes differ at different elevations. This is primarily because air temperature decreases about 6°C for every 1,000-meter increase in altitude and because, especially in desert areas, rainfall increases with altitude.

This brief survey of biome characteristics should make it obvious that various regions differ in their ability to return to an ecologically stable condition once they have been disrupted by human activities. Thus it should not be surprising that certain practices are far more devastating to the local ecology in some areas than they are in others. For example, strip mining in the flat or gently rolling lands of Illinois, Indiana, and Ohio is certainly disruptive to the environment, yet with proper soil reclamation practices the land can be restored to productive uses once mining has ceased. In the arid regions of the High Plains and Southwest, however, exploitation of fossil fuel reserves by strip mining presents a real threat that the acres thus despoiled could never recover and would remain permanent wastelands.

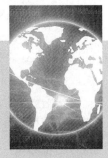

········ 1-3 ········

A New Lease on Life for the Everglades

Once degraded, can an ecosystem ever truly be restored? Federal and state officials in Florida, working in cooperation with conservation groups, are convinced the answer to this question is a resounding "yes" as they move forward on the **Comprehensive Everglades Restoration Plan (CERP)**. Authorized by Congress in 2000, the mammoth $8 billion, 30-year project now underway represents the most ambitious, far-reaching environmental restoration effort ever attempted anywhere. Among its prime objectives are reestablishing the area's natural water flow patterns to the greatest degree possible; improving wildlife habitat to protect biodiversity; ensuring a safe, reliable public water supply; and providing flood protection. Another essential element in protecting and restoring the Everglades ecosystem is curbing urban development in rapidly growing South Florida. By 2010 planners had anticipated a population of 8 million in the Miami area, up from 6 million in 2000. In the absence of wise-growth policies, urban sprawl and the water demands of additional millions will severely jeopardize Everglades restoration efforts. Currently a regional program called "Eastward Ho!" is striving to redirect new growth toward vacant land in already-developed areas and to alter building and zoning codes to require higher-density housing in new suburban developments.

The Everglades ecosystem, Florida's legendary "River of Grass," originally extended from the Kissimmee Chain of Lakes to Lake Okeechobee in the central part of the state southward more than 100 miles to Florida Bay, encompassing close to 8.9 million acres. Under incremental attack by human development for more than a century, the Everglades today is one of the most threatened ecosystems in the United States. Progressively dredged, drained, and diked, this once-vast swampland has shrunk to little more than half its original size. Flood control and other water management projects launched in 1948 under the Army Corps of Engineers' **Central and South Florida (C&SF) Project** made it possible for over 7 million people to live and work in the 18,000 square mile area, but the consequence of these efforts was ecologic disaster. The water demands of irrigated agriculture and of cities lining the Sunshine State's "Gold Coast," along with flood control projects and natural droughts, disrupted the natural sheet flow of water that for millennia sustained the natural rhythms of life throughout the Everglades. The environmental damage caused by this disruption has been compounded by serious degradation of water quality due to fertilizer-laden drainage from sugar cane fields since the early 1930s. Phosphate pollution in particular has precipitated massive fish kills and algal blooms, as well as the explosive growth of cattails.

Another major threat to ecosystem stability in the Everglades has been the melaleuca tree, an exotic Australian species introduced in 1906 to help drain the swamp; it did its job only too well and, in the absence of natural enemies, has displaced many of South Florida's native plant and animal species. As a result of drainage projects, pollution, and melaleuca, wildlife populations in the Everglades have plummeted in recent decades; breeding pairs of waterbirds are down 90% from former levels and 68 species of indigenous plants and animals are listed as threatened or endangered. Degradation of the Everglades threatens not only wildlife but Floridians as well, since the groundwater on which the southern part of the state depends, naturally replenished through hydrologic contact with the Everglades, is not being recharged as rapidly as in the past. Soil resources also are threatened as drainage projects and intensive agricultural production have exposed the rich topsoil to oxidation and erosion.

The slow ecological decline of this invaluable wetland resource has not gone unnoticed; since the early 1900s, activists have loudly protested the activities which, they warned, would destroy the very features that attracted people to South Florida in the first place. In 1947 preservationists convinced Congress to set aside the southern portion of the giant marshland as Everglades National Park. Several decades later, environmentalists began pressing toward a far more ambitious goal—re-engineering, and in some places undoing, the elaborate plumbing system that makes the Everglades the most intensively managed region on earth. In 1992 Congress authorized a comprehensive review of the C&SF Project and the following year established the South Florida Ecosystem Restoration Task Force. The state of Florida remained an active partner in these efforts, passing the 1994 Everglades Forever Act establishing a multifaceted program to restore large portions of the Everglades. Studies conducted throughout the 1990s under the joint direction of the U.S. Army Corps of Engineers and the South Florida Water Management District (SFWMD) culminated in passage of the federal legislation that in 2000 created CERP.

Unfortunately, progress toward meeting CERP's objectives has been agonizingly slow, largely due to inadequate funding. Much to the disappointment of conservationists, the restoration project has had to be scaled back several times, most recently in August 2010, when the SFWMD voted to purchase just 26,790 acres of land from U.S. Sugar Corporation, down from the 73,000 acres the state had announced it would buy in 2009 (two years earlier, the original deal with U.S. Sugar called for purchase of 187,000 acres, plus all the company's assets). The water district intends to use the newly acquired land to increase water storage and treatment for the Everglades and reserves the option to buy additional company acres included in the original deal sometime in the years ahead, if and when funds become available. Future federal dollars to augment state monies could be instrumental in obtaining the land environmentalists insist is essential if full restoration goals are to be realized.

Achieving all these objectives will be challenging and expensive, but the cost of allowing continued ecosystem degradation would be even higher. Years ago, author Marjorie Douglas, a tireless crusader for preservation of Florida's wetlands, aptly described the situation in a stirring call to action. "The Everglades is a test," she proclaimed. "If we pass, we get to keep the planet" (Derr, 1993).

ECOLOGICAL NICHES

Within any biotic community each species is defined by its own unique position, or **niche,** different from that of any other member of the community and determined largely by its size and food habits. Through the processes of evolution and natural selection, plants and animals have become increasingly better adapted to the specific environments in which they live. In order to reduce competition among species for food and living space, organisms have become more specialized in terms of the foods they utilize, period of the day or night during which they are active, and/or the types of microhabitats they exploit. Thus, in an ecological context, the term niche denotes not simply the physical space that a species occupies but, more importantly, what that species *does* (Pianka, 1988). The **Principle of Competitive Exclusion,** basic to ecological theory, holds that when two species are competing for the same limited resources, only one will survive. Only when the environmental resources in a given community are partitioned among the coinhabiting species by means of niche diversification is direct competition minimized, thus permitting coexistence of species.

The benefits of niche diversification can be well illustrated by several species of lice, which peacefully coexist on a human host by restricting their activities to different anatomical regions. The body louse, notorious in history as the vector of typhus fever, feeds on parts of the body below the neck; the closely related head louse confines its activities to the head and neck. The fact that the two are quite similar in appearance and occasionally interbreed indicates their close relationship, but niche diversification is quite apparent in their different behavioral patterns. Head lice cement their eggs ("nits") to hairs of the scalp, while body lice usually glue theirs to fibers of clothing; in fact, body lice spend most of their time on clothing, coming into contact with the human body only when taking a blood meal. A third type, the crab louse, is morphologically specialized for life among the widely spaced, coarse hairs of the pubic areas. Unlike body and head lice that constantly move about, crab lice tend to settle in one spot and feed off and on for many hours at a time. Through behavioral and territorial specialization, these species avoid competition and thrive in their own unique ecological niche.

In other situations, species may utilize the same physical space but minimize competition by restricting their feeding activities to different times of the day. Within any given area one can find some species that are diurnal (active during the day), such as most birds, grazing animals, primates, and so on; other species that are nocturnal (active at night), including most snakes, many predators such as lions, foxes, owls, and so on; and still others such as deer and rabbits that prefer the in-between hours of dawn and dusk. Structural modifications among species allow animals inhabiting the same general area to utilize different foods. The finches of the Galapagos Islands, immortalized by Charles Darwin, were very similar in appearance and obviously evolved from the same parental stock, but modifications in their beak structure permitted each species to utilize a different type of food—insects, small seeds, medium-sized seeds, or large seeds, depending on the size and shape of beak—and thus to coexist within the same geographic area.

Examples of niche diversification illustrate the fact that throughout evolutionary history ecosystems have become exceedingly complex through increasingly effective adaptation of organisms within any natural community. Such a complex ecosystem is generally quite stable unless something happens to change that environment. The processes of natural selection and adaptation are too slow to permit the vast majority of organisms to adjust quickly to radical changes in their surroundings. When such changes occur, the animal and plant populations generally die out or move elsewhere and the previously stable ecosystem collapses or, at a minimum, becomes less varied and less stable.

LIMITING FACTORS

Most of us intuitively realize that a specific plant, animal, or microbe can live in some places but not others. Corn plants, for example, thrive in central Illinois but not in Norway; ferns are abundant in Appalachian forests but not in the Mohave Desert; the bacterium responsible for botulism (*Clostridium botulinum*) may produce its poison in home-canned green beans but never in fresh ones. The reason why living things occur and thrive where they do depends upon a variety of conditions. Sometimes those conditions are quite obvious: summer temperatures in Norway are not hot enough nor is the growing season long enough to produce a bountiful corn harvest; lack of water and shade make survival of ferns impossible in a desert environment. In other cases the factors that control where a plant or animal lives are not quite so apparent: *Clostridium botulinum* can multiply and produce its deadly toxin only in an environment where oxygen is absent; hence it may present a threat in improperly canned foods, but seldom in fresh ones.

Environmental conditions that limit or control where an organism can live are called **limiting factors.** Obviously not every factor in an organism's environment is equally important in determining where that plant or animal can live. Components that are relatively constant

in amount and moderately abundant are seldom limiting factors, particularly if the individual in question has a wide limit of tolerance. On the other hand, if an individual has a narrow limit of tolerance for a factor that exists in low or variable amounts, then that factor might indeed be the crucial determinant in where the organism can live. For example, most higher forms of life require a plentiful supply of oxygen to carry out their metabolic activities. Nevertheless, even though oxygen is essential, because it is so abundantly present and readily available to most land plants and animals it is almost never a limiting factor in terrestrial communities. On the other hand, lack of oxygen can definitely be a limiting factor for a number of aquatic organisms. The larvae of certain insects such as mayflies and caddis flies, as well as important game fish such as brook trout, simply die or move elsewhere when levels of dissolved oxygen in a waterway drop below a critical point.

Although the Native Americans who taught the Pilgrims to bury a dead fish in each hill of corn must have intuitively understood the concept, the idea of limiting factors was first formulated in 1840 by the German biochemist Justus Liebig while studying problems of fertility in agricultural soils. Liebig was experimenting with the use of inorganic chemical fertilizers in place of manures then currently in use and found that crop yields were affected not so much by the nutrients needed in large quantities—such as carbon dioxide and water, since these were generally present in plentiful supply—but by some mineral, such as copper, needed in minute amounts but lacking from particular soils. From this observation he proclaimed his famous **Law of the Minimum**, stating that "the growth of a plant is dependent on the amount of foodstuff which is presented to it in a minimum quantity." Succeeding generations of ecologists have expanded Liebig's concept to include not only mineral nutrients but also such things as light, temperature, pH, water, oxygen supply, and soil type as possible limiting factors to the distribution of organisms.

Further investigations revealed a complicating fact: when some factor other than the minimum one is available in very high concentrations, this may moderate the rate at which the critical one is used. For example, plants growing in the shade require less zinc than those growing in the sun. Thus shade-grown plants are less affected by a zinc-deficient soil than are plants of the same species growing in full sunlight. Also, some organisms can substitute a chemically similar nutrient for one that is deficient, as can be seen in certain mollusks that partially substitute strontium for calcium in their shells when amounts of calcium are low.

To make matters more complex, by the early 20th century it became clear that the old adage, "If a little bit is good, then more must be better," was quite untrue so far as the needs of living things were concerned. The concept of the Law of the Minimum was broadened by the American ecologist Victor Shelford, who demonstrated that too much of a limiting factor can be just as harmful as not enough. Organisms have both an ecological maximum and minimum, the range in between these two extremes representing that organism's limits of tolerance.

LIMITS OF TOLERANCE

Subsequent investigations in regard to tolerance ranges have revealed a great deal about why certain species live where they do. Not surprisingly, those plants and animals that have a wide range of tolerance for all factors are the ones that have the widest distribution. However, some organisms can have a wide tolerance range for some factors but a narrow range for others, and thus their distribution will be accordingly more limited. Not all stages of an animal's or plant's life cycle are equally sensitive to the effect of limiting factors. Among many spore-forming bacteria, for example, high temperatures that would be almost instantly fatal for actively growing cells have no effect on the spore stage unless the duration of exposure is fairly long. In general, the most critical period when environmental factors are most likely to be limiting (i.e., when the range of tolerance is narrowest) is during the reproductive period. Susceptibility of the young to conditions that adult organisms could tolerate with little difficulty is well established in regard to acid rainfall. The low pH levels that are blamed for the near-total disappearance of many species of fish in lakes throughout eastern Canada, northeastern United States, and parts of Scandinavia have been shown to be lethal to fish eggs and fingerlings, but not to adult fish. Thus the effects of acid rain on aquatic life are much less dramatic than the effects of, for example, a chemical spill into a river. Rather than a massive, immediately visible (and smelly!) fish kill, the fish in an acidifying lake simply fail to reproduce and become less and less abundant, older and older, until they die out completely.

Other examples of the vulnerability of the reproductive stage include the observations that while adult cypress trees can grow either on dry ground or with their bases continually submerged in water, cypress seedlings can only develop in moist, unflooded soil. Similarly, some adult marine animals such as blue crabs can tolerate freshwater that is slightly salty and so are frequently found in rivers some distance upstream from the sea. Their young, however, can thrive only in saltwater, so reproduction and permanent establishment of these organisms in rivers cannot occur. Among humans, the very young also display less tolerance to environmental extremes than do adults. Many widespread environmental toxins have been shown, some in tragic ways, to have a much more devastating effect on developing fetuses and young children than on adults. The drug thalidomide and organic mercury are just two substances that have been ingested by pregnant women with no harmful effects on themselves but with disastrous results on their unborn children. Levels of air pollution that are largely ignored by the adult population can cause severe respiratory distress in infants and children. It's important for us to keep in mind the qualifications to the range of tolerance concept when we hear official assurances that exposure to this or that substance is "safe." What is safe for one segment of the population may be far from safe for others.

ENERGY FLOW THROUGH THE BIOSPHERE

Living things are dependent for their existence not only on proper soil and climate conditions but also on some form of energy. A basic understanding of the flow of energy through an ecosystem is fundamental to the study of how that system functions.

The ultimate source of all life activities, from the unfolding of a flower bud to the 100-meter dash of an Olympic athlete is, of course, the sun. Some 93 million miles (150 million km) from the earth, the sun emits vast amounts of electromagnetic radiation which, traveling through space at a rate of 186,000 miles (300,000 km) per second, takes about nine minutes to reach the earth's surface. There is no energy loss as the sun's radiation travels through space, but since its intensity decreases inversely as the square of the distance from the sun, the amount of solar radiation intercepted by the earth is but one two-billionth of the sun's total energy output. On this seemingly tiny portion all life on earth depends.

More than half the incoming radiation is unusable by living things, however. Electromagnetic radiation consists of several different wavelengths. Of the total amount of energy received from the sun, 9% is in the form of short-wave, high-energy ultraviolet rays; 53% is in the form of long-wave, infrared waves (heat waves); and 38% is visible light (Smil, 2002). Only those wavelengths within the visible spectrum, particularly those in the red and blue range, can be absorbed and utilized by green plants. These, through the process of photosynthesis, convert solar energy into the energy of chemical bonds. The complex and still not fully understood mechanism whereby plants harness certain wavelengths of sunlight and use this energy to join molecules of carbon dioxide and water to form the simple sugar glucose, releasing oxygen in the process, makes possible the existence of all higher forms of life. The transfer of this captured energy from organism to organism is basic to the functioning of ecosystems. Before examining the paths of energy flow, however, let us take a brief look at some physical laws that control and limit the amount of energy available to living things.

Laws of Thermodynamics

An understanding of many problems in both environmental science and energy technology depends on a basic conception of the principles that govern how energy is changed from one form into another. Known as the first and second laws of thermodynamics, these principles can be summarized as follows.

The First Law of Thermodynamics

Sometimes called the Law of Conservation of Energy, it states that energy can neither be created nor destroyed, even though it may be changed from one form into another. **Solar energy** that is absorbed by rocks or soil or water on the earth's surface is converted into **heat energy** which, because of temperature differentials and the earth's rotation, gives rise to winds and water currents that are a form of **kinetic energy.** When such kinetic energy accomplishes work such as the raising of water by wind, then it has been changed into **potential energy,** so-called because the latent energy of a water droplet in a cloud or at the top of a dam can be converted into some other kind of energy when it falls. In the same way, light energy absorbed by the chlorophyll molecules in a leaf is converted into the potential energy of chemical bonds within carbohydrates, proteins, and fats. As light energy passes from one form to another, it may appear that most of it is eventually lost or consumed (how often have we heard references to that misnomer, "energy consumption"?). This is a misconception, however, for if one maintained a global balance sheet it would show that all the energy that enters the biosphere as light is reradiated and leaves the earth's surface in the form of invisible heat waves. The form of energy leaving the system is different from the incoming radiation, but no energy has been either created or destroyed during its passage through the biosphere.

The Second Law of Thermodynamics

This law states that with every energy transformation there is a loss of usable energy (that is, energy that can be used to do work). Put another way, all physical processes proceed in such a way that the availability of the energy involved decreases (note that the *availability*, not the *total amount*, of energy is what decreases—the latter would be a violation of the First Law). The Second Law introduces the concept of **entropy,** the idea that all energy is moving toward an ever less available and more dispersed state. This process will continue until all energy has been transformed to heat distributed at a uniform temperature throughout the solar system—at which point the stable state will have been achieved.

The Second Law has some interesting implications concerning ecological relationships. Perhaps the most important of these is the fact that no type of energy transformation is ever 100% efficient—there will always be a significant loss of usable energy whenever energy is transferred from one organism to another. This explains why we need a continued input of energy to maintain ourselves and why we must consume substantially more than a pound of food in order to gain a pound of weight. In addition, because a given quantity of energy can be used only once, the ability to convert energy into useful work cannot be "recycled." Thus energy, unlike the essential minerals and gases, moves in a unidirectional way through ecosystems, becoming ever more dispersed and eventually being degraded to heat. Bearing these fundamental physical laws in mind, let's now take a more detailed look at the flow of energy through the biotic community.

Food Chains

Although overly simplistic, the concept of a **food chain** is useful for conveying a general understanding of how energy moves through ecosystems. Basically, a food chain involves the transfer of food energy from a given source through a series of organisms, each of which eats the next lower individual in the chain. In terms of energy flow, the living components of the ecosystem can be subdivided into three broad categories:

1. Producers—the green plants that convert the sun's energy into food energy. On land the major producers are the flowering plants and the conifers; in water they are mainly the diatoms, microflagellates, and green algae.

2. Consumers—animals; primary consumers are the herbivores and secondary consumers are the carnivores.

3. Decomposers—primarily bacteria and fungi, some insects. Decomposers are essential for recycling detritus back into the soil where it is once again available for use by producer organisms. No community could exist very long without decomposers.

There are basically three types of food chains. The most familiar of these, called a **grazing food chain** (or "predator chain"), may be typified by a grass → rabbit → fox association that starts with a plant base and proceeds from smaller to larger animals. Less conspicuous but equally important is the **detritus food chain,** where dead organic matter (detritus) is broken down by microorganisms, primarily bacteria. Small animals eat particles of this detritus, securing energy largely from assimilation of the energy-rich bacteria. The small animals, in turn, become a source of energy for larger consumers. A prime example of a detritus food chain accounting for a substantial portion of an ecosystem's energy flow can be found in the salt marsh habitat of many coastal areas. Here plants such as marsh grass die and are washed into estuaries where they are decomposed by microbes into finely divided particles which are then consumed by such primary consumers as fiddler crabs and mollusks. These, in turn, may be eaten by secondary consumers such as raccoons, water birds, or other crabs.

A variation on grazing food chains can be seen in certain **parasitic chains,** in which energy flows from larger to smaller animals (e.g., dogs that provide an energy source for fleas that in turn are fed upon by parasitic protozoans). In energy terms, however, there is no fundamental difference between a parasitic food chain and a grazing food chain, since a parasite is basically a "consumer."

Ecological Pyramids

Through the interactions of the community, a unidirectional flow of energy occurs from producers to primary consumers to secondary consumers, and so on. Each of these stages in a food chain is called a **trophic level.** It should be noted that placement of an organism into one trophic level or another depends on what that organism *does,* not to which species it belongs, since individuals of the same species may feed at different trophic levels, depending on factors such as age or sex. A male mosquito, for example, is an herbivore (primary consumer), dining on plant juices and nectar, while his mate would be classified as a carnivore (secondary consumer) when she takes the blood meal essential for egg laying. Similarly, while grazing animals such as cattle and horses are strict vegetarians as adults, their young thrive on a diet of mother's milk, making them, in effect, secondary consumers.

To describe the relationships among members of various trophic levels, ecologists frequently use the concept of **ecological pyramids.** If we examine a food chain in terms of its animal and plant constituents, it becomes apparent that these forms can be arranged into what is called a "pyramid of numbers." At the bottom of the pyramid are multitudes of energy-producing plants, then a smaller number of herbivores that feed upon them, then a still smaller number of primary carnivores, followed by an even smaller number of secondary carnivores. The animals at the top of the heap, the final consumers, are usually the largest in the community, while those organisms at the bottom of the pyramid, the producers, are usually the smallest, but much more abundant. In addition, the organisms at the lower trophic levels usually reproduce more rapidly and more prolifically than those higher up, so there is seldom danger of a predator eating itself out of its food supply. It should be noted, however, that in those cases where the size of the producer organisms is very large and the size of the primary consumers is small (e.g., a cherry tree being munched upon by hundreds of caterpillars), the shape of the pyramid of numbers may be inverted.

Just as the number of individual organisms in a community is generally greatest at the lower trophic levels, so the living weight, or **biomass** (measured as dry weight per unit area), is generally greatest at the producer trophic level. In the same way, biomass of the primary consumers will be greater than that of the secondary consumers, so the ecological biomass pyramids used to portray weight relationships among trophic levels will often look identical to numbers pyramids. Biomass, which in effect is an indicator of the amount of energy stored within an ecosystem, varies widely from one type of biotic community to another. For example, the amount of biomass in a tropical rain forest far exceeds that in a comparable area of abandoned field, while open ocean water is relatively poor in terms of biomass.

Although biomass pyramids, like numbers pyramids, usually have a broad base and tapered apex, in those situations where the organisms at the producer level are much smaller than the consumers, the shape of the biomass pyramid may be upside-down. This occurs because the "standing crop biomass" (the total dry weight of organisms present at any one moment in time) that can be maintained by a steady flow of energy in a food chain depends to a large extent on the size of the individual organisms. The smaller the organisms, the greater their metabolic rate per gram of biomass. Thus the smaller the organism, the smaller the biomass that can be supported at a given trophic level; in the same way, the larger the organism, the larger the amount of biomass at any one point in time. This is why in, say, an aquatic ecosystem the biomass of the blue whale would be far greater than the biomass of the microscopic diatoms and zooplankton on which it feeds. The biomass pyramid that illustrates the energy relationships in such a situation would be an inverted one. This doesn't mean that the producer organisms are defying the laws of nature; it simply reflects the fact that the tiny phytoplankton have very high metabolic rates and that they reproduce much more rapidly than do whales, having complete turnovers in their populations within very short time periods.

Whereas pyramids of numbers tend to exaggerate the importance of small organisms and pyramids of biomass often understate their role, **pyramids of energy** give the best picture of energy flow through a food chain, showing what actually is happening within the biotic community. As was mentioned earlier, light energy from the sun is captured by green plants and stored in the form of chemical bonds in the molecules of starch, glucose, fats, and so forth. However, as the Second Law of Thermodynamics states, only a portion of the energy stored by one trophic level is available to the next higher one, since a considerable amount is lost at every stage of transformation. Thus when cows graze in a pasture, some of the chemical bond energy in the grass is converted into the muscle tissue that represents stored food in the cow. The largest portion of energy derived from the grass, however, is lost in the form of waste heat during respiration. A lesser amount is lost as unassimilated food materials in feces or urine and as organic material that is not eaten by the next higher trophic level (i.e., just as people do not eat every part of a cow or pig, so many animals leave certain parts of their prey unconsumed; such "rejects" constitute an energy loss to the food chain).

At each transfer within a food chain, most of the chemical energy stored in organisms of the lower level is lost and therefore unavailable to those at the higher level. The magnitude of such energy losses ranges from a high of 99% (i.e., an energy transfer efficiency of just 1%) for most warm-blooded animals to approximately 85% for many species of insects and other small invertebrates (Bush, 2000). Since the total amount of energy entering the food chain is fixed by the photosynthetic activities of plants (and plants are less than 1% efficient, on the average, in converting solar energy into chemical energy), obviously more usable energy is available to organisms occupying lower positions in the food chain than to those at higher trophic levels. This basic fact of life explains why countries like China and India are largely vegetarian. In order to produce enough food to sustain many millions of people, such nations cannot afford the luxury of wasting the amount of energy involved in raising animals for meat. The constraints of energy transfer also explain why populations that are almost exclusively dependent on meat as a food source cannot permit their numbers to grow very large. One important factor contributing to the small population size of Eskimo groups is that these people exist as top carnivores of a relatively long food chain:

diatoms → zooplankton → fish → seals → Eskimos

The preceding observations should make it readily apparent that food chains are limited by energy considerations to no more than four or five trophic levels. A food chain of unlimited length is a physical impossibility, because the higher the feeding level, the less energy there is available within a given area. An animal that is a high-level consumer must range over wide areas in order to find enough food to support itself. Eventually the point is reached where the energy required to secure the food is greater than the energy obtained by eating it. At such a point no more organisms can be supported and the upper limits of the food chain have been reached.

Of course in most real communities the actual structure of trophic levels is much more complex than the food chain concept portrays. A "food web" would be a more accurate depiction, since many organisms feed on many different species and in some cases on more than one trophic level. Humans, for example, can be quaternary or tertiary consumers by eating fish, secondary consumers when dining on roast turkey, or primary consumers when munching on peanut-butter sandwiches. The many interlocking food chains tend to promote stability for organisms at the higher levels, providing them with alternative food sources should one or more of the prey species become less abundant. In general, the more complex the food web, the more stable the ecosystem is likely to be.

BIOGEOCHEMICAL CYCLING

Every home gardener who maintains a compost pile in the backyard intuitively understands the basic principles of biogeochemical cycling. All living organisms are dependent not only on a source of energy, but also on a number of inorganic materials that are continuously being circulated throughout the ecosystem. These materials provide both the physical framework that supports life activities and the inorganic chemical building blocks from which living molecules are formed. When such molecules are synthesized or broken down, changed from one form into another as they move through the ecosystem, their components are not lost or degraded in the same way in which energy moving through a food chain becomes unusable. Indeed, the manner in which inorganic materials move through ecosystems differs fundamentally from the movement of energy through those same systems in that matter, unlike energy, is conserved within the ecosystem, its atoms and molecules being used and reused indefinitely.

The cycling of earth materials through living systems and back to the earth is called **biogeochemical cycling.** Of the 92 naturally occurring chemical elements, about 40 are essential to the existence of living organisms and hence are known as **nutrients.** Some of these nutrients are fairly abundant and are needed in relatively large quantities by plants and animals. Such substances are termed **macronutrients** and include carbon, hydrogen, oxygen, nitrogen, phosphorus, potassium, calcium, magnesium, and sulfur. Others that are equally necessary but are required in much smaller amounts are called **trace elements.** These include such substances as iron, copper, manganese, zinc, chlorine, and iodine. The perpetuation of life on this planet is ultimately dependent on the repeated recycling of these inorganic materials in more or less circular paths from the abiotic environment to living things and back to the environment again. Such cycling involves a change in the elements from an inorganic form to an organic molecule and back again. Biogeochemical cycles are important because they help retain vital nutrients in forms usable by plants and animals and help maintain the stability of ecosystems.

Organisms have developed various adaptations to enable them to capture and retain nutrients. As we have seen in our discussion of biomes, plants in both the tropical rain forest and in desert regions have widespread, shallow root systems that permit them quickly to absorb water and the mineral nutrients that it carries in dissolved form before these can be lost through rapid runoff, competition from other organisms, or evaporation. In the tropical rain forest, for example, virtually all the mineral nutrients are retained in plant tissues and the topsoil of this biome is extremely nutrient-poor. If nutrient cycling did not occur, amounts of necessary elements would constantly decrease and would make the development of stable plant and animal populations impossible, since there is no constant addition to the source of nutrients from outside (as there is of energy in the form of sunlight).

There are basically two types of biogeochemical cycles—gaseous and sedimentary—depending on whether the primary source for the nutrient involved happens to be air and water (gaseous cycle) or soil and rocks (sedimentary cycle).

Gaseous Cycles

The elements moved about by gaseous cycles, primarily through the atmosphere but to a lesser degree in water, recycle much more quickly and efficiently than do those in the sedimentary cycle. Gaseous cycles pertain to only four elements: carbon, hydrogen, oxygen, and nitrogen. These four constitute about 97.2% of the bulk of protoplasm and so are of vital importance to life. An examination of two of these, the carbon and nitrogen cycles, gives an idea of the complexity of gaseous cycles.

Carbon cycle

Carbon atoms are the basic units of all organic compounds and hence, along with water, could be considered the most important component of biological systems. The principal inorganic source of carbon is the carbon dioxide found in the atmosphere and dissolved in bodies of water (the concentration of carbon dioxide dissolved in water is about 100 times greater than the amount present in the atmosphere; for this reason, carbon dioxide is much more accessible to aquatic organisms than to species living on land). Another large source of inorganic carbon lies in storage within deposits of fossil fuels—coal, oil, gas—but the largest amount of all occurs in the form of carbonate sediments such as limestone, formed under the seas and gradually uplifted during slow geologic processes.

Carbon is made available to living organisms through the process of photosynthesis, whereby green plants utilize solar energy to combine carbon dioxide and water, ultimately producing carbon-containing simple sugars. These constitute the basic building blocks for the synthesis of all other organic molecules. Animals obtain the carbon they need by eating plants and resynthesizing these into new carbon-containing compounds. Completion of the cycle, the breakdown of organic molecules to release inorganic carbon dioxide, is accomplished by several different pathways: (1) through the processes of respiration, whereby plants and animals take in oxygen and release carbon dioxide as a waste product; (2) through the decay of dead organisms or animal wastes, whereby bacteria and fungi decompose the carbon-containing organic molecules, releasing large amounts of carbon dioxide through their respiratory activities; (3) natural weathering of limestone; and (4) by the combustion of organic fuels (coal, oil, gas, wood). The last of these sources of inorganic carbon is causing growing concern among scientists who note that while the amount of atmospheric carbon remained relatively stable for millions of years, it has been rising significantly since the onset of the Industrial Revolution. Accelerating rates of increase in atmospheric carbon levels, especially during the past half century, have prompted warnings of worldwide climate change as the so-called "Greenhouse Effect" intensifies (see chapter 11).

Nitrogen cycle

The major reservoirs of nitrogen in the ecosystem are the 78% of free nitrogen gas that makes up our atmosphere and the nitrogen stored in rock-forming minerals. Atmospheric nitrogen, however, is biologically inert and cannot be utilized as such by most green plants. In nature, gaseous nitrogen is returned to the soil and converted to a form accessible to plants in one of two ways.

1. Lightning passing through the atmosphere can convert nitrogen to nitrogen oxide; when nitrogen oxide is dissolved in water it can be acted upon by certain bacteria in the soil which convert it into nitrate ions that can be absorbed by plant roots.

2. Fixation of atmospheric nitrogen by Rhizobium sp. bacteria that live in symbiotic association with leguminous plants inside root nodules, converting nitrogen to nitrates; certain species of free-living soil bacteria (Azobacter, Clostridium) and some cyanobacteria (Anabaena, Calothrix, Nostoc) also have the ability to fix free nitrogen into nitrates.

Of these two methods, fixation of atmospheric nitrogen by bacteria is by far the most significant way of making nitrogen available to other organisms. To complete the nitrogen cycle, nitrogenous wastes in the form of dead organisms, feces, urine, and so forth, are decomposed to ammonia by other types of soil bacteria; ammonia in turn is acted upon by nitrifying bacteria that form more nitrates. Such nitrates may be taken up again by plants or further broken down by another group of microorganisms called de-nitrifying bacteria, which act upon nitrates to produce free nitrogen that is once again returned to the atmosphere.

Since the early 20th century, natural processes of cycling nitrogen have been supplemented by human activities, which have more than doubled the annual rate at which fixed nitrogen enters the land-based nitrogen cycle (little is known about nitrogen cycling in the oceans). Industrial nitrogen fixation for fertilizer production constitutes the largest human addition of new nitrogen to the global nitrogen cycle; burning of fossil fuels releases gaseous forms of nitrogen into the atmosphere from their long-term storage in geological formations; and still-expanding cultivation of such leguminous crops as soybeans and alfalfa further increases nitrogen releases to the global environment (Vitousek et al., 1997). The adverse ecological consequences of such massive new additions of nitrogen will be discussed in subsequent chapters.

Sedimentary Cycles

Many of the elements that are essential for plant and animal life occur most commonly in the form of sedimentary rocks from which recycling takes place very slowly. Indeed, such sedimentary cycles may extend across long periods of geologic time and for all practical purposes constitute what are essentially one-way flows. In comparison with gaseous cycles, sedimentary cycles seem relatively simple. Iron, calcium, and phosphorus are examples of nutrients whose cycling occurs via the basic sedimentary pattern. A brief look at the phosphorus cycle will give an idea of the transformations involved.

Phosphorus cycle

Phosphorus, a key element in the nucleic acids DNA and RNA, as well as a component of the organic molecules that govern energy transfer within living organisms, occurs principally in the form of phosphate rock deposits. Smaller, though locally significant, amounts occur where quantities of excrement from fish-eating birds accumulate or in deposits of fossil bones. When such phosphate reservoirs are exposed to rainfall, phosphorus ions dissolve and can be absorbed by plant roots and incorporated into vegetative tissue. At the same time, much phosphorus is effectively lost from the ecosystem through runoff to the sea. Animals obtain the phosphorus they need by eating plants. When animals excrete waste products or when they die and decay, phosphates are returned to the soil where they once again become available for uptake by plants or are lost by downhill transport into the sea. Within shallow coastal areas some of this phosphorus is taken up by marine phytoplankton, which constitute the

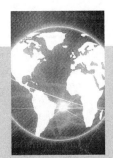

· · · · · · · 1-4 · · · · · · ·

Tourism: Environmental Boon or Bane?

Tourism has been a mixed blessing for nations striving to diversify local economies by marketing the charms of their sun-swept beaches, verdant rain forests, or native wildlife. Tourist dollars (and Euros and yen) have been pouring into exotic locales from Belize to Bali as developing countries vigorously promote international tourism as a means to stimulate investment and earn foreign currency. At first glance, their efforts appear stunningly successful. Travel and tourism is estimated to be the world's largest industry, employing one out of every twelve people. In the least-developed countries, tourism ranks second only to oil as a source of foreign exchange, while in some small island nations in the Caribbean and South Pacific, fully 40% of total earnings comes from international tourism. Yet such gains come at a price. The foreign investment needed to create the tourism infrastructure (e.g., upscale hotels, recreational facilities, modern airports) has increased the overall cost of living for local residents while providing mainly low-wage service jobs. Governments themselves frequently reap fewer benefits than expected because the foreign operators who control the tourist industry in many developing nations send most profits back to their home countries.

More obvious are tourism's negative environmental impacts. Some of the world's most unique and scenic tourist destinations are increasingly at risk of being "loved to death," degraded and polluted by the very visitors who come to enjoy their natural beauty. In many poor countries where public services such as sewage treatment, garbage collection, and provision of safe drinking water were already inadequate, the upsurge in demand by tourists who take such amenities for granted has only made matters worse. In tourist locales throughout the developing world, discarded plastic bottles and bags, soda cans, and food containers litter beaches and other tourist attractions. Untreated wastewater discharges from cruise ships and hotels add to the burden of pollution in coastal waters and local streams. In some chronically water-short regions, available supplies are diverted to fill resort swimming pools, launder tourists' clothes and bedding, or maintain lush golf courses, while local people may experience water shortages and rising utility prices. Excessive water demand can cause long-term ecological damage as well. In Israel, water levels in the Dead Sea have dropped more than 100 feet in the last 50 years, due in part to withdrawals to serve the tourist industry; some observers predict that if present trends continue, the famous inland sea could dry up completely by 2050. In numerous tropical seaside resorts such as Cancún, Mexico, construction of resort hotels, marinas, and docking facilities has destroyed coastal mangrove forests, salt marshes, and other wildlife habitats. Coral reefs are being crushed by the massive anchors of cruise ships, while careless breakage by the estimated 6 million snorkelers and scuba divers adds to reef destruction. At many prime tourist destinations, the sheer number of visitors is the main problem. Some governments have tried to minimize human pressures on ecologically fragile sites by limiting the number of tourists permitted at any given time, but whether the limits set are sufficiently protective is open to debate.

Reacting against the despoliation and commercialization so evident at many popular vacation spots, a growing segment of the traveling public has begun to embrace the less-frequented, more pristine locations where efforts are being made to keep the "human footprint" as light as possible. Since the mid-1990s, **ecotourism**, as this new trend is called, has become the fastest-growing segment of the travel and tourism industry. Defined by the International Ecotourism Society as "responsible travel to natural areas that conserves the environment and sustains the well-being of local people," ecotourism is closely related to the concept of sustainable development, requiring that the impact of travel on the environment and people of the host country be a positive one. Genuine ecotourism seeks to practice what it preaches, striving to minimize energy use, waste, and pollution. It also involves local people in the management of tourist enterprises, thereby channeling a substantial portion of tourism earnings back to the community. Doing so gives local people a sound economic reason to protect the land and wildlife they might otherwise exploit, since they realize they can earn more money guiding tour groups or catering to other tourist needs than they ever could by hunting, poaching, or subsistence farming.

Today ecotourists can be found trekking in the mountains of Nepal, bird-watching in a Costa Rican rain forest, taking lessons in reef ecology while scuba diving off Australia, or cruising to Antarctica to view penguins in their icy habitat. The burgeoning interest in ecotourism has already prompted environmentally positive governmental actions, such as giving protected status to valuable natural areas threatened by logging, mining, or agricultural development and has created employment opportunities and training for people living nearby.

The growing popularity—and profitability—of ecotourism has resulted, predictably, in a watering-down or outright corruption of the concept by some operators. Claiming adherence to the principles of ecotourism, some providers limit their environmental commitment to using low-flow shower heads and refraining from laundering visitors' sheets and towels on a daily basis. Others stress their "green" values in promotional advertising but not in their facilities and programs. The situation has prompted a growing demand for a clear set of codified standards—a green certification program—that prospective ecotourists can rely upon to choose a travel package or resort destination that does, in fact, provide the environmentally friendly experience they seek. Currently there are more than 100 tourism certification programs worldwide, but they are based on widely differing standards, with no international guidelines to provide tourists with trustworthy, reliable information. A move is now underway to create a global accreditation body to certify the green tourism certification programs.

In the meantime, would-be ecotourists can make a personal contribution to environmental preservation by choosing to stay in lodgings that minimize use of electricity, water consumption, and waste generation; they can scrupulously follow rules and regulations for visitors, refrain from buying souvenirs made from endangered species, and respect local customs and manners. Tourists can be a positive force for safeguarding the world's remaining natural areas if they travel with a keen awareness of their impact on natural ecosystems and a commitment to "tread lightly on the Earth."

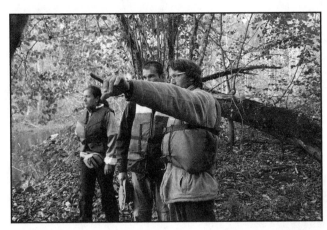

Genuine ecotourism requires that the impact of travel on the environment and people of the host country be a positive one. [*Courtesy of The International Ecotourism Society*]

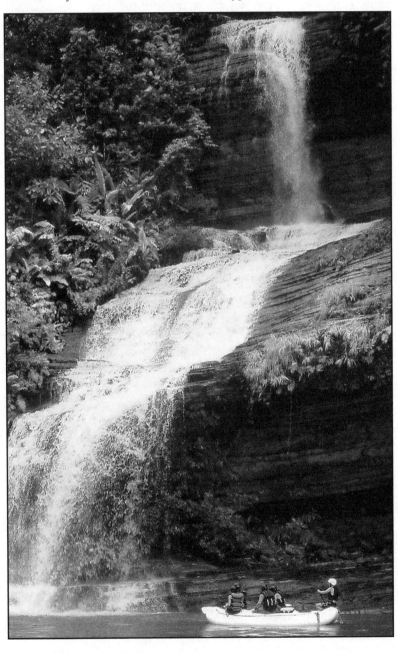

ultimate source of phosphorus for fish and sea birds. However, much of the phosphorus entering the sea is carried by currents to the deeper marine sediments where it is inaccessible to living organisms and may remain locked up for millions of years until future geologic upheavals. The large amounts of phosphate being produced commercially today for use as fertilizers come from the mining of phosphate rock. Unfortunately, much as in the case of oil or coal, such phosphate deposits constitute an essentially nonrenewable resource, since the processes responsible for their creation occurred millions of years in the past.

The fact that the general pattern in sedimentary cycling is a downhill one, where materials tend to move through ecosystems into relatively inaccessible geologic pools, poses some interesting implications for the stability of ecosystems. The loss of soluble mineral nutrients from upland areas to the lowlands and oceans is curbed only by local biological recycling mechanisms that prevent downhill loss from outpacing the release of new materials from underlying rocks. Such local recycling depends upon the return of dead organic material to the soil where breakdown and reuse of materials can occur. Human disruption of this process through wide-scale removal of potential nutrients (e.g., by logging, which removes trees that would otherwise have died and decayed in place; grazing of livestock that consume local resources but whose flesh, wool, bones, and so on will be disposed of elsewhere) accelerates the impoverishment of certain ecosystems where essential mineral nutrients are already in short supply. In such situations the lowlands have not benefited either, for the increased flow of materials they receive generally pass into the sea and out of biological circulation before they can be assimilated. Concern about the long-range stability of ecosystems demands that we begin to pay more careful attention to the biological recycling of inorganic materials that move in sedimentary cycles.

CHANGE IN ECOSYSTEMS

The fact that ecosystems undergo dramatic change over vast periods of time is now well accepted. Geologists have shown us how mountains are worn down and washed to the seas, forming thick layers of underwater sediments that eons later may be uplifted by immense tectonic pressures to form new mountains; deserts expand and retreat as rainfall patterns shift; and periodically great glacial ice sheets move southward, changing the face of the earth. As landforms and climates change, the biotic communities within the affected ecosystems change also. It is now recognized that the biotic communities in past geologic eras differed greatly from those existing today. What is less well understood is that present ecosystems

have a dynamic quality of their own, their component communities changing in an orderly sequence within a given area, a process known as **ecological succession.**

Succession

On May 18, 1980, Mount St. Helens volcano in southwestern Washington State exploded in a blast that obliterated the lush fir and hemlock forests that had blanketed its slopes for centuries. The collapse of the mountain's north face triggered an avalanche of mud and rocks that swept 15 miles down the Toutle River Valley, burying everything in its path under a 140-foot layer of volcanic debris. Observers surveying the scene at the time might understandably have wondered whether life could ever return to a scene of such devastation, yet within a year perennial wildflowers such as fireweed were blooming on the ash-laden mountainside. Year by year, the avalanche-affected area has become progressively greener. By the early 1990s, ecologists studying the area reported that 83 of the 256 plant species known to have been present prior to the eruption were once again thriving. While researchers concede that a return to anything resembling normal conditions will take more than a century (the area in the vicinity of the crater itself still remains virtually barren), the process of regeneration is well underway (Wilford, 1991).

The gradual, step-by-step changes over time in the relative abundance of dominant species within a biotic community following a disturbance are termed **succession** (Huston and Smith, 1987). While the sequence of events following the Mount St. Helens eruption provides one of the most dramatic recent illustrations of the process, numerous examples of succession in action can be seen all around us. While a casual glance at the plants and animals living together on a vacant city lot or an abandoned pasture may suggest an environmentally stable situation, such an impression is deceptive. If one could observe the same scene over a period of many years, it would be obvious that the composition of the area's biotic community, as well as the physical environment itself, is slowly changing in a directional manner toward a relatively stable, self-perpetuating stage called the **climax community.** Depending on the particular location involved, the changes might take thousands of years or be completed within decades, but in any case the process of change would follow a definite sequence.

The concept can be more easily understood by examining, step by step, the mechanisms of succession in a specific situation. Imagine that a retreating glacier has left behind a barren landscape of scoured bedrock or glacial till. Will the surface of the rock remain lifeless forever? Of course not; over a period of time, perhaps thousands of years if the climate is cold and dry, faster if it is warm and wet, changes in the biotic community occupying the surface of the rock will change it beyond recognition.

At first the only factors that can change the nature of the rock's surface are physical ones. Rain falls, combining with carbon dioxide in the air to form a dilute solution of carbonic acid. Bit by bit, this gradually begins to wear down the rocky surface. If the climate is a northern or temperate one, freezing and thawing may occur, helping to split the rock further. Wind erosion may also play a part. Algal and fungal spores or plant seeds will be carried to the site by air currents or by animals passing through the area, and colonies of lichens or other hardy plants establish themselves on the rock surface. The life processes of these organisms hasten the deterioration of the rock, and when the plants die, their dead organic matter contributes toward building up a thin layer of soil. These **pioneer plants** of the first stage of succession generally are small, low-growing species that can tolerate

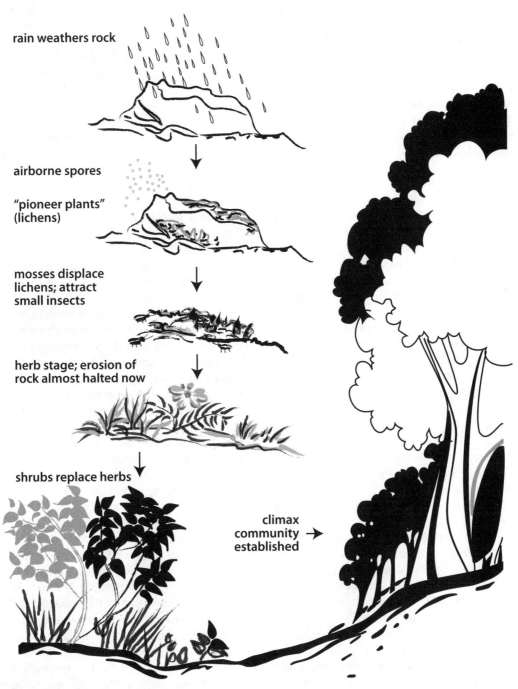

rain weathers rock

airborne spores

"pioneer plants" (lichens)

mosses displace lichens; attract small insects

herb stage; erosion of rock almost halted now

shrubs replace herbs

climax community established →

Figure 1-1   Primary Succession

severe climatic conditions (e.g., intense sunlight, wide fluctuations in daily temperature, periodic wetting and drying), produce large numbers of spores or seeds annually, grow rapidly, and have short life cycles. While pioneer plants are quite tolerant of adverse physical conditions, they are generally intolerant of other organisms. For example, once lichens have helped to corrode rock, create a small amount of soil, and maintain better moisture conditions, mosses take over and crowd out the lichens. These may form a dense cover, attracting insects and other small invertebrates. The mosses continue to build up deposits of organic matter and soil as more rock is broken away and as the old mosses and lichens die. The most significant change these organisms can produce in an environment is that created by their own dead bodies. As decayed organic material accumulates, erosion of the rock slows down, but herbaceous plants move in and assume dominance. Insects and other arthropods will be the main form of animal life at this stage, but some small mammals and reptiles may be present also.

As succession continues, shrubs and tree saplings eventually establish themselves, and since the taller plants furnish shade and act as a windbreak, the moisture conditions of the soil and near-soil atmosphere improve and temperature fluctuations at soil level become less extreme. Gradually the shrubs become the dominant plants, shading out many of the annual herbaceous species. Corresponding animal types change also, insects perhaps becoming fewer but bird species increasing in number. As the shrub stage matures, sapling trees begin to predominate. Shade-loving plants proliferate under the canopy. The large trees that characterize the late stages of succession in forest ecosystems are long-lived species that grow slowly and tend to persist for an indefinite period of time if environmental conditions of the area remain more or less constant. This relatively stable, self-perpetuating assemblage of species represents the climax community. Of course in reality a change in environmental conditions, especially climate, is not unusual, and natural events such as fires, high winds, earthquakes, or pest outbreaks (or unnatural events such as lumbering or grazing) can create a mosaic of successional stages within a given region. It is important to note that during the successional process it is not only the composition of the biotic community that is constantly changing through time—the physical environment is being substantially altered as well. Thus succession represents a dynamic process in which abiotic factors influence the plants and animals of the community, and these, in turn, modify the physical habitat.

The preceding example of succession beginning when pioneer organisms colonize an area formerly devoid of life is referred to as **primary succession.** A less extreme but far more common situation is that of **secondary succession.** In this case, succession proceeds from a state in which other organisms are still present; new life doesn't have to start from scratch, so to speak. Even in cases where the disturbed area may appear quite barren, roots, rhizomes, or dormant seeds lying underneath the soil surface quickly initiate the process of revegetation, joined by migrant species from outside the area taking advantage of the altered conditions. In the case of Mount St. Helens, for example, buried seeds and roots gave rise to new shoots pushing through the volcanic debris as erosion thinned the overlying ash. Examples of secondary succession are legion—abandoned Vermont farmland reverting to forest, revegetation of Yellowstone National Park after the devastating fires of 1988, untended suburban lawns growing up in weeds. In such cases succession begins at a more advanced stage but proceeds, like primary succession, in a directional, more or less predictable manner toward the climax community (Stiling, 1992).

Thus far we have only referred to terrestrial succession, but the same concept applies to most enclosed bodies of water as well. A newly formed lake (e.g., one left behind by a retreating glacier) will generally have clear water with little or no vegetation or debris. Gradually silt and dead materials are deposited on the lake bottom. The sides of the lake may also be eroded by wave action and thus help fill in the deeper parts of the basin. Around the edges of the lake rooted aquatic plants such as water lilies and pickerel weed, rushes, cattails, and so forth, become established. With the accumulation of dead organic material, the supply of nutrients necessary for the growth of algae and microorganisms is increased and they flourish accordingly, providing a food source for fish and other large animals. This process of nutrient enrichment is called **eutrophication.** The speed with which this phenomenon occurs is greatly accelerated when human-produced substances such as phosphate detergents, chemical fertilizers, or sewage are introduced. Eventually, as the lake becomes more completely filled with sediment, the whole area is converted into a marsh. Terrestrial grasses and moisture-tolerant plants subsequently move in, converting the marsh into a meadow, and finally the grasses are displaced by trees, resulting in a climax community. The length of time required for such succession to take place varies widely, depending on such variables as the original depth of the basin, the rate of sedimentation, and other physical conditions that affect the growth of organisms. It should be mentioned in passing, however, that not all aquatic succession results in the establishment of a terrestrial climax community. In cases where the body of water is very large and deep or where there is strong wave action, a stable aquatic community may form and undergo no further change.

Although the later stages of succession are characterized by biotic communities better able to withstand adverse environmental conditions and more stable in terms of species composition and population, humans have generally preferred to utilize the types of communities characterized by the earlier stages of succession. In aquatic ecosystems, for example, the desirable food and game fish such as trout, bass, and perch are all found in the clear, well-oxygenated water of deep, non-eutrophic lakes or in swiftly flowing streams. The carp that thrive in waters at a more advanced successional stage are less highly regarded. In relation to land communities, the development of agriculture and pastoralism has resulted in humans exerting increasingly effective efforts to main-

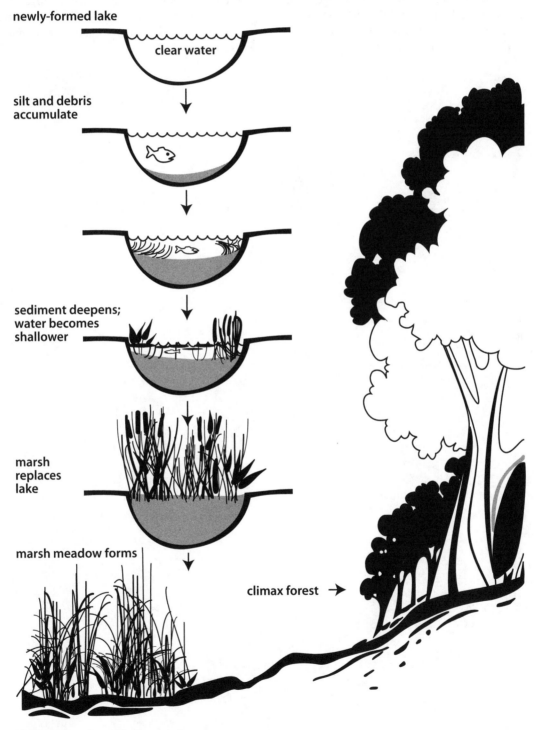

newly-formed lake

clear water

silt and debris accumulate

sediment deepens; water becomes shallower

marsh replaces lake

marsh meadow forms

climax forest →

Figure 1-2   Aquatic Succession

tain succession at an early, simplified stage. By replacing natural biotic communities with large expanses of just a few species of crop plants and through the attempt to eliminate such competitors as insects, rodents, and birds, agricultural humans have further simplified biotic communities, often undermining the stability of ecosystems in the process.

The stresses that humans are today imposing upon natural ecosystems extend far beyond the biological simplification of agricultural communities. Toxic pollutants being discharged into the air and water in unprecedented amounts are subjecting biotic communities to pressures with which they are evolutionarily unequipped to cope. In addition, the sheer increase in numbers of humans and their domestic animals creates physical pressures that degrade ecosystems. Of all threats to ecological stability, however, none is more serious than human-induced climate change—a phenomenon that, in the absence of effective international action, will change ecosystems in ways that are severely detrimental, not only to the biological communities which inhabit them, but to human interests as well.

The command "Be fruitful and multiply" was promulgated,
according to our authorities, when the population
of the world consisted of two people.
—William R. Inge (1931)

Population Dynamics

"Standing room only" is a phrase used only half in jest to describe the possible human predicament on this finite planet if present growth rates continue unchecked indefinitely into the future. Population projections based on a continuation of current growth rates reveal that within a few centuries, every human on the planet would have just one square meter of land, excluding polar ice caps, on which to live; if the world's present population size were to double twenty times, each individual would have to make do with just 0.7 millionth of an acre of arable land (Rohe, 1998). Obviously such figures represent an exercise in the absurd. Common sense observation of the world around us reveals that when populations of any organism explode, be they swarms of migratory locusts, tent caterpillars, or lemmings marching toward the sea, something, sooner or later, brings that population back into a state of relative equilibrium with its environment. There is no reason to suppose that humans, any more than locusts, caterpillars, or lemmings, can defy the laws of nature by multiplying indefinitely. Certain ecological principles govern the ways in which populations change in size. The study of such changes, or population dynamics, is of great practical importance to those who wish to predict or control the population size of other organisms or, even more important today, to forecast trends in human population growth and, if possible, guide such growth into ecologically sustainable patterns.

POPULATION ATTRIBUTES

As we saw in chapter 1, a biotic community is made up of populations of a number of different species that are bound together by an intricate web of relationships, interacting with each other and with the physical environment. Any population exhibits certain measurable group attributes that are unique to that population. Such group attributes include birth and death rates, age structure, population density, spatial distribution, and so forth. Knowing what these characteristics are for any given population is helpful in predicting how that population will change in response to changes in the environment.

Basically, assessing dynamic changes within a population largely revolves around keeping track of additions to that population from births and immigration and of losses from the same group due to deaths and emigration. Age structure of the population also must be taken into account in those species, such as *Homo sapiens*, where generations tend to overlap.

Limits to Growth

Nearly 150 years ago Charles Darwin observed in his *Origin of Species* that all organisms have a tendency to produce many more offspring than will survive to maturity. Indeed, in nature a given population of organisms tends to maintain relatively stable numbers over a long period of time. Although a single oyster may produce up to 100 million eggs at one spawning, an orchid may release a million seeds, or one mushroom may be responsible for hundreds of thousands of fungal spores drifting through the air, nevertheless, the world has not yet been overwhelmed with oysters, orchids, or mushrooms. Even much less prolific species theoretically could give rise to staggering numbers of offspring. Darwin himself cited the example of the slow-breeding elephant (gestation period of 600–630 days), showing that the progeny from a single pair would number 19 million after 750 years, assuming that all survived to reproductive age.

Obviously the increase of populations as described above could only occur in a situation where no forces act to slow the growth rate—a scenario that is virtually nonexistent in the real world, at least for any extended period of time.

The maximum growth rate that a population could achieve in an unlimited environment is referred to as that population's **biotic potential.** In reality, of course, no organism ever reaches its biotic potential because one or more factors limit its growth. Such limiting factors include food shortages, overcrowding, disease, predation, and accumulation of toxic wastes. Taken together, the environmental pressures that limit a population's inherent capacity for growth are termed **environmental resistance.** Environmental resistance is generally measured as the difference between the biotic potential of a population and the actual rate of increase as observed under laboratory or field conditions (Odum, 1959).

POPULATION GROWTH FORMS

In the early 1900s a number of population biologists were curious to discover what would happen to a population if most of the usual factors of environmental resistance were removed. They devised carefully controlled laboratory experiments to chart growth curves for populations where limitation of resources, predation, parasites, and other factors that normally contribute to high death rates would not come into play. Their findings revealed that populations exhibit characteristic patterns of increase that biologists call **population growth forms.** Experimentation with a wide variety of organisms has revealed two basic patterns, described as the S-curve and the J-curve.

S-Curve

A classic study in population dynamics was carried out by Russian biologist G. F. Gause in 1932 using a population of the protozoan, *Paramecium caudatum.* Gause placed one paramecium into an aquarium with a broth of bacterial cells suspended in water to provide a food supply and then carefully observed the subsequent growth of

that population. He found that numbers of paramecia increased rather slowly for the first few days, then increased very rapidly for a period; finally the rate of increase began to slow and gradually leveled off as the upper limits of growth were reached and a steady-state equilibrium was achieved. The growth pattern thus revealed is that of an S-curve (sigmoid curve). The upper limit of such a curve, called the **upper asymptote,** indicates that point at which increased mortality has brought birth and death rates into balance once again (in the case of Gause's paramecia, increased mortality was due to overcrowding in the culture and the inability of the constant food supply to support all the organisms). The population density at the upper asymptote thus represents an equilibrium level between the biotic potential of that population and the environmental resistance. Thus the upper asymptote of the S-curve is often referred to as the **carrying capacity** of that environment—the limit at which that environment can support a population.

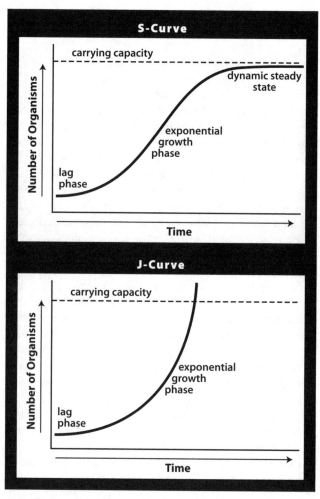

Figure 2-1   Population Growth Forms

J-Curve

The sigmoid growth pattern just discussed, typical of populations as diverse as microorganisms, plants, and many types of birds and mammals as well, results from the gradually increasing pressures of environmental resistance as the population density increases. Another type of population growth form, more dramatic because it frequently results in the population "crashes" that attract widespread journalistic attention, can be represented by a J-curve. In this situation population growth increases at rapid exponential rates up to or even beyond the carrying capacity of the environment. The environmental resistance becomes effective only at the last moment, so to speak, and as a result populations that have overshot the carrying capacity suffer severe diebacks. This pattern is frequently seen in many natural populations such as lemmings, algal blooms, and certain insects. It should be apparent that the early phases of growth represented by S- and J-curves are identical: a preliminary "lag" phase, during which time the rate of increase is relatively slow, followed by a logarithmic, or exponential, growth phase during which not only do the actual numbers grow rapidly, but the rate of increase also increases (in the manner of compound interest). Thus, a J-curve basically can be considered an incomplete S-curve since the sudden imposition of limiting effects halts growth before the self-limiting effects within a population become apparent.

HOMEOSTATIC CONTROLS

Food shortage, excess predation, and disease are not the only factors that can cause populations to decline. Extensive research has shown that a number of self-regulating factors, or **homeostatic controls,** in the form of behavioral, physiological, and social responses within a population are also very important in controlling its size. Each population appears to have an optimal density, and if this optimum is exceeded a number of stress-related responses become evident. For example, it has been observed that among the snowshoe hares of northern Canada, population crashes occur at regular 9–10 year intervals even in the absence of predators, disease, or human hunting pressures. Researchers have found that during the rapid die-off phase of these oscillations, large numbers of hares suffer a stress-induced degeneration of their livers, resulting in inadequate glycogen reserves. The animals may then exhibit "shock disease," lapsing into convulsions, coma, and ultimately death (Farb, 1963).

Classic studies on the effects of overcrowding in rats have shown that even when abundant food is present, self-regulating mechanisms induce population crashes when rat populations exceed a certain density. When crowded, rats begin to exhibit abnormally hostile behavior; social interactions become pathological and fighting intensifies, often with fatal results to one of the combatants. Some individual males become hyperactive and hypersexual, attempting to mate without the customary courtship rituals and often mounting males, nonreceptive females, and juveniles indiscriminately. Pregnant females under crowded conditions frequently abort; if the young are born alive they are frequently killed by the mother or die as a consequence of neglect. It has been suggested that the cause of such deviant behavior can be traced to the effects of crowding-induced stress on the functioning of the endocrine system, which regulates hormone levels in animals. Whether the rats' response to crowding is indicative of what we can expect among human populations as our species continues to increase is open to question, but there are those who point to rising levels of violence and aggression in many parts of the world as ominous portents.

HUMAN POPULATION GROWTH

Insights gained from laboratory studies of microbial populations have an importance far transcending mere academic interest. The exponential curves tracking the growth of, say, paramecia or migratory locusts have a parallel in the growth patterns that typify many human societies today. The fact is that since the mid-20th century the human species has experienced an unprecedented population explosion, with growth rates resembling those depicted on a J-curve. Although the average *rate* of growth is now decreasing after reaching a peak in the early 1970s (perhaps indicating that humans are S-curve rather than J-curve organisms?), in terms of absolute numbers the annual increase to the world's total population is now over 80 million [Population Reference Bureau (PRB), 2009]. The explosive growth of the human species is arguably the most significant development of the past million years. No other event, geological or biological, has posed a threat to earthly life comparable to that of human overpopulation. We have little hope of significantly reducing other types of environmental degradation if present rates of population increase are not reversed.

In the past, people who warned of an impending population/resource crunch or advocated even the mildest measures to restrain birth rates were either ridiculed, castigated, or ignored. One of the earliest to voice alarm was British clergyman-economist Thomas Malthus who, some 200 years ago, argued that the rapid population growth his country was then experiencing was a prelude to mass misery. Demonstrating that population grows geometrically (2, 4, 8, 16, 32) while agricultural production increases only arithmetically (1, 2, 3, 4, 5), Malthus contended that population would always tend to outpace additions to the food supply, thereby condemning the bulk of humanity to a marginal standard of living and frequent bouts of famine, war, and disease. Although Malthus' "dismal theorem" stimulated a great deal of discussion at the time, his views were soon discounted when improvements in British agricultural technology and the opening of the American prairies to grain production resulted in food supply increases far exceeding the number of new mouths to be fed. As a result, Malthus' warnings were largely dismissed and forgotten. The prevailing attitude throughout the 19th and well into the 20th century viewed population growth as a desirable phenomenon, enhancing a nation's productivity, wealth, and power. Indeed, as late as the 1930s, the main population concern in the United States was that the temporary

dip in the American birth rate experienced during the Depression years might indicate a worrisome *shrinking* of U.S. population size!

However, after World War II, and especially since the 1960s, concerns that population growth rates were excessive began to be expressed, first by a handful of far-sighted individuals and private organizations, later by national governments and international agencies. Such concern was precipitated by the awareness that intensive efforts to improve living standards and ensure national stability in the newly independent developing nations were largely being nullified by the rapid population growth they were experiencing. Today the governments of most developing countries regard their rate of population increase as too high and have adopted policies aimed at stabilizing numbers as quickly as possible. Unfortunately, such efforts should have been launched decades earlier; the momentum of growth is now so enormous and the existing population base so large, that the ability of some countries to curb growth before national carrying capacity is surpassed is very much in doubt. In order to understand why the seriousness of our current population crisis was recognized so belatedly and why there's such a sense of urgency now, we need to look at some demographic facts.

Historical Trends in Human Population Growth

Assuming that the first humans appeared on Earth between 1.5 million and 600,000 years ago, we can estimate that somewhere between 60 and 100 billion people have inhabited the planet at some time. Today the earth supports almost 7 billion human inhabitants—close to 7% of all who have ever lived. We don't have enough information to estimate accurately what populations were before AD 1650, but we can make some educated guesses based on circumstantial evidence (e.g., number of people who could be supported on X square miles by hunting and gathering, by primitive agriculture, and so on). On this basis, it's been calculated that the total human population in 8000 BC was about 5 million people. By the beginning of the Christian Era, when agricultural settlements had become widespread, world population is estimated to have risen to about 200–300 million, and increased to about 500 million by 1650. It then doubled to one billion by 1850, to two

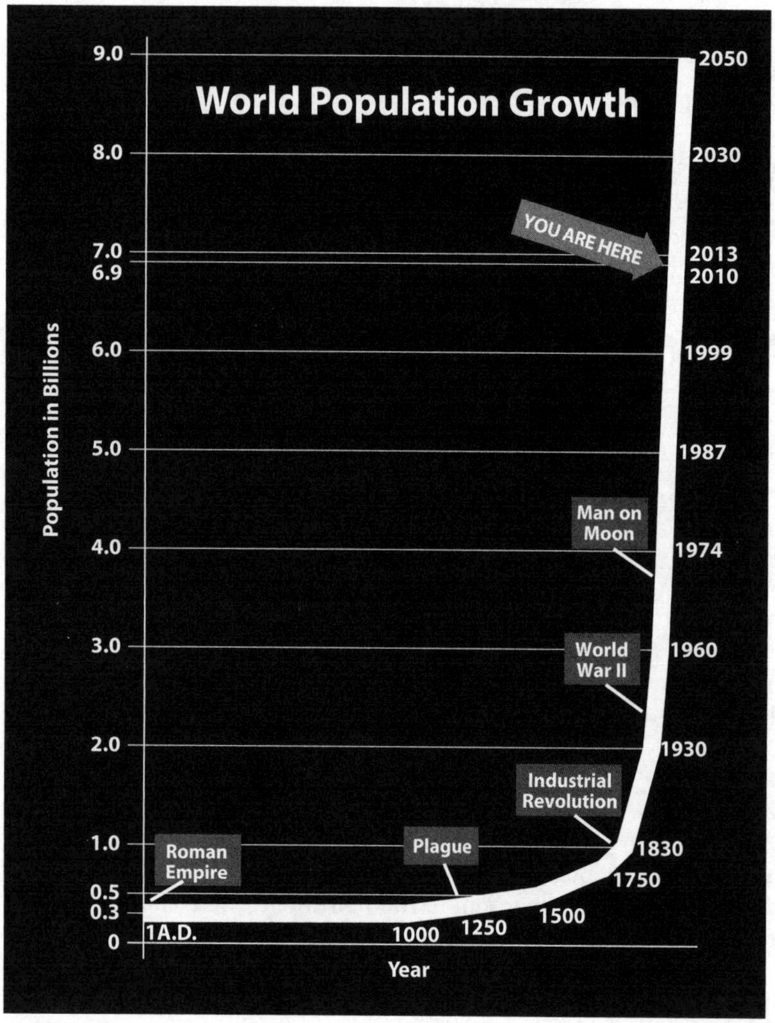

Source: Population Connection. Used with permission.

Figure 2-2   World Population Growth

billion by 1930, and to four billion by 1975. By 1999 world population hit 6 billion and continues to climb. Thus not only has world population been increasing steadily (with minor irregularities) for the past million years, but the rate of growth also has increased.

Doubling Time

Perhaps the best way to describe growth rate is in terms of **doubling time**—the time required for a population to double in size. During the period from 8000 BC to AD 1650, the population doubled about every 1,500 years. The next doubling took 200 years, the next 80 years, and the next, 45 years.

Historical evidence indicates that the increase in human numbers did not occur at a steady pace but rather that three main surges occurred. The first took place about 600,000 years ago with the evolution of culture (developing and learning techniques of social organization and group and individual survival); the next occurred about 8000 BC with the agricultural revolution; and the most recent began about 200 years ago with the onset of the industrial-medical-scientific revolution (Ehrlich, Ehrlich, and Holdren, 1977). Bearing in mind that changes in the size of populations occur when birth and death rates are out of balance, one can reasonably conclude that each of these spurts indicates that the story of human population growth is not primarily a story of changes in birth rates, but of changes in death rates. Let's now take a closer look at some of the demographic facts that help to explain our current population dilemma.

Birth Rates, Death Rates, and Fertility Rates

Birth rates are generally expressed as the number of babies born per 1,000 people per year. Prior to the Industrial Revolution, birth rates in every society typically were in the 40–50 per 1,000 range. Today the birth-rate gap between nations has widened dramatically, exemplified by Germany and Taiwan's 8, among the world's lowest, compared to 52, the highest, in the West African nation of Niger. Indeed, in recent years a nation's birth rate can be looked at as a crude barometer of its level of economic development, since the most prosperous, most

technologically advanced countries generally are characterized by low birth rates.

Death rates are calculated in the same way as birth rates, representing the annual number of deaths per 1,000 population. Birth and death rates are frequently referred to as "crude" rates because they don't reflect the wide variations in age distribution within a population—a fact that might result in misleading conclusions when comparing statistics from different countries. For example, the fact that the Palestinian Territory has a death rate of 4 per 1,000 population while the death rate in Italy is 10 might lead one to assume that Palestinians enjoy better health care and a higher standard of living than do Italians. Such an assumption would be erroneous, however, since the reason for the Palestinian Territory's apparent advantage is that 44% of the Palestinian population is under the age of 15—an age cohort everywhere typified by a low likelihood of death. Italy, on the other hand, is characterized by an aging population; only 14% of Italians are under 15, while 20% are over age 65 (compared to just 3% among Palestinians). Even with excellent medical care, death rates are bound to be higher in a predominantly middle-aged to elderly population than in one primarily composed of the very young.

Total fertility rate (TFR), representing the average number of children each woman within a given population is likely to bear during her reproductive lifetime (assuming that current age-specific birth rates remain constant), perhaps gives a clearer picture of reproductive behavior than does crude birth rate. Although *world* TFR has been gradually falling in recent decades to its present level of 2.5, the wide discrepancies in national fertility rates are illustrated by countries such as Niger, whose total fertility rate of 7.4 is currently the world's highest, and by Taiwan, whose total fertility rate of 1.0 suggests a preference for one-child families on that crowded island (PRB, 2010).

Growth Rates

Since birth rates represent additions to a population and death rates represent subtractions, a change in population size is represented by the difference between the two, that is, the **growth rate** (sometimes called the **rate of natural increase**). Growth rates, which do not take migration into account, can be calculated quite simply by subtracting the death rate from the birth rate. Take the case of Pakistan, for example: with a 2010 birth rate of 30 and a death rate of 7, the growth rate of Pakistan's population will be 30 minus 7, or 23 per 1,000 population. However, because growth rate is expressed as a percentage (i.e., per 100), not per 1,000 as in birth and death rates, Pakistan has an annual growth of 2.3%.

Table 2-1	**Doubling Time of World Population**	
Date	Estimated Human Population	Doubling Time (in years)
8000 BC	5 million	1500
AD 1650	500 million	200
AD 1850	1 billion	80
AD 1930	2 billion	45
AD 1975	4 billion	36
AD 2042	8 billion	67

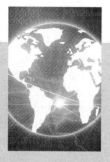

········ 2~1 ·······

Will AIDS Defuse Africa's Population Explosion?

It is a generally accepted fact that human population growth can't continue indefinitely. Sooner or later the increase in human numbers must level off or decline as the forces of environmental resistance intensify—or when couples everywhere voluntarily limit their number of children to one or two. In recent years the grim toll exacted by the HIV/AIDS epidemic has prompted some observers to question whether rising death rates due to this disease could bring a halt to population growth, at least in the regions now most affected.

The statistics are horrifying; by the end of 2007 there were approximately 33 million people worldwide infected with the human immunodeficiency virus (HIV), the pathogen that causes AIDS; more than 25 million have died of the disease since it was first recognized in 1981. In addition, the average age of new victims appears to be falling; in 2007, 45% of all newly infected individuals 15 or older were youths between the ages of 15–24. The number of AIDS orphans is also growing, with more than 15 million children under the age of 18 having lost one or both parents to AIDS. An estimated 11.6 million of these children live in sub-Saharan Africa. Moreover, in hard-hit countries like Botswana and Namibia an estimated 20% of children are AIDS orphans.

Fortunately, after two decades of rapid increase, the *percentage* of the world's people living with HIV has stabilized since 2000; nevertheless, the overall *number* of people infected continues to increase each year, owing both to new infections and to the fact that many victims are now living longer, thanks to more widespread availability of antiretroviral drugs. However, in spite of a 10-fold expansion in the availability of life-prolonging antiretroviral medicines in low- and middle-income countries since 2001—almost 3 million people were receiving them by 2007—globally, for every three people who receive treatment, five more become infected (UNAIDS, 2008).

HIV/AIDS is now a **pandemic**—global in scope—affecting almost every country in the world. In regions such as the Caribbean, North America, and central Africa the disease has been well-established since the early 1980s. Sub-Saharan Africa remains the region most devastated by the disease, accounting for 67% of all HIV-infected individuals and 72% of all AIDS deaths in 2007. Although the early focus of infection was limited to settlements along major truck routes, the range of HIV/AIDS in sub-Saharan Africa has now broadened to include both urban centers and the rural hinterlands of all countries in the region, with prevalence of the disease significantly higher in urban areas.

In recent years the nations of eastern Europe and central Asia, especially Russia and Ukraine, have experienced an explosive increase in HIV-infection rates. According to AVERT, an international AIDS charity based in the United Kingdom, the number of people in this region living with HIV reached 1.5 million in 2007, double the figure for 2001, with 58,000 AIDS deaths that year. While the prevalence rate for the area as a whole is 0.8%, it is significantly higher in Ukraine (1.6%) and Russia (1.1%)—two nations that account for 90% of all HIV infections in that region of the world. While the percentage of infections worldwide seems to be stabilizing, the HIV/AIDS epidemic continues to expand more rapidly in eastern Europe than anywhere else in the world, primarily due to increasing rates of intravenous drug use. Some health officials fear the worst is yet to come and predict that Russia will experience the greatest number of AIDS-related deaths between 2009 and 2015.

Next to sub-Saharan Africa, Asia currently ranks second in numbers of adults and children living with HIV/AIDS—an estimated 5 million throughout the region. India alone is thought to have 2.5 million HIV-infected people—the third-highest HIV-positive population in the world. China, largely unaffected until relatively recently, is now thought to have a prevalence rate of 0.1%, with 75,000 AIDS patients and 700,000 more living with HIV. In Thailand, approximately 1% of adults is HIV-positive and AIDS has become a leading cause of death in spite of the government's widely acclaimed and generally effective preventive efforts focused on the commercial sex industry.

Just as the geography of HIV/AIDS has been expanding, the sociology of the pandemic has been dynamic as well. Population subgroups once thought to be at low risk of infection have experienced an alarming increase in disease rates in recent years. Once confined mainly to homosexual men and intravenous drug abusers, HIV/AIDS prevalence has risen dramatically among women and infants as heterosexual contact became the main route of transmission in many countries, particularly in sub-Saharan Africa. Increased infection rates among women mean that, in the absence of effective therapy, more children are born HIV-positive. In several African countries, 5% or more of pregnant women attending prenatal classes test HIV-positive—a proportion that rises to over 15% in South Africa and 23% in Swaziland. In the absence of services to prevent mother-to-child transmission, as many as 4 out of 10 women will transmit the infection to their babies. Though such preventive services have expanded significantly since 2002, an estimated 370,000 children under the age of 15 became HIV-infected in 2007. Worldwide, the number of children younger than 15 living with HIV increased from 1.6 million in 2001 to 2 million in 2007—90% of them in sub-Saharan Africa (UNAIDS, 2008).

As Africa continues to suffer disproportionately from the ravages of HIV/AIDS—with prevalence rates among the adult population (15–49 years) as high as 15–20% in South Africa, Zambia, and Zimbabwe, and exceeding 20% in Botswana, Lesotho, and Swaziland—it seems relevant to question whether AIDS may represent one of those forces of environmental resistance acting to bring a halt to a runaway rate of population growth on that continent. Since heterosexual relations constitute the major route of transmission in African countries, the demographic implications of HIV/AIDS are a subject of considerable speculation. If women of childbearing age sicken and die while still relatively young, total fertility rates obviously will be lower. Similarly, if child mortality rises because HIV-positive mothers are transmitting the virus to their babies *in utero* or in breast milk, overall growth rates should be affected.

Whether AIDS-influenced declines in growth rates will be large enough to cause an actual decrease in population size—or even a leveling off—in African countries is doubtful, however. Data from Uganda, one of the first countries to be hard-hit by the HIV/AIDS epidemic, yield no evidence the disease is having any noticeable influence on that nation's fertility rate, at 6.5 children per woman in 2010. Uganda reported a 3.4% population growth rate for that year, a figure which, if maintained, would lead to a doubling of the population in just 20 years. This situation can be explained, at least in part, by the fact that death due to AIDS generally doesn't occur until 8–10 years after infection with the virus—and may now be delayed for decades, thanks to wider access to antiretroviral drugs. If a woman acquired her infection soon after becoming sexually active in her teens or early twenties, she could still live long enough to bear a number of children. Although AIDS-related mortality may reduce total fertility to some extent, demographers predict that the impact of such a decline will simply be to lower growth rates in certain African countries to somewhere between 0.5% to 2.0%—rates that still represent relatively rapid growth.

While much remains to be learned about the association between HIV/AIDS and fertility, population experts generally agree that in spite of the tragic humanitarian aspects of the disease, African populations will continue to grow for the foreseeable future—perhaps not quite as rapidly as they would in the absence of AIDS, but grow nevertheless.

Growth rate is the critical factor from which to get a quick impression of what is happening to a particular population. It is entirely possible that a country could have a traditionally high birth rate and still have a relatively low growth rate if the death rate is high also. In fact, just such a situation was characteristic of most human societies in the world until only a few hundred years ago.

When the average person hears that Pakistan has a population growth rate of 2.3%, the number may fail to make an appropriate impact, since most of us find it difficult to conceptualize what a 2.3% growth rate means in human terms. Besides, 2.3% really doesn't sound like very much! However, when expressed in terms of doubling time, the importance of growth rates takes on a new perspective. By calculating the annual growth rate of a population and then referring to a conversion table, we can learn what the doubling time of that population will be:

Growth Rate	Doubling Time
0.5%	140 years
0.8%	87 years
1.0%	70 years
2.0%	35 years
3.0%	24 years
4.0%	17 years

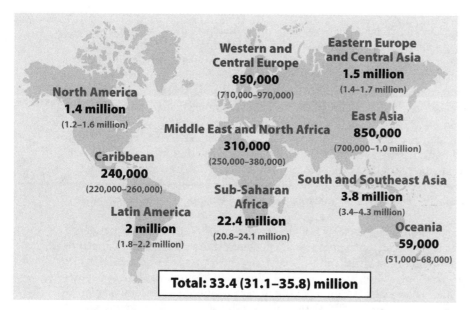

Western and
Central Europe
850,000
(710,000–970,000)

Eastern Europe
and Central Asia
1.5 million
(1.4–1.7 million)

North America
1.4 million
(1.2–1.6 million)

Middle East and North Africa
310,000
(250,000–380,000)

East Asia
850,000
(700,000–1.0 million)

Caribbean
240,000
(220,000–260,000)

South and Southeast Asia
3.8 million
(3.4–4.3 million)

Sub-Saharan
Africa
22.4 million
(20.8–24.1 million)

Latin America
2 million
(1.8–2.2 million)

Oceania
59,000
(51,000–68,000)

Total: 33.4 (31.1–35.8) million

Source: *2009 AIDS Epidemic Update*, UNAIDS. Reprinted with permission of UNAIDS. www.unaids.org.

Figure 2-3   Adults and Children Estimated to be Living with HIV as of 2008

Thus, with an annual growth rate of 2.3%, the population of Pakistan, already at 185 million, will double in just 30 years. In human terms this means that *just to maintain present standards of living* everything in Pakistan needs to be doubled in 30 years—food production, provision of jobs, educational facilities, medical personnel, public services, and so forth. Whether such a Herculean task can be accomplished remains to be seen; certainly the leaders of Pakistan (and of a great many other nations whose doubling times are similarly brief) face a formidable challenge in the decades ahead, especially at a time when the "revolution of rising expectations" has created a grassroots demand for improved living standards, not just maintenance of the status quo.

POPULATION EXPLOSION

With a basic understanding of what birth, death, and growth rates imply, let us now turn to the crucial question of why growth rates have so accelerated during the past several generations. Surveying the history of human population growth (an admittedly risky enterprise, particularly for the prehistoric period), we can say with a fair degree of certainty that birth rates throughout the world were uniformly high until relatively modern times. (Some anthropologists doing research among contemporary hunter-gatherer societies have forwarded the idea that, prior to the agricultural revolution, birth rates among primitive peoples were lower than among subsequent agricultural societies. This they attribute to environmental restraints causing such groups to attempt to

space the births of their children.) Even today, while birth rates in most parts of the world are gradually declining, women in most sub-Saharan African nations continue to bear children at traditionally high levels.

With birth rates having apparently held steady during most of human history, we must look then to changes in death rates to explain why growth rates have shot upwards. Each of the three major changes in human lifestyle mentioned earlier effected a decline in the death rate. Cultural advances among prehistoric humans probably reduced the death rate to some slight degree, but the consequences of this cultural evolution were minor compared with the changes wrought by the agricultural revolution. The increase in food supply, the more settled mode of existence, and the general rise in living standards are thought to have reduced mortality rates and increased life expectancy to some degree over that of primitive peoples.

Even so, the gains were gradual until about 200–300 years ago, when improvements in public sanitation, advances in agriculture, and the control of infectious disease resulted in a precipitous decline in death rates, particularly in regard to infant and child mortality.

The growth in human numbers that resulted from these improved conditions was not, of course, a steady, uninterrupted rise. Wars, famine, and disease provoked periods of sharp population declines among localized groups. Certainly the most spectacular reversal of the overall growth trend was the impact of bubonic plague (the notorious "Black Death" of the Middle Ages) on the societies of Europe. Plague first reached the Continent in AD 1348 and within two years had killed approximately 25% of the total population. Successive outbreaks of the disease continued to sweep across Europe during the next several decades, during which time the population of England dropped by nearly one-half, and many regions in both Europe and Asia were similarly decimated. Nearly constant warfare and the disease and famine that frequently accompanied such conflict also had a negative influence on population growth. Particularly devastating in terms of civilian suffering was the Thirty Years' War (1618–1648), during which time it is estimated that as many as one-third of the inhabitants of Germany and Bohemia died as a direct result of the war.

Outside of Europe, warfare, even prior to the World Wars of the 20th century, resulted in enormous loss of life. Conquest and subjugation of Native American civilizations by European colonizers, tribal warfare in Africa, the Moghul invasion of Hindu India, and centuries of internal strife in China resulted in high death rates and sometimes severe depopulation within the affected groups. Perhaps the most extreme example of a population being decimated by warfare involves the most bloody, savage war ever fought in South America. This five-year conflict, which ended in 1870, pitted the combined forces of Brazil, Uruguay, and Argentina against

Table 2-2   2010 Population Data for Selected Countries

Region or Country	Population* (millions)	Birth Rate	Death Rate	Growth Rate, %	Projected Population (millions) mid-2050
WORLD	6892	20	8	1.2	9,485
AFRICA	1,030	37	13	2.4	2,084
Egypt	80.4	27	6	2.1	137.7
Ethiopia	85.0	39	12	2.7	173.8
Ghana	24.0	31	9	2.2	44.6
Niger	15.9	52	17	3.5	58.2
Nigeria	158.3	42	17	2.4	326.4
South Africa	49.9	21	12	0.9	57.4
Kenya	40.0	37	10	2.7	65.2
Congo, Dem. Rep. of	67.8	47	17	2.9	166.2
ASIA	4,157	19	7	1.2	5,424
Afghanistan	29.1	39	18	2.1	53.4
China	1,338.1	12	7	0.5	1,437.0
India	1,188.8	23	7	1.5	1,748.0
Iraq	31.5	32	6	2.6	64.0
Japan	127.4	9	9	0.0	95.2
Philippines	94.0	26	5	2.1	140.5
Thailand	68.1	15	9	0.6	73.4
Turkey	73.6	18	6	1.2	94.7
Vietnam	88.9	17	5	1.2	113.7
LATIN AMERICA	585	19	6	1.3	729
Argentina	40.5	18	8	1.0	52.4
Brazil	193.3	17	6	1.0	215.3
Colombia	45.5	20	6	1.4	61.3
Cuba	11.2	11	8	0.3	9.7
Mexico	110.6	19	5	1.4	129.0
Panama	3.5	20	5	1.6	5.0
Peru	29.5	21	6	1.6	39.8
Venezuela	28.8	21	5	1.6	41.7
NORTH AMERICA	344	13	8	0.6	471
Canada	34.1	11	7	0.4	48.4
United States	309.6	14	8	0.6	422.6
EUROPE	739	11	11	0.0	720
France	63	13	9	0.4	70.0
Germany	81.6	8	10	−0.2	71.5
Ireland	4.5	17	6	1.0	6.4
Italy	60.5	10	10	0.0	61.7
Poland	38.2	11	10	0.1	31.8
Russia	141.9	12	14	−0.2	126.7
Spain	47.1	11	8	0.3	49.1
United Kingdom	62.2	13	9	0.4	77.0
Ukraine	45.9	11	15	−0.4	35.3

*(mid-2010)
Source: Extracted from *2010 World Population Data Sheet*, July 2010, Population Reference Bureau.

those of Paraguay. The result was virtual extinction for the Paraguayans, whose army was outnumbered 10 to 1 and included 12-year-old boys fighting alongside their grandfathers. Within a five-year period, the population of Paraguay dropped from an estimated 525,000 to 221,000, of whom slightly less than 29,000 were men. A new generation of Paraguayans was sired courtesy of the Brazilian army of occupation (Herring, 1960).

Such examples, while tragic in terms of individual suffering and occasionally disastrous to certain ethnic groups or nationalities (e.g., the total extermination of native Tasmanians by white settlers), nevertheless represented only minor aberrations from the general upward trend. In general, world population has increased more or less steadily, at first quite slowly but subsequently faster and faster from ancient times right up to the present.

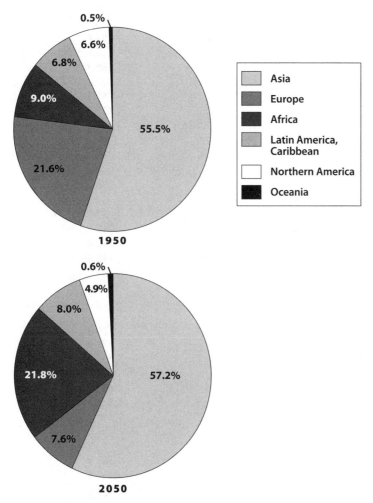

Source: Adapted from *World Population Prospects: The 2008 Revision*, United Nations Population Division, 2009. Used with permission.

Figure 2-4   Share of World Population by Major Geographical Region, 1950 and 2050

Demographic Transition

By the latter half of the 19th century, western Europe began to witness a demographic phenomenon unlike any that had occurred previously anywhere in the world. Toward the end of the 1700s and early in the 1800s, as the Industrial Revolution began transforming an entire way of life, death rates started to fall gradually in response to a more adequate food supply, improved medical knowledge, better public sanitation, and so forth. As a result, growth rates predictably accelerated, and during the early years of the 19th century western Europe experienced a population boom. This led, among other things, to massive emigration to the Western Hemisphere. By approximately 1850 another rather surprising trend became apparent: throughout the industrializing nations of that era, birth rates began to fall for the first time since the agricultural revolution. The Scandinavian countries (which were among the first to compile accurate demographic records) provide a good example of the changes that were occurring. In Denmark, Norway, and Sweden the combined birth rate was about 32 in 1850; by 1900 it had dropped to 28 and today stands at 12, among the lowest in the world. Elsewhere in western Europe similar declines were becoming apparent. This phenomenon—declining birth and death rates following industrialization—marked the onset of the **demographic transition**, a trend that accelerated throughout the 20th century. By the 1930s, decreases in the birth rates in some countries had outpaced decreases in death rates, though actual birth rates remained somewhat higher than death rates.

Reasons for the demographic transition are still being debated, but the cause for declining birth rates probably centers on the realization by married couples that in an industrial society children are an economic liability; they are expensive to feed, clothe, and educate; they reduce family mobility and make capital accumulation more difficult. In rural areas of Europe, population pressures on a finite amount of land and the modernization and mechanization of farming techniques, which reduced the amount of manual labor needed, combined to bring about a reduction in rural birth rates also. In addition, during the late 1800s and into the 20th century, a trend toward marrying at a later age undoubtedly contributed to the decreasing birth rates.

The decline in both birth and death rates that marked the demographic transition in western Europe became noticeable in both eastern Europe and North America several decades later. Today Russia and most of the formerly Communist nations of eastern Europe have some of the lowest birth rates in the world, attributed in large part to poor economic conditions that have convinced young women that now is not the time to start a family. Recently, however, in Russia and several other former Soviet republics, the decline in mortality rates experienced almost everywhere else in the world has been reversed. Due largely to rampant alcoholism, the spread of HIV/AIDS, and a deteriorating health-care system, death rates, especially for Russian men, have risen dramatically since the mid-1960s; life expectancy for Russian men in 2010 was the lowest in Europe, just 62 compared with a continent-wide average of 72 and a high of 80 for Iceland and Switzerland. Mortality rates for Russian women are somewhat better at 74, but still well below the European average of 80. Infant mortality also is considerably higher than that of other industrialized countries. According to the 2009 *CIA World Factbook* figures, 10.56 out of every 1,000 Russian babies were dying before their first birthday, compared to 6.3 in the United States and just 2.75 in Sweden. This situation of falling birth rates and rising death rates has resulted in an unprecedented population decline in that region of the world. In North America today, Canada's demographic statistics mirror those of western Europe. The United States, by contrast, outpaces all other industrialized countries in its rate of population growth, in part due to a slightly higher birth rate and record-high levels of immigration.

In the nations of Asia, Africa, and Latin America where traditional societies were only marginally influenced by the dynamic economic and social changes occurring in Europe and North America, demographic patterns changed very little until early in the 20th century. In the areas under the control of imperial powers, improvements in public sanitation and an imposed peace between formerly warring factions within the subject nations permitted a gradual increase in population levels. This gradual decline in death rates took a quantum leap in the years immediately following World War II as modern drugs and public health measures were exported from the industrialized nations to the developing countries. Virtually overnight, the widely applauded introduction of "death control" into traditional cultures produced the most rapid, widespread change known in the history of population dynamics, as wide-scale spraying with the chemical insecticide DDT brought rapid, albeit temporary, control over mosquito-borne killers such as malaria

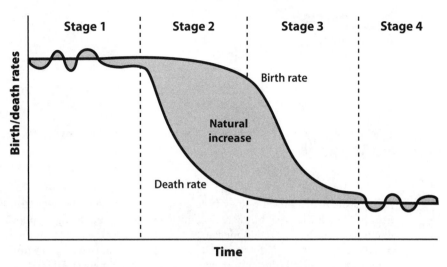

Source: "Population: A Lively Introduction" by Joseph A. McFalls, Jr., *Population Bulletin* 58, no. 4 (Dec. 2003). Used with permission of the Population Reference Bureau.

Figure 2-5   The Classic Stages of Demographic Transition

and yellow fever. Similar victories over smallpox, cholera, polio, and other infectious diseases caused death rates to plummet throughout most of the developing world during the 1950s and 1960s.

This trend has been most pronounced among children and young adults. Since 1960, according to a World Bank report, the number of children who die before reaching their fifth birthday has declined by two-thirds, thanks to greater public access to standard immunizations and oral rehydration therapy for treating diarrheal diseases (Altman, 1993). In spite of this notable achievement, child mortality still accounts for a large proportion of all deaths in low-income countries, making additional gains in eliminating childhood infectious diseases the most effective way of further lowering mortality rates in poor countries. By contrast, in wealthier nations, where the largest proportion of deaths is among the elderly, the notable gains in life expectancy witnessed during the past several decades are largely a result of reduced death rates among middle-aged and older people. In these societies, the greatest potential for increasing life expectancy lies in improved treatment for adult health problems (Bremner et al., 2009).

The rapid fall in death rates experienced by developing nations in the years immediately following World War II was qualitatively different from the slow, long-term decline that occurred throughout most of the world following the agricultural revolution. It was also different in kind from the comparatively more rapid decline in death rates in the Western world over the past century. The difference is that it came about in response to a spectacular environmental change in the nations of Asia, Africa, and Latin America largely through the control of infectious

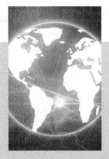

· · · · · · · 2-2 · · · · · · ·

Europe's Demographic Dilemma

Europe today is grappling with a demographic conundrum as its leaders confront a continent-wide "birth dearth" that promises inevitable population decline in the decades ahead. With fertility rates in most European countries well below replacement level and a rapidly aging population, Europe's demographic dilemma raises serious economic issues, since the current worker-to-retiree ratio of 4:1 will shrink to just 2:1 by 2050 if present trends continue. Officials estimate that two decades from now the European Union (EU) could face a shortfall of 20 million workers. In such a situation, EU nations would find it extremely difficult to finance the retirement benefits of so many retirees and would either have to reduce pensions or raise the retirement age. Some Europeans voice concerns that too few young men are produced for military service and fear loss of world influence, while others foresee the likely collapse of Europe's elaborate social welfare system. Efforts to forestall such problems have focused largely on incentives to boost birth rates and/or on augmentation of the labor force through "guest worker" programs. Unfortunately, the former have been largely unsuccessful, while the latter have been highly controversial, provoking a right-wing backlash among native Europeans fearful of becoming ethnic minorities in their own homelands.

In general, politicians find it easier and more palatable to tackle Europe's demographic challenge through policies aimed at providing "baby bonuses" and subsidized day care to encourage couples to produce more children. Among the most generous is France, which not only gives direct per-child payments to families but also allocates funds for clothing and school supplies. In Austria, women receive the equivalent of nearly $600/month for three years after a birth. Such policies have helped to maintain fertility at near replacement level in the Scandinavian countries and France, but notwithstanding these financial incentives, young women from Paris to Prague are opting for careers in preference to tending a houseful of children.

Immigration thus remains the most realistic option for rejuvenating Europe's aging societies, since few European countries are maintaining their population through births. However, the number of new immigrants necessary to prevent population decline is so large that political realities make such an influx highly unlikely. Opinion polls in most EU countries, as well as in Russia, reveal strong opposition to increasing immigration as a means of maintaining current population levels.

The continent's current immigration headaches can be attributed in large part to the shortage of workers in the 1960s, when western Europe's post-World War II export industries were booming. When an influx of labor from Italy and other southern European countries proved insufficient to meet the demand, France and Germany began recruiting "guest workers" from North Africa and Turkey. It was assumed that these foreign laborers would eventually return home, but as observers have wryly remarked, "Nothing is more permanent than temporary workers." As the years passed, these first cohorts of migrants settled in and were joined by family members, showing little inclination to return to less-prosperous homelands, even when host countries offered unemployed migrants "departure bonuses" as an alternative to social welfare benefits during hard economic times. Today, half a century after the influx began, European governments are still struggling to integrate these guest workers and their offspring, stymied both by the unwillingness of native citizens to welcome alien newcomers as equals and by the reluctance of many immigrants to relinquish their own culture and adopt the values and customs of their new country of residence.

In recent years, immigration to western Europe has grown to 300,000–500,000 legal new arrivals annually, plus up to a half million illegal migrants each year. By 2005 the foreign-born percentage of the population totaled 9% in Germany and Belgium, 10% in Austria, 20% in Switzerland, and 40% in tiny Luxembourg. If the European-born children of immigrant families are included, the percentage of residents of foreign *origin* in some countries is considerably higher. In the Netherlands, for example, the percentage of residents born in another country is just 4%, but those of foreign origin total 19%. Since Europe has traditionally been a region of *emigration*, experiencing an outflow of more than 60 million people between 1820 and 1914, its new role as a *destination* for international migrants has generated rising concern and some degree of antagonism among the host population. Such concerns have been intensified by the fact that most of the immigrants are from non-EU countries—66% of migrants to the United Kingdom, 62% in the Netherlands, 55% in France (Martin and Zürcher, 2008). The impact on the ethnic composition of the receiving nations is provoking worries that the flood of alien newcomers could have a deleterious impact on local economies and culture, particularly since many come from Muslim countries, provoking fears that immigrant ghettos could be breeding grounds for Islamic fundamentalism and terrorist incidents within Europe.

As the immigrant population continues to increase, some observers question whether a new type of demographic transition is now underway in wealthy, low-fertility countries, characterized by a radical and probably permanent alteration in the ethnic and racial composition of once-homogeneous societies. They use the term "replacement migration" to describe the situation occurring throughout western Europe, where increasing numbers of young immigrants are out-producing the natives and constitute a growing percentage of the population—one of the most radical demographic shifts ever seen over such a large geographic area in the absence of force or military invasion (Coleman, 2006).

Immigration has, not surprisingly, become a hot domestic policy issue in several European countries and has given rise to far-right political movements with a distinctly anti-foreign flavor. The fact that unemployment rates among foreign-origin residents are often twice as high as those for native-born citizens is another reason for many Europeans to object to prevailing immigration policies. They are also demanding stronger measures to discourage illegal immigration; in response, the European Union Commission and individual EU member states are establishing "mobility partnership agreements" with certain nations of origin for illegal migrants. A case in point involves the agreement between the West African nation of Senegal and Spain, in which the former agreed to patrol its harbors to prevent migrants from embarking in small boats headed for Spain's Canary Islands—a major European entry point for illegal migrants—while Spain, in return, pledged to admit several thousand Senegalese to work legally in that country for a year or two.

Given that over a million migrants, both legal and illegal, are entering Europe each year, recent estimates by the UN Population Division on the number required to solve Europe's future demographic problems are sobering. According to the UN, in order to maintain Europe's population size at its 1995 level, EU countries as a whole would need to quadruple the number of immigrants admitted each year; to maintain the size of the labor force, immigration would have to increase six-fold; and to preserve the 1995 ratio between those aged 15–64 vs. those over 65, 50 times more migrants would need to be granted entry than was the case in 1995. There is no evidence that Europeans are willing to open their doors to such a massive influx, especially in light of growing hostility to those already settled in but not assimilated. Thus it is likely that a long-term population decline for most of the continent's nations—and a gradual shift in their ethnic makeup as established migrant communities continue to out-breed their hosts—is now irrevocable and well underway (Martin and Zürcher, 2008).

diseases, not through a fundamental change in their institutions or way of life. Furthermore, the change did not originate in these countries themselves, but was introduced from the outside. The importation of death control without corresponding adoption of birth control in the mid-20th century resulted in a large portion of humanity moving rapidly from a situation of high birth and death rates to one of low death rates but still-high birth rates—and a corresponding explosive increase in total population size. By the 1960s and 1970s, alarmed observers like population biologist Paul Ehrlich were referring to this phenomenon as the "population bomb" and forecast dire consequences for scores of developing nations.

However, by the 1980s and 1990s, a steady decline in fertility in almost all developing nations—except those in sub-Saharan Africa—was well underway, signaling that

the demographic transition was indeed a near-universal phenomenon. Today, even in nations where levels of economic development remain low, access to modern contraceptives and greater employment opportunities for women have resulted in larger-than-expected fertility declines within the past two decades. Nevertheless, it will take at least another generation or two for most developing nations to complete their demographic transition, characterized by replacement-level fertility and a stable population size. In the meantime, the demographic gap between developed and developing nations continues to widen. Just as developing nations were responsible for 90% of the population growth during the 20th century, demographers predict that virtually all the increase in human numbers likely to occur over the next several decades will be in less-developed countries. While some industrialized nations will continue to experience modest growth due to immigration from the developing world (indeed, 40% of U.S. population growth in recent years is a result of immigration), only in the United States does natural increase—the excess of births over deaths—account for more than half of annual population growth (Bremner et al., 2009).

Age Structure

It's relatively easy to comprehend the significance of birth and death rates so far as population growth is concerned, but there are other characteristics of a population that are important also. Age structure refers to the number of people in different age categories within a given population. In countries where populations are growing rapidly because of high birth rates and declining death rates, a large percentage of the population is made up of young people; in many African countries, 43% of the population is under the age of 15. In western Europe, by contrast, there are proportionately many more people in the middle and older age groups. In countries where children comprise a large segment of the population, there hasn't been time yet for individuals born during the period of "death control" to reach the older age groups where death rates are higher than those of the younger age categories. In most of these countries the greatest decreases in death rates among infants and children occurred in the late 1940s and the large numbers of children born in that period reached their peak reproductive years in the 1970s. Their children, in turn, are further inflating the lower tiers of the population structure. The extraordinarily large percentage of children that characterizes the current population of most developing countries accounts for the fact that their death rates today are as low as, or lower than, death rates in the industrialized countries where a significantly larger percentage of the population is elderly.

One of the most significant features of age structure in a population is the proportion of people who are economically productive (arbitrarily considered to be those persons between 15 and 59) in relation to those who are dependent on them. The proportion of dependents in the underdeveloped countries is much higher than in the developed nations, presenting an additional heavy burden to those countries as they struggle for economic development. The high percentage of people under 15 is also indicative of the explosive growth potential of their populations. In most developing nations this percentage is 30–40%, while in Uganda and Niger children comprise fully 49% of the population! By contrast, the percentage under 15 in most industrialized countries is 17%. In the United States, for example, there are two people of working age for every one who is too young or too old to work; in Mexico and Nigeria there is only one. Thus, underdeveloped countries have a much greater proportion of people in their pre-reproductive years. As they grow up and marry, the size of the childbearing fraction of the population will increase tremendously and their children will further inflate the size of the youngest age groups. The existence of such large numbers of young people means that even if great progress were made immediately in reducing the number of births per female in those countries, it would still be some 30 years before such birth control could significantly slow down population growth (PRB, 2010).

For those nations that have recently experienced rapidly declining fertility, there may be some positive short-term economic consequences resulting from their shifting demographic profile. As their large current crop of youngsters enters the workforce and is replaced at the bottom of the age structure pyramid by a much smaller cohort of "baby-busters," economic development could soar, just as it did in South Korea, Taiwan, and Thailand when their fertility rates began a free-fall a few decades ago. Economists are urging leaders in these countries to

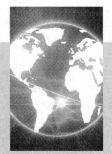

· · · · · · · 2-3 · · · · · · ·

Global Graying

While leaders of the developing nations struggle to meet the needs of still-growing populations, their counterparts in the industrialized world are facing an entirely different problem: a disproportionate and rapidly increasing percentage of elderly citizens as the "baby bust" generates ever-smaller cohorts of young people. Thanks to improved health care, nutrition, and general standard of living, today's elderly are experiencing an unprecedented degree of longevity. Indeed, it's estimated that in all of human history, two-thirds of all the people who have ever reached age 65 are living today. Global life expectancy has lengthened more in the last 50 years than it did throughout the previous 5,000. Until the onset of the industrial era, only 2–3% of people born lived beyond age 65; today in developed countries that figure is 15% and rising. By 2030, the UN estimates that fully one-quarter of the planet's population will be in the "senior" category.

This "global graying" is especially pronounced in Japan and Europe. Characterized by plummeting birth rates and excellent health care, those countries have been witnessing a steady decline in the proportion of young people and a simultaneous swelling of the ranks of the elderly. Italy now has more citizens over 60 years old than it has under the age of 20—the first nation in history to experience such a transformation in age structure. In what one commentator refers to as the "Floridazation" of the developed world, many countries have already or will soon attain the 19% elderly population that already characterizes the "Sunshine State." Germany, Italy, Greece, and Japan have already reached or surpassed that benchmark and will soon be joined by Belgium and Spain; by 2016 France and the United Kingdom will be added to the list (higher fertility rates in the U.S. and Canada should postpone their year of reckoning until 2021 and 2023, respectively).

So why should these trends cause any concern? After all, humans have always considered long life among the greatest of blessings, and for years environmentalists and population control advocates have preached the virtues of small family size. Now that these goals have been attained, at least in some countries, why isn't there universal rejoicing? Certainly from an ecological standpoint the news *is* good, since all of the countries in question could be considered overpopulated in terms of their environmental impact. Any reduction in population size can only improve congestion, levels of pollution and consumption, and impact on ecosystems. Worries about global aging trends focus primarily on economic and socio-political considerations, with some analysts predicting that this unprecedented demographic age shift promises to become the overriding economic and political issue of the 21st century.

Paramount among the issues involved is the impact on retirement benefit systems. Like the U.S. Social Security System, the "safety net" social programs in place in most industrialized nations were created at a time when average life expectancy was less than the legal retirement age and when the ratio of young workers to retired persons was heavily weighted toward the former group. Most social security schemes, in essence, borrow from today's workers to support today's retirees. However, as the retired population grows larger and the proportion of young people in the population shrinks, the economic burden on working-age men and women will become increasingly heavy. Today throughout the industrialized world there are three working taxpayers for every retired person. However, unless national retirement systems are radically reformed, by 2030 there will be only 1.5 workers for every pensioner. In negative-growth countries like Italy and Germany the ratio will be just 1:1. While American politicians debate how to save Social Security, the dilemmas confronting leaders in Europe and Japan are even more urgent. With lower birth rates, more rapidly aging populations, larger public pension benefits, and weaker private pension systems than in the U.S., Europeans and Japanese will be hard pressed to preserve social programs and a high standard of living. Health-care costs in an aging world will be even more burdensome than pensions. Since the elderly consume three to five times more health-care services per person than do younger citizens, health-care spending is likely to soar. Experts predict that to meet existing old-age benefit commitments, within the next 30 years developed nations cumulatively will have to spend an extra 12–13% of GDP. Fears are that this unprecedented burden could destabilize the global economy, threatening financial and political institutions worldwide.

Global graying presents national security concerns as well. Whether developed countries remain able to maintain their military commitments in light of a shrinking pool of potential soldiers and sailors is as yet an unanswered question. Pressure to relax immigration restrictions to ease worker shortages could mount in some countries, in turn creating more strife and political turmoil in areas where an ethnic imbalance is already provoking nationalistic resentment.

Whether or not current developed-world attitudes become more pronatalist in the future (and there's no indication they will), global graying is inevitable in the decades ahead because the elderly of 2050 have already been born. The implications of this trend—for society, the economy, and for the environment—will be profound in ways we can now only dimly foresee. As Nicholas Eberstadt, a demographer at the American Enterprise Institute remarked: "What is happening now has simply never happened before in the history of the world. . . . If these trends continue, in a generation or two there may be countries where most people's only blood relatives will be their parents" (Peterson, 2002; 1999).

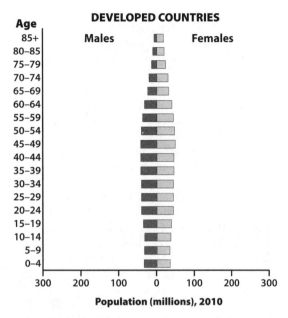

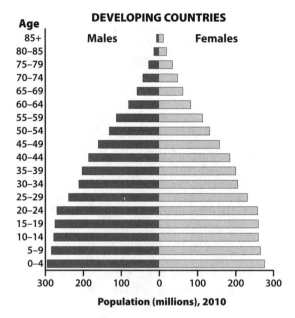

Source: Carl Haub, *2010 World Population Data Sheet*. Permission granted by the Population Reference Bureau, www.prb.org.

Figure 2-6   Population Pyramid of Developed versus Developing Countries

take advantage of this "demographic dividend"—a narrow window in time when the working-age population will be at an all-time high in relation to the number of young children and elderly citizens. A lower dependency load during this once-only opportunity will facilitate higher savings and investment, providing that governments develop wise economic policies and invest adequate resources to improve education, health care, and the status of women. If they let this opportunity pass, the "window" will close as the ranks of the elderly steadily climb (Sheehan, 2003; "Economics Focus," 2002).

URBANIZATION

The "urban explosion," referring to the tremendous population increase in metropolitan areas, has been one of the most marked phenomena related to the overall growth of human populations during the past century. Urbanization is, of course, one of the oldest of demographic trends, having its roots in the small settled communities made possible by an agricultural way of life. The first true cities are believed to have arisen in Mesopotamia about 5 or 6 thousand years ago, but growth of urban areas proceeded rather slowly during the millennia that followed. Increase in urban populations depended almost entirely on an influx of new residents from the surrounding countryside. Due to extremely poor sanitary conditions and crowded living conditions, mortality rates in these urban centers were higher than birth rates, and

not until recent times have urban centers become self-sustaining in terms of population growth.

The advent of the Industrial Revolution gave a tremendous impetus to the growth of cities, and the rate of increase has continued to accelerate ever since. As an example of the population shift that has occurred, consider the change in rural-urban ratios in the United States: in 1800 a mere 6% of all Americans lived in an urban area; the number of city dwellers increased to 15% by 1850 and to 40% by 1900. In 2010, 79% of the U.S. population lived in cities. [Note: in the United States, "urban" is defined as any community with a population of 2,500 or more. Different countries use different cutoff points to distinguish urban from rural populations, complicating the comparison of urbanization statistics from various parts of the world. For example, while American demographers utilize the 2,500 figure, their colleagues in Iceland consider a village of 200 as urban; in Italy the corresponding number is 10,000, while in densely populated Japan, a community is considered urban only when its population surpasses 50,000! (Haub, 1993).]

In the world as a whole, population increased by a factor of 2.6 during the years between 1800 and 1950; during that same time period the number of people living in cities over 20,000 population grew from 22 million to over half a billion—a factor of 23. In the largest cities (100,000 or more) of the industrialized countries, the growth was even more rapid, increasing by a factor of 35. By 1950, 29% of the world's people lived in cities; in early 2008 city dwellers surpassed 50% of world population for the first time in history, reaching 3.3 billion. By 2050 that number will nearly double to 6.4 billion.

In recent years this urban expansion in the developed world has slowed somewhat, but since 1900 has accelerated at a great rate in the nations of Asia, Africa, and Latin America, fueled both by natural population growth within cities and by in-migration from rural hinterlands. By 2030, according to United Nations (UN) projections, over half the developing world's population will live in urban areas (44% in 2009); by 2050, two-thirds will be city dwellers. In fact, virtually all the increase in world population between now and mid-century will occur within urban areas of developing countries, at which time the UN projects their numbers to swell to 5.26 billion, up from slightly over 2 billion in 2009.

The phenomenal rate of urban growth during the past century has given rise to a new term—**megacity**—coined to describe any urban area with a population of 10 million or more. In 1900 there were none; at that time London, with a population of 5 million, was the world's largest city. One hundred years later, the UN estimated there were 19 megacities, 13 in the developing world, and predicted that by 2015 an additional 15 would be added to the list, all of them in less-developed countries. Nevertheless, in spite of this spectacular growth in a number of major metropolitan areas, only about 12% of urban residents in the developing world live in megacities. The great majority reside in smaller towns and cities where provision of basic services is scarcely better than it is in the countryside (Montgomery, 2008). Such growth is already having a staggering impact on the ability of those municipalities to provide even the rudiments of a decent standard of living. Much of the population growth in Third World cities

occurs in so-called "illegal settlements"—slum areas and shantytowns built without regard to local regulations, often on land illegally occupied or illegally subdivided. These squatter settlements continue to spread like ugly cancerous growths around the periphery of almost every large city in the developing world. Estimates indicate that between 30–60% of the people in developing world cities

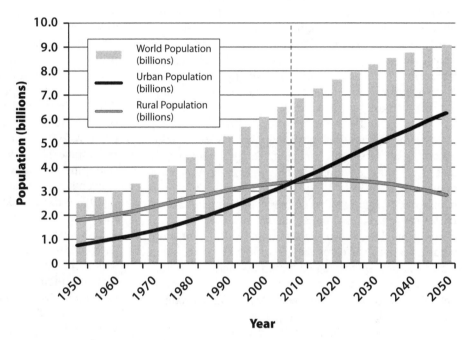

Source: Data from *World Urbanization Prospects: The 2009 Revision*, United Nations Population Division, 2010; *World Population Prospects: The 2008 Revision*, United Nations Population Division, 2009.

Figure 2-7   World Urban and Rural Population, 1950–2050

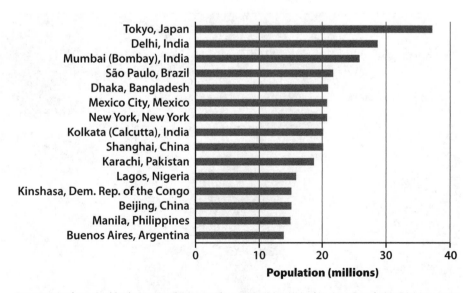

Source: Data from *World Urbanization Prospects: The 2009 Revision*, United Nations Population Division, 2010.

Figure 2-8   15 Largest Cities in the World in 2025

currently live in substandard housing (World Resources Institute, 1996). These uncontrolled settlements are growing even faster than the urban areas as a whole, with the consequence that in the years ahead an ever-larger segment of city dwellers in developing countries will be living in the squalor and hopelessness that characterize these shantytowns.

In most cases the urbanization trend seems to be driven by the hope for a better, more comfortable life, and though most migrants continue to live in abject poverty, nearly all seem to prefer to remain there rather than return to the deprivation of their rural home villages. Ironically, recent studies have shown that, contrary to migrant expectations, the quality of life in many developing world cities today is worse than it is in the rural areas they left behind (Brockerhoff and Brennan, 1998). Throughout the developing world, poverty is increasingly becoming an urban phenomenon. Today approximately half of the world's poorest people are living in urban settlements and the World Bank predicts that by 2025 most people in developing world cities will be living in poverty. Historically, urbanization seems to have the universal effect of breaking down the traditional cultures of those who migrate to the cities, where anonymity is the main feature. A large percentage of urban dwellers in developing countries are migrants who have brought their peasant culture with them. They generally lack the specialized education and skills required to penetrate the city's complex social web. Migrants inevitably find that their limited skills make them incapable of contributing to the economy and consequently they are scarcely any better off than before.

The rapid growth of urban populations in less-developed countries has profound public health implications, particularly for residents of the informal settlements and shantytowns. Although city dwellers in the developing world generally tend to enjoy a "health advantage" compared to rural villagers, those living in urban slums are often no better off—and sometimes worse—than their country cousins in terms of health risks. Inadequate access to reliable supplies of safe drinking water and the provision of sanitary services constitute major problems affecting the health and well-being of millions of poor urban residents in the developing world. In spite of the UN's Millennium Development Goal of reducing by half the proportion of people lacking safe water supplies by 2015, it's estimated that over the last decade the number of city dwellers in this category *increased* by 60 million (Barlow, 2006). In many developing-world slums, a large percentage of residents obtain their water from shared standpipes that may serve hundreds or even thousands of residents, necessitating long waits for their turn at the tap. Even those lucky enough to have a water tap inside their home face sporadic cutoffs in supply; in Chennai, India's fourth-largest city, a prolonged drought during the early 1990s resulted in the restriction of tap water provision to just two hours every two days. Even under normal conditions, residents of many cities throughout the developing world must cope with an intermittent water supply on a daily basis, utilizing the few hours when water is flowing to fill every available storage vessel.

Inadequate—or nonexistent—sanitation systems affect an even larger proportion of city dwellers in poor countries. In slum areas it's common for families to share

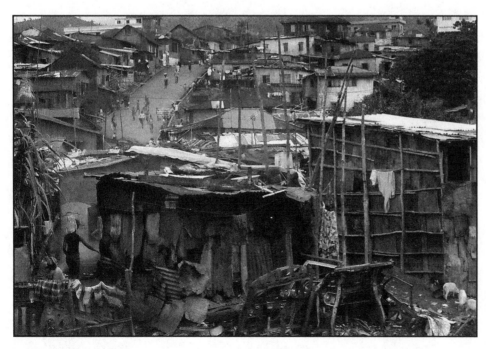

Much of the urban population growth in the least developed countries occurs in slum areas that lack even the most basic rudiments of a decent standard of living.

poorly maintained, often overflowing public latrines with 100 or more neighbors. Millions of urban residents in developing countries don't have access even to simple latrines, having to resort to roadside ditches or open spaces (Hardoy et al., 2001). Exposed, untreated human wastes constitute a serious water pollution problem when stormwater washes fecal material into adjacent waterways. In many developing world cities, rivers and canals are little more than open sewers and constitute a direct public health threat. An example of the magnitude of this problem is China, where approximately 200 million people live in communities that lack any sanitation system whatsoever other than pipes carrying wastewater to the nearest ditch. Not surprisingly, it's estimated that fully 60% of the rivers flowing through Chinese cities fail to meet minimum drinking water standards (Economy, 2004; Jiang et al., 2008).

As urban populations continue to expand, the ability of governments to provide such basic services will undoubtedly lag even further behind, increasing the threat of epidemic disease. In addition to water supply and sanitation problems, air quality continues to worsen as the number of private automobiles, trucks, buses, and motorbikes rises exponentially. Poorly regulated industrial emissions further contribute to the unhealthy urban atmosphere. The proliferation of motor vehicles has spawned a new hazard in developing-world cities; due to nonexistent or poorly enforced driving regulations, traffic

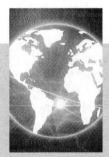

• • • • • • • 2-4 • • • • • • •
Failed States

Each year since 2005, *Foreign Policy* magazine, in collaboration with independent research organization The Fund for Peace, publishes the "Failed States Index" in its July/August issue. Based on information gathered from over 30,000 publicly available sources, the authors of the report examine indicators of national performance and cohesion such as public services, human rights, refugee flows, economic decline, and so forth. Among these key indicators of instability and impending crisis in the world's most fragile countries, demographic pressures head the list. High rates of unemployment in the swollen ranks of teenagers and young adults that characterize age structure in most developing countries are inextricably linked to the high birth rates still prevailing in those societies. Studies have shown a direct link between youthful populations and outbreaks of civil unrest, documenting a 15% greater risk of conflict in societies where young people make up more than 35% of the population, as compared to those with a more evenly balanced age ratio. Poverty, environmental degradation, and competition for dwindling resources are all made worse by high rates of population growth and contribute to conflict, chaos, and, in some cases, institutional collapse. Little wonder, then, that the top ten countries in the most recent "Failed States Index" are all nations characterized by exceptionally high birth rates and a high percentage of their population under the age of 15. (For reference, recall that the average birth rate in developed countries is 12, with just 17% of the population below the age of 15.)

RANKING OF "FAILED STATES"

Rank	Country	Birth Rate	Percent of Population <15
1	Somalia	45	45
2	Zimbabwe	32	40
3	Sudan	33	41
4	Chad	43	46
5	Dem. Rep. of the Congo	47	47
6	Iraq	32	41
7	Afghanistan	39	44
8	Central African Republic	38	41
9	Guinea	39	43
10	Pakistan	30	38

For these countries, as well as numerous others slightly lower on the list, rapidly increasing population size isn't the only factor thrusting them into the "failed" category, but it certainly makes all their other problems more difficult to solve. Approximately 57% of the world's people today live in countries where the population is still growing, and although UN population projections assume that fertility everywhere will eventually drop slightly below replacement level, such an assumption may be overly optimistic. During the past decade, fertility declines in sub-Saharan Africa have stalled at 4 children/woman or higher and poor developing nations are expected to see their already-bulging populations grow by almost 3 billion by 2050 (Leahy and Peoples, 2008).

The potential for such rapid population growth to overwhelm existing resources, thereby threatening livelihoods and sparking conflict, has already been recognized as a threat to global security. The director of the U.S. Central Intelligence Agency (CIA), General Michael Hayden, in 2008 cited population growth as among the top three destabilizing trends facing the world community. A case in point is Somalia, #1 on the list of failed states, where a total breakdown of governance, intertribal strife, flight of refugees, collapse of public services and security—exacerbated by rapid population growth—has provoked fears within the international community that al Qaeda or other terrorist organizations could emerge as the dominant force controlling the country. (Other sources, however, contend that Somalia is "too failed even for al Qaeda"!) Global security experts are also watching the nation of Yemen with considerable trepidation. Located at the southwestern tip of the Arabian peninsula, Yemen's population (3% annual rate of increase) of 23 million is projected to double in just 24 years; by 2025 its population will be almost equal to that of its geographically much larger neighbor, Saudi Arabia, and by 2050 will exceed that of the Saudis. Yemen is currently the main destination for Somali refugees, with 50,000 entering the country in 2008 alone. Absorbing such a large—and continuing—influx of migrants is putting further stress on Yemen's already overtaxed land and water resources. High rates of extraction are causing water tables to fall by 6 feet annually and experts predict the country's groundwater supply will be totally exhausted within a generation or two. Decreasing availability of water for irrigation is naturally having an impact on food production; Yemen's grain harvest has fallen by 50% over the last 35 years and the country now imports most of its food. As a result of spiraling population growth and a declining rural economy, Yemen's capital city, Sana'a, is now one of the fastest-growing urban areas in the world, expanding at a rate of 4% annually (Brown, 2009). With a rapidly growing, well-armed but poorly educated aggressive tribal society confronting escalating environmental and social pressures in a geographic region rife with political turmoil and extremist ideology, the potential for serious trouble in the years ahead is high. No wonder Yemen currently ranks #18 on the list of failed states.

One indicator *not* included in the *Foreign Policy*/Fund for Peace rankings is the potential for state failure due to impending climate change. Nevertheless, a number of observers have commented that the increasing frequency of droughts, floods, severe weather events, and, particularly, sea level rise could lead to collapse of some states. High on the list of those likely to be most affected as the world's climate heats up is Bangladesh, currently tied with Yemen for a #18 ranking. Flooding caused by warming-induced cyclones and rising sea levels could provoke a catastrophic humanitarian crisis, with mass migration of millions of refugees from that low-lying country into neighboring—and also overcrowded—India, Burma, and other nearby countries. In all likelihood, such population shifts will lead to clashes and rioting as native residents protest the incoming surge of environmental refugees. Perhaps the worst-case scenario involves Pakistan, now #10 on the list, where climate change is likely to devastate that nation's ability to feed itself. As disappearing Himalayan glaciers fail to replenish the rivers flowing from India's Kashmir State, irrigated agriculture in Pakistan, 90% of which relies on rivers with headwaters in Kashmir, will be devastated. Any efforts by India to dam Kashmiri rivers for its own use could result in armed conflict between two rival nations with a long history of enmity—and nuclear weapons (Faris, 2009).

Obviously, rapid population growth is not the only factor responsible for state failure—corrupt governance, a faltering economy, prolonged drought, global recession—all have a role to play. Nevertheless, for those trying to forecast the world's likeliest trouble spots in the years ahead, a brief comparison of national population growth statistics provides a good place to start.

accidents have become a leading cause of death and disability in many urban areas. The World Health Organization (WHO) estimates that, globally, 1.2 million people are killed each year in road traffic accidents, with an additional 20–50 million injuries; of these, the majority occur in poor countries. Among those aged 5–25, traffic accidents are among the three leading causes of death worldwide, with pedestrians facing the greatest risk in African countries, while bicycle and motor-scooter riders are the most common victims in Southeast Asia.

Other factors associated with the overcrowding and stress of millions of poor urban residents in the developing world are high levels of violence, including gang violence, criminal assault, and domestic violence—particularly physical and mental abuse of women. Although the latter can be an issue at any level of society, it seems to be more frequent in slum communities where male partners are often upset by their inability to find work, so indulge in heavy drinking and vent their frustrations by beating or verbally abusing their wives or girlfriends. As a result, studies of mental health in poor countries indicate that up to 51% of urban adults suffer from some type of depression, with women more likely to be affected than men, and poor women more so than those living in better neighborhoods.

Despite the ever-present risk of epidemic disease in crowded, unsanitary slums, access to health care for the poor is also problematic. Although most cities in the developing world have no shortage of doctors or health-care facilities, the fee-for-service system makes good medical care unaffordable for many poor residents. Although many countries provide government-subsidized health care for the poor, studies focusing on the level of medical skill among providers have shown wide discrepancies in the quality of care available in slum vs. non-slum sections of the same city, with significantly less-qualified doctors serving poorer neighborhoods (Montgomery, 2009). The imperative to ameliorate such conditions, along with pressures on municipal authorities to provide jobs, better housing, public transportation, and schools will mount inexorably in the years ahead and will present those societies with economic and environmental challenges which may prove impossible to meet.

POPULATION PROJECTIONS

The obvious question to anyone looking at a graphic representation of population growth such as that in figure 2.2 is "How long will growth continue?" and "At what level will population ultimately stabilize?" The implicit assumption, and one that is validated by the results of numerous animal experiments, is that human population growth cannot continue indefinitely. Statistical evidence indicates, in fact, that the world population annual growth rate peaked at about 2% in the early

1970s, declining gradually since then to its present 1.2%. Nevertheless, although a growth rate decrease is good news, in terms of absolute numbers population size will continue to increase for many decades, due to the world's enormous population base and the large proportion of young people in developing countries.

The United Nations, an organization logically quite interested in future world growth patterns, regularly publishes projections of population size for the next several decades. Such projections are not just extrapolations of present trends, but take into consideration trends in fertility, mortality, migration, and so on (they do not consider the possibility of major disasters such as a nuclear war, however). The UN Population Division presents several sets of projections, all of which assume that there will be some lowering of fertility rates (a substantial drop in fertility is assumed for the low projection, a less significant decline for the high projection) in regions where these are currently quite high. The most widely used medium range projection anticipates a world population of 9.2 billion by 2050, a figure that reflects a drop in fertility rates to replacement level or below in most countries (a group of high-fertility African nations, plus Afghanistan and Yemen, are exceptions to the general downward trend) and a rise in HIV/AIDS-related mortality rates in a number of severely impacted countries. Under the high-growth scenario, with fertility at 2.5 children per woman instead of 2.0 as assumed under the medium projection, world population size in 2050 would be approximately 10.5 billion. Under the UN's low projection, in which worldwide fertility rates rapidly drop below replacement level to just 1.5 children per woman, world population would peak in 2042 at 8 billion and then begin a gradual decline (UNFPA, 2009). Quite obviously, the childbearing decisions of millions of individual couples will have an enormous impact on total world population size at the time growth eventually levels off. Of course, widely divergent fertility patterns in different areas of the world guarantee that some regions will achieve population stability long before others do. Austria, Italy, and Japan have already reached zero population growth (ZPG), while such countries as Germany, Russia, Ukraine, Belarus, Hungary, Serbia, Croatia, Romania, Portugal, and Bulgaria actually have negative growth rates (PRB, 2010). By 2050 the UN projects that the populations of 30 developed nations, including Japan and most of the European countries, will be smaller than they are today, as deaths among the large cohorts of elderly outnumber births.

Looking at population projections on a regional basis, Asia, thanks to its already huge population base, will experience the largest increase in total numbers in spite of declining fertility levels. India alone, growing by about 20 million annually, is expected to surpass China to become the world's most populous country within the next few decades. With the world's highest birth rates and a large percentage of its children under 15, Africa currently has the world's highest growth rates and will see its current population of nearly 1 billion more than double by 2050. Together, Africa and Asia will account

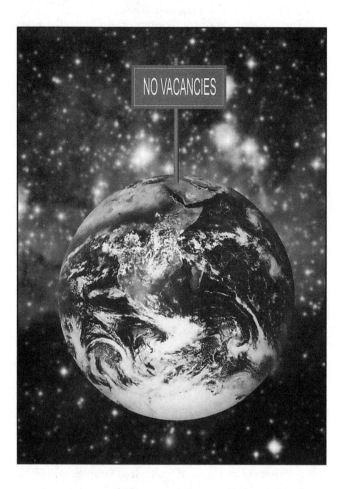

for fully 80% of the world's total population at the time of stabilization. Latin America and the Caribbean nations, with a current combined population of 580 million, continue to grow at a rate second only to Africa. In 1960 there were approximately equal numbers of Latin Americans and North Americans; by 2050 there will be 724 million people living south of the Rio Grande, 481 million to the north. Only Europe, among major geographical regions, is projected to experience population decline in the years ahead, falling from 739 million in 2010 to 720 million in 2050 (PRB, 2010).

Obviously, making global population projections is a risky business, with accuracy of forecasts depending not only on the childbearing decisions of millions of individual couples but also on trends in mortality rates. While most long-range projections show global population growth halting between 2050–2100, the ability of natural ecosystems to support additional billions of people has been questioned. Since almost all of the expected increase will occur in the poorest countries where people are most dependent on natural ecosystems for their survival and well-being, many observers insist that population growth needs to be stabilized long before it reaches the theoretical levels projected by the United Nations. Recognizing the enormous cooperative effort needed to resolve humanity's demographic dilemma, 1,670 scientists from 70 countries have signed a population stabilization statement drafted by the Union of Concerned Scientists, declaring that:

> Fundamental changes are urgent if we are to avoid the collision our present course will bring about . . . if vast human misery is to be avoided and our global home on this planet is not to be irretrievably mutilated. (Tobias, 1998)

······· 3 ·······

We want better reasons for having children
than not knowing how to prevent them.
—Dora Russell, English feminist (1925)

Population Control

Apocalyptic visions of a planet imploding under the sheer weight of human numbers, so prevalent just a few decades ago, are now giving way to the realization that the "population bomb" has largely been defused. Thanks in part to the alarms raised during the 1960s and 1970s when the world population growth rate was at its peak, the introduction of family-planning programs and modern means of contraception into high-fertility developing nations has had a profound impact in reducing runaway population growth. Indeed, a number of developing countries are now close to achieving population stability, having completed their demographic transition far more rapidly than experts had predicted. However, media reports alleging that overpopulation is no longer a problem mistakenly assume that the decline in growth rates implies a leveling-off in total population size. In fact, owing to an already-enormous population base, today's 1.2% population growth rate, down from the 2% prevailing at the peak of the "population explosion," translates to a world population increase of more than 80 million annually—about the same as the yearly increment in the early 1970s when alarm bells were ringing. Also, as mentioned in the preceding chapter, high fertility and correspondingly high rates of population growth continue to be the norm in most nations of Africa and the Middle East. These countries, among the world's poorest, could see their populations more than double in size by 2050. Even in the Asian and Latin American nations hailed as success stories for rapidly reducing birth rates, fertility remains above replacement level; these countries will continue to experience significant population increase in the decades immediately ahead.

As described in chapter 2, studies of population dynamics clearly demonstrate that no species can sustain limitless growth. Just as declining *death* rates caused the population explosion, it is widely assumed that a decrease in *birth* rates will humanely bring a halt to future growth. The accuracy of that assumption hinges on the success of both governments and the private sector in providing family-planning services to all who desire them and on the childbearing decisions of millions of individual couples.

EARLY ATTEMPTS AT FAMILY LIMITATION

Although most traditional cultures have consistently encouraged prolific childbearing, records indicate that during stressful periods of famine, war, or civil upheaval many couples throughout history have attempted in various ways to prevent unwanted births. While some of the methods employed were based on nothing more than superstition, others were moderately effective and continue to be used today.

One of the oldest documented means of contraception, referred to in the Old Testament story of Onan (Genesis 38:9), is that of withdrawal (*coitus interruptus*), whereby the man withdraws his penis from the vagina prior to ejaculation. Since a keen sense of timing is essential to the success of this method, withdrawal has the highest failure rate of any major method of birth control, but it does have the advantage of requiring no drugs or devices nor access to medical personnel for its use—and it costs nothing. Where couples are highly motivated not to have children, it can be fairly successful and, in fact, is believed to be the method by which European couples substantially reduced birth rates in that part of the world during the early years of the demographic transition. Even today, according to Planned Parenthood, approximately 35 million couples worldwide continue to rely on withdrawal for preventing unwanted births. In several countries of eastern Europe and the Middle East—Ukraine, Romania, Albania, Bosnia, Armenia, Azerbaijan, and Turkey—it remains the most common means of birth control even today, with 20–30% of contracepting couples relying on this age-old method (PRB, 2002). Among American women, according to CDC data, just 3% in the 15–44 age cohort rely on their partners to practice withdrawal as their primary means of contraception, though others may use it as an occasional back-up method in combination with other contraceptive devices.

Crude barriers to the cervix, similar in concept to the modern diaphragm or cervical cap, were used by women in ancient Egypt who fashioned such devices out of leaves, cloth, wads of cotton fibers, or even crocodile dung!

Herbal concoctions have been used for both contraceptive and abortive purposes for thousands of years. The modern era's contraceptive pill, along with hormonal patches and injectables, are but the most recent in a venerable line of antifertility drugs widely employed in ancient and medieval societies as well as in folk cultures right up to the present time. Although it long was fashionable to dismiss such brews as totally useless, recent research has found that some of the plants used are, in fact, remarkably effective in preventing pregnancy, while others are powerful abortifacients. The contraceptive properties of drugs extracted from pomegranate rind, black pepper, ivy, cabbage flowers, and willow bark were described in Greek and Roman medical literature almost 2,000 years ago. Pennyroyal (*Mentha pulegium*), a member of the mint family, was widely used for centuries to induce abortions, as was rue (*Ruta graveolans*), which has both abortifacient and contraceptive properties. In recent decades the results of a number of studies and field observations confirm that certain plant substances do indeed exert an antifertility effect (a phenomenon first noticed in relation to spontaneous abortions or a failure of ovulation among grazing animals when feeding on certain plants). Preliminary research has confirmed many of the claims made by ancient medical authorities and efforts are now ongoing in a number of countries, especially India and China, to conduct clinical and laboratory tests of traditional drugs believed to possess contraceptive properties (McLaren, 1990; Riddle, 1992).

The use of condoms dates back at least to the 16th century when a fine linen sheath worn on the penis during intercourse was recommended as a means of preventing the spread of venereal disease. By the 17th century condoms made of lamb intestines, tied shut at the end with a ribbon, were introduced for the express purpose of preventing conception and by the 18th century were reportedly available for use by patrons at all the finer houses of prostitution in Europe (some versions were also made of silk!). With the advent of vulcanized rubber in 1844, a truly effective and relatively cheap (advertised at $5 per dozen in 1850) male contraceptive became available for the masses. Nevertheless, rubber condoms were not widely used until World War I, when they were distributed among the troops as protection against venereal disease (Stokes, 1980; McLaren, 1990).

Other birth control practices with a similarly long history include douching (flushing out the vagina with a water solution immediately after intercourse), almost totally ineffective in spite of its popularity; and breast-feeding of infants, quite an effective means of suppressing the onset of ovulation following childbirth and thereby helpful in spacing pregnancies. In fact, prior to the advent of modern contraceptives, breast-feeding was the chief tactic employed by women to prevent an unwanted second pregnancy soon after childbirth. A survey conducted in Bangladesh revealed that, on average, each month of breast-feeding increased the birth interval between babies by about 0.4 months (Weiss, 1993; Kleinman and Senanayake, 1984).

When such birth control methods failed, as they frequently did, women commonly resorted to abortion, a very ancient practice believed to have been the most prevalent method of family limitation throughout history.

As a last resort, unwanted children in past centuries frequently fell victim to infanticide—the deliberate killing of babies, particularly female babies, immediately after birth. This practice was quite common in ancient Greece and in several Asian countries up until fairly recent times, especially during periods of famine or civil upheaval.

MODERN FAMILY-PLANNING MOVEMENT

The origins of the modern family-planning movement in the United States can be traced to the publication in 1832 of a contraceptive textbook, *Fruits of Philosophy,* written by Dr. Charles Knowlton. Dr. Knowlton won renown as the first person in the United States to be jailed for advocating birth control. The development of the diaphragm in the 1840s further stimulated public interest in contraceptive techniques and although proponents of birth control were viciously persecuted by so-called "societies for the suppression of vice," the resultant notoriety only enhanced sales of birth control literature. Open discussion of sex or reproductive matters was still taboo during those years of Victorian morality, however, and an "establishment" backlash against the growing birth control movement was reflected in the passage in 1873 of the Comstock Law, a federal mandate that prohibited sending birth control information or devices through the mail, such items being defined as "obscene."

Toward the end of the 19th century, the burgeoning feminist movement lent support to the concept of family planning, stressing the health burdens imposed on women by too many children born too close together. An outstanding pioneer of family planning in America was Margaret Sanger, a nurse in New York City who was appalled by the extent of poverty due to over-large families and the rate of maternal death due to abortion among the people with whom she worked. Recognizing that the Comstock Law prevented such people from obtaining the contraceptive information they needed, she launched a personal crusade to overturn that legislation. In 1914 Sanger founded the National Birth Control League and began publishing a monthly magazine, *The Woman Rebel,* containing birth control information—which the Post Office therefore refused to distribute. The following year she circulated a more comprehensive birth control pamphlet, *Family Limitation,* which also violated the Comstock Law. Sanger was indicted for this action, but the indictment was subsequently dropped. In 1916 Mrs. Sanger opened the first birth control clinic in America, in a section of Brooklyn, New York. For this offense she was arrested and served 30 days in prison, but the resulting public outcry led to a gradual easing of legal restrictions against the family-planning movement.

Mrs. Sanger traveled extensively throughout the country, seeking to persuade both the medical profession and the public at large of the importance of facilitating access to birth control. By 1932 the Birth Control League had established 80 clinics throughout the United States; in 1937 the American Medical Association officially endorsed birth control; finally, by 1938, two major court cases resulted in the overthrow of the Comstock Law and, in effect, made it possible for doctors to prescribe contraceptives to patients (except in Connecticut and Massachusetts where contraceptives remained illegal under state law until the 1960s). In 1942 the National Birth Control League and its affiliated clinics became Planned Parenthood Federation, with Margaret Sanger as honorary chairperson (League of Women Voters Education Fund, 1982).

BIRTH CONTROL— ITS HEALTH IMPACT

Over the years the services offered by Planned Parenthood have expanded to include premarital counseling and fertility assistance in addition to the original intent of providing birth control information to married women. However, the basic rationale of all family planning work in America—today as in 1916 when the first clinic opened its doors—is to promote the health and well-being of mothers and children by preventing unwanted births. Because of the threat that uncontrolled fertility poses, both to maternal health and to that of infants, it is generally accepted today that no community health program can be considered complete if it fails to provide ready access to birth control devices and information.

Enhancement of maternal and child health through family planning is largely related to one of three basic parameters: (1) age of the mother, (2) interval between births, and (3) total number of births during a woman's reproductive lifetime. A brief examination of each of these factors reveals how uncontrolled fertility has a major impact on mortality and morbidity rates among both women and infants.

Age of Mother

Although the average woman is fertile from her early teens until her late 40s, the biologically optimum period for childbearing is much shorter, extending from approximately 20 to 30 years of age. In fact, research suggests that becoming pregnant is increasingly difficult as women approach middle age. The ability to conceive appears to peak at age 31 and declines steadily every year thereafter. From a safety standpoint, mothers either younger or older than this optimum age span run an increased risk of difficulties or death during pregnancy and childbirth, and their infants are statistically more likely to die than are babies of mothers in their 20s.

Girls in their early teens whose pelvic bones and reproductive organs are not yet fully developed are more likely to suffer obstructed or prolonged labor and to die during childbirth than are women in their prime reproductive years. In addition, babies of young mothers have a tendency to be born premature or underweight, factors that greatly increase their susceptibility to infectious diseases and malnutrition. Studies have revealed consistently higher infant mortality rates among babies born to mothers under age 20 as compared to those born to mothers in their late 20s. In addition, even when healthy at birth, babies born to mothers 15 or under are much more likely to die before their first birthday than are babies whose mothers are in their 20s. Reasons for this discrepancy are unclear, but may be due to neglect,

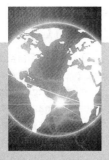

· · · · · · · 3-1 · · · · · · · ·

When All Else Fails . . .

When contraceptives are unavailable, not used, or fail, abortion remains today, as it has for millennia, the birth control method of last resort. Even in this modern age of the Pill and the Patch, accidents still happen; as a result, about half of all pregnancies in the United States are unplanned and, of these, approximately half end in abortion (Jones et al., 2008).

Controversy over the legalization of abortion has been raging in the U.S. for more than a century and shows no signs of mellowing. By the mid-1800s American physicians had launched a vigorous lobbying effort to outlaw abortion, a practice unaddressed by either state or federal laws up to that time. Motivated in part by a belief that abortion was morally wrong, but also by a desire to put "quack" doctors out of business and by opposition to new social roles for women, anti-abortion lobbyists had succeeded in making the procedure illegal everywhere in the U.S. by 1900 (outlawing abortions didn't end them of course—it simply made them more dangerous).

This situation prevailed until the 1960s, when public attitudes toward abortion began to shift. Concerns about the "quality of life" as opposed to mere biological existence were voiced, as was the view that anti-abortion statutes discriminated against poor women, since the wealthy could, and did, travel abroad to obtain an abortion. By 1970, the states of Alaska, Hawaii, New York, and Washington had completely legalized first-trimester abortions and one-third of all states permitted first-trimester abortions in situations where (1) continuation of the pregnancy might endanger the life or health of the mother; (2) when the child might be born severely deformed or intellectually disabled; or (3) when an unmarried girl under 16 became pregnant due to rape or incest. In 1973 the U.S. Supreme Court stunned the nation by issuing its historic *Roe v. Wade* decision, ruling that states cannot place any restrictions on abortion during the first trimester other than to require that the procedure be performed by a physician. During the second trimester the state can regulate abortion only in ways to protect maternal health; only during the last trimester, said the Court, may the state prohibit abortion unless the life of the mother is in danger.

The Court's 1973 landmark ruling invalidated all remaining state anti-abortion laws but it did nothing to end the controversy surrounding the issue. If anything, the debate has only grown more heated during the decades since *Roe v. Wade*, polarizing both society and politics.

During the 1980s the number of abortions in the U.S. held relatively steady at about 1.6 million annually. By the early 1990s, surgical abortions began a gradual decline, down to 1.21 million in 2005—an 8% decline since 2000 (the all-time high was 1.6 million in 1990) and the lowest number recorded in the U.S. since 1976. The abortion *rate* has also dropped, from 27 per 1000 women aged 15–44 in 1990 to 21 per 1000 in 2000. A number of factors have contributed to this trend, among them a decline in sexual activity among adolescents; that, plus more consistent and effective use of contraceptives by those teens who do engage in sex has cut the number of unwanted teenage pregnancies, thereby reducing the demand for abortions. Changes on the "supply side" are significant as well. For the past several decades pro-life groups have lobbied vigorously at every level of government to make legal abortion more difficult to obtain and have pressured hospitals and health-care providers not to offer abortion services. As a result, by 2005 the number of abortion providers in the United States had declined to 1,787—down from a high of 2,900 in 1982.

The vast majority of all abortions (95%) are now being performed in clinics or by family doctors rather than in hospitals, most of them in large metropolitan areas; in rural areas, fully 97% of counties lack any abortion providers. Laws in various states mandating waiting periods prior to obtaining an abortion, as well as restrictions on minors' access to abortion and on insurance coverage for the procedure, have also discouraged women from seeking services. The near-total ban on federal funding to poor women wanting abortions similarly has made legal abortion unaffordable for many who would otherwise have opted for the procedure. It is impossible to say how many abortions these restrictions have prevented, but there is no question that they have had a disproportionate impact on women living in poverty, women in underserved rural areas, and on young women.

To some extent, the decline in *surgical* abortions reflects a rise in *medical* abortions. In September 2000, after years of controversy as to whether its use should be permitted in the U.S., the so-called "French abortion pill," originally known as RU-486 but now referred to as **mifepristone** (brand name Mifeprex), was approved by the FDA. Used in combination with **misoprostol**, a form of prostaglandin, mifepristone has been shown to be both safe and 95–97% effective when taken within 8 weeks after a woman's last menstrual period. A woman opting for medical abortion must visit a doctor to receive counseling and a mifepristone pill; 24–72 hours later, a second pill, this time misoprostol, is taken at home. For most women, bleeding and expulsion of the fetus then occurs within 6–8 hours. In the small percentage of cases that fail, a standard suction procedure must be performed to complete the abortion. By 2005, the abortion pill accounted for 13% of all U.S. abortions and 22% of abortions earlier than nine weeks of gestation. An estimated 57% of all abortion providers reported performing one or more medical abortions that year—a 70% increase since 2001 (Jones et al., 2008). The fact that medical abortion is noninvasive, removing any risk of uterine perforation, and that it requires no anesthesia makes it more appealing than surgical abortion to many women.

Most recently, a significant factor in reducing abortion demand in the U.S. has been the growing use of **emergency contraception**. Unlike mifepristone, the so-called "morning-after pill," Plan B™, is *not* an abortifacient as some opponents allege. Instead, it works by preventing or delaying ovulation or by inhibiting the implantation of a fertilized egg. Essentially a high-dose birth control pill, Plan B provides protection against unwanted pregnancy for women who engaged in sex without using birth control or used it incorrectly, such as the accidental break of a condom during intercourse. To be effective, Plan B must be used within 5 days of having sex (the sooner, the better); Plan B's manufacturer claims 95% effectiveness of its product if taken within 24 hours of intercourse. Although originally available by prescription only—a problematic situation when time is of the essence—in the United States today, Plan B is available over the counter at drug stores and health centers for anyone aged 17 or older. For those under 17, however, a prescription is still required. Plan B can be taken either in one dose, with two pills swallowed simultaneously, or in two doses, with the second pill taken 12 hours after the first. In addition to Plan B, several brands of standard birth control pills can be used in concentrated dosages for emergency contraception, as can the intrauterine device, ParaGard, which, if inserted within 120 hours after unprotected sex, can reduce the risk of pregnancy by 99.9%.

abuse, or inadequate parenting skills on the part of very young mothers (Phipps, Blume, and DeMonner, 2002).

Among women over 35, pregnancy poses an increased risk of complications during childbirth. Studies of pregnant women aged 44 and older reveal considerably higher rates of medical complications such as high blood pressure and diabetes compared to women in their 20s and 30s; women in the over-44 cohort also are much more likely than younger mothers to have a Caesarean delivery (Dulitzki et al., 1998). Mothers over 35 are more likely than younger women to bear a child with congenital disorders such as Down syndrome (however, a Canadian study of more than half a million births revealed no greater risk of nonchromosomal birth defects among babies born to older mothers than among infants whose mothers were younger). In addition to concerns regarding birth abnormalities, mothers in their 30s and 40s have reason to worry about the general health of their babies. Up to age 30, a pregnant woman has an 89% likelihood of delivering a healthy baby; this level of assurance diminishes by 3.5% for each additional year of maternal age (Baird, Sadovnick, and Yee, 1991; van Noord-Zaadstra, 1991).

Interval between Births

Short birth intervals have long been recognized as an important factor contributing to infant mortality. Studies conducted in rural India demonstrated that babies born less than two years after a previous birth were 50% more likely to die before their first birthday than were babies born after a birth interval of more than two years. Researchers working with the U.S. Agency for International Development in Bangladesh report that efforts to encourage women to space their pregnancies had a greater impact on reducing infant mortality than did childhood immunization campaigns or oral rehydration therapy.

For years public health workers assumed that short birth intervals were equally harmful to the health of the mother. A condition called "maternal depletion syndrome," characterized by premature aging, weakness, and anemia, is frequently observed among undernourished women in poor societies, where teenage marriage is often followed by about 20 years of uninterrupted pregnancy. Anemic women may indeed be at heightened risk of dying during or soon after childbirth due to their lower tolerance for blood loss. If one pregnancy quickly follows

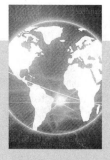

······· 3-2 ·······

The Perils of Pregnancy

While motherhood can be a woman's greatest blessing, it also entails serious health risks, particularly if the woman is young, poor, and living in a developing nation. Each year an estimated half-million women in the developing world die as a result of pregnancy or childbirth; another 15–20 million survive but incur injuries or illness that seriously affect their health and well-being for years afterwards. Childbirth-related disabilities are tragic for many reasons: they blight the lives of young women during what should be their most productive years; they impose serious financial and psychological stress on the affected families; they affect the quality of care the sick mother is able to give her children; and they are largely preventable.

For the most part, maternal death or disability is a result of inadequate or nonexistent medical care during pregnancy, labor, and immediately following childbirth. While most women in rich nations have regular prenatal checkups, poor women in developing countries may never see a doctor prior to delivery—and half don't have medical care even then. In Africa and Asia, many pregnant women see no reason to visit a doctor unless they have a specific complaint, not realizing the importance of good prenatal care. Others live in remote areas where no doctor is available, while some simply can't afford medical care. In Muslim countries, scarcity of female physicians may prevent women from accessing health care, since cultural taboos forbid a female patient being examined by a male doctor.

Poor-quality medical facilities in many parts of the developing world constitute another obstacle to adequate medical attention. Women who arrive at such hospitals or clinics in urgent need of emergency obstetric care often fail to receive proper or timely treatment because of inadequate staffing, lack of equipment, and a chronic shortage of surgical supplies. Unsafe abortions pose yet another health hazard. Though accurate figures are hard to come by, the World Health Organization estimates that as many as one out of every ten pregnancies in developing countries is terminated by abortion, many of them self-induced or performed by unskilled providers, and all-too-frequently ending in death or disability for the desperate woman.

Among the more tragic consequences of pregnancy and childbirth in areas where good prenatal health care is lacking is a condition known as **obstetric fistula**, one of several potential consequences of obstructed labor. Occurring most commonly among young women who marry and conceive a child before their pelvic bones are fully grown, fistula constitutes what one physician calls "a comprehensive social and psychological disaster." Once common worldwide, obstetric fistula today is virtually unknown in developed countries where high-quality medical services are widely available and marriage of very young girls is illegal. Among impoverished communities in Asia and sub-Saharan Africa, however, the lives of an estimated two million or more women are blighted by obstetric fistulas and another 50,000–100,000 join their ranks each year.

A fistula, or hole, in the birth canal forms as a result of prolonged labor, caused by constant pressure of the baby's head against the mother's pelvis. This pressure gradually cuts off the blood supply to the surrounding tissue, causing it to rot away and leaving a hole between the vagina and the bladder, the vagina and the rectum, or both. As a consequence, the woman experiences uncontrollable leakage of urine and feces and becomes a social pariah, constantly wet and foul-smelling. Frequently rejected by their husbands, avoided by friends and relatives, and plagued by feelings of self-loathing and depression, women suffering from fistula often die prematurely due to infection-induced kidney failure.

Ironically, obstetric fistula is both preventable and curable. Postponing marriage and pregnancy for very young girls and ensuring access to facilities providing Caesarean sections could largely eliminate the problem of obstructed labor. For women already suffering from this condition, reconstructive surgery is successful for approximately 90% of women seeking such treatment. Unfortunately, most sufferers are unaware that treatment exists; those who *do* know often cannot afford the cost of the operation, plus the approximately two weeks of post-operative care needed to prevent subsequent infection (UNFPA, 2003b).

Unfortunately, fistula is but one of many debilitating, even life-threatening, disabilities that typify the perils of pregnancy in less developed countries. While some of these problems are of an acute nature, affecting the mother during or immediately after childbirth, others may negatively impact her health and quality of life for months or years afterward. Included among the most serious are (1) **postpartum hemorrhage**, the leading cause of maternal death; (2) **blood poisoning (sepsis)** resulting from unsanitary conditions during delivery or abortion, sometimes leading to pelvic inflammatory disease; (3) **anemia**, low levels of iron in the blood, which is a major contributor to postpartum maternal death or illness; (4) **pregnancy-induced hypertension**, a complex of symptoms which, if not detected and treated, can result in seizures or convulsions leading to death of the mother or chronic disabilities; and (5) **obstructed labor**, a situation in which labor may be prolonged for days because the mother's pelvis is too narrow to permit easy passage of the fetus through the birth canal.

Preventing problems such as these can be achieved through greater efforts to ensure that poor women in developing countries have the same access to good nutrition, family planning, prenatal care, obstetric care, and postnatal care that women in wealthier nations already enjoy. Given the human misery and suffering caused by such largely preventable complications of pregnancy and childbirth, providing such assistance should be a moral imperative for the international health community.

another, the intervening period may be too short for an anemic woman to make up the blood loss experienced during the earlier birth, thus increasing her risk of death due to hemorrhage or childbed fever during the next delivery. However, a study conducted in Bangladesh could find no evidence to support general claims of a direct link between birth intervals of less than two years and enhanced risk of maternal mortality. Short birth intervals, without question, pose real concerns regarding survival prospects of the baby; however, contrary to popular belief, it cannot be demonstrated that having several babies close together increases a woman's own likelihood of dying during pregnancy or childbirth (Ronsmans and Campbell, 1998).

Total Number of Births

Contrary to the popular notion that mothers with large numbers of children give birth "as easy as rolling off a log," statistics reveal that such women are especially prone to problem pregnancies and death during child-

Table 3-1   Complications of Pregnancy and Childbirth: Estimates for Less Developed Countries

Complication	Maternal Disabilities that May Result
Severe bleeding (hemorrhage)	• Severe anemia • Pituitary gland failure and other hormonal imbalances • Infertility
Infection during or after labor (sepsis)	• Pelvic inflammatory disease • Chronic pelvic pain • Damage to reproductive organs • Infertility
Obstructed or prolonged labor	• Incontinence • Fistula • General prolapse • Uterine rupture, vaginal tears • Nerve damage
Pregnancy-induced hypertension (preeclampsia and eclampsia)	• Chronic hypertension • Kidney failure • Nervous system disorders
Unsafe abortion	• Reproductive tract infection • Damage to uterus • Infertility • Pelvic inflammatory disease • Chronic pelvic pain

Source: Adapted from C. Murray and A. Lopez, eds., *Health Dimensions of Sex and Reproduction*, vol. 3 (Boston: Harvard Univ. Press, 1998), as summarized in L. Ashford, *Hidden Suffering: Disabilities from Pregnancy and Childbirth in Less Developed Countries* (Washington, DC: Population Reference Bureau, 2002).

birth. Indeed, the total number of babies born to a woman during her lifetime can have a significant impact on her general state of health.

Generally speaking, a woman's second and third births are the safest; the first birth carries slightly greater risk statistically because it will reveal any physical or genetic abnormalities in the parents that could cause problems. With the fourth pregnancy, risk of maternal death, stillbirth, and infant death begins to rise, increasing sharply with the birth of the fifth and every succeeding child. Degree of risk depends to a considerable extent on the socioeconomic status of the mother, the greatest hazards being faced by women from the lowest income groups. However, even among well-nourished, affluent women, every birth after the fourth involves an increased degree of danger for both mother and child.

Significantly higher rates of infant and child mortality among higher-order births in poor families seem to be due primarily to poor nutrition, as the limited amount of food available must be divided among many mouths. Unlike their older siblings, the latest born children must survive on reduced average portions during those early years when they are most susceptible to the effects of nutritional deficiency. In addition, mothers who have already borne a large number of children are likely to be physically run down during their pregnancy, making it more likely that higher-order babies may suffer fetal growth retardation and low birth weight (Pandey et al., 1998).

Thus a family-planning program that provides contraceptive protection for teenage women, women over 35, mothers who have already borne three or more children, and women who have recently given birth can make a very positive contribution to improving public health.

CONTRACEPTIVE SAFETY

In assessing the health impact of family planning, one must of course take into account possible risks posed by contraceptive use. Questions have been raised regarding the safety of the birth control pill and the intrauterine device (IUD), prompting public concerns and causing potential contraceptors to turn to less reliable methods or to abandon attempts at birth control altogether. What indeed are the risks and benefits of the most commonly used contraceptives? A brief summary of the most popular methods used in the United States indicates that although various adverse side effects may accompany the use of contraceptives for some women, all common means of contraception entail fewer risks than do pregnancy and childbirth.

Hormonal Contraceptives

Such contraceptives are made of synthetic substances similar to the hormones that occur naturally in women's bodies. They prevent pregnancy by inhibiting ovulation.

Birth Control Pill

Among American women aged 15–44 currently practicing contraception, 28% use "the Pill," making this the most popular method of birth control among American women in their prime reproductive years (Mosher and Jones, 2010). Available in a number of different brands either as a combination pill (containing both estrogen and a progestin) or as a "mini-pill" containing progestin only, oral contraceptives, when used correctly, are 97–99% effective in preventing pregnancy.

Since the early 1960s when the birth control pill first became available, safety concerns centered around a possible increased risk of cardiovascular disorders such as blood clots, which could lead to a stroke or heart attack. For this reason medical authorities feel that a decision to use oral contraceptives should be made only after consultation with a health professional, and currently in all Western nations a doctor's prescription is required for the purchase of birth control pills. Nevertheless, the results of extensive epidemiological research on oral contraceptive safety over five decades of pill use indicate that women over 40 are the only group for whom pill use poses a greater health threat than does childbearing; among this group an increase in cardiovascular problems suggests the advisability of discontinuing pill use in favor of other contraceptive methods. However, for younger women, with the exception of those who smoke or have certain medical conditions (e.g., a history of blood clots, heart problems, cancer of the breast or female organs), medical

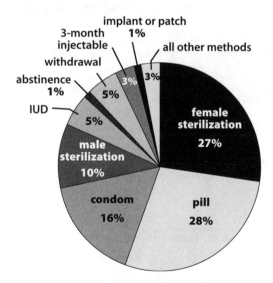

Source: Mosher, W. D. and J. Jones, "Use of Contraception in the United States: 1982–2008." National Center for Health Statistics, *Vital Health Statistics* 23, no. 29, August 2010.

Figure 3-1   Percentage of U.S. Women Ages 15–44 Currently Using Contraception by Method, 2006–2008

evidence supports the view that the Pill is quite safe. Moreover, during the period they are taking contraceptive pills, users experience certain health benefits, including significant long-term protection against ovarian cancer (Riman et al., 2002), as well as reduced risk for ovarian cysts, endometrial cancer, pelvic inflammatory disease, iron-deficiency anemia, and fibrocystic breast disease. Persistent fears that women who use contraceptive pills might be at greater risk of developing cancer later in life were laid to rest in 1999 with the publication of results from a 25-year investigation of British women who had used oral contraceptives. The study convincingly demonstrated that ten years after they stopped taking contraceptive pills, the women experienced no higher risk of dying of cancer or stroke than did women who had never used oral contraceptives—good news for the hundreds of millions of women worldwide who have used the Pill at one time or another (Beral et al., 1999).

Depo-Provera

After more than 20 years of use in over 90 countries worldwide, Depo-Provera won FDA approval in 1992 and is now the most popular non-oral hormonal contraceptive in the United States, used by 3.2% of contracepting women between 15–44 years of age. Administered as an injection in the arm or buttocks every three months, Depo-Provera fills a need for women who want the reliability of hormonal contraceptives without having to worry about forgetting to take a daily pill. Depo-Provera is a synthetic form of progesterone that works by inhibiting ovulation and is 99% effective in preventing pregnancy, so long as the user is conscientious about getting the shot regularly every 12 weeks. Worldwide, millions of women have taken the drug since it was first introduced in 1969 and its overall safety record is good. Common side effects for women receiving a Depo-Provera injection include cessation of the menstrual period or irregular menstruation and modest weight gain. One potential disadvantage for those considering this method of birth control is that it may take up to a year or more after discontinuing Depo-Provera shots to get pregnant if the woman decides she wants a baby.

Birth Control Implant (Implanon)

In 1990 the first birth control implant approved for use in the United States was introduced in the form of six small progestin-containing capsules inserted by a health-care professional just below the skin of the upper arm. Marketed under the trade name Norplant, this contraceptive implant was hailed as the most radical new form of birth control since the Pill, continuously releasing a small amount of contraceptive hormone into the user's body over a period of several years and providing a consistently high level of protection without any further action on the part of the woman or her partner. However, even though Norplant was a safe and extremely effective method of contraception, many women encountered difficulties with having the capsules removed—a process requiring the services of a trained physician—in most cases because medical personnel lacked the skill to perform the removal efficiently and without pain. Because of this problem, usage declined and subsequently a new, single-rod version of Norplant called Implanon has now replaced the original 6-rod implant. A special insertion device has also been developed for Implanon, making both insertion and removal much easier than was the case with Norplant. Like Norplant, Implanon is one of the most reliable contraceptives on the market today, 99% effective for a period up to 3 years. A completely reversible method, Implanon begins providing protection within 24 hours after insertion; if at any time during the three-year period of use a woman decides she would like to have a baby, the capsule can be removed and fertility is immediately restored. In spite of its excellent record in terms of safety (the implant can be used safely by mothers who are breast-feeding), effectiveness, and convenience, Implanon is currently the method of choice for only about 1% of contraceptive users in the United States; interestingly, however, it is almost four times as popular among American Hispanic women as it is among other ethnic groups (Mosher and Jones, 2010).

Contraceptive Patch, Vaginal Ring

Two non-oral hormonal contraceptives, both the patch and the vaginal ring, deliver hormones through the skin of the user. Both are self-administered, precluding regular visits to a clinic or health-care provider and thus enhancing their appeal for some women. The Ortho-Evra™ patch, containing the same estrogen and progestin compounds found in birth control pills, is applied once a week for three consecutive weeks, then removed for the fourth week, at which time menstruation begins. The patch can be worn on the abdomen, the outside of the upper arm, the buttocks, or anywhere on the upper torso except for the breasts. Available only by prescription, the patch is 99% effective at preventing pregnancy when used correctly; it is somewhat less effective, however, when used by women weighing more than 198 pounds. It is also very important to apply the patch on the same day each week—otherwise pregnancy may result.

Unlike the patch, which must be changed weekly, the vaginal ring is inserted by the user once a month; after 21 days she removes it for the last 7 days of her cycle and then inserts a new ring. The NuvaRing™ delivers a lower dose of estrogen than do other hormonal contraceptives, but, like them, is 99% effective in preventing conception (Dieben, Roumen, and Apter, 2002).

Sterilization

The second-most widely adopted method of family limitation in the United States among women aged 15–44, sterilization is a logical alternative for those who have already attained their desired family size. Indeed, for women 35 and older, female sterilization is the most popular contraceptive choice. Among the 40–44 age cohort, 50% of women have been sterilized, while an additional 18% have a partner who has undergone a vasectomy. Vasectomy, or male sterilization, is a simple operation involving an incision in the scrotum to cut or block the vas deferens (tubes that carry semen from the testes to the penis). Vasectomy most often is performed under local anesthesia in a doctor's office, the entire procedure generally taking less than 30 minutes. In 2003 an alternative approach to male birth control was approved by the FDA. Vasclip, a tiny clamp attached to each vas deferens to block the flow of sperm, has several advantages over a typical vasectomy. Vasclip is cheaper, less painful, and quicker (about 10 minutes) than the standard surgical procedure; the company that manufactures Vasclip is hopeful that future studies will demonstrate greater potential for reversibility as well, since it doesn't involve cutting or cauterizing the vas deferens (Good, 2003). In rare cases, minor postoperative infections may develop, but in general male sterilization is among the safest of all birth control methods.

Female sterilization, or tubal ligation, entails a slightly higher degree of risk since it involves sealing off the fallopian tubes—an operating room procedure done under general anesthesia. Although major complications are rare, they occur in an estimated 1.7% of cases. A newer, incision-free form of female sterilization called Essure™ was approved by the FDA in 2002 and now provides an alternative to tubal ligation. This method, which can be performed in a doctor's office using only a local anesthetic, involves inserting a small metal coil into each fallopian tube, accessed through the cervix using a narrow catheter. Over a period of three months following insertion, the coils stimulate the formation of enough scar tissue to hold the coils in place and completely block the passage of eggs through the fallopian tubes (Minkin and Hanlon, 2003). Sterilization, both male and female, is more than 99% effective in preventing pregnancy and ends any further expense or bother related to contraceptive use. However, sterilization is a permanent method of birth control and such a decision should not be made lightly. Efforts to date at reopening the vas deferens or fallopian tubes have met with minimal success, so sterilization should be regarded as irreversible.

Intra-uterine Device (IUD)

Once among the most popular forms of contraception in the United States and still widely relied upon by women in other countries (particularly in China and Russia where it is the most common method of birth control), the IUD today is the method of choice for only about 5.5% of contracepting American women. Indeed, by the mid-1980s IUDs had nearly disappeared from the marketplace, withdrawn by manufacturers fearing legal liability for alleged harmful side effects of the device (a situation brought about by thousands of lawsuits against the A. H. Robins pharmaceutical firm, charging that the company's Dalkon Shield had caused numerous cases of bleeding, pelvic infections, and resultant infertility among users). Nevertheless, physicians and manufacturers consider most IUDs both safe and reliable. Currently two types of IUD are being marketed in the U.S.—ParaGard™, containing copper and effective for 12 years, and Mirena™, an IUD that releases a small amount of the hormone progestin and is intended to last 5 years. Among mal-

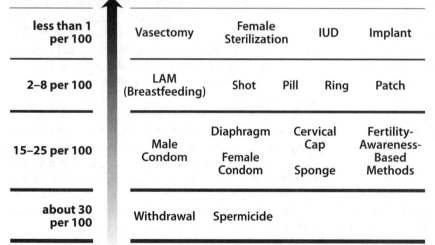

MORE EFFECTIVE

**less than 1 pregnancy
per 100 women each year**

less than 1 per 100	Vasectomy	Female Sterilization	IUD	Implant
2–8 per 100	LAM (Breastfeeding)	Shot	Pill	Ring	Patch
15–25 per 100	Male Condom	Diaphragm / Female Condom	Cervical Cap / Sponge	Fertility-Awareness-Based Methods
about 30 per 100	Withdrawal	Spermicide		

LESS EFFECTIVE

**about 30 pregnancies
per 100 women each year**

Source: Adapted from plannedparenthood.org.

Figure 3-2   Comparing Effectiveness of Birth Control Methods

nourished, anemic women IUD use has sometimes been correlated with increased blood loss during menstruation. For healthy, well-nourished women, however, IUDs are as safe as the Pill and nearly as dependable; they are also among the least-expensive and longest-lasting forms of birth control available. IUDs are not recommended for women who have never been pregnant and in general are considered most suitable for young women in mutually monogamous relationships who want no more children but are not yet ready for an irreversible surgical sterilization.

Spermicides

Spermicidal foams, creams, suppositories, or gels must be inserted into the vagina within an hour before intercourse and must be replenished if intercourse is repeated. They act to form both a physical and chemical barrier to sperm and are available without a prescription. While few problems are associated with spermicides (those who experience a burning sensation or irritation should avoid them), their effectiveness when used alone is only 70–80%.

Barrier Methods

Barrier methods employ some device that prevents the egg and sperm from uniting, thus preventing fertilization.

Vaginal Contraceptives

Diaphragms, cervical caps, sponges, and the female condom all work by keeping egg and sperm apart. (The polyurethane female condom is also intended to provide some protection against sexually transmitted disease, but medical authorities caution that for best protection, male latex condoms are preferable.) When used with spermicides, vaginal contraceptives have few, if any, adverse effects and are moderately effective at preventing pregnancy. Both the sponge and the female condom have an estimated failure rate of about 1 in 4; the cervical cap and diaphragm are somewhat more trustworthy, with failure rates ranging from 6% for a diaphragm used with spermicide to 18% for the cervical cap.

Condoms

Like the vaginal contraceptives, condoms cause no adverse health effects other than an occasional allergic reaction to rubber among some individuals. Used alone, their reliability is significantly less than pills or IUDs, but in combination with vaginal contraceptives and in situations where legal, early abortion is available, they offer the safest means, other than sterilization, of totally effective fertility control. The third most commonly used contraceptive method in the United States and Canada, the condom is being actively promoted by health agencies in many countries not only for birth control reasons but also as an effective prophylactic against the spread of AIDS and other sexually transmitted diseases (STDs). As a case in point, efforts to promote condom use in Thailand have reduced the incidence of new HIV infections in that country's sex industry by 85% within the last few years, according to the director of the United Nation's AIDS program. A comprehensive report by the National Institutes of Health on the efficacy of male condoms for preventing such infections concluded that they are indeed effective in preventing transmission of HIV, gonorrhea, and chlamydia, so long as they are used correctly and consistently. The report emphasized the need for public health agencies to reinforce the message that condoms *do* work in preventing STDs and pregnancies and that the overwhelming issue affecting condom failure is non-use (NIAID, 2001).

Periodic Abstinence

Frequently referred to as the "rhythm method," this approach to birth control carries no health risk but has a consistently high failure rate. To utilize this method, a woman attempts to determine when she is ovulating by charting daily bodily functions such as basal temperature (i.e., temperature when the body is at its lowest level of metabolic activity, usually measured before getting out of bed in the morning) and by examining her cervical mucus. The problem is that many women experience monthly variations in their menstrual cycle, making accurate calculation of the fertile period problematic. In addition, the abstinence from sexual activity during fertile periods which must be rigorously observed by couples using natural family planning requires a high degree of motivation and cooperation between partners and can significantly limit the number of days each month when couples can have intercourse free from fear of unwanted pregnancy.

The success of the family-planning movement in the United States is evident from surveys which reveal that among sexually active women at risk of an unwanted pregnancy, fully 93% are using some method of birth control (Mosher and Jones, 2010). In an age when sexual activity seems to be as popular a pastime as it ever was, an even more convincing indicator is the fact that the average number of children per U.S. couple is now just two, one of the lowest figures in our history.

FAMILY PLANNING IN THE DEVELOPING WORLD

Whereas the birth control movement in the United States and Europe grew out of the conviction that health and social considerations demanded that women receive help in regulating their fertility, the impetus for family planning in most developing countries grew directly out of concerns over the high rates of post-World War II population growth and the awareness that this "population explosion" would impede their rate of economic development. Only after family-planning programs had been launched did governments in the developing world attempt to justify their support for such efforts on the basis of protecting maternal and child health and of guaranteeing couples the means for regulating the spacing and number of their children. This superficial shift in emphasis constituted a publicly acceptable rationale for reconciling the interests of the nation with those of individuals.

In most cases, the initial promoters of family planning in less-developed countries were private organizations such as International Planned Parenthood Federation, the Ford and Rockefeller Foundations, and the Population Council. By the 1960s, however, even earlier in some countries, national governments were becoming increasingly active in establishing their own family-planning programs, usually in conjunction with their ministries of health. Generally they were assisted by the private organizations mentioned and, in later years, by the U.S. Agency for International Development and such United Nations agencies as the World Bank and the UN Fund for Population Activities (UNFPA). Funds, both governmental and private, allocated for family-planning work increased sharply after the mid-1960s, but even today constitute a very small percentage of most national budgets. Today the vast majority of developing countries have some sort of family-planning program in operation. How effective those programs are in reducing national birth rates will in large part determine the success of such countries in raising living standards and ensuring a brighter future for their people.

Spreading the Word

Since the main impetus for implementing family planning came from central governments or outside agencies rather than reflecting grassroots interest, as was the case in North America and Europe, success required intensive efforts to reach all elements of society, the majority of whom lived at subsistence level in rural areas, often isolated from adequate medical care and frequently illiterate. Such people had to be made aware of the existence of fertility-regulating methods, provided with regular access to the same, and convinced that it was in their own best interest to use them.

In pursuing this goal, family-planning workers in less-developed countries adopted methods radically different from those used in Western nations. Mobile units in the form of specially equipped vans or buses have been essential in carrying health workers and equipment into villages far from any hospital. Trained field workers actively attempt to recruit contraceptive acceptors, meeting with women's groups, farmers, and so on, to persuade them of the advantages inherent in limiting family size. Considerable reliance has been placed on mass media communications. Advertisements in newspapers, on radio, and in cinemas regularly stress the benefits of small families while roadside billboards or posters on buses, in train stations—even painted on the hides of farm animals—proclaim such messages as "Two or Three—Enough!"

One of the most successful approaches to rapid attitudinal change on matters pertaining to contraception and desired family size was pioneered by Mexican TV producer Miguel Sabido in the late 1970s. Sabido introduced a long-running television soap opera called *Acompáñame* (Come With Me) to demonstrate the personal benefits of family planning. During the decade that this show and several others with a similar theme were on the air (1977–1986), the Mexican birth rate plummeted by 34%. The dramas prompted a flood of phone calls—up from zero to an

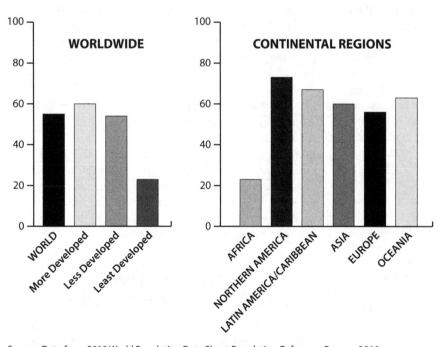

Source: Data from *2010 World Population Data Sheet*, Population Reference Bureau, 2010.

Figure 3-3   Percent of Married Women 15–49 Using Modern Contraception Methods Worldwide by Development and by Continental Region

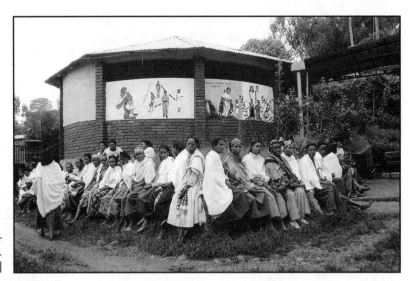

Women wait their turn for services at a family-planning clinic in West Shoa, Ethiopia.
[*Melesse Desalgn, USAID*]

average of 500 per month—to Mexico's national population council, a significant increase in the number of women enrolled at family-planning clinics, and a surge in contraceptive sales. As a result, in 1986 Mexico was awarded the United Nations Population Prize for the world's most outstanding population success story.

In the decades that followed, Sabido's model of entertainment-education has been adapted by the U.S.-based Population Media Center (PMC), which now has projects in 15 countries and plans to expand to several more. In 2002 PMC launched a major effort in Ethiopia, utilizing radio soap operas to deal with a number of reproductive health issues; two years later, 63% of the new clients seeking contraceptive services at regional service centers reported that they had listened to these dramas. Similar testimonies to the persuasive power of entertainment-education programs are coming from new contraceptive acceptors from Nigeria and Rwanda to Brazil. Soap operas featuring positive role models with whom audiences can form a lasting bond help viewers make informed decisions without telling them what to do. They are also far more cost-effective than traditional methods of spreading the word because they attract a mass audience and have an enormous impact, motivating millions of women to seize control of their own reproductive destiny (Connolly, Elmore, and Ryerson, 2008; Brown, 2009).

Most family-planning programs in developing countries, like those in the West, offer a choice of birth control methods and generally include information on spacing births, nutrition, and child care along with contraceptive services. Some also enlist the services of midwives, teachers, or other respected community leaders to act as distributors of contraceptives, particularly pills and condoms, thereby giving these influential individuals a vested interest in the success of such programs.

Motivation—The Key to Success

Efforts to reduce birth rates in developing nations have met with mixed results, though general trends have been encouraging. With the exception of the countries of sub-Saharan Africa, where fertility remains at traditionally high levels (a current average of 6 children per mother), birth rates have declined significantly in recent decades. Today in the less-developed nations as a whole, average family size is 2.7 children and nearly 60% of all married couples employ some form of contraception; if only modern methods of contraception are considered, this figure falls to 54%. In those countries categorized as "least developed," family size is considerably higher, with an average of 4.5 children per woman and just 29% using some form of birth control (PRB, 2010).

A number of surveys conducted over the past several decades have shown that the vast majority of women in the developing world are aware of the existence of at least one modern method of contraception. Nevertheless, a sizable proportion of these women—including many who told interviewers they wanted no more children—were, for one reason or another, not practicing contraception. As a result, in almost every country surveyed, women were having more babies than they said they wanted. To some extent, failure to use contraceptives is related to easy access; not surprisingly, contraceptive use was higher in communities where a family-planning clinic or other source of contraceptive supplies was close by—a particularly important factor among people using either pills or condoms. Cost can also be a major deterrent to poor women; even when they have access to contraceptives, many cannot afford to buy them. A British physician visiting Sri Lanka reported meeting women desperate to control their fertility but too poor to buy more than 5 contraceptive pills at a time, rather than a full month's supply of 21 (Potts, 2000).

A far more important determinant of contraceptive practice, however, is motivation—the desire of couples to limit family size. In many parts of the developing world economic and social factors interact to perpetuate traditional attitudes toward childbearing. For very practical reasons, many couples in the developing world have concluded that although two or three children per family might be in the best interest of society, they want and feel they need a significantly larger number themselves. In the absence of coercion, when individual and societal needs conflict, personal desires generally prevail. Factors contributing to this continued preference for large families among many couples in developing countries include high infant mortality rates, the view of children as "social security," the desire for sons, and the low educational and economic status of women.

High Infant Mortality Rates

Although the drop in infant and child death rates in large part fueled the explosive growth of developing world populations, such rates are still substantially above the levels prevailing in developed countries. In parts of Africa, for example, infant death rates are more than 100 per 1,000 live births, compared to 6.4 in the United States, 5.1 in Canada, and 2.6 in Japan (PRB, 2010). At the personal level, surveys have found that wherever childhood deaths are common, it is extremely difficult to convince parents to limit themselves to two births. For this reason, sharply lowering infant and child mortality rates is regarded as one of the key components in any population control program.

Children as "Social Security"

In most developing countries, lack of extensive social welfare programs means that most parents are dependent on their grown children for financial support in their post-retirement years. In such cultures, responsibility for elderly parents falls primarily on the sons; thus a couple may feel the need to produce at least two or three boys to ensure their being adequately provided for in old age. In addition, even young children may be regarded as financial assets, since their labor is needed on the farm or around the home. In such situations an additional baby is not viewed as another mouth to feed but rather as an additional pair of hands to gather wood, tend livestock, haul water, and so forth (Dasgupta, 1995).

Desire for Sons

Many family-planning program administrators fear that the preference for sons rather than daughters will keep fertility rates high in many developing countries. Son preference is apparent in surveys of American couples but is even more pronounced among parents in most developing world nations. In such cultures, doubt about whether they will have enough boys concerns parents who are asked to produce no more than two or three offspring. A woman's status, even the stability of her marriage, is dependent on her having sons. To some extent, such preferences are based on economic concerns: sons can support parents in old age while daughters are a financial liability, often requiring an expensive dowry at time of marriage. A fertility preference study conducted in Nepal found that although more than 80% of the couples surveyed named two to three children as the ideal family size, a substantial majority of both husbands and wives would opt for one extra child in order to achieve their preferred number of sons; almost half of the husbands and a third of the wives indicated their willingness to have more than twice the number of children they really wanted in order to attain the desired number of sons (two was the most commonly designated number of boys wanted). While over two-thirds of the couples questioned said they'd like to have one daughter, none had any desire to go beyond their stated ideal family size if the first two children were boys (Mahler, 1997). China has recently begun offering financial incentives to couples who have daughters in order to narrow the current gap in sex ratio at birth (120 boys for 100 girls), the result of its one-child policy (Hvistendahl, 2009).

Low Educational and Economic Status of Women

Birth rates today are highest in those parts of the world where women have little schooling and few opportunities for paid employment outside the home. In such societies, a woman's worth is measured in terms of her childbearing abilities. Such women, striving to maintain favor with their husbands and in-laws, are unlikely to respond favorably to the idea of family limitation. In addition, illiterate women or women with only an elementary education are less likely than better educated women to have heard about modern contraceptive techniques or to know how to use them. Surveys indicate that providing women with at least a secondary school education is one of the most effective ways of reducing the birth rate in developing countries. In general, fertility drops noticeably as the level of female education increases, primarily because educated women tend to marry later, have greater opportunity for employment outside the home, are more aware of the advantages of smaller family size, and understand how to practice contraception more effectively. The mother's education level is even more strongly correlated with improved childhood health and nutritional status. Women who have primary schooling or higher are much less likely to see their children die than are women who never attended school; children whose mothers completed high school or college are much less likely to be underweight or short for their age in comparison with children whose mothers are less educated (Riley, 1997).

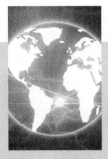

· · · · · · · · 3-3 · · · · · · ·

Missing Girls

Census results from the world's two most populous nations, China and India, reveal a worrisome trend—a steady decline in the proportion of baby girls to baby boys. For human societies everywhere, the normal sex ratio at birth is 105–106 boys for every 100 girls (or, viewed in reverse, 94–95 girls for every 100 boys). Since the mortality rate for males is slightly higher than that for females in every age group, this gender imbalance at birth seems to be Nature's way of ensuring approximately equal numbers of young men and women during the prime reproductive years. However, the gender discrepancy revealed by Chinese census reports showed 120 boys for every 100 girls, indicating a deficit of at least 980,000 girls (Hvistendahl, 2009). Similarly, in India, the 2001 census showed that for every 1,000 boys born, the corresponding number for girls was 927.

This recent unnatural widening of the gender gap suggests that something out of the ordinary is going on in countries where parental preference for sons has always been a fact of life. Both India and China are highly patriarchal societies, where sons are valued as a means of support for parents in their old age and for perpetuating the family line. A daughter, by contrast, leaves home to join her husband's family when she marries (in rural China a married daughter is no longer considered a member of her birth family) and thus represents more of a financial burden than an asset to her parents. This burden is particularly onerous today in India, where the custom of providing daughters with a huge cash dowry at the time of marriage imposes a crushing debt on many families. Dowry concerns don't trouble Chinese parents, but constraints imposed by China's strict family-planning laws do. In most parts of that country, severe penalties are imposed on couples having more than one, or at most two, children (in some counties parents are permitted to have a second child only if the first one is a girl); more than two, regardless of sex, is prohibited. These new legal realities impose added pressure to ensure that the one child is a son.

For centuries strong son preference in Chinese and Indian society occasionally manifested itself in the form of female infanticide. Even today, among poor families in some rural areas of India, the killing of female babies immediately after birth remains far too common. One young mother, interviewed during a UN-sponsored study conducted in northwestern India, was unrepentant about killing her first two baby girls and said she would kill any others she might bear because she had hardly any money to give them at the time of their wedding. In China, the age-old practice of killing or abandoning unwanted baby girls was stamped out by the Communist government during the early decades of that regime, but following the 1979 introduction of China's "one-child policy," numerous cases were reported of newborn girls being murdered by parents who hoped that a second try would produce a boy.

More recently, the advent of modern medical technology and the legalization of abortion in both countries have given Indian and Chinese parents an effective new approach for ensuring they have a son. Amniocentesis was introduced decades ago as a means of prenatal determination of a wide variety of genetic disorders. However, the chromosomal analysis also revealed the unborn child's sex and as early as the 1970s was being used by some couples specifically for sex-selection purposes; if amniocentesis showed the fetus to be female, the mother frequently chose to terminate her pregnancy. One survey conducted in Mumbai hospitals revealed that of 8,000 abortions performed, all but one were of female fetuses.

However, the fact that amniocentesis must be performed in a modern medical setting and is relatively expensive limited its use to urban areas and more affluent patients. Only with the introduction of ultrasound technology in the mid-1980s did the possibility of sex-selection become a reality for the masses—and the birth ratio of girls to boys began its steady downward slide. Ultrasound imaging for gender detection has several distinct advantages over amniocentesis: it presents no risk to the fetus or mother; can be performed earlier in the pregnancy (13–14 weeks vs. 18–20 weeks), costs half as much, and is widely available. By the 1990s, ultrasound technology had spread from urban areas into the countryside. At public hospitals and proliferating for-profit maternity clinics, demand for sex-determination services has continued to grow. Providing gender information has proven to be quite profitable for doctors, clinic operators, and the manufacturers of ultrasound scanners—a fact that helps to explain the spread of sex-determination services to the remotest corners of both countries, despite laws prohibiting the use of ultrasound for such purposes. Although medical practitioners in India are legally proscribed from telling expectant mothers what ultrasonography revealed about the sex of the fetus, the law is almost never enforced.

In China the likelihood that an abortion will follow determination that the fetus is a girl varies depending on the order of the pregnancy and the sex of previous children. Surveys in a rural area of that country suggest that if a couple has one daughter already and finds that a second pregnancy would result in another girl, chances are overwhelming that the mother will opt for abortion. Since the Chinese don't regard the fetus as a person, believing that human life begins at birth, the act of abortion itself raises no moral qualms. However, if the first child is a son, odds of an abortion to prevent the birth of a little sister are considerably less. By contrast, research in India reveals numerous first-pregnancy abortions of female fetuses, as well as among women who already had one living son.

The issue of sex-selective abortions has become increasingly controversial in both India and China, as concerns grow about the widening gender gap. Emotionally conflicted feminist groups in India deplore the situation as yet another example of the victimization of women in that male-dominated society, yet they strongly defend a woman's right to abortion as a matter of free choice and control over her own reproduction. Some commentators in India defend the practice on the grounds that it is preferable for a woman to abort unwanted daughters rather than produce six or seven children in order to have one or two boys. Others justify the practice on the grounds that the girls who *are* born will suffer less discrimination, while some predict that over the long term, a declining sex ratio will improve women's status in society as they become an increasingly scarce commodity. Unfortunately, the latter conjecture is contradicted by the reality in certain rural areas of China today where the paucity of young women in relation to young men has caused severe disruptions in the "marriage market." Rather than being accorded greater respect and better treatment, young women in that region are now at heightened danger of being kidnapped by criminal gangs and sold to village men desperate for wives.

The widespread practice of sex-selective abortion has prompted soul-searching discussion among Indian and Chinese policy makers and academicians about what, if anything, can be done to end this perverse use of medical technology. Imposing legal prohibitions obviously is not the answer; although India and China both have strict laws regulating the use of ultrasound scanners, the devices are now so widespread, corruption so rampant, the profit motive among service providers so strong, and the desire for sons so overwhelming that curbing the abuse of medical technology through legislation is likely to prove impossible. Given these realities, there is general agreement that the only lasting solution to the problem is a fundamental shift in societal attitudes toward women and the wide-scale implementation of economic, social, and legal measures to promote gender equity. Until the status of women is improved to the point that the birth of a baby girl is welcomed as joyously as the birth of a boy, millions more girls are fated to "go missing" (Chu, 2001; Ooman and Ganatra, 2002; UNFPA, 2003a).

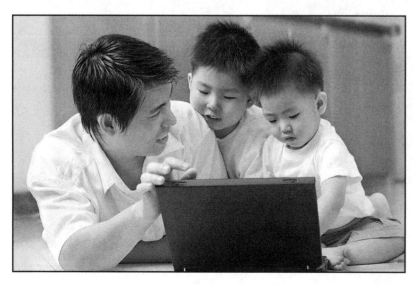

The age-old desire for sons among Chinese couples, coupled with modern ultrasound technology, has produced a gender ratio of 120 boys for every 100 girls, indicating a deficit of nearly one million girls.

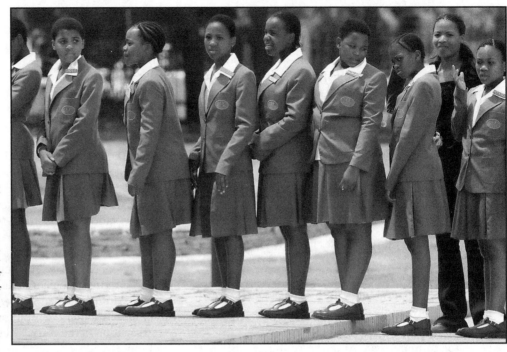

Girls line up for the opening of the Oprah Winfrey Leadership Academy for Girls in a small town in South Africa. Providing young women with at least a secondary school education is one of the most effective ways of reducing birth rates in developing countries. [*AP Photo/ Denis Farrell*]

Such factors support the contention of many demographers that broad-based social and economic changes must precede or accompany population programs in developing nations if population growth is ever to be stabilized; simply making contraceptives more widely available will not be enough to overcome traditional biases that favor large families.

POPULATION POLICY: MOVING BEYOND BIRTH CONTROL

Since the inception of both private and government-sponsored family-planning programs in the 1950s and 1960s, efforts have focused on increasing the availability of contraceptives while simultaneously trying to encourage their use. Numerous surveys conducted in many countries during these years demonstrated that many women were having more children than they desired, often because of misperceptions about the health effects of certain contraceptives, the cost of contraceptives, insufficient choice of contraceptive methods, or other problems related to access. Building new clinics and expanding social outreach programs seemed like the most straightforward approach to dealing with a problem that government leaders were beginning to view as increasingly urgent. By the 1980s, public opinion in many developing countries supported efforts to stabilize growth rates and governments began implementing vigorous efforts to increase the percentage of couples practicing contraception. A declaration by delegates to the UN-sponsored International Conference on Population, held in Mexico City in 1984, for governments to make family-planning services "universally available" was hailed as a significant achievement by population control advocates.

During those same years, however, feminists and others concerned about women's health issues and civil rights were growing increasingly critical of the single-minded focus on distributing contraceptives, often with no follow-up and little concern for the welfare of the women they were recruiting as contraceptive acceptors. Particularly in Asian countries (India and China being notable examples), family-planning programs were target-driven, with administrators' job security based on how many IUDs their staffs inserted within a month or how many sterilizations they performed. Such quota systems inevitably lead to violations of patients' rights—sometimes to outright coercion—and critics charged that the emphasis on numerical goals diminished the quality of services provided.

In 1994 when the United Nations convened the International Conference on Population and Development (ICPD) in Cairo, Egypt, a grassroots insistence that contraceptives alone are not the answer to the world's population dilemma persuaded planners of the need for a broad-based development initiative to improve health, reduce poverty, and improve the status of women. Attracting delegates from 180 different countries, as well as representatives of 1,200 nongovernmental organizations, many of them women's advocacy groups, the Cairo conference was the most comprehensive international meeting ever held on the population issue. While agreeing that both family planning *and* economic development are essential for reducing population growth rates, delegates for the first time acknowledged that empowerment of women will be a crucial factor in stabilizing world population size. The Programme of Action coming out of Cairo was based on the premise that population programs should focus on individual needs, not on numerical targets. Endorsed by all but a few of the 180 national delegations participating, the Programme of Action lists 243 goals to be achieved by 2015. Among the most important are the following:

1. To provide universal access to a full range of safe and reliable family-planning methods and related reproductive health services.

2. To reduce infant mortality rates to below 35 per 1,000 live births and child mortality rates (i.e., deaths of children under age 5) below 45.

3. To achieve a maternal mortality rate below 60 deaths per 100,000 live births.

4. To increase life expectancy at birth to more than 75 years (or to more than 70 in the countries currently experiencing high mortality rates).

5. To achieve universal access to and completion of primary education; ensure the widest and earliest possible access by girls and women to secondary and higher levels of education.

This ambitious program requires a sustained commitment by national governments, as well as billions of dollars, to implement the called-for reproductive health programs. Unfortunately, in the years following proclamation of the Cairo conference's lofty goals, the share of global health aid targeted for population and reproductive health programs has decreased sharply, from 30% in 1994 to 12% in 2008, with many countries diverting their attention from reproductive health to the problems of HIV/AIDS, malaria, and tuberculosis. There are some signs that priorities may be swinging back to a more balanced approach to international health aid funding, with President Obama in 2009 allocating $50 million for the United Nations Population Fund—but much more is needed to help poor women get access to reproductive health services. Achievement of the designated goals is also incumbent on wrenching changes in lifestyle and cultural norms in societies reluctant to alter age-old traditions regarding gender roles (Ashford, 1995). It remains to be seen whether the promise of Cairo (and subsequent reaffirmation of these goals at the 2004 ICPD conference in France) will be realized in an era of dwindling development dollars, when women's opportunities remain severely constrained in many countries, and at a time when the developing world is beset by pressing economic problems.

Famine seems to be the last, the most dreadful resource of nature.
The power of population is so superior to the power in the earth to
produce subsistence for man, that premature death must
in some shape or other visit the human race.
—Thomas Malthus, "An Essay on the
Principal of Population" (1798)

The People-Food Predicament

The fierce debate sparked by Malthus' gloomy pronouncements over two centuries ago continues to reverberate today as policy makers and scientists argue about the planet's ability to meet the nutritional needs of additional billions of people in the decades ahead. Viewpoints vary widely, with many experts expressing cautious optimism that improvements in agricultural technology, coupled with declining birth rates, guarantee that future generations will be adequately fed. Other observers insist that current trends are already seriously undermining the long-term sustainability of world agriculture and fisheries while simultaneously increasing the number of mouths to be fed.

The wide divergence in outlook stems from personal assumptions regarding future trends in human fertility, world economic growth, environmental degradation, and agricultural productivity—assumptions that may ultimately prove correct or radically off base. Until relatively recently, remarkable gains in agricultural productivity worldwide provided ample grounds for optimism that one day in the not-too-distant future, no child would go to bed hungry. From 1950 until 1984 the world's farm-ers were successful in producing increased quantities of food more rapidly than the world's parents were producing babies. During this period world grain consumption per person increased by 38% in spite of spiraling population figures, resulting in impressive nutritional gains in many formerly food-short regions of the world.

Global trends were somewhat misleading, however, since the world food production averages to a large extent reflected an enormous and disproportionate increase in North American crop yields during those years. These figures masked grimmer statistics showing that in many of the rapidly growing developing nations, per capita increase in food production had halted by the late 1950s due to high rates of population increase. Until the mid-1980s, global averages continued to convey the impression that all was rosy on the food front. Throughout this period, world grain harvests increased by almost 3% annually (compared with a world population growth rate at this time of about 2%). During the 1970s the resource-intensive technologies of the Green Revolution resulted in a major boost in agricultural production in the developing world; by the early 1980s news of huge crop surpluses dominated the farm pages of newspapers and laments of a worldwide "grain glut" were heard from Chicago to Melbourne. Even western Europe, reliant on food imports for the past 200 years, became a grain exporter during those golden years.

By the mid-1980s, however, some worrisome trends were becoming evident, as rapid yearly increases in world harvests began to slacken. Between 1990–2008, total world grain production grew by just 1.3% annually, barely enough to keep pace with population growth. On a per capita basis of 350 kg/person in recent years, annual global grain production appears adequate to sustain the world's current population. However, output per person varies widely in different parts of the world, ranging from approximately 1,230 kg/person/year in the United States (with the lion's share of this amount diverted to livestock feed) to just 90 kg/person/year in Zimbabwe. Nearly half the world's harvest—46%—is produced by China, India, and the United States, with European countries (including Russia and the former Soviet republics) accounting for an additional 21%.

Trends in global grain production vary also in terms of specific crop species. Wheat, rice, and corn constitute fully 85% of the world's grain harvest by weight, with minor grains such as barley, oats, sorghum, millet, and several others comprising the remainder. Of these, only corn, barley, sorghum, and other grains fed to animals (collectively referred to as "coarse grains") have experienced a significant upswing in production in recent years and can claim credit for most of the increase in total grain harvest. The United States is the world's leading corn producer, accounting for more than 40% of the global harvest (and half of all corn exports), with China in second place. Compared to corn, world wheat and rice production have been relatively stagnant, increasing marginally during years when weather conditions are favorable, but falling when they are not. In terms of production, the United States and China rank number 1 and 2, respectively, for wheat, just as they do for corn, while China, India, and several other Asian countries collectively account for 90% of the world's rice harvest.

Because their large populations generate a high level of consumer demand for domestically grown food supplies, major grain producers like China and India are not among the ranks of leading grain exporters. When it comes to supplying the needs of countries that are not self-sufficient in food grains, the world must rely on just a handful of countries with surplus food for export. The United States, Canada, Argentina, Australia, and the European Union account for 80% of all wheat exports, while 80% of the corn in international trade originates in the United States, Argentina, and the EU. One troubling trend evident during the past decade is the decline in grain reserves held by governments as a cushion against poor harvests and rising prices. At the end of 2007 the amounts in storage represented only 14% of annual consumption, well below their record highs in the mid-1980s and late 1990s—and reserves continue to dwindle (Halweil, 2009a).

Of course, livestock production and fisheries also contribute significantly to human diets. Mirroring the per capita increase in grain harvests, production of beef and mutton tripled between 1950 and 1990; since then, a lowering of rangeland productivity due to overgrazing has resulted in a leveling off in production, with future increases unlikely unless more feed grains are diverted to livestock. Meat production overall has continued to grow, exceeding 280 million tons in 2008, thanks largely to big increases in poultry production, as well as to a continued expansion in the market for pork, the world's most popular red meat. While meat currently comprises a much larger proportion of the daily diet in rich countries than in the developing world, meat consumption is rising more rapidly in developing nations, which now account for at least 60% of world meat production. China has now become the leading producer and consumer of pork, accounting for half the world's supply (Halweil, 2009b). Growth in world fisheries, which witnessed a near-quintupling of the annual catch between the early 1950s and the early 1990s, now appears to be at or near its maximum sustainable yield; many stocks of preferred table fish species have already been fished to commercial extinction and marine biologists fear we may have already exceeded the carrying capacity of the world's oceans (Watson and Pauly, 2001).

While many national leaders tend to blame adverse weather conditions for food shortfalls, the true causes are more complex: loss of good cropland to erosion and nonfarm uses, diversion of food crops to biofuels production, inefficient agrarian structures, lack of investment in agriculture by city-oriented government officials, cutbacks in agricultural research, and *too many people*.

FACTORS INFLUENCING FOOD DEMAND

While it is obvious that the total yield of the world's croplands, pasturelands, and fisheries constitutes the world's food *supply*, assessing food *demand* is slightly more complicated. **Population growth,** not surprisingly, is the single largest factor in determining food demand. Since almost all of the world's population increase is occurring in the countries of Asia, Africa, and Latin America, food supply problems currently are most acute in these regions. An additional factor must be considered in assessing food demand, however. **Rising personal incomes** that have characterized the economic

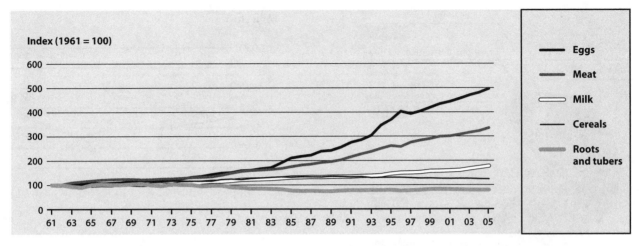

Source: *The State of Food and Agriculture 2009: Livestock in the Balance.* Food and Agriculture Organization, January 2010.

Figure 4-1   Per Capita Consumption of Major Food Items in Developing Countries, 1961–2005

development of most industrialized countries since World War II have greatly added to world food demand. This is not because the typical American, Swede, or Japanese eats tremendously greater quantities than the average Peruvian, Pakistani, or Sudanese, but because higher incomes generally translate into an increased demand for high-quality foods, particularly meat and dairy products. As you will recall from our discussion of trophic levels and energy transfer (chapter 1), it requires several times as much grain to produce a pound of human flesh from meat as it would if that same grain were eaten directly, due to inescapable inefficiencies of energy conversion. (Some animals are more efficient converters than others, however. The grain demand imposed by eating poultry or fish is far less than that of eating beef, for example, since producing a pound of chicken or farmed catfish requires just two pounds of feed grain, while it takes seven pounds of grain to produce a pound of beef.) Currently 36% of world grain production is utilized for livestock feed. Between 1950–2007, world meat consumption soared from 44 million tons to 260 million tons, with corresponding increases in the consumption of eggs and dairy products as well. Experts foresee world meat production doubling by 2050, further increasing the pressure on grain supplies (Halweil, 2009b).

Perhaps nowhere does the pent-up consumer craving for animal protein have more explosive potential than in China, where rapid economic growth is bringing hitherto undreamed-of prosperity to the world's most populous nation. Meat-eating has now become a status symbol in China, a way for Chinese to demonstrate their embrace of a modern lifestyle and a repudiation of past poverty that imposed a largely vegetarian diet (Gardner and Halweil, 2000). The rapid rise in personal incomes in East Asia and in many developing nations during the past decade is having a profound impact on both the type and amount of food people in those countries eat. As the people of China—and elsewhere—shift from primarily vegetarian to more heavily meat-based diets, world grain demand will grow even faster than mere population figures would suggest.

EXTENT OF HUNGER

Determining the number of hungry people in the world today is an inexact science. Certainly there is a quantum difference between the teenager coming home from school complaining, "When's dinner, Mom? I'm starving!" and a Somali child with stick-like limbs and protruding abdomen, dying of acute malnutrition. In an attempt to establish some basis for comparison, the Food and Agriculture Organization (FAO) of the United Nations has devised a concept called the **basal metabolic rate (BMR).** The BMR is defined as the minimum amount of energy required to power human body maintenance, not including energy required for activity. On this basis, the FAO considers anyone receiving less than 1.2 BMR food intake daily to be undernourished. Using this rather conservative figure (some authorities feel the cut-off point should be raised to 1.5 BMR), the FAO in 2009 estimated that just over a billion people in the world were undernourished, receiving insufficient food to develop their full physical and mental potential. Hunger, of course, is not equally shared among nations or even within nations. The vast majority of the world's hungry people inhabit the South Asian countries of India, Pakistan, and Bangladesh, parts of Southeast Asia, Africa south of the Sahara, and the Andean region of South

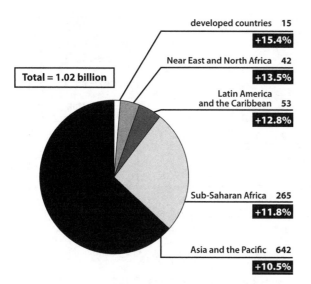

Source: *The State of Food Insecurity in the World 2009*, Food and Agriculture Organization, October 2009.

Figure 4-2   Undernourishment in 2009 by Region (millions) and Increase from 2008

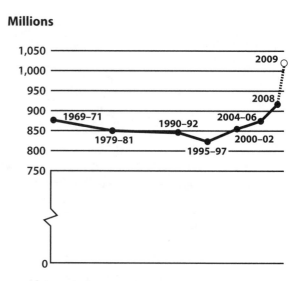

Source: *The State of Food Insecurity in the World 2009*, Food and Agriculture Organization, October 2009.

Figure 4-3   Number of Undernourished in the World, 1969–71 to 2009

America—all regions where rates of population growth continue to be high. Nevertheless, pockets of hunger can be found even within many affluent societies. In the United States malnutrition is distressingly common among the poor, the elderly, migrant farm workers, and Native Americans.

In developing nations as a group, as many as one-third of all children under 5 years old are malnourished, a figure that rises as high as two-thirds in India and Bangladesh. The World Health Organization (WHO) estimates that every day 19,000 children (over 6 million a year) die as a result of malnutrition and related ailments; malnutrition is the direct or indirect cause of more than half the deaths of children under age 5 in less-developed countries. Women, too, are at disproportionate risk of malnutrition. This situation exists because within households in many cultures men, being the primary workers and providers, are served the best food before the rest of the family eats. Children and women, including both pregnant and nursing mothers, whose nutritional needs in proportion to their size exceed those of men, subsist on whatever remains. In such situations, girl children frequently receive less than boys, since males are more highly regarded (Riley, 1997).

The hunger issue most frequently impinges on the public consciousness during periods of severe famine, generally caused by prolonged droughts, floods, or wartime upheavals. During recent years, media coverage of starving children and anguished parents in Somalia, Zimbabwe, Congo, and Ethiopia have kept us grimly aware of human suffering during times of calamity elsewhere in the world. Such periodic episodes of famine, tragic though they are, do not represent the world's major hunger problem, however. Rather, a "covert famine"—the chronic, undramatic, day-after-day undernutrition of those who know that, good harvest or poor, their bellies will never be full—constitutes today's most serious food supply dilemma.

CAUSES OF HUNGER

The existence of more than a billion severely malnourished people in a world where a roughly equivalent number are overweight or obese, suffering health problems due to too much food, seems obscene. Although threats to future food supplies loom on the horizon, most commentators conclude that at present the world's farmers, ranchers, and fishers are producing enough food to supply every human on the planet with a healthy diet. If this is true, why are so many people today suffering from hunger? The current situation is caused largely by two factors: **uneven distribution** of food and **poverty**.

Although global averages suggest that there should be enough food for everyone, many of the areas where hunger is endemic are regions where there is a widening gap between food production and population growth; only imports from food-surplus areas prevent the problem from worsening further. However, as human numbers continue to climb, more equitable distribution of existing resources may not suffice—particularly if a high-quality diet rather than caloric content alone is the goal. Estimates as to how many people the earth can support vary widely, depending on the prevailing type of diet. Assuming that the world grain harvest remains at its present annual level of approximately 2 billion tons, 2.5 billion people could enjoy a typical North American diet, rich in animal protein; if, by contrast, everyone were to consume a Mediterranean-style diet, featuring more moderate amounts of meat along with vegetables, cheese, pasta, and seafood, the world's harvest could adequately support about 5 billion people. Only a strictly vegetarian diet such as that consumed by the average Indian could meet the food needs of 10 billion people (Brown, 2009).

On a more practical level, however, the most basic explanation for the prevalence of hunger is poverty. Even in chronically food-short countries, the rich eat quite well. By contrast, even in the wealthiest nations, where markets bulge with a veritable cornucopia of foods, people who lack money to purchase groceries go hungry. The sudden surge in food prices that occurred in late 2007–2008, when wheat prices almost doubled and rice prices nearly tripled, provoked food riots and protests in more than 60 countries and was the major factor responsible for the increasing incidence of malnutrition.

According to World Bank estimates, over one billion people live in absolute poverty, earning less than the equivalent of $1 per day. These "poorest of the poor" include farmers whose land holdings are too small to be economically viable, rural landless laborers, and urban residents of the rapidly growing squatter settlements ringing many developing world cities. For these people, and for 2 billion more who are only marginally better off, an increase in world food production will mean little unless corresponding social and economic improvements increase their ability to purchase food for their families.

Most observers are confident that until 2025 at least there will be adequate food to meet the demand of those who can afford to pay for it. For those who cannot, the outlook is dismal. In a number of the poorest countries, food production is falling farther and farther behind increasing food demand as their populations continue to grow. If their economies are unable to generate the foreign exchange necessary to purchase food from abroad, nutritional levels are likely to suffer. Free food aid and other forms of development assistance from the wealthy industrialized countries have declined substantially in recent years, further increasing the vulnerability of the world's poorest people. Food insecurity is expected to increase significantly in sub-Saharan Africa and South Asia in the years immediately ahead, with large proportions of the population in those regions too poor to purchase food at prevailing prices. Political instability, regional conflicts, greater variability in agricultural production due to climate change—all could have an impact on food price fluctuations that will determine who eats and who goes hungry.

HEALTH IMPACT OF HUNGER

> The most serious energy crisis in the world is the depletion of human energy—a depletion that comes about because the brain receives too few calories or too few proteins to think, and the body too few to act.
> —Richard J. Barnet, *New Yorker*, March 31, 1980

Malnutrition

Hunger is more than a state of physical discomfort and a cause of political unrest. Even in the absence of acute famine, inadequate food intake has a profound impact on human health. Among the poor in developing countries, **protein-energy malnutrition** (PEM) is a leading cause of death and disease; numerous studies have shown that protein-energy malnutrition is responsible, directly or indirectly, for 50–60% of all childhood deaths in developing countries. Such deaths are seldom due to outright starvation, but rather to a chronic deficit of calories and essential nutrients that leave a child underweight, weak, and vulnerable to infection (FAO, 2002a). If children receive less than 70% of the daily standard food requirement, their growth and activity fall below normal levels; if food deprivation is prolonged, stunted physical development becomes irreversible. The World Health Organization estimated that in 2000 malnutrition affected one out of every three children worldwide to some extent, with 70% of those affected living in Asia, 26% in Africa, and 4% in Latin America and the Caribbean.

Even more ominous than the link between malnutrition and decreased physical development, however, is the finding that severe malnutrition in children, especially very young infants, results in a permanent stunting of brain development, characterized by a decrease in the number of brain cells and an alteration of brain chemistry. Studies have shown that if a nutritional deficiency occurs just before or immediately after birth, the baby will suffer a 15–25% reduction in number of brain cells. If malnutrition afflicts the developing fetus and continues to persist in the postnatal period, the child's complement of brain cells will be lowered by 50–60%.

Two clinical manifestations of PEM, occurring most commonly among children in famine-stricken areas or under conditions of limited food supply, are **kwashiorkor** and **marasmus**. The former is a protein deficiency disease that affects millions of children in tropical areas, particularly in Africa. Although usually associated with food supply emergencies (drought, floods, or violent conflict),

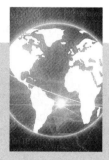

········ 4-1 ········

Eating Close to Home

In March 2009 when Michelle Obama and a group of eager schoolchildren broke ground on the White House lawn to plant a vegetable garden, promoters of locally grown food, as well as millions of backyard gardeners (this author included!) cheered the First Lady's good example. Enthusiasm for eating food grown close to home, with a minimum of chemical inputs, harvested in season and only when ripe, has been growing by leaps and bounds in recent years. Home gardening is reputed to be Americans' favorite pastime, while the rapid proliferation of farmers' markets provides a popular alternative for those with neither the space nor the energy for tending a backyard vegetable patch.

Devotees of the local food movement, so-called "locavores" (the New Oxford American Dictionary's "Word of the Year" for 2007!) who try to restrict their diet to foods harvested within a 100-mile radius of where they live, point to many benefits of opting for alternatives to the industrialized agriculture products now dominating supermarket shelves. (*Note:* the definition of "local" in the case of "local foods" is controversial, but food grown within 100 miles of home seems to be the accepted standard.) Since it doesn't have to be transported thousands of miles from field to consumer, locally grown produce is both fresher and more nutritious (since nutrient value declines with time after harvesting), is less likely to be contaminated with pesticide residues, and certainly tastes better, as anyone who has eaten a fresh-from-the-vine tomato on a hot summer day can attest! In addition to these obvious advantages, locavores now emphasize a feature of locally grown food that has global environmental implications—significantly lower greenhouse gas (GHG) emissions at a time when climate change is the primary environmental threat to the planet.

Research on the climatic impact of the modern food system focused initially on the concept of "food miles"—that is, the distance food travels from farm to dinner table. Studies conducted at Iowa State University concluded that the average food item purchased in a U.S. supermarket travels 1,500 miles before reaching the consumer; locally grown food, by contrast, is transported just 44.6 miles, on average. Since fewer miles traveled translates into less fuel burned and thus lower carbon emissions, the obvious implication is that eating food grown close to home is better for the planet. Results of a Canadian study quantified these benefits, showing that if all the imported foods in the Waterloo, Ontario, area were replaced by similar locally grown products, the drop in transportation-related emissions would be equivalent to taking 16,191 cars off the road.

As the researchers admit, however, such calculations can be a bit misleading, since in looking only at food *miles* traveled, they don't consider the *method* of transport. Since the energy efficiency of railroads is approximately 10 times greater than that of trucks, a train carrying a ton of oranges from Florida to New York would generate fewer GHG emissions than would a truck transporting a similar load to consumers just 100 miles away. In determining the environmental benefits of locally grown food, therefore, the method by which food is brought from field to market is significant.

Similarly, *how* a particular food item is grown can make a big difference in terms of its impact vis-à-vis carbon emissions. In northern Europe, consumers in countries such as Sweden and Russia typically enjoy locally grown tomatoes and other fresh produce throughout the winter, thanks to production in fossil-fuel-heated greenhouses. If curtailing GHG emissions were the top priority, it would be more ecologically correct to ship in field-grown Spanish tomatoes, despite the significant increase in food miles.

Only when comparisons of locally grown vs. conventionally produced food examine exactly the same crops, grown and transported to market in the same way, does the concept of food miles acquire relevance, demonstrating that local foods have a smaller "carbon footprint." In any other situation, it's necessary to take a broader view of GHG emissions, examining each stage of a food's production, transport, packaging, and consumption. One life-cycle analysis of the average American diet published by researchers at Carnegie Mellon University in 2008 revealed that food miles constitute a mere 4% of all the GHG emissions from the U.S. food system. When considering all forms of transport in the food supply chain (e.g., bringing fertilizers and pesticides to the fields, transporting livestock feed, etc.), transport is responsible for 11% of total food system carbon emissions. By contrast, 83% of GHG emissions associated with the food supply chain is generated by planting, cultivating, and harvesting the crop. Locavore skeptics thus can legitimately question whether it really makes much difference in terms of climate change to restrict one's diet to locally grown foods.

What *does* seem to matter a great deal in terms of carbon footprint is *what* one eats. The higher an item is on the food chain, the more energy it takes to produce that food and the more GHGs are emitted in the process. Red meat and dairy products rank at the top of the food list in terms of their contribution to global warming, not only because of the energy consumed in growing the grain to feed livestock, but, perhaps most importantly, because cattle and other ruminants constantly belch copious amounts of methane, a greenhouse gas that is 23 times more potent than carbon dioxide in terms of its impact on climate change. In one study conducted in the United Kingdom, researchers calculated that meat and dairy products are responsible for half of all the GHG emissions associated with the food system. The Carnegie Mellon team concurred with their British colleagues, pointing out that red meat, on average, is more carbon-intensive than any other food (responsible for 150% more emissions than fish or poultry), with dairy products in second place. Opting for a vegetarian diet just one day a week, they concluded, would reduce GHG emissions as much as would driving 1,160 miles less per year.

The environmental impact of food choices, of course, involves more than just carbon emissions; locally produced foods are often grown organically or with significantly lower inputs of chemical fertilizers and pesticides than is the case for commercial agriculture. Small local farms and home gardens often feature a much wider diversity of crops, as well as bordering wild plants or flowers that provide food and habitat for beneficial insects and other wildlife (DeWeerdt, 2009).

For these reasons and more, the local foods movement is steadily gaining adherents. The trend is exemplified by the one million community gardens in cities and small towns across the country, where for a small rental fee municipal governments provide garden plots to residents who lack sufficient land of their own. The potential for further expansion of urban gardening is enormous, since there are hundreds of thousands of vacant lots in cities across the country, just waiting to be transformed into bountiful gardens. Farmers' markets have an even wider appeal, providing a means for small local growers to bring their fresh produce directly to consumers. Between 1994 and 2009, the number of farmers' markets in the United States nearly tripled, growing from 1,755 to more than 4,700 during that 15-year period.

Just as the main purpose of the new White House vegetable garden is to educate children about healthy, locally grown foods as a way to combat childhood obesity and diabetes, so many schools, particularly in urban settings, are establishing their own gardens. California is a national leader in this movement, with approximately 6,000 school gardens where city children learn that food doesn't grow in cans and where they have the opportunity to plant, tend, and harvest the vegetables they can subsequently eat in their school cafeteria. A number of upscale restaurants have also become enthusiastic promoters of locally grown food, emphasizing such fare on their menus and providing a lucrative market for local farmers (Brown, 2009).

The ultimate in locally grown food, of course, is to grow it yourself in your own backyard, eliminating any food miles whatsoever, other than those you expend walking from house to plot, and enjoying the fruits (or veggies!) of your labor within minutes after the harvest. Though the nation has a long way to go to equal the 40% of all fresh produce grown in U.S. "victory gardens" during World War II, the potential is immense. If even a small portion of the estimated 18 million acres now occupied by turfgrass lawns were converted to vegetable gardens, the nutritional rewards to Americans would be tremendous—not to mention the exercise benefits! With county-based Master Gardener volunteers across the nation ready and eager to help gardening neophytes with advice and moral support, there's seldom been a better time to take up home gardening. To sum up the message: eat food that's fresher, tastier, and healthier; fight climate change; protect the environment; plant a garden—and become a locavore!

kwashiorkor can develop in babies who are weaned early and given only starchy, low-protein foods such as rice, cassava, or bananas to eat—common baby foods in many tropical regions. Symptoms of mild kwashiorkor include discoloration of the hair (in dark-haired children, hair may assume a reddish cast), white patches on the skin, retardation of physical growth, development of a protruding abdomen due to accumulation of fluids, and a loss of appetite. In more severe cases the hair may fall out painlessly in tufts, digestive problems arise, fluid collects in the

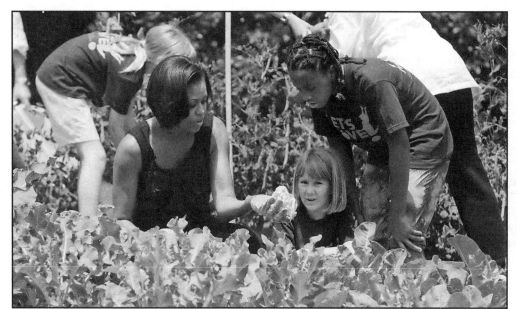

First Lady Michelle Obama and local schoolchildren harvest vegetables from the garden planted on the South Lawn of the White House in this June 2010 photo. The First Family is promoting the consumption of locally grown food that's fresher, healthier, free of pesticides, and incurs a smaller carbon footprint than processed foods. [*AP Photo/ Alex Brandon*]

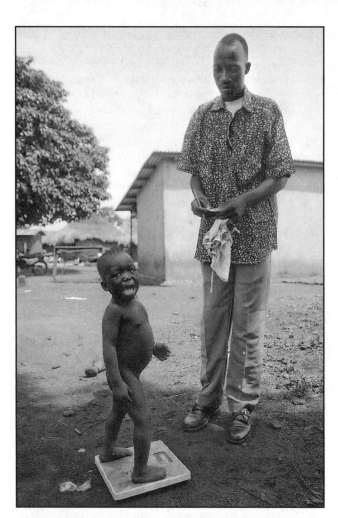

A nurse weighs a young boy who exhibits the protruding abdomen characteristic of kwashiorkor sufferers. [*AP Photo/Marco Chown Oved*]

legs and feet, muscle wastage and enlargement of the liver may occur, and the child becomes listless and apathetic. Once this stage of the disease is reached, shock and coma leading to death are likely unless the child receives medical attention. Victims who recover from severe cases of kwashiorkor never attain their full height and growth potential. In its milder forms, however, the effects of kwashiorkor are reversible and generally disappear as the child becomes older and is given a more varied diet.

Marasmus, the second of the two most commonly observed deficiency diseases among children, is an indication of overall protein-calorie deprivation—in essence, the child is starving. Most frequently striking babies under one year of age, especially those no longer being breast-fed, marasmus often occurs after the child has been suffering from diarrhea or some other disease. Victims of marasmus can be distinguished by their thin, wasted appearance, with skin hanging in loose wrinkles around wrists and legs and eyes appearing unusually large and bright because of the shrunken aspect of the rest of the body.

In addition to its direct impact on growth and mental development, malnutrition also greatly increases a child's susceptibility to infectious disease by reducing bodily defenses. Even mild levels of malnutrition can increase a child's risk of dying from common childhood ailments such as diarrhea, measles, or acute respiratory infections. As the severity of malnutrition (measured in terms of a child's weight-to-age ratio) increases, so does the risk of death due to infectious disease, from 2.5 times higher for mildly malnourished children to 4.6 times for those moderately underfed to 8.4 times excess risk for severely malnourished youngsters (FAO, 2002a).

Malnutrition takes its toll among older children and adults as well. Undernourished people lose weight and become less able to combat infections or environmental stress. They thereby become less economically productive and less able to care for their families. Surveys in developing countries have shown that nutritionally deprived adults who are smaller and slighter than normal earn lower wages than their better-fed colleagues when employed in jobs requiring physical labor—proof that while poverty may be a cause of hunger, hunger can also cause poverty (FAO, 2002a). However, while adults suffering temporarily from severe food deprivation may become listless and apathetic, unable to engage in strenuous physical labor, they seldom experience the permanent damage characteristic of childhood malnutrition. At greatest risk, of course, are pregnant and lactating women. Such women, if malnourished, run a significantly higher risk of miscarriage or premature delivery than do adequately fed mothers. If they manage to carry their babies full-term, the child is likely to suffer from low birth weight (one of the most frequent causes of infant mortality) or to be stillborn. The old myth that nursing mothers draw on their own nutritional reserves to provide top-quality food for their infants is untrue—the milk of undernourished mothers is lower than normal in vitamins, fat, and protein content.

Micronutrient Deficiencies

A large portion of the world's undernourished population suffers as well from an inadequate intake of essential vitamins and minerals. This situation is largely a reflection of the lack of variety in the diet of the poor, who may subsist on little but rice, tortillas, or chappatis. However, micronutrient deficiencies are not limited to chronically hungry populations; many people receiving an adequate, even excess, daily intake of calories may still be malnourished in terms of vitamin or mineral deficiencies if their diets are heavily skewed toward starchy, low-nutrient foods. The WHO estimates that some 2.0–3.5 billion people worldwide are currently affected by micronutrient deficiencies that make them more susceptible to disease, stunt their mental and physical development, and sap their energy. Of particular concern because the condition is so widespread is insufficient intake of vitamin A, iron, and iodine.

Vitamin A Deficiency (VAD)

A public health problem among the poor in over 100 countries, VAD is the single most important cause of childhood blindness in low-income countries. VAD, seldom a concern among those whose diet includes eggs, dairy products, and green leafy vegetables, can result in a drying of the eye membranes or a softening of the cornea. Such conditions lead first to night-blindness and, if

not treated, to total blindness of its victims. In areas such as South and Southeast Asia, Africa, Central America, Haiti, and northeastern Brazil, an estimated 100–140 million children suffer from VAD and 250,000–500,000 will go blind as a result. Scientists have confirmed that VAD not only can lead to blindness, but also is an important determinant of mortality in children and pregnant women due to its deleterious effect on the immune system. Vitamin A stimulates maturation of white blood cells, which aid the body in fighting infection; its deficiency provokes changes in the mucous membranes lining the respiratory, gastrointestinal, and urinary tracts, rendering them less effective in protecting the body against invading pathogens.

Efforts by the World Health Organization to combat VAD focus on several complimentary approaches. Promoting breast-feeding of infants is regarded as the best way to protect babies against VAD, since breast milk is a natural source of vitamin A. For children already suffering from VAD, one of the most widely adopted approaches has been administering mega-doses of vitamin A in capsule form twice a year, often in conjunction with polio eradication campaigns. However, because the effects of the capsules last only 4–6 months and because breast-feeding is time-limited as well, neither can be considered a long-term solution. Yet another approach involves fortifying some common dietary constituent such as sugar with vitamin A, a strategy that has been pursued with some success in parts of Central and South America for several decades. Educating parents to provide their children with foods rich in vitamin A seems to offer the best solution to the problem; such an approach can include promotion of home gardening to grow vitamin A-rich foods in regions where they aren't locally available in the marketplace or are too expensive. In the long run, however, eliminating VAD depends on reducing levels of poverty and raising living standards so that all families can enjoy an adequate and nutritious diet (WHO, 2009).

Iodine Deficiency

The incidence of Iodine Deficiency Disorders (IDD), a serious public health problem that in the early 1990s affected an estimated 2 billion people, today is estimated at approximately 400 million, half of them in India. Other regions where IDD is most common include Southeast Asia, Africa, and the Western Pacific, where it is particularly prevalent among pregnant women, preschool children, and the poor. Associated in the public mind with a condition called **goiter** (a disfiguring enlargement of the thyroid gland on the neck), IDD has far more serious health implications; regarded by public health agencies as the world's single most important cause of preventable brain damage and mental retardation, IDD can reduce a victim's IQ by 15 points. The World Health Organization estimates that almost 50 million people currently suffer from some degree of IDD-related brain damage and that 38 million children are born at risk of iodine deficiencies each year. If a pregnant woman is iodine-deficient, her fetus can incur irreversible brain damage, resulting in the baby being born dwarfed and intellectually disabled, a condition referred to as cretinism. Serious iodine deficiency during pregnancy can also result in miscarriage or stillbirth. For those less severely afflicted, IDD's impairment of mental ability lowers the intellectual capacity of millions of people, with a corresponding impact on the economic productivity of regions most affected.

Fortunately, prospects for eradicating IDD worldwide now appear bright. In 1993 the World Health Organization launched its Universal Salt Iodization campaign, providing technical tools and guidance to countries wishing to create their own salt iodization programs. Because salt is widely available, eaten in consistent amounts year-round, and cheap to iodize (about 5 cents per person per year), it provides an ideal vehicle for international efforts at fortification, just as it did in the United States decades earlier. Progress in reducing IDD since initiation of the WHO effort has been dramatic. The number of countries with salt iodization programs has soared since the program was initiated; 70% of the world's households now use iodized salt, up from less than 20% before the Universal Salt Iodization campaign was launched. As a result, global rates of goiter, mental retardation, and cretinism are falling rapidly, offering hope that one day in the not-too-distant future, iodine deficiency disorders will be regarded as ancient history, much like scurvy, beriberi, and pellagra.

Iron Deficiency

Iron deficiency anemia, the most common of all nutritional deficiency diseases, afflicts more people worldwide than any other single condition and may well be regarded as a public health epidemic. The WHO estimates that between 4–5 billion people (66–80% of the world's population) currently suffer from iron deficiency. Of these, 2 billion are anemic, at least half of them because of inadequate dietary intake of iron, especially among those subsisting on vegetarian diets, but also exacerbated in many tropical countries by malaria and parasitic worm infections. Anemia is surprisingly common in the United States as well, though for different reasons. Over-consumption of calorie-rich "junk foods" instead of nutritionally superior fare has contributed to a situation where almost 20% of premenopausal American women are iron-deficient—a figure that rises to 42% of pregnant African-American women living in poverty (Gardner and Halweil, 2000).

Anemia is characterized by lack of energy and low levels of productive activity. It is especially dangerous—and especially common—in pregnant women, where it increases the likelihood of maternal death, premature delivery, or stillbirth. Repeated pregnancies rapidly drain a woman's reserve supplies of iron; in India, where the problem is more severe than anywhere else in the world, the WHO reports that almost 70% of women and 75% of preschool-age children suffer from insufficient iron intake. Iron deficiency anemia is held responsible, at least in part, for the high female mortality rate in that country. While women need three times as much iron as men to replace losses during menstruation and pregnancy, their food intake is generally lower than that of their husbands, sons, and brothers. Various strategies have been tried to ameliorate iron deficiency anemia. These include providing iron supplements to population subgroups at particular risk, such as pregnant women and teenage girls; encouraging people to diversify their diets, including more iron-rich foods; and fortifying common food staples with iron. Among the most promising options is the recent introduction of Double Fortified Salt (DFS), containing an encapsulated iron compound, ferrous fumarate, as well as iodine. Groups such as Canada's Micronutrient Initiative are hopeful that DFS will be as effective in reducing the incidence of iron deficiency in poor countries as the widely hailed Universal Salt Iodization campaign has been in reducing IDD (Micronutrient Initiative, 2009).

PROSPECTS FOR REDUCING WORLD HUNGER

Certainly there has been no shortage of suggestions as to what might be done to ease the population-food crunch. Some of the approaches being tried have real merit, as well as limitations, while others are merely wishful thinking. It's important that people have some understanding of the key elements in the ongoing debate as to how best to eradicate hunger, since this issue is certain to assume even greater urgency in the years ahead. Some of the most frequently mentioned ways of increasing the world food supply are discussed in the following sections.

Expanding the Amount of Land Under Cultivation

From the beginning of the Agricultural Revolution right up to the early 1950s, increasing acreage put to the plow was the major, often the only, way of increasing food supply. Expanding the amount of cultivated land was accomplished by clearing forests, terracing mountainsides, or building irrigation systems—all of which permitted hitherto unproductive lands to be farmed. During the 1950s the Soviet Union vastly increased its agricultural acreage by opening up the "virgin lands" of Kazakhstan; at the same time the Chinese completed some major irrigation networks, substantially expanding their cultivated acreage and making it possible to raise two to three crops per year on the same land. Since that time, significant increases in highly productive farmland have been quite limited. Worldwide, total acreage devoted to agriculture expanded by just 8% since the mid-1960s, with almost all of this increase in developing countries, particularly in sub-Saharan Africa where almost 90% of the increase in food production since 1990 has been achieved by expanding the area under cultivation (FAO, 2009a).

The hard truth is that the world's prime farmland is in finite supply, and after approximately 10,000 years of agricultural expansion most good land is already being cultivated. Since the 1950s most of the additional land cleared for farming has been so-called "marginal land"—land that is incapable of sustaining moderately good yields over any extended period of time due to its poor soil, erodability, or steep slope. Farmers who today move onto marginal lands, desperate to eke out a living for their families, do so only because the better lands are already overcrowded. The additional food that such lands will contribute to world harvests is negligible and the long-term ecological damage caused by removing the natural vegetative cover from such lands may eventually have an adverse impact on better lands elsewhere.

Some optimists look hopefully to regions of South America and Africa where nearly half of the yet-undeveloped land suitable for agriculture is located. However, such lands are far from current markets and lack the transportation infrastructure necessary for viable agricultural development. The huge amount of capital investment that would be required appears at present to be far beyond the financial capabilities of the nations involved. Moreover, increasing cultivated acreage in a few land-abundant regions is unlikely to provide additional food or benefits for land-scarce countries. In the world's two most populous nations, China and India, opportunities to expand farmland acreage are virtually nonexistent (Bender and Smith, 1997).

The other side of the coin, often overlooked by commentators, is the substantial amounts of good cropland that are lost every year to erosion, desertification, salinization and water-logging of irrigated fields, and urban development. It is now recognized that the increase in world food production witnessed during the 1970s and early 1980s was achieved in part by plowing marginal lands unsuitable for sustained cultivation and by over-irrigating, which has resulted in drastic drawing-down of groundwater reserves in many areas. Today in many of the major grain-producing areas of the world, the cropland base is beginning to shrink as highly erodible lands

are abandoned—including 40% of Kazakhstan's once-lauded "virgin lands" (Brown, 2009). The World Resources Institute reports that approximately two-thirds of the world's crop and pasturelands have suffered some degree of degradation over the past half century, with 40% of agricultural lands rated as strongly or very strongly degraded. The situation is sufficiently severe and widespread to reduce productivity on 16% of farmlands, particularly in Africa and Central America. While crop yields on a worldwide basis are expected to increase over the next few decades, the results of soil degradation surveys suggest that the long-term productivity of more than half the world's agricultural lands is being undermined by erosion and nutrient depletion (WRI, 2000). The following chapter will examine these trends in more detail, but it is important to bear in mind that while most of the lands currently being added to our agricultural base are marginal acres, those being lost are, for the most part, prime croplands that will never be returned to production.

Increasing World Fish Catch

When one considers that 71% of the earth's surface is water, it's understandable that many people look to the oceans as the source of apparently limitless high-quality animal protein. Such optimism seemed justified during the years between 1950–1989, when total world fish catch soared from about 22 million tons annually to 89 million tons—a four-fold increase that, even at a time of unprecedented population growth, resulted in a doubling in the per capita availability of seafood. Since fish provide at least 15% of the animal protein consumed by almost 3 billion people worldwide—and as much as 50% for those in some countries like Bangladesh and Indonesia—this bounty from the sea raised hopes for substantial progress in combating malnutrition.

Since the 1990s, the world's capture fisheries (i.e. those taking wild fish by line, net, or trap) have stabilized at between 90–95 million tons per year and future increases beyond this level are considered unlikely. Large predator fish, once the mainstay of ocean fisheries, have declined precipitously in recent decades, as overexploitation by industrial fishing fleets has reduced stocks of some species to a mere 10% of their former levels (Myers and Worm, 2003). As a result, stocks of species regarded as desirable table-grade fish—swordfish, haddock, hake, toothfish (aka Chilean sea bass), orange roughy—are now in sharp decline. For some species the situation is even more dire; the International Union for Conservation of Nature and Natural Resources (IUCN) *Red List* now includes such overfished species as the Atlantic cod, Atlantic halibut, yellowtail flounder, and five species of tuna as headed toward extinction, at least over large expanses of their original range (WRI, 2000).

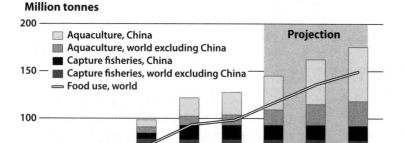

Source: Adapted from www.fishfarming.com; data from *The State of the World's Fisheries and Aquaculture 2008*, Food and Agriculture Organization, 2009.

Figure 4-4   World Fish Production and Food Use Consumption 1976–2030

The fact that the total annual catch hasn't dropped precipitously is due to what some researchers refer to as "fishing down the food web" (Pauly et al., 1998), maintaining tonnage by hauling in many lower-trophic level species, such as anchovetas, herring, and mackerel, formerly regarded as "trash fish." Since the 1980s, low-value fish species have accounted for almost three-quarters of the overall increase in world fish catch. The FAO reports that approximately 52% of the major marine fish stocks are now fully exploited, yielding catches at or close to their maximum sustainable limits and therefore offering little hope for increased future harvests. Another 19% of stocks are already overexploited, making it likely that in the years ahead catches of these species will be further reduced unless remedial action is taken soon to lessen the pressures of overfishing. Eight percent of stocks are already significantly depleted, while 1% is recovering from depletion but far less productive than formerly. Fish stocks that are still underexploited or only moderately exploited, the group representing the greatest potential for increasing world marine fish catch, comprise just 20% of the major fish stocks for which information is available (FAO, 2009b).

Ocean fisheries, of course, don't account for the world's entire fish catch. Inland capture fisheries supply about 12% of all fish consumed by people. Like their marine counterpart, however, inland fisheries are now being exploited at nonsustainable levels. Only through restocking and by introducing more productive fish species (a practice restricted to a few countries such as China) has it been possible to maintain some growth in inland fisheries (WRI, 2000). The declining capacity of the world's coastal and marine ecosystems to meet the growing demand for seafood will inevitably lead to higher prices. Already a major share of the world's marine fish harvest is exported to affluent consumers in Japan, the U.S., and other industrialized nations. In the years ahead, rising prices sparked by rising demand will further boost fish exports from developing nations, leaving fewer fish for local consumers and making fish protein less affordable for low-income families.

While the main factor affecting sustainability of capture fisheries is overexploitation, pollution is having an impact as well. It has not yet been possible to demonstrate a decline in the abundance of entire species in the open sea due solely to pollution, but experiments have shown that toxic contaminants such as hydrocarbons, heavy metals, and synthetic organic compounds—all common water pollutants—can kill or injure aquatic organisms. In the coastal waters that constitute some of the world's most productive fishing grounds, nutrients, primarily nitrates and phosphates from sewage discharges or farmland runoff, constitute the most extensive and serious pollution problem. A large area of sea bottom in the Gulf of Mexico offshore from New Orleans is now a virtual "dead zone," thanks largely to agricultural runoff from Midwest farmlands.

Fears about Gulf Coast fisheries escalated in the summer of 2010 when the offshore Deepwater Horizon oil rig exploded, killing 11 workers and releasing nearly 5 million barrels (almost 185 million gallons) of oil from BP's Macondo 252 well into the Gulf. Alarms were raised that Gulf fisheries would be devastated and that coastal marshes serving as nurseries for many commercially important species would suffer massive long-term damage. Thousands of seabirds were killed and extensive areas of the Gulf declared off-limits to fishers and shrimpers. To the surprise of scientists, however, by the time the well was finally sealed in mid-September, the environmental impact, though certainly not negligible, appeared to be far less than originally expected. According to the National Oceanic and Atmospheric Administration (NOAA), the oil from the spill had rapidly broken down, probably due to the relatively warm water temperature, and, thanks to a fortuitous shift in ocean currents, much of it remained well offshore from sensitive wetlands. Although subtle effects could still be manifested over time, scientists estimate the environmental toll will be considerably lower than that of the much smaller Exxon Valdez oil spill in Alaska in 1989 and are cautiously optimistic that the Gulf ecosystem will soon recover (Kaufman and Dewan, 2010).

Elsewhere, the decline of Chesapeake Bay's crab and oyster harvest, once among the world's richest, can be traced to contamination from runoff. Shellfish are particularly susceptible to pollution of near-shore areas; if not directly killed by toxic contaminants, they are often declared unmarketable because of the health threat they pose to human consumers.

Development activities that destroy coastal habitats, particularly coastal marshes, mangroves, and sea grasses, also play a role in reducing populations of ocean fish because many commercially important species depend on coastal or estuarine waters for survival during some phase of their life cycle. Burgeoning urban populations along most of the world's coastlines are rapidly increasing development pressures in these areas, yet few countries are managing such growth in a manner that will protect the ocean's biotic resources.

Aquaculture

In contrast to the rather gloomy outlook for the capture fisheries, fish harvests from **aquaculture** (fish farming) have been the fastest-growing source of animal protein since 1990, with production rising from 13 million tons that year to over 50 million tons in 2007 (Brown, 2009; FAO, 2009b). Growth of aquaculture has been particularly rapid in China, the source of 70% of aquaculture production and more than half the total value; Chinese are also the world's most avid fish-eaters, consuming an average 25.8 kilograms live weight per person annually, compared to 18.6 kg for the average Canadian or American. India ranks a distant second among the leading aquaculture producers, followed by Vietnam, Thailand, and Indonesia; in the Western Hemisphere, only Chile ranks among the world's top ten (McKeown and Halweil, 2009).

Table 4-1   Top 15 Countries in Aquaculture Production

Producer	2006 (tonnes)
China	34,429,122
India	3,123,135
Vietnam	1,657,727
Thailand	1,385,801
Indonesia	1,292,899
Bangladesh	892,049
Chile	802,410
Japan	733,891
Norway	708,780
Philippines	623,369
Egypt	595,030
Myanmar	574,990
South Korea	513,568
U.S.	465,061
China (Taiwan)	310,216

Source: Adapted from "Aquaculture Production 2006," *Yearbook of Fishery Statistics*, table A-4. Food and Agriculture Organization of the United Nations.

While fish farming in the United States still accounts for less than 2% of world production, it already supplies most of the catfish sold in American supermarkets. While as much as a third of the wild fish catch is used to make fish meal and fish oil, farmed fish go directly to human consumers. Aquaculture now provides 47% of all the fish on human dinner tables and it is assumed that any future increases in fish consumption will have to come from aquaculture, since there is little hope of further increasing ocean fish catch (FAO, 2009b). Unlike capture fisheries, however, aquaculture demands significant resource inputs. Freshwater fish farms require considerable amounts of land and water, both of which must be diverted from other types of agricultural production. Concerns over cropland loss to fish production have already prompted Chinese authorities to restrict future farmland conversion to aquaculture. Additionally, farmed fish, unlike those caught on the open seas, must be fed by those who raise them. Fortunately, fish are among the most efficient energy converters, requiring less than 2 pounds of feed to gain one pound of flesh.

Few serious problems are associated with aquaculture production of herbivorous fish species such as tilapia, carp, and catfish, but aquaculture operations focused on more profitable carnivorous species such as salmon and shrimp raise legitimate environmental concerns. Salmon are less efficient protein converters than their herbivorous cousins because they must be fed pelleted feed made of fish meal or fish oil, produced by grinding up enormous numbers of so-called "industrial fish," mainly small, oily deep-sea species harvested from already over-exploited marine fisheries. Excess pellets not eaten by the caged salmon, along with fish feces, drift downward from the pens to the ocean floor, where they decompose and release nutrients that contribute to algal blooms and lead to the creation of oxygen-deficient "dead zones" in the vicinity of salmon farms. Crowded conditions in the salmon pens can lead to disease outbreaks that infect not only the farmed fish but nearby wild salmon populations as well, while the profligate use of vaccines, antibiotics, and parasiticides by farm managers to keep such problems under control poses a threat to the marine environment.

Shrimp farming also has an ecological downside, since coastal mangrove forests are often destroyed to make room for shrimp ponds. The 2004 tsunami that devastated several Southeast Asian countries caused much greater damage along sections of the Thai coast where shrimp farms had proliferated than in undisturbed areas where the mangrove ecosystem was still intact and capable of buffering inland areas against the fury of the waves. Like every other enterprise, aquaculture has its economic and environmental costs.

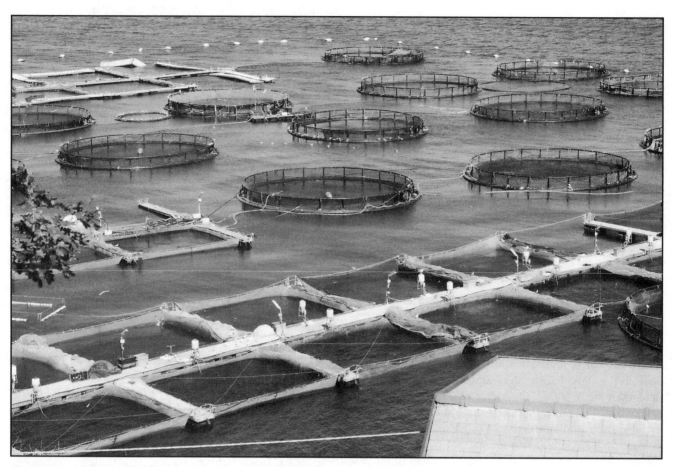

Since 1990, fish harvests from aquaculture have been the fastest-growing source of animal protein.

Reducing Post-Harvest Food Losses

Implementation of better methods of handling and protecting food between the time it is harvested and the time it appears on the consumer's plate may, in the short-run at least, help increase the availability of food in the marketplace. Each year enormous amounts of harvested foods are lost to pests and spoilage, particularly in tropical countries. Rats, birds, insects, and molds all consume or render unfit for human use large amounts of stored foods that would otherwise have been available for people. Cultural practices are partially responsible for such losses. In many countries grains are stored in the open or in easily penetrated sacks or bins. Lack of adequate refrigeration promotes spoilage, while poor transport facilities delay rapid movement of food from fields to consumers.

In wealthier countries, consumers' insistence that food be cosmetically perfect results in substantial wastage of harvested crops, particularly fruits and vegetables. Tiny blemishes that in no way affect a food's taste or nutritional value frequently result in its being discarded because it doesn't meet market standards of aesthetic acceptability. Retailing, food service, and personal consumption habits also result in considerable wastage of food. Just these three stages of the marketing process account for the loss of almost 95 billion pounds of food annually in the United States—27% of all food available for consumption (Kantor, 1997).

Eating Lower on the Food Chain

Humanitarians are frequently troubled by the apparent inefficiency of converting a substantial portion of the world grain harvest into meat or poultry to satisfy consumers' carnivorous cravings. The same amount of corn, wheat, or oats, they argue, could satisfy the caloric needs of millions of additional people dining on vegetarian fare. (To be consistent, they might also target the 10% of the U.S. corn crop diverted to the manufacture of corn syrup, much of which is used for sweetening soft drinks.) On the other hand, proponents of a vegetarian diet overlook the fact that most of the world's beef and mutton is produced on grasslands that are too dry or mountainous for farming; if not used for grazing to produce meat and dairy products, these vast areas—at least twice as extensive as

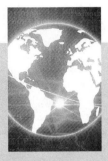

$\cdots\cdots\cdots$ 4-2 $\cdots\cdots\cdots$

Looking Abroad for Food Security

What can a food-deficit nation do when commodity prices soar and the cost of grain imports climbs sky-high? If the country in question is oil-rich but water-poor, it can outsource farmland in another country and grow its own food abroad. That's exactly what Saudi Arabia, Libya, and several of the Persian Gulf states are now doing, as are China and South Korea, where falling water tables have prompted government concerns about long-term food security. A number of observers insist that water shortages are the main impetus behind farmland outsourcing, since water rights accompany land deals; one corporate executive has dubbed the recent trend "the great water grab."

The current rush for overseas land acquisitions was sparked by a 78% increase in world food prices in late 2007–2008 (soybean and rice prices during this period experienced an even larger increase, soaring by 130%), followed by the imposition of temporary trade bans by a number of food-exporting countries hoping to forestall food price hikes at home. Even rich countries like Saudi Arabia and China who could afford to pay the higher cost of food imports feared the supplies they needed might not be available at any price. The default solution to this dilemma was to purchase or lease farmlands abroad, grow their own crops there, and ship the harvest back home. Libya was among the first to pursue this option, reaching an agreement with Ukraine in the spring of 2009 to grow Libyan wheat on 100,000 hectares (almost 250,000 acres) of Ukrainian cropland. Subsequently there have been approximately 50 agreements for outsourcing domestic food production to other countries, primarily to poor nations that need capital and are willing to make land available. Included among the deals recently finalized or in negotiation is an initiative in Ethiopia, where Saudi businessmen are investing $100 million to cultivate wheat, rice, and barley on land leased to them by the Ethiopian government with the understanding that they can ship the entire harvest back to Saudi Arabia. Saudi investors have also been granted access to 2 million hectares (4.9 million acres) of land for rice cultivation in Indonesia. Not to be outdone, the Chinese have been granted rights to 2.8 million hectares (6.9 million acres) in the Democratic Republic of the Congo to establish the world's largest palm oil plantation, destined for biofuels production. China is also negotiating with Zambia for an additional 2 million hectares where jatropha—another biofuels crop—will be planted if the deal moves forward. South Korea is making massive investments in Sudan, where it plans to grow wheat on 1.7 million acres of Sudanese farmland, and in eastern Siberia where it intends to raise corn and soybeans. Kuwait is now growing rice in Cambodia, and the United Kingdom has jatropha plantations in Mozambique; altogether, the International Food Policy Research Institute (IFPRI), a Washington think-tank, estimates that foreign land acquisitions for crop production, including those still under negotiation, involve 15-20 million hectares of land in deals worth an estimated $20–30 billion.

Ironically, several of the countries where these land acquisitions are taking place are desperately poor nations with high rates of hunger and malnutrition, as well as being major recipients of international food aid. A case in point is Ethiopia, where the World Food Programme is now providing food for 4.6 million Ethiopians at a cost of $116 million—almost the same amount the Saudis are paying to lease farmland for their own use. Sudan, which receives more food aid than any other country in the world, has announced its intention to reserve approximately 20% of its cultivated land for foreign investors—and has agreed to allow 70% of the crops grown on those acres to be exported to the investors' countries.

Why are poor nations so willing—even eager—to negotiate deals that appear exploitative, allowing foreigners to take control of land resources that should benefit their own people? Officially, such deals are justified as a way for the host countries to access badly needed new farm technologies that could help them modernize their own agricultural economies. In Africa particularly, growth in grain yields has stagnated since the 1970s and agricultural output per worker is among the lowest in the world. Foreign investors have sweetened the deals with promises of new seed varieties, new marketing strategies, new roads, schools, and clinics. On a continent where investment in agricultural research has lagged badly, China has established 11 new African research facilities aimed at developing improved varieties of staple crops.

Critics, however, question whether the technically sophisticated, highly mechanized, large agricultural operations being established are appropriate for African conditions. In a region where unemployment is widespread, they also worry about the impact on local employment, not only because of mechanization but also because some investors, most notably China and South Korea, are bringing in their own workers; some estimates put the number of Chinese farm workers in Africa in 2009 at approximately one million.

Although some of the land acquisition agreements have involved private investors, the majority have been government-to-government, with host countries dealing directly with foreign regimes or with foreign government-owned corporations. In many cases, the negotiations have lacked transparency, with only a few high-ranking officials aware of what was happening and the terms of any agreements kept confidential. While host governments generally insist that the land they offer foreigners is "vacant" or publicly owned, it frequently supports subsistence-level farmers or herders who have lived there for generations and consider it theirs by customary rights, if not by law. Not surprisingly, this can provoke widespread popular resentment or even violence when farmers or herders displaced by such deals learn what has transpired; on several occasions, signed agreements have had to be cancelled due to public backlash. In Madagascar, outrage over a deal in which a South Korean company was granted rights to half the country's arable land—over a million acres—contributed to the overthrow of the government and ultimate cancellation of the agreement; similar public opposition led to failed acquisitions by China in the Philippines and by the Saudi Binladin Group in Indonesia.

Outsourcing food production raises environmental concerns as well; the huge biofuels plantations envisioned in the Congo, Zambia, Indonesia, and Brazil target lands now covered by tropical rain forest and threaten the rich biodiversity characteristic of this ecosystem. Destruction of these forests will result in more greenhouse gas emissions, since enormous amounts of carbon are now sequestered in tropical forest soils and biomass. Concerned observers also raise several ethical/political issues—what would happen if the host country should experience a severe harvest shortfall and rising levels of hunger among its people? Would the food grown on foreign-used lands still be shipped back to the investing country? Will it be necessary for the host country to provide security for alien landholders in such a situation? Anticipating such an eventuality while attempting to strike a deal with Persian Gulf investors for close to 100 million acres, Pakistani officials have volunteered to provide a security force of 100,000 men to protect investors' land and assets in case of trouble.

Only time will tell whether outsourcing food production is a "win-win" situation—secure supplies for investor nations, improved agricultural technology for host countries—or a new form of colonialism, with foreigners appropriating the land and water resources of needy developing nations for their own benefit. Groups such as IFPRI, the African Union, and other international bodies are advocates for an investment code of conduct to govern land acquisition. Such a code would include provisions for respecting the customary rights of local people as well as those of the investors, making deals more transparent to the public, and agreeing not to export food if the host country is experiencing famine. Several versions of a proposed code are now being drafted, but whether its terms would be respected by all parties involved remains to be seen. Outside observers can only hope that the growing number of land acquisitions live up to their promised benefits rather than leading to increased levels of hunger and political instability in poor host countries (Brown, 2009; "Buying Farmland Abroad," 2009).

the world's croplands—would contribute nothing to humanity's food supply (Brown, 2009).

The impact of diverting feed to food, even if fully implemented, might not be as great as proponents suggest. It has been estimated that abandoning the use of grain for feed entirely would increase market supplies of food by 20–30% at most (Ehrlich, Ehrlich, and Daily, 1993). If world population continues to grow as projections indicate, the one-time gains achieved by going vegetarian would soon be erased by the food demands generated by more and more people.

Regardless of whether promoting meatless diets would be an advisable or effective approach to increasing food availability, it is not a realistic option. While health concerns are prompting some individuals to reduce their consumption of high-fat animal products, no society in modern times has voluntarily reduced meat-eating by any significant amount. Indeed, as we have seen, trends in newly affluent areas of the world are in exactly the opposite direction as their citizens enthusiastically begin to ascend the "protein ladder." While consumers might simplify their diets in response to scarcity-induced higher prices, an appeal to altruism—asking diners to forego their steaks and sauerbraten so that strangers far away could enjoy a temporary increase in food supplies—is unlikely to meet with a positive response.

Improving Yields per Acre

Since the 1950s the largest gains in world food supply have been obtained not by expanding our cropland base but by dramatically increasing per acre or per hectare (metric unit for land measurement, equivalent to 2.47 acres) yields on existing farmlands. In the United States, corn yields, which had remained stable for almost 70 years, more than quadrupled from 1940 to 1985. Impressive increases were also achieved for wheat, rice, barley, rye, peanuts, and sorghum. In Great Britain, where wheat yields are the world's highest, per hectare wheat production tripled from 1940 to 1984. These enormous gains were accomplished through the application of research and technological improvements gradually developed and perfected since the late 1800s, the major elements of which included new hybrid crop varieties, better farm machinery, tremendous expansion in the use of chemical fertilizers and pesticides, and increased use of irrigation.

The developed nations were not alone in realizing major gains in agricultural productivity during this period. In the late 1960s, twenty years of plant breeding experiments to improve grain yields in tropical and semi-tropical regions resulted in the development of several strains of so-called "miracle wheat" and "miracle rice" which heralded the advent of what commentators have dubbed "The Green Revolution." Within a few years of its introduction, the new hybrid wheat was giving farmers from Mexico to India yields two to three times greater than the best formerly obtained from traditional strains. Since the introduction of the first miracle wheat in India in 1966, that country has more than doubled its wheat production. Pakistan, Turkey, and Mexico were among more than 30 other countries whose farmers eagerly adopted the new technology and witnessed a corresponding surge in their wheat production statistics. Similarly, the miracle rice varieties developed at the International Rice Research Institute in the Philippines have approximately doubled the yields of this grain in situations where the hybrid seeds, along with proper fertilization and adequate irrigation, were employed. By 2007, hybrid rice varieties that yield up to 20% more than traditional inbred varieties accounted for 65% of China's rice harvest and were being planted on 57% of that country's total rice area. The fact that they haven't totally replaced non-hybrids is largely due to the fact that Chinese consumers complain the new rice varieties don't taste as good—a factor that has limited their adoption in other countries as well (Normile, 2008).

The spectacular gains of the Green Revolution led many political leaders during the early 1970s to relax on the population issue, assuming that continued dramatic increases in food production had erased the Malthusian image of starving millions. Agricultural experts, however, were less sanguine regarding the food-population crunch and warned that it would be a fatal mistake to assume that plant scientists would be able to achieve another quantum leap in crop yields in the foreseeable future. Agronomist Norman Borlaug, "Father of the Green Revolution" and recipient of the 1970 Nobel Peace Prize for his key role in developing miracle wheat, cautioned dignitaries assembled for the awards ceremony in Oslo that his contribution would, at best, buy humankind about 30 years of food security—years during which they must tame the population monster, he warned.

Unfortunately, Borlaug's gift of time has largely been squandered; in developed and developing nations alike the gains of the Green Revolution are losing momentum even as population figures continue to climb. The fact that many of the world's farmers are already fully exploiting modern technologies means that future gains will come in ever-smaller increments and will be increasingly difficult to achieve. Throughout the 1990s, increases in per acre grain yields averaged barely 1% annually, with analysts lamenting the "yield plateau" that now seems to characterize cereal production in most of the world's major grain-growing areas. Of the major food grains, only corn is still experiencing modest increases in yields, thanks to massive research investments in corn breeding programs by private seed companies. Chinese researchers have recently developed some new hybrid rice strains that offer promise of better yields, but the gains are markedly less than those reaped by the Green Revolution's "miracle rice" (Brown, 2009).

One alternative approach to increasing harvests without expanding existing acreage is to produce two or even three crops per year on the same piece of land. So-called "double-cropping" has become more widely practiced in recent years, thanks to the development of new grain cultivars that mature earlier than older varieties, making it possible to harvest one crop and then immediately plant another. By double-cropping winter wheat, followed by corn, farmers in northern China can now produce 10 tons of grain/hectare each year—5 tons of wheat followed by 5 tons of corn. In northern India, double-cropping of wheat and rice has become the norm, while in southern India and southern China, farmers commonly reap two or even three rice crops per year. The increased per-hectare yields due to double-cropping have made a substantial contribution to ensuring that food production keeps pace with population growth in these two countries, as well as in Brazil and Argentina, where wheat or corn are routinely double-cropped with soybeans (Brown, 2009).

Nevertheless, the potential for future increases in world harvests is not limitless. Some observers predict that in the not-too-distant future we are likely to encounter an absolute yield ceiling imposed by plants' photosynthetic efficiency. The plant breeders who developed the miracle strains of wheat and rice created these high-yielding genetic cultivars by boosting the proportion of sugars produced by photosynthesis that are diverted to seed production. While traditional varieties converted roughly 20% of these sugars into seeds, Green Revolution cultivars are able to convert over 50%. Scientists estimate that the absolute upper limit of sugar production that could go into seed formation without depriving the plant of energy needed for other vital functions is about 60%. Therefore, the opportunity for further yield gains through conventional breeding programs is extremely limited (Brown, Flavin, and French, 1999).

Similar limits are becoming apparent regarding fertilizer applications. Use of nitrogen fertilizers grew from 14 million tons in 1950 to 175 million tons in 2008, and, along with hybrid seeds, receives much of the credit for the crop yield increases of the past 60 years. However, there are now signs that the Law of Diminishing Returns has set in and crops that have been receiving higher and higher levels of fertilizer applications for many years are approaching the limits of their physiological capacity to utilize nutrients. As an example of this, take the case of fertilizer use in America's "Corn Belt." During the 1950s and 1960s, for every extra pound of nitrogen applied a farmer could expect a yield increase of 15–20 extra bushels of corn. By the late 1970s, that increment was 5–7 bushels and falling. By the 1990s, growth in fertilizer use in the U.S., Japan, and Western Europe had virtually halted, partly due to more efficient application methods but also in response to farmers' recognition that additional fertilizer inputs were not economically justified by the minimal boosts in yields per acre.

The same trend is likely to be repeated soon in China and India, since farmers there now use more fertilizer than do American farmers. In other developing regions, particularly in Africa, where reliance on nitrogen fertilizer is more recent and less intensive, potential for increasing yields through additional fertilizer application still exists. In the longer term, however, the same laws of nature will impose an upper ceiling on production there as well. Unless plant scientists can develop new cultivars of wheat,

rice, and corn that are even more responsive to heavy fertilization than those currently being grown, it is unlikely that the slowdown in annual growth of world harvests witnessed during the past decade will be reversed.

Other components critical to the success of Green Revolution technologies—irrigation and chemical pesticides—also may be approaching practical limits. High-yielding varieties can only achieve their maximum potential when supplied with abundant water. Today 40% of all crops harvested come from the 17% of world cropland under irrigation (WRI, 2000). During the last half of the 20th century, the world's croplands under irrigation almost tripled, from 94 million hectares in 1950 to 278 million in 2000. Since then, however, there has been little further increase and any hopes for improving yields through irrigation lie in improving the efficiency of irrigation technologies (e.g., switching from flood or furrow-type irrigation to sprinkler or drip irrigation systems) rather than seeking to exploit new sources (Brown, 2009). Unfortunately, as will be discussed at greater length in the Water Resources chapter, in many of the world's prime agricultural areas overpumping of groundwater for irrigating crops has resulted in a rapid lowering of water tables at the same time that impending climate change threatens long-term declines in annual rainfall—both trends that suggest increasing pressures on water supplies in the years ahead. In the absence of irrigation, miracle grains perform less well than lower-yielding traditional varieties—another reason why the recent slowdown in grain production is likely to continue. Chemical pesticide use is another factor critical in optimizing yields from new crop strains since they are highly susceptible to insects and fungal pathogens, but it is proving less effective than it was several decades ago. Overuse of these products has promoted development of resistant pest populations that are once again having an adverse impact on agricultural production.

Many people optimistically assume that biotechnology will soon present us with a new generation of super-high-yielding crop plants (see box 4-3). In the short term, biotechnology's main contribution to world agriculture is likely to be the introduction of disease- and insect-resistant crop varieties, as well as crops more tolerant of

Table 4-2   Sample of Genetically Modified Organisms

GMO species	Genetic modification	Purpose of genetic modification	Primary beneficiaries
Maize	Insect resistance	Reduced insect damage	Farmers
Soybean	Herbicide tolerance	Greater weed control	Farmers
Cotton	Insect resistance	Reduced insect damage	Farmers
Carnation	Alteration of color	Production of different flower varieties	Retailers and consumers
Rice	Pro-Vitamin A	Increase Vitamin A supply	Consumers

Source: Adapted from "Biotechnology and Food Security," Food and Agriculture Organization of the United Nations, www.fao.org.

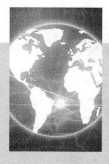

· · · · · · · 4-3 · · · · · · ·

GMOs: A "Second Green Revolution" or "Frankenfoods"?

As the quantum leaps in world grain production witnessed in the late 1960s tapered off and population in the developing world continued to soar, agricultural scientists began to ask "What's next?" in terms of a magic bullet for increasing global food supplies. By the mid-1970s remarkable progress was being made in DNA sequencing, making it possible to consciously design new forms of life; that is, to insert a gene from one organism (most commonly a virus or bacterium) into another species, thereby producing a GMO—"genetically modified organism." With the 1980 Supreme Court ruling (*Diamond vs. Chakrabarty*) confirming patent rights for living organisms, what some commentators have dubbed the "Second Green Revolution" was off and running.

This landmark Court decision made the resource-intensive laboratory work profitable and during the 1980s the new field of biotechnology grew by leaps and bounds. Giant corporations, most notably St. Louis-based Monsanto, poured millions of investment dollars into the race to market the first genetically engineered crop varieties. Competition was fierce, with seed companies and chemical manufacturers on both sides of the Atlantic scrambling to secure patents and get their products commercialized before their rivals beat them to the marketplace (Charles, 2003).

In 1996 GMO crops went commercial, introduced into a number of countries around the globe. Today genetically modified crops are cultivated on approximately 10% of the world's agricultural lands, with the United States the leading producer, followed by Argentina, Brazil, Canada, India, and China, in order of production. The first widely planted transgenic crops were varieties that featured resistance to herbicides and specific insect pests—features that offered farmers savings in labor and chemical costs but held few apparent benefits to the general public. By the late 1990s vast acreages across the American Midwest and South were being planted in Roundup-Ready corn, cotton, soybeans, and canola (these four cash crops still accounted for almost the entire GMO harvest in 2009; a Roundup-Ready variety of sugar beets has been developed but still awaits final approval from the U.S. Department of Agriculture). Roundup-Ready crops provide growers with an easy method for controlling troublesome weeds: just spray the field with Monsanto's non-selective Roundup (glyphosate) herbicide to kill the vulnerable weeds while sparing the now genetically resistant Roundup-Ready crop plants. Other GM crops engineered to defend themselves against plant-devouring caterpillars soon followed the introduction of herbicide-resistant varieties. A gene from the bacterium *Bacillus thuringiensis (Bt)*, an organism that secretes a toxin lethal to larvae of many lepidopterous insects (moths and butterflies), was introduced into corn and cotton to protect those crops from pests such as the European corn borer and the tobacco budworm, a major pest of cotton, while simultaneously reducing use of environmentally damaging chemical insecticides. Worldwide, the dominant GM crop traits today remain herbicide tolerance (63%), insect resistance (18%), and a combination of the two (referred to as "stacked") making up the remainder (McKeown, 2009).

Unfortunately, earlier hopes that the new GMOs would include crop varieties that were higher-yielding, more nutritious, or tolerant of adverse weather conditions have yet to be realized, though field trials of a GM rice variety high in vitamin A—the so-called "golden rice"—are expected to begin soon in Bangladesh. However, any GMOs with nutrition-related traits aren't expected to be on the market for at least five years (McKeown, 2009). The public image of GMOs as crops whose benefits accrue almost exclusively to a small number of huge, private corporations that jealously guard their patent rights and act aggressively to control any products they commercialize has generated a backlash against genetic modification among some consumer and environmental groups.

Since the mid-1980s, anti-GMO activists have been warning that tinkering with plants' genetic material amounts to "playing God" by regarding life forms as mere commodities to be altered at will. They warn that insufficient research has been conducted on the possible harmful impacts of wide-scale release of GMOs into the general environment, suggesting that cross-breeding between Roundup-Ready crops and their wild relatives could produce new strains of "superweeds" or that the prevalence of *Bt* crop varieties will eventually lead to insects resistant to the *Bt* toxin, the primary weapon now used by organic farmers to protect their crops. GMO critics point out that almost all the safety testing for transgenic organisms has been done by the companies themselves and urge governments to require independent testing of the products' safety and environmental impact. They raise fears about the potential for allergens from one species to be introduced unintentionally into another, jeopardizing the health of consumers of genetically modified foods (to date there is no evidence that this has happened in any commercialized transgenic product). In general, the response among American consumers has been rather "ho-hum," with most expressing confidence that such food is safe and only a small minority perceiving GMOs as a serious food risk. Indeed, the fact that transgenic products have been present since the late 1990s in many of the foods Americans eat on a daily basis suggests that there is little to worry about so far as human health is concerned.

The public reaction in Europe and elsewhere has been far different, however. By chance misfortune, the European Commission had voted to accept Roundup-Ready soybeans in March 1996, just five days before the British Prime Minister announced that at least 10 people had died from a human variant of "mad cow disease." Reassurances to a skeptical public that the government could be relied upon to guarantee food safety carried little weight at that point and Greenpeace activists enthusiastically entered the fray to halt a threatened GMO invasion of Europe. By and large, the European media, especially in the U.K., supported those campaigning against so-called "Frankenfoods." The scientific communities in Europe and the U.S. were unable to convince European consumers that they should welcome genetically altered foods into their kitchens and the European Union subsequently instituted a ban on GM crops (Charles, 2003).

So how valid are concerns that "Frankenfoods" pose genuine long-term health and environmental risks? Most scientists, including those in Europe, are convinced that the danger is minimal—certainly no greater than threats posed by conventional foods, many of which contain natural toxins that seldom worry many consumers. Similarly, fears raised about pollen from transgenic crops contaminating conventional fields or harming wildlife seem exaggerated; the impact to date appears negligible—certainly far less than the impact traditional agricultural operations have had on wildlife, soil, and water quality. By reducing the quantities of chemical insecticides needed to control crop pests, GMOs may leave, on balance, a slightly positive environmental footprint.

From the standpoint of global food security, however, the promise of transgenic foods as a solution to world hunger has largely been squandered. The European ban on GMOs bears some of the responsibility for this situation. Not only has productivity growth in European agriculture been retarded by the ban (experts think grain yields in Europe could be boosted by 15% if the ban were lifted), but the pace of research on GM technology on the continent has also declined sharply. Without public funding and lack of incentive for private companies to engage in research (since there would be no domestic market for any new GM seeds), scientific advances on GMOs in Europe are at a standstill. More troublesome is the fact that the official European stance has intimidated many African governments into prohibiting the use of GM crops by their own farmers, due to concerns that exports of such food crops to Europe would be blocked. The predictable result of this self-denial is that badly needed research on crops vital to African food self-sufficiency—crops such as yams and cassava—is not being funded because there is currently no market for any new discoveries. With African grain yields stagnant, mouths to be fed still increasing, and climate change likely to intensify drought conditions, Africa desperately needs the biological revolution promised by GM crops. For some time the UN's Food and Agriculture Organization (FAO) has been warning about the growing "molecular divide" between developing countries and the industrialized world in terms of agricultural research and development, but until the ban on GM crops in Europe and Africa is lifted, a substantial narrowing of this divide is unlikely. In the meantime, progress has been inching forward on research by several large agribusinesses on several so-called "climate-ready" GM crops suitable for African growing conditions, particularly on drought-tolerant corn and a new GM corn variety resistant to a beetle now responsible for post-harvest losses in storage of 15–40%. Although promising, these new GMOs are not expected to be widely available for at least 5–10 years, even if researchers can overcome a number of technical obstacles to successful genetic modification of these traits (Collier, 2008; McKeown, 2009). Enthusiastic claims by GMO boosters that genetic engineering is humanity's "last, best hope" for ending world hunger sound rather dubious in light of marginal progress toward that goal thus far.

GMOs are clearly here to stay, but the distrust and antagonism they arouse in many quarters show few signs of dissipating any time soon. Greater efforts on the part of the biotechnology industry to develop crops that meet real consumer needs and a willingness to share their expertise with poor nations could go a long way to redeeming the now-dubious promise of genetic engineering as a force for good in the world.

drought, heat, or salt. Such cultivars may boost current yields somewhat, but do not represent the quantum leap in production represented by the Green Revolution's miracle grains.

For all these reasons, experts seriously doubt that a doubling or tripling of world harvests can be repeated. In most of the world's major agricultural areas farmers have already reaped the full potential offered by miracle crops; in regions not yet touched by the Green Revolution, natural conditions such as lack of water resources or inadequate technology transfer may preclude them from ever enjoying its fruits. Even within countries where the new technologies have boosted food self-sufficiency, large areas remain mired in poverty and backwardness—northwest China, the Andean Mountain area, the highlands of Mexico, and large areas of central India are all notable examples. The outlook for improvement is perhaps most clouded in the semiarid regions of sub-Saharan Africa where yields of maize, the most important cereal crop, have remained stagnant at about one ton per hectare since 1961. Food production in these chronically

food-deficit areas could improve, despite maximum *genetic* yield barriers, if the use of existing production technology is further expanded. More on-site research to develop seed varieties adapted to local growing conditions, more attention to efficient water use and proper planting dates, greater emphasis on educational outreach programs to transfer the latest agricultural developments to cultivators in the field, adoption of government financial and economic policies that make it profitable for farmers to adopt new technologies—all offer potential for boosting currently modest yields in some less-developed countries. However, population growth rates in those same areas demand that the governments of those nations give priority to modernizing their agricultural sectors in order to realize this potential. In addition, bountiful harvests alone will not eradicate hunger among those too poor to buy food for their families.

At a time when more than a billion people are suffering from malnutrition—and with demographic projections indicating that world population will continue to climb by 80 million or more annually—the fact that per

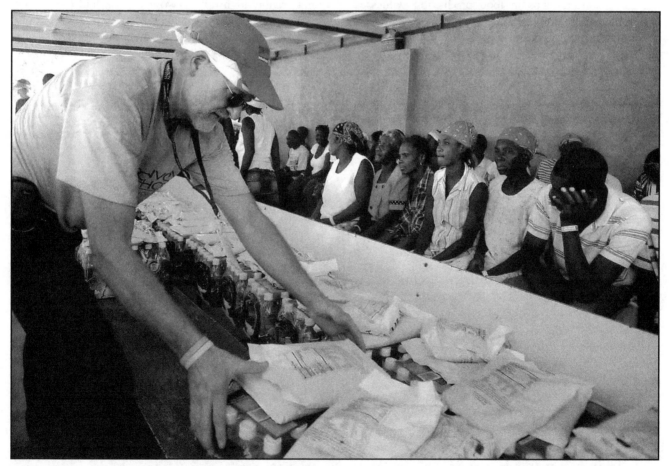

With world population projected to climb by 80 million annually and a leveling off of per capita growth in the food supply, scenes like this of aid workers distributing emergency provisions of food and water will become increasingly common as more and more people join the ranks of the hungry. [*Justin E. Stumberg, USAID*]

capita growth in food supply has leveled off or even declined in some areas of the world is alarming. The International Rice Research Institute (IRRI), based in the Philippines, reports that for the past several years more rice has been consumed than grown, with world stockpiles making up the difference. Since rice provides 20% of all the calories consumed worldwide, stagnant rice yields are extremely worrisome; the IRRI warns that rice production must grow by 50 million tons/year by 2015 if production is to match demand. Doing so will require increasing yields by more than 1.2% annually—a challenging task, given current trends.

Food prices have dropped slightly since their 2008 high, but in many developing countries the cost of feeding one's family remains well above earlier levels. With a shrinking cropland base, falling water tables, diminishing impact of chemical fertilizers, and the long-term prospect of drought and crop-withering heat waves due to climate change in some of the world's most productive agricultural regions, farmers will be hard-pressed to meet future food demand at prices the world's poor can afford. Currently there are no new technologies on the horizon offering the quantum leaps in food production witnessed during the latter half of the 20th century. To some degree, this situation reflects the sharp reduction in both public and private investment in agricultural research and development (R&D) by the United States, the European countries, and Japan since the 1980s. Numerous cost-benefit studies have shown that investments in agricultural R&D have yielded impressive returns in the past and were largely responsible for the rapid gains in crop productivity after 1950. Unfortunately, such investment has tapered off in recent decades, not only affecting research programs in the U.S. and other developed countries, but also cutting funding for vital farm extension programs that provide improved seeds and information on new technologies to farmers in many poor countries. In addition, a significant proportion of the funds that *have* been allocated for agricultural research have been directed towards concerns unrelated to increased grain yields—concerns such as food quality and safety, environmental impacts of agriculture, and energy uses of agricultural commodities. For productivity growth to be restored and sustained over the long term, a renewed commitment by developed countries to agricultural R&D investment is essential. In its absence, world food production will continue to lag behind demand, food prices will remain unaffordably high for the world's poor, and the proportion of humanity categorized as "hungry" will continue its upward trajectory (Alston et al., 2009).

The one process now going on that will take millions of years to correct is the loss of genetic and species diversity by the destruction of natural habitats. This is the folly our descendants are least likely to forgive us.
—E. O. Wilson, *Biophilia* (1984)

Impacts of Growth on Ecosystems

Certainly the issue of how to feed additional multitudes in the years ahead, when a billion of the earth's current inhabitants are malnourished, looms as a monumental task for future world leaders. However, population growth exerts many other socioeconomic and environmental impacts that may be less publicized than famine, yet have a profound impact on human well-being and on the sustainability of planetary life-support systems. In many parts of the world today evidence is mounting that large and still-growing human and livestock populations have already exceeded the carrying capacity of the land itself. In effect, at a time when we are trying to produce more and more from a given land area, the activities of those people are damaging natural ecosystems to the extent that they are becoming incapable of supporting their present population, much less future billions.

Giving evidence of the fact that population growth and ecological degradation are inextricably interrelated are growing numbers of **"environmental refugees"**— people seeking refuge abroad due to environmental problems at home. Over the past several decades, millions of people have been forced to leave their place of birth due to water scarcity, depleted soils, deforestation, desertification, or other calamities. Intensification of such problems due to climate change threatens to swell these numbers in the years immediately ahead. In its Fourth Assessment Report, issued in 2007, the Intergovernmental Panel on Climate Change projected there could be 50 million environmental refugees by 2010 and as many as 200 million by mid-century. Regions most affected include Central America, the Indian subcontinent, China, the Horn of Africa, and the Sahel. Such vast movements of environmentally displaced persons could become one of the major political and national security issues in the years ahead.

DEGRADATION OF LAND RESOURCES

We abuse land because we regard it as a commodity belonging to us. When we see land as a community to which we belong, we may begin to use it with love and respect.
—Aldo Leopold, *A Sand County Almanac*

The disruption of natural cycles resulting from human pressures on land resources is undermining the sustainability of ecosystems in many parts of the world today. In reference to agricultural lands, scientists at the International Food Policy Research Institute warn that, worldwide, close to 40% is seriously degraded; as a result, productivity has already been adversely affected on about 16% of global farm acreage. Land degradation is most severe in Central America, where approximately 75% of croplands are seriously degraded; in Africa, with close to 20%, mostly pasturelands, affected; and in Asia, with 11%. Although much of this land is still being cultivated, some of its natural productivity has been lost and could be restored only through implementation of expensive national programs to provide farmers with technical assistance and financial incentives. In the absence of such efforts, the condition of these lands will only deteriorate further. The factors responsible for land degradation include overgrazing of livestock herds, faulty agricultural practices, and deforestation. While the environmental damage provoked by such activities theoretically could occur anywhere, certain natural areas are more vulnerable to long-lasting destruction than others. Tundra, desert, tropical rain forest, and arid grasslands are more easily impaired and take much longer to recover from disruption than does, for example, temperate deciduous forest. Because several of these areas today encompass

the homelands of many millions of people whose well-being, and indeed survival, depends on the continued productivity of their land, it is important for us to take a closer look at some specific ways in which humans, consciously or not, are radically undermining the stability of natural ecosystems.

Overgrazing

Of the various activities contributing to soil degradation, none is more significant than overgrazing. Rangelands occupy approximately 40% of the earth's land surface—four times as much area as croplands—primarily in semi-arid or mountainous regions not suitable for sustained crop production. Today approximately half of these pasturelands are affected by light to moderate degradation, with 5% categorized as "severely degraded"; on such lands restoration, for all practical purposes, is impossible (Brown, 2008). Under natural conditions, grassland communities are well-adapted to a moderate level of grazing; herds of bison, antelope, wild horses, and so forth have for millennia been the dominant animals in the grassland biome, evolving and adapting in conjunction with the native plants on which they are

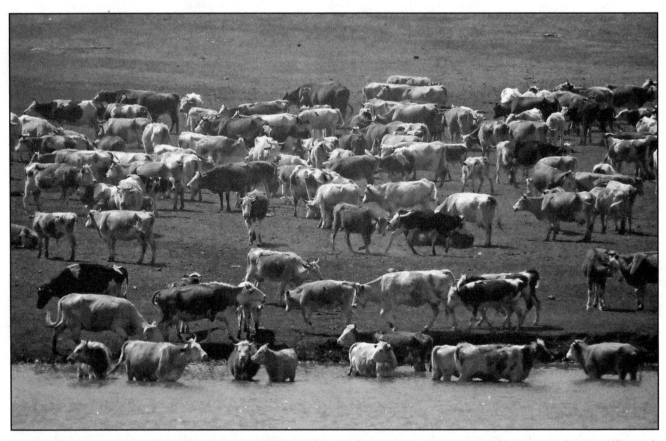

Overgrazing is the most significant contributor to soil degradation, placing pressures on plant populations, stream bank stability, and riparian habitats.

dependent. However, when livestock managers increase the number of livestock beyond a certain size or when they introduce types of grazing animals foreign to a particular plant community, the resulting pressure on that community often leads to an unraveling of the ecosystem.

The effects of overgrazing are first seen in the declining populations of those plant species least able to tolerate the increased cropping. As these plants disappear, species more tolerant of heavy grazing are then relieved of competition and expand to fill the niche vacated by the more vulnerable types. The loss of the latter, however, results in an overall reduction in the height, biomass, and total coverage of the grassland. If overgrazing persists, even the more resistant native plants will be unable to withstand the pressure and give way to invader weed species that were not members of the original community. Such plants are generally much inferior to the native plants in nutritive qualities and, as a result, the vitality of the herd is adversely affected. Eventually the weeds themselves may be trampled to such an extent that they, too, are reduced in coverage. The soil, thus exposed to the forces of wind and water, may be worn away, leaving a barren mud flat or rocky hillside, devoid of any plant community (Whittaker, 1975).

While land degradation due to overgrazing is most pronounced in Australia (80%) and in Africa (49%), severe problems of overgrazing are all too evident in the Middle East, northern India, Central Asia, Mongolia, and much of northern and western China. In many of these regions, deterioration of rangelands is directly linked to population growth. As the numbers of human pastoralists multiplied, so did the size of the herds on which their livelihoods depend. In 1950, for example, African herders numbered approximately 238 million, with 273 million livestock; by 2006 there were 926 million pastoralists and 738 million animals (Brown, 2008).

Extensive areas of rangeland in the American West are severely affected as well. Of the approximately 270 million acres of publicly owned rangeland in 16 western states, over 60% are considered to be in unsatisfactory condition, degraded by years of overgrazing and mismanagement. The many native species of fish and wildlife inhabiting these rangelands have been severely affected by the deteriorating ecological conditions; close to 90 animal species on federal lands are now listed as endangered or threatened because of environmental damage provoked by overgrazing. Rangeland riparian habitats—the narrow bands of lush vegetation bordering streams and lakes—have been particularly hard-hit. When oversized herds of cattle or sheep congregate in or along the edge of waterways, they trample and eat vegetation, pollute the water, and damage stream bank stability. The resulting soil erosion and sedimentation may result in streambeds becoming shallower, warmer, and

more turbid, negatively affecting aquatic life. Overgrazing is now regarded as the leading culprit blamed for the decline of native trout populations in western states.

Soil Erosion

Throughout much of the world, including the rich farmlands of the American Midwest, the fertile topsoil that is the basis of agricultural productivity is thinning at an alarming rate. Around the globe, experts estimate that one-third or more of the world's agricultural land is losing soil faster than it is being replenished (Brown, 2008). Given the fact that under normal agricultural conditions it takes from 200 to 1,000 years to form an inch of topsoil, such losses could well undermine the productive capacity of farmlands if effective conservation strategies are not implemented. The UN's Food and Agriculture Organization (FAO) has warned that unless developing countries give much higher priority to soil erosion control efforts, they could witness a 30% reduction in harvests by the end of the 21st century—at which time their populations will have increased by as much as sixfold over current levels.

Some degree of soil loss is, of course, a natural process and occurs even in the absence of human intervention. Poor agricultural practices, however, greatly increase the rate of erosion, and when the amount of topsoil lost exceeds that of new soil formed through the gradual decomposition of organic matter (an amount referred to in agricultural circles as **T-value** or, more simply, **"T"**), then the layer of topsoil becomes thinner and thinner until it disappears completely, leaving only the unproductive subsoil or, in extreme cases, bare rock. Topsoil loss has a direct negative impact on cropland productivity, though in recent decades the relationship between soil erosion and diminishing yields has been largely masked by the greatly expanded use of chemical fertilizers. We have, in a sense, been substituting chemical nitrogen and potash for topsoil in order to maintain good harvests. However, while chemicals can replace nutrients lost through erosion, they can't substitute for the lost organic material necessary for maintaining a porous, healthy soil structure. Some studies suggest that heavy fertilizer use can actually damage the soil by disrupting natural nutrient cycles and predict that future per-acre yields, even on lands receiving chemical inputs, will begin to drop if erosion trends aren't reversed (Smil, 1991).

Serious erosion control efforts in the United States grew out of the disastrous Dust Bowl years of the mid-1930s, when millions of tons of rich Great Plains topsoil were literally "gone with the wind" as a result of drought and unwise cultivation practices. In 1935 the Soil Conservation Service (SCS) was created and Congress funded a major research effort to learn more about the processes of erosion and effective methods of control (in 1994 the name of this agency was changed to Natural Resources Conservation Service, or NRCS). By the 1940s and 1950s soil loss on U.S. farmlands was declining noticeably as American farmers followed the advice of Cooperative Extension advisors (county agents) or SCS personnel to install terraces, plant windbreaks, contour strip-crop, build grass waterways—whatever method or combination of methods was most suitable to reduce erosion rates on the lands they were cultivating.

By the 1970s, however, soil loss due to farmland erosion once again began to accelerate, reversing the gains of the previous two decades. High commodity prices and the demand for agricultural exports to feed growing populations overseas combined to boost farm production—and promoted record levels of erosion. Citing the link between farm exports and land degradation, an official at the Illinois Department of Agriculture remarked at the time that " . . . for every bushel of corn we ship overseas, we send 1½ bushels of topsoil down the Mississippi River." In the push for expanded production, the traditional practice of crop rotation was abandoned in favor of continuous cropping of corn or soybeans, a practice that greatly increases erosion rates since this leaves the soil surface without any plant cover during a considerable portion of the year. Strong export demand prompted farmers to plow "from fencepost-to-fencepost" to reap the maximum possible profit. By doing so, however, they brought into production much highly erodible land that would have been better left in pasture—and it promptly began to wash away. In the Midwest, fall plowing came into vogue and contributed to substantial amounts of erosion by both wind and water during winter and early spring when fields are bare.

By the late 1970s it was evident that soil loss was once again becoming a serious national problem. In 1981 the USDA estimated that the inherent productivity of fully one-third of American farmlands was declining because of high rates of erosion. Efforts were launched at both the state and federal level to reduce soil loss to tolerable levels (i.e., to T-value). The main strategy for achieving this goal was the promotion of **conservation tillage**, a cultivation practice that involves leaving 30% or more of the soil surface covered with the previous year's crop residue. Variants on conservation tillage include **no-till**, in which crops are planted in the undisturbed residue of an old crop; **mulch-till**, a situation where crops are planted in a field where the entire surface has been disturbed, but at least the minimum amount of residue remains after planting; and **strip-till**, a variant of no-till, in which narrow (10–12″), raised (3–4″) strips are plowed the length of the field, leaving the soil on either side of the strips untouched. Seeds are planted in the center of these strip rows and fertilizer applications are efficiently targeted to these areas. Strip-till cultivation is rapidly winning adherents in the midwestern Corn Belt, since the removal of a narrow band of crop residue in the seed bed promotes warming and drying of the soil during cool, wet spring weather, thus making it possible for farmers to plant earlier than they could under a conventional no-till system. These crop residues perform a number of protective functions: cushioning the impact of falling raindrops, decreasing wind access to bare soil, serving as mini-dams to restrict overland runoff from fields, and improving soil characteristics that resist erosive forces. Alone or in combination with such soil conservation measures as terracing or construction of grass waterways, conservation tillage can substantially reduce

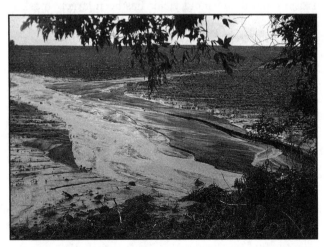

Sheet erosion after heavy rain robs farmland of valuable topsoil and causes water pollution and sedimentation problems in nearby streams and ditches. [*Lynn Betts, Natural Resources Conservation Service*]

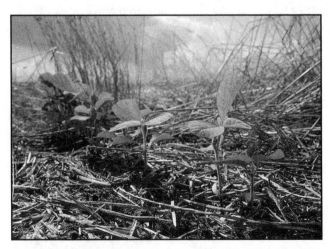

No-till farming: young soybean plants thrive in the residue of a wheat crop. This method of planting protects the soil from erosion and helps retain moisture for the new crop. [*Tim McCabe, Natural Resources Conservation Service*]

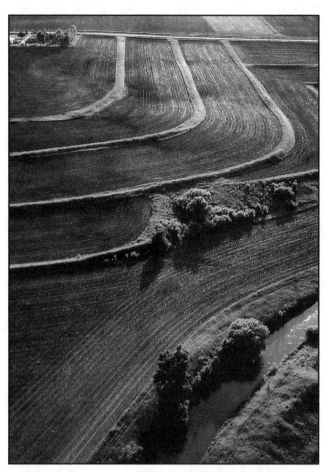

Terraces, conservation tillage, and filter strips help reduce erosion rates while maintaining or even increasing crop yields.
[*Lynn Betts, Natural Resources Conservation Service*]

erosion rates while maintaining or even increasing crop yields. While conservation tillage is not appropriate for all crops, the practice has expanded rapidly since the early 1980s, particularly in corn-and soybean-producing areas of the Midwest.

Erosion control efforts in the United States were given a major boost when Congress passed the **Food Security Act of 1985**, creating the **Conservation Reserve Program (CRP)**. Under this landmark program, excessive production and soil loss are being curbed by offering farmers financial incentives to take highly erodible or environmentally sensitive land out of production for 10 to 15 years, converting them to pastures or woodlands. Surveys by the NRCS indicate a 19-ton per acre reduction in soil loss from lands under CRP contract. Modifications to the CRP since its inception in 1985 have broadened the focus of conservation activities. Though CRP's original goal of controlling soil erosion remains a top priority, improving wildlife habitat and water quality are now important components of the program. Landowners are encouraged to sign up for high-priority conservation projects such as developing filter strips (areas of grass or other vegetation at the low end of fields that can filter out soil particles or other pollutants suspended in farmland runoff) or windbreaks. The magnitude and far-reaching scope of the Conservation Reserve Program makes it the federal government's single largest environmental improvement program and represents a major success story in reversing soil loss on U.S. agricultural lands (USDA, 1997).

Similar efforts to reduce excessive soil erosion are desperately needed in many developing countries where the situation is even more serious. In Ethiopia, erosion is depriving that nation's hard-pressed farmers of 1.5 to 2 billion cubic meters of topsoil every year; as a result, 4 million hectares (about 10 million acres) of Ethiopian highlands are now termed "irreversibly degraded." In central Africa, the dramatic effects of wind erosion are exemplified by huge dust storms that have become common occurrences across the Sahel, stripping an estimated 2–3 billion tons of soil from the continent and transporting it westward across the Atlantic, sometimes as far as Caribbean waters where the fallout of African sediment is damaging coral reefs (Brown, 2008). In China, soil erosion is endangering increases in crop production desperately needed to feed a still-growing population. In China's northwestern Gansu Province, half or more of all arable land has already been lost to erosion and encroaching deserts.

Although soil erosion is the most obvious form of land degradation, other processes may play a role as well. Improper methods of mechanical tillage may cause compaction or crusting of soils. Repeatedly growing crops on the same land without sufficient fallow periods depletes soil nutrients, though this can be mitigated through the use of manure, cover crops, or appropriate amounts of chemical fertilizers. Extensive land degradation in arid regions of the world has been caused by poor water management on irrigated fields. Failure to drain such areas adequately can result in the salinization or waterlogging of soils. The former process occurs when salts naturally present in certain soils are dissolved by rising water tables under poorly drained irrigated fields and eventually accumulate at the soil surface, poisoning crop roots. Currently between 10–15% of all irrigated lands are plagued by waterlogging or salinization. In the case of salt-affected lands, restoration efforts may take generations, with some lands never recovering. In Australia, 10% of the land area is now suffering from salinization and experts there worry that the percentage could grow to 40% within the next 50 years. Other regions threatened by salinization include irrigated areas of Iraq, Turkey, Pakistan, northern India, China, and the American Southwest.

Deforestation

For the last ten thousand years humans have been cutting and burning woodlands at an ever-increasing pace in their quest for additional farmland, fuel, and building material. Forests still cover approximately 30% of the world's land area, but recent decades have witnessed a significant decline in both the area covered by forests and in the quality of remaining woodlands. In spite of increased forest protection efforts in many parts of the world, as well as afforestation projects and natural regrowth on abandoned lands, each year an additional 13 million hectares of forests are lost, primarily through conversion to agricultural uses. Balancing these gains and losses, the net change in forest lands from 2000–2005 was a loss of 7.3 million hectares per year—a bit better than the decade of the 1990s when net forest loss totaled 8.9 million hectares annually.

Forests have shrunk the most in Africa and South America, while they have been slowly expanding in Europe. According to the FAO, by 2005 only 36% of the lands categorized as "forested" were classified as **primary forests**—relatively undisturbed, extensive areas that remain ecologically intact—down from 40% in 2000. The remaining so-called "forested" areas include secondary forests, tree plantations, open woodlands, and brushlands. Primary forests today are largely limited to the northern boreal forests of Russia, Canada, and Alaska and to the tropical forests of the northwestern Amazon basin and the Guyana Shield along South America's northern coast. These remaining primary forests cover scarcely one-third the areas they occupied before human activities set in motion the processes of deforestation that have markedly accelerated within recent decades. As the rate of forest loss accelerates, so do pressures on ecosystems in the form of species loss, soil erosion, and climate change.

Deforestation, defined as the permanent decline in crown cover of trees to less than 10% of its original extent, is particularly worrisome in regard to tropical forests, where most of the deforestation of the past 60 years has occurred. Unfortunately, rates of loss continue to accelerate. Between 1960–1990, one-fifth of tropical forests were destroyed, including over 30% of those in Asia and approximately 18% in Latin America and Africa (Abramovitz, 1998). FAO statistics suggest that the rate of tropical deforestation began to slow somewhat during the 1990s, a decline that accelerated slightly during the period from 2000–2005, but the UN agency admits that its estimates are questionable, since reliable direct measurements are scarce. Indeed, more recent studies suggest that forest loss in Brazil and Indonesia is more extensive than FAO estimates indicate.

Elsewhere, in the semiarid regions of Asia, Africa, and Latin America where forests have always been scanty, existing forests have almost entirely vanished. Only in Europe and, quite recently, in North America are forests being managed on a sustained-yield basis. In the United States, wooded areas have expanded significantly over the past 50 years, as once-cleared marginal farmlands revert to forest. The FAO estimates that forested areas in the industrialized countries as a whole expanded by 2.7% between 1980–1995 (FAO, 2001). However, this overall increase in forest biomass obscures the fact that large areas of temperate old-growth forest have been replaced by tree plantations, often comprising but a single species that is grown and harvested within a relatively short time period. Such plantations can be ecologically beneficial for reducing erosion, regenerating degraded soils (e.g., pulpwood plantations in the U.S. Southeast now thriving on abandoned cotton acreage), or providing fuelwood for local consumption. Nevertheless, they are

Table 5-1   Ten Countries with Largest Annual Net Forest Loss, 1990–2010

Country	Annual change 1990–2000 thousands hectares/yr	Country	Annual change 2000–2010 thousands hectares/yr
Brazil	−2,890	Brazil	−2,642
Indonesia	−1,914	Australia	−562
Sudan	−589	Indonesia	−498
Myanmar	−435	Nigeria	−410
Nigeria	−410	United Republic of Tanzania	−403
United Republic of Tanzania	−403	Zimbabwe	−327
Mexico	−354	Democratic Republic of the Congo	−311
Zimbabwe	−327	Myanmar	−310
Democratic Republic of the Congo	−311	Bolivia (Plurinational State of)	−290
Argentina	−293	Venezuela (Bolivarian Republic of)	−288
Total	**−7,926**	**Total**	**−6,040**

Source: *Global Forest Resources Assessment 2010: Main Report.* FAO, 2010.

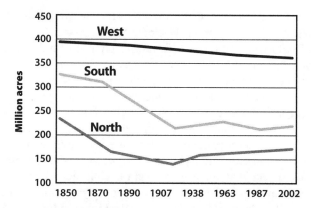

Source: Smith, W. Brad and D. Darr, *U.S. Forest Resource Facts and Historical Trends*, USDA Forest Service, 2005.

Figure 5-1   Forest Trends in the United States, 1850–2002

much less biologically diverse than the primary forest ecosystems that once flourished in those regions.

The largest single cause of deforestation, particularly in Africa, Amazonia, Malaysia, and Indonesia, is the **clearing of land for agriculture**. The population pressures behind this trend and the ecological damage caused by exploitation of marginal lands not suited for sustained cultivation have already been described. The Cote d'Ivoire (Ivory Coast) provides a classic example of such pressures. With an annual population growth rate averaging between 3–4% until quite recently, slash-and-burn farmers have destroyed fully 95% of the forest cover in that West African nation (Tobias, 1998).

Contributing to the degradation of forests in Africa, the Indian subcontinent, and many other poor countries is the **gathering of wood for fuel**. The FAO estimates that approximately half of all wood cut in the world today is used for firewood or for making charcoal. For approximately 90% of the people in the world's less-developed nations, today's true energy crisis is the scarcity of firewood. In most tropical countries wood is used largely for cooking, but in colder climates and mountainous regions it's used for heating as well. While nearly two-thirds of fuelwood is being gleaned from trees along roadsides, small woodlots, or from wood industries, the remainder comes from forest resources. The problem is particularly acute in semiarid regions where removal of vegetation leaves land at the mercy of wind and water. In once heavily forested lands such as Nepal, whole mountainsides are being stripped by villagers who now spend most of the day searching for a supply of firewood that a few decades ago could have been gathered in an hour. The investment in time and physical energy required just to obtain enough fuel to cook the family meal has thus increased tremendously in just one generation.

Of greater concern to Nepali officials, however, and to their counterparts in the vast Indian subcontinent to the south is the fact that the progressive denudation of the Himalayan slopes is resulting in a massive increase in soil erosion in this ecologically fragile mountain region. As a result, not only is the productive capacity of the land rapidly decreasing, but also much more frequent and severe flooding is occurring downstream in the river valleys of northern India, Pakistan, and Bangladesh due to greatly increased amounts of runoff in the headwaters area of the Ganges, Indus, and Brahmaputra rivers. The devastating floods that regularly leave millions homeless and kill thousands during the subcontinent's monsoon season represent an "unnatural disaster" caused by increased runoff from the denuded Himalayan watershed upstream and increased rates of siltation in lowland deltas that diminish their water-holding capacity. While severe flooding used to occur perhaps twice in a century, "50-year floods" have become regular events, thanks to progressive deforestation in the Himalayas.

Table 5-2   Ten Countries with Largest Annual Net Forest Gain, 1990–2010

Country	Annual change 1990–2000 thousands hectares/yr	Country	Annual change 2000–2010 thousands hectares/yr
China	1,986	China	2,986
United States	386	United States	383
Spain	317	India	304
Vietnam	236	Vietnam	207
India	145	Turkey	119
France	82	Spain	119
Italy	78	Sweden	81
Chile	57	Italy	78
Finland	57	Norway	76
Philippines	55	France	60
Total	**3,399**	**Total**	**4,414**

Source: *Global Forest Resources Assessment 2010: Main Report*. FAO, 2010.

Even today, in more than 40 countries fuelwood provides more than 70% of total energy consumption. As populations continue to grow, demand increases, supplies diminish, and fuelwood prices rise. In many developing world countries, fuelwood is more expensive than food; some urban households spend anywhere from 20–50% of their income for wood to cook their meals and warm their homes (Williams, 2006). Where people can't afford the high cost of wood, women and children spend much of their time scrounging the countryside for anything burnable—dry grass, fallen leaves, animal dung, garbage—a practice that in the long run further degrades the soil by robbing it of these natural fertilizers. In the industrialized nations, which until about 100 years ago had been just as dependent on wood for fuel as the developing countries are today, the substitution of coal, petroleum products, and natural gas for wood forestalled a growing pressure on their forests. In the developing world, increasing use of kerosene or bottled gas stoves has slightly eased the burdens on those nations' timber resources. Unfortunately, for millions of the world's poorest people such wood substitutes remain priced out of reach.

In Southeast Asia, Central Africa, and tropical South America, **commercial lumbering** has become a major cause of deforestation, decimating valuable tropical hardwood reserves in order to supply the increased demands of industrial nations for furniture, plywood, and paper pulp. Until relatively recently, tropical forests largely escaped the logging pressures that earlier had decimated the virgin forests of Europe and North America, primarily because they were sparsely populated and not easily accessible. In addition, in tropical forests commercially valuable tree species are widely dispersed over a broad geographic area, interspersed with many less-desired species, a fact that made large-scale exploitation economically unfeasible. This situation changed dramatically in the 1960s when mechanization of the timber industry and the arrival of giant multinational lumber companies made possible the ever-more-rapid felling of tropical forests. The methods employed by these companies have been particularly destructive and wasteful; in a typical operation only 10–20% of the trees are cut and removed (i.e., those species with commercial value), but 30–50% of non-target trees are destroyed in the process. On many tracts, trees are felled by utilizing giant tractors, working in tandem, to drag huge link chains across the forest floor, pulling down everything in their path. This process causes such extensive soil damage that the land may never fully recover.

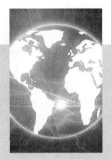

········ 5-1 ········

Eco-Certification of Coffee: A New Approach to Saving Tropical Forests

Want to help save Latin America's tropical forests? If so, insist that your next cup of coffee bear the Rainforest Alliance Certified (formerly "ECO-O.K.") stamp of approval!

Throughout the highlands of Central America, Colombia, and the Caribbean, coffee cultivation has been a mainstay of the economy for almost 200 years. Introduced to New World settlements by European colonial powers (who had themselves been introduced to the stimulating brew several centuries earlier by Arab traders), coffee was well-suited to growing conditions in the mountainous terrain stretching from southern Mexico to Colombia. A shade-loving, small evergreen tree, coffee thrives on steeply sloping hillsides where temperatures are consistently mild, rainfall abundant, and the rich volcanic soil well-drained. As coffee farms proliferated throughout the region during the 19th and 20th centuries, extensive areas of primary forest were cut to make room for coffee plants. However, in contrast to the devastating ecological impact of clearing forests for cattle ranching or banana plantations, the traditional method of coffee cultivation was relatively benign in terms of its environmental "footprint." Individual coffee farms tended to be relatively small, with coffee trees spaced at intervals among dozens of other tree species—some indigenous to the original forest, others planted to provide the grower with supplemental income from fruit, fuelwood, or fiber. This method of production was beneficial both to the crop plant, providing essential shade and protection from the wind, and to the environment. The overarching canopy of diverse tree species and the leaf litter below provided abundant habitat for a wide variety of tropical birds, mammals, insects, and other wildlife.

Traditional coffee farms, in fact, function ecologically in much the same way as the forests they replaced and are considered the least disruptive form of agriculture currently practiced.

Unfortunately, in recent years market forces and technological advances have been changing the way coffee is grown, undermining the ecological balance of coffee-producing regions. Seeking to maximize production and boost earnings, commercial coffee growers have been planting more sun-tolerant coffee tree varieties, adopting high-density methods of cultivation in which plants are closely spaced in hedge-rows in vast open fields. This technique has increased yields by approximately 50%, but at a severe cost to the environment. Converting to sun-grown coffee plantations, growers have bulldozed millions of acres of traditional coffee farms, transforming them into what some observers call "biological deserts." The new coffee monocultures, unlike traditional shade-grown farms, are heavily dependent on chemical inputs to maintain high levels of productivity and to ward off insects, weeds, and fungal diseases. The proliferation of sun-grown coffee farms has been devastating to local biodiversity, with the number of species plummeting as a once richly varied habitat is rapidly simplified to broad expanses of nothing but coffee.

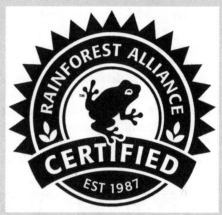

[*Courtesy of Rainforest Alliance, www.rainforest-alliance.org*]

In 1987, concerns about worldwide tropical forest loss prompted formation of the Rainforest Alliance, an international nonprofit organization whose mission centers on developing and promoting economically sound and socially responsible alternatives to tropical deforestation. In 1991 this group created an eco-labeling program that focuses specifically on agricultural crops whose production has had a major negative impact on tropical ecosystems, with sun-grown coffee a prime target (bananas and oranges have also been subjects for Rainforest Alliance production standards). The concept of eco-labeling is a well-established method for encouraging "green" purchasing decisions by providing consumers with the assurance that the item in question has been produced in an environmentally sustainable manner. To ensure that such eco-labels represent more than just a promotional gimmick, certification programs have been established to evaluate the accuracy of environmental claims. The Rainforest Alliance's sustainable coffee-labeling program has developed a list of stringent standards that must be met by every farm they certify. A team of conservationists, scientists, representatives of relevant government agencies, and coffee farmers work together to develop certification criteria. Among the basic principles with which any certified farm must comply are agreements to: avoid any further deforestation; protect native plants and wildlife; prohibit hunting; protect streams and wetlands; maintain tree canopy cover; minimize applications of chemical fertilizers and pesticides; follow sound soil conservation practices; treat workers fairly and adhere to local labor laws; provide workers with safe and sanitary working conditions; and avoid racial discrimination. Farms desiring eco-certification must submit to a field evaluation by a team of Rainforest Alliance technicians who write a report specifying any changes that must be made in order to comply with certification criteria. A follow-up visit to confirm compliance will subsequently be made and a detailed report prepared for examination by a review board. If approved, coffee from the now-certified farm can be labeled with the Rainforest Alliance seal of approval, distinguishing it from other brands in the marketplace. To guarantee that a certified grower doesn't fail to uphold high standards, an annual audit is required to maintain certification.

What motivates growers to devote the effort it takes to earn certification? In part it is pride in their work and love of the land that many of them have cultivated for generations—coffee farmers, too, can be ardent conservationists. It can also be a sound business decision. At a time when world commodity prices for coffee are at record lows due to overproduction, shade-grown eco-certified brands occupy a unique market niche in the upscale gourmet coffee world. Known for superior flavor and carrying a cachet of social and environmental responsibility, shade-grown coffee bearing the Rainforest Alliance label guarantees growers a higher price than they could hope to earn from a higher-yielding but inferior quality sun-grown crop.

The ultimate success of this novel approach to saving forests depends, of course, on the willingness of coffee consumers to "vote with their pocketbooks" and opt for eco-certified brands. These are sold through an increasing number of online and retail outlets, an updated listing of which can be found on the Internet at Rainforest Marketplace, http://www.rainforest-alliance.org/marketplace/index.html.

During the 1990s, the use of fire to clear vast tracts of land became the principle means of deforestation in the Amazon and was widely employed in Indonesia as well. In late 1997, fires set to clear new land for rice cultivation and tree plantations burned out of control, spreading through at least 2 million hectares of forest and igniting underground deposits of peat. The fires cast a pall of smoke across much of Southeast Asia for several months, creating serious air quality problems as far away as Malaysia, Singapore, the Philippines, and Thailand (Abramovitz, 1998). The denuded landscapes left when vast tracts of forest are burned over or extensively logged are frequently subject to severe erosion, leading to flooding and landslides during the rainy season. In August 1998, the Chinese government prohibited all logging in the upper Yangtze River basin after weeks of heavy rain-

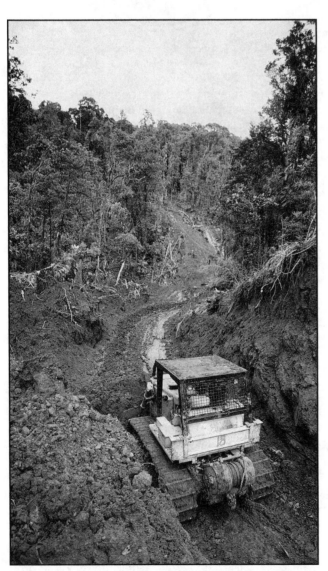

Bulldozer at work carving out access roads for lumbering enterprises on the Solomon Islands, east of Papua New Guinea.

fall resulted in $30 billion worth of damage due to record-breaking floods. While this ban has been effective in helping to protect China's remaining forests, it has only encouraged over-cutting elsewhere. China's insatiable demand for wood to produce furniture, flooring, and particle board destined for its booming export market has driven Chinese logging companies into neighboring countries such as Myanmar, Indonesia, Papua New Guinea, and Siberia, felling timber at such a rate that experts estimate that natural forests in those regions will be gone in another decade or two—and Chinese firms are now moving into the Amazon and Congo River basins (Brown, 2008).

While commercial lumbering in the tropics has taken its greatest toll thus far in Southeast Asia, the near-exhaustion of primary forests in that region has prompted timber barons to shift their attention to South America, particularly to Bolivia, where logging concessions have been granted for more than half that nation's forest lands; to Guyana, where more than 80% of government-owned forests have been leased to wealthy Korean and Malaysian timber companies on terms extremely generous to the Asian firms; and to Chile, where the world's largest remaining expanse of still-pristine temperate rain forest is being felled at an alarming rate to meet the insatiable demands of Japanese paper producers for wood chips. Environmentalists fully expect to see the same well-documented pattern of land degradation and abuse that has accompanied logging operations in Africa, Malaysia, Indonesia, and Papua New Guinea repeated in South America.

In countries where politicians control the distribution of timber concessions, bribery and corruption ensure the overexploitation of forest resources with minimal regulation of environmental damage. Careless logging practices frequently result in permanent ecological degradation and those charged with enforcing sound forest management practices are either bought off or become totally frustrated by their inability to prosecute loggers whose political connections insulate them from any enforcement actions. Land rights of indigenous forest peoples, 50 million of whom still make their home within the tropical rain forest, are another casualty of commercial logging operations in the tropics. Preexisting tribal claims are seldom considered when timber concessions are granted; a case in point was the Bolivian government's give-away of logging rights within Guarayo and Chiquitano de Monte Verde indigenous territories in the late 1990s. Native peoples frequently suffer total impoverishment after logging destroys the forest resources that sustained these groups for millennia (Ayres, 2004; Colchester, 1994).

In Latin America, **cattle ranching** has imposed additional pressures on threatened forests. In such Central American nations as Costa Rica and Panama, cattle

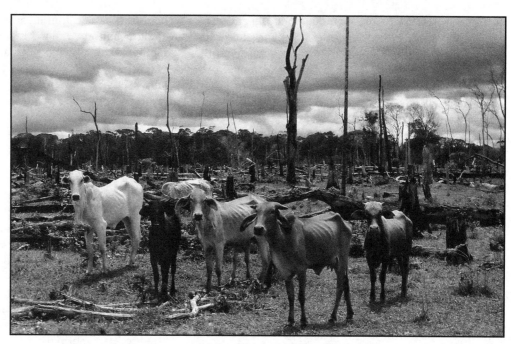

Cattle graze where the Amazon was once fertile. Cattle farmers in the Brazilian Amazon have used a slash-and-burn method to clear millions of acres of rain forest for pastureland. [*AP Photo/Ron Haviv/VII*]

ranching has destroyed more hectares of tropical forest than any other activity—70% of the land formerly covered by trees in both countries is now utilized as pastureland (Coffin, 1993). During the 1980s much of this destruction was driven by the demand for cheap beef to supply fast-food chains in the United States. In Brazil, cattle ranching is a major cause of deforestation in the Amazon basin, the largest continuous tract of tropical forest in the world. Since the 1970s, ranchers have cleared more than 10 million hectares of rain forest for pastureland, a practice originally encouraged by generous tax breaks and subsidies from a Brazilian government eager to develop the vast interior of that nation while providing an abundant supply of inexpensive meat for working-class consumers in the country's large coastal cities. In recent years subsidy programs have been terminated, but ranchers continue to clear new pasture as a form of land speculation—a means of obtaining legal title to such lands at a time of rapidly rising property values. Unfortunately, as in the case of agricultural exploitation in Amazonia, grazing pressures on these deforested tracts can be sustained profitably for only a few years. When the fragile tropical soils wear out, their content of phosphorus and other nutrients depleted, ranchers simply move on, burn or cut down more trees, and thus perpetuate the destructive cycle.

Within the past few years commercial **soybean production** has emerged as yet another key factor fueling deforestation in Amazonia. To meet escalating global demand for soy, large areas of previously untouched jungle are being cleared for cultivation of Brazil's newest cash crop. In 2002, soybean fields were responsible for a 40% jump in the rate of Amazonian deforestation. Similarly, since the late 1990s large areas of forest in Borneo have been converted to palm oil plantations; booming worldwide demand for biodiesel and the desire by Malaysian and Indonesian business interests to increase their export earnings make it likely that palm oil acreage will continue to grow rapidly in the years ahead, while tropical forests correspondingly shrink (Brown, 2008).

That destruction of the earth's forest cover will have a serious and adverse impact on terrestrial ecosystems—and on their human inhabitants as well—is undisputed. Past history should have taught us that heedless deforestation can lead to excessive erosion rates, decrease the soil's water-absorbing capacity, increase the amount of runoff and flooding, and lead to the transformation of once-productive environments into desert-like conditions. Today we have growing evidence to indicate that loss of forest cover also can lead to local climatic changes, with an increase in temperature and drop in annual rainfall when large expanses of woodland are cleared. More ominous is the possibility that deforestation will hasten the onset of global warming, due to the pivotal role forests play as a "carbon sink," absorbing CO_2 and thereby counteracting the so-called "Greenhouse Effect."

One might suppose that since the consequences of deforestation are well understood, a serious attempt to reverse current trends would be well underway. Unfortunately, in many of the countries most seriously affected reforestation efforts are negligible. Even where the political will exists and funds are available, large-scale tree-planting programs encounter serious difficulties that are inextricably related to the cultural, political, and economic facts of life in rural societies. In many areas saplings planted with high hopes are promptly devoured by overabundant and freely roaming goats, sheep, and cattle. In some places nomads passing through an area may decimate a village's efforts at reforestation, while in still other areas villagers themselves may uproot young trees because they simply have no other source of fuel. Successful reforestation efforts require extensive administrative efforts to protect the plants for years. There have been some reforestation success stories, most notably in India where approximately four hectares of trees are being planted for every one that is deforested. Although these tree plantations, which consist primarily of fast-growing eucalyptus or pine, lack the diversity of the native forest cover, they nevertheless provide soil and watershed protection while serving as windbreaks and a renewable source of fuel for local residents.

Ultimately the most serious obstacle to curbing forest loss is the continued rapid growth of human populations in the countries most affected. As a Costa Rican squatter on a partially forested ranch poignantly stated, "By subsisting today I know I can destroy the future of the forest and the people. But I have to eat today" (Hamilton, 1989).

Desertification

That humans can create desert-like conditions on once-productive land has been known, though largely ignored, since the time 2300 years ago when Plato bewailed the ecological fate of his native Attica, writing that "our land, compared with what it was, is like the skeleton of a body wasted by disease. The soft, plump parts have vanished and all that remains is the bare carcass." This sorry situation was brought about by the cutting of forests and overgrazing of livestock, which in that semiarid climate inevitably resulted in topsoil erosion and springs that dried up because they were no longer being recharged (due to rainwater runoff). The formation of agricultural wastelands, which occurred in ancient Greece and the lands around the eastern Mediterranean, is a process that so increased in extent during the 20th century that it was graced with the somewhat unwieldy, though descriptive, term **desertification**. Defined by delegates at the 1992 UN Conference on Environment and Development (UNCED) as "land degradation in arid, semiarid, and dry sub-humid areas resulting from various factors including climatic variations and human activities," desertification today is adversely affecting the lives and economic well-being of an estimated 900 million people in over 100 countries.

Contrary to the prevailing image of sand dunes relentlessly sweeping down over green fields and pastures, desertification seldom involves the steady influx of sands along a uniform front. Most often the process is set in motion when climatic fluctuations and abusive land-use practices interact to extend desert-like conditions irregularly over susceptible land. Spots of extreme degradation are especially likely to form around water holes when nearby pastures are heavily grazed and trampled and around towns when people denude adjacent lands in their search for fuelwood. Since desertification first captured world attention in the 1960s and 1970s, it has generally been assumed that population pressures have been the primary cause. More recently, however, data obtained from a decade's worth of satellite photos indicate that climatic variations exert a much more pronounced influence on the expansion of desert-like conditions than do human pressures. In the world's arid grasslands and semi-desert regions, year-to-year fluctuations of rainfall can be moderately destructive to biotic communities even under natural conditions, but natural processes can correct the imbalance in the long run. However, when environmental stresses due to normal climatic variation are coupled with such activities as overgrazing, gathering fuelwood, and poor cultivation practices, problems of land degradation are seriously aggravated. If such human pressures persist and intensify, they can sharply limit the regenerative capabilities of the land, hindering its recovery even after climatic conditions improve (Hulme and Kelly, 1993).

Whatever its cause, desertification is a process occurring today on an unprecedented scale. The human tragedy embodied in the great dust storms that blackened the skies in the American prairie states during the 1930s is being repeated today in dryland ecosystems that occupy more than 40% of the earth's land surface and are home to over two billion people. Desertification has already degraded between 10–20% of these lands and threatens to extend its reach as population growth continues and global warming accelerates. Some of the regions most adversely affected include sub-Saharan Africa, where nomadic herdsmen and their oversized flocks have exceeded the sustainable yield of grasslands from Ethiopia and Somalia in the east to Senegal and Mauritania in the west. In northern Nigeria, Africa's most populous country, agricultural lands are gradually converting to desert under the pressure of too many people tending too many sheep, goats, and cattle. In the Middle East, more than a hundred Iranian villages have been buried by sandstorms and abandoned, while in neighboring Afghanistan more than 80% of the land is experiencing degradation as deserts expand rapidly in the northern, eastern, and southern regions of that country—in part because fuelwood gathering has stripped the land of the woody plants that once provided a buffer against shifting sands.

Desertification is perhaps most rampant in northwestern China, where once-productive rangelands are now blowing away and turning to desert due to overgrazing. During the 1990s China was losing 3,600 square kilometers of land to desertification annually. Although the Chinese government is urging herders in the area to reduce their flocks by 40% in a desperate effort to combat desertification, China's Gobi Desert continues to expand eastward, forcing villagers to flee their homes to escape the encroaching sands. Huge dust storms in late winter or early spring occur with increasing frequency, producing "brown rain" as far afield as Korea and Japan and creating fears that northern China is turning into a "Dust Bowl." In the Western Hemisphere, desertification is affecting land resources and local economies in both northeastern Brazil and in Mexico, prompting massive human migration as croplands deteriorate (Brown, 2008, 2003; MOAF, 2007). Many of these areas still have the potential to reestablish their former grassland ecosystems if the constant pressure of overgrazing and overplowing could be lifted, but some have been irreversibly degraded by complete loss of topsoil. If human pressures continue to mount, degradation of arid lands will result in the permanent destabilization of existing ecosystems and a continuing impoverishment of both ecological and cultural conditions. Ecosystems, like civilizations, can decline and fall if pushed too far.

Wetlands Loss

Swamps, bogs, fens, tidal marshlands, pocosins, estuaries, ponds, river bottoms, flood plains, and prairie potholes all fall under the designation of **wetlands**, ecosystems characterized by soils that are inundated or water-saturated for at least a portion of the year and by the presence of certain water-loving plants (hydrophytes). In the not-too-distant past, most people viewed wetlands as a nuisance, useful only to frogs and mosquitoes, and thus prime candidates for draining or filling to convert them into more "profitable" areas for farming, mining, or urban development. As a result, over half the wetlands that existed in the contiguous 48 states at the time European settlers first arrived (estimated at about 247 million acres in AD 1600) have now disappeared. Fortunately, the rate of loss has declined significantly in recent years, thanks to federal legislation protecting wetlands. In its most recent *Status and Trends* report, issued in 2006 for the period covering 1998–2004, the U.S. Fish and Wildlife Service published data showing that wetlands gains in the United States have now surpassed wetland losses,

for an average annual net gain of 32,000 acres during the reporting period. Most of the gains were achieved by the creation of numerous artificial freshwater ponds (even though these don't provide the full range of ecological functions as do natural marshlands, they nevertheless are defined as "wetlands") and through agricultural conservation programs aimed at wetlands restoration.

Unfortunately, largely due to continued urban expansion and rural development, high-quality U.S. wetlands continue to decline in extent, albeit at a much slower pace than in past decades. Today wetlands cover 5.5% (107.7 million acres) of the land surface in the lower 48 states. Alaska has another 160 million acres, with wetlands extending across half the North Star State. Outside Alaska, Florida and Louisiana have the largest remaining expanses of wetlands, though they are also among the states with the highest rates of wetlands loss in recent years. California has lost a greater percentage of its original wetlands than any other state (91%), but Florida has lost the largest number of acres (WRI, 1992). In recent decades, belated recognition of the importance of wetlands has resulted in efforts at both the federal and state level to control wetlands conversion. In 2004, President George W. Bush established a new federal policy

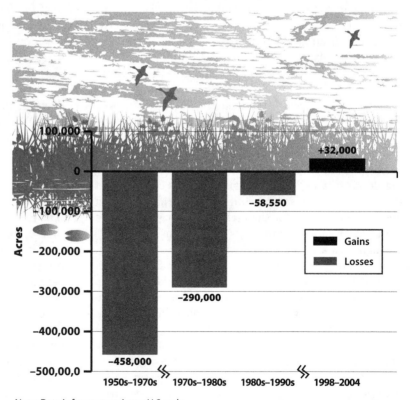

Note: Data is for conterminous U.S. only.

Source: Dahl, T. E. *Status and Trends of Wetlands in the Conterminous U.S., 1984–2004*, 2006.

Figure 5-2 Average Annual Net Loss and Gain Estimates for Wetlands in the U.S., 1954 to 2004

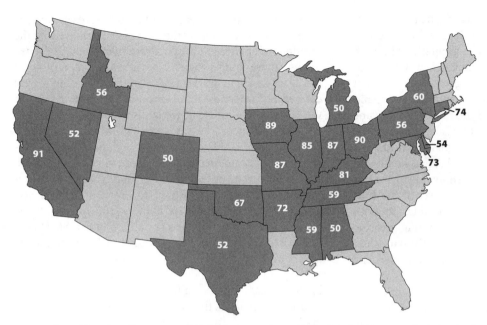

Source: Adapted from EPA, "Percentage of Wetlands Acreage Lost, 1780s–1980s." www.epa.gov/type/wetlands

Figure 5-3   States with 50% or Greater Wetlands Acreage Lost, 1780s to 1980s

into the ground. Indeed, taking advantage of wetlands' capacity to act as "nature's kidneys," some communities are now utilizing constructed marshes to treat stormwater or secondary wastewater effluent by directing the flow through **engineered wetlands**, where living organisms remove pollutants efficiently and inexpensively. The sustained productivity of commercial fisheries is also heavily dependent on the existence of wetlands. Between 60–90% of fish caught along the Atlantic and Gulf coasts spend at least some portion of their life cycle, usually the vulnerable early stages, in coastal marshes or estuaries. Further inland in the Midwest, the system of lakes, marshes, and prairie potholes extending from the Gulf of Mexico north into Canada provides the major life-support system for millions of migratory waterfowl (half of all ducklings in North America are hatched in the prairie potholes of the Dakotas and Canada). A $1 billion recreational hunting industry, attracting 2.5 million duck hunters each year, is thus totally dependent on preservation of these vital wetlands breeding areas. Wetlands provide a habitat not only for ducks and geese but also for many other bird and mammal species—whooping cranes, river otters, black bears, and so on.

Although some wetlands are lost due to natural causes such as erosion, land subsidence, storms, or saltwater intrusion (the U.S. Geological Survey estimates that Hurricanes Katrina and Rita destroyed about 100 square miles of southeastern Louisiana coastal marshes, converting them to open water), human activities are the primary culprit. Draining swamps or bottomlands for agricultural purposes is the leading cause of freshwater wetlands loss, with development and silviculture taking a lesser toll. Coastal development also has taken a heavy toll of wetlands, particularly along estuaries that provide vital habitat and breeding grounds for many commercially valuable fish and shellfish species. Dredging for canals and port construction, flood control projects, and road building have all had a negative impact on wetlands, as has urban sprawl. In the southeastern states, deep-soil swamps were cleared and drained for conversion to pine plantations, resulting in extensive wetlands loss until the EPA banned such activities in 1994. While there are no

aimed at increasing both the quantity and quality of U.S. wetlands, moving beyond the "no net loss" objective set in 1988, and proclaiming the goal of "restoring, improving, and protecting" more than 3 million acres by 2009. Globally, the loss of wetlands has mirrored that in the United States and is estimated at about 50%; in France and Germany the loss is even higher, with wetlands destruction totaling 80% (Hinrichsen, 2003).

Today the importance of wetlands in both ecological and economic terms is unquestioned. Their ability to retain large amounts of water makes them extremely valuable as nature's own method of preventing devastating floods. Many knowledgeable observers contend that the devastation caused by Hurricane Katrina in August 2005 would have been significantly less had Louisiana not lost more than a third of its natural coastal wetlands through decades of channel dredging, levee construction, and damming of upstream tributaries in the Mississippi River delta. These activities, intended to aid navigation and control floods, prevented millions of tons of sediment from reaching the delta and replenishing the wetlands that formerly provided a buffer against storm surges and rising sea levels. Similarly, the impact of the December 2004 South Asian tsunami was much worse in areas where coastal development had destroyed native mangrove swamps than in areas where such wetlands were still intact (Leahy, 2005).

Wetlands provide the major recharge areas for groundwater reserves and also serve as "living filters" for purifying contaminated surface waters as these percolate federal laws expressly prohibiting the draining, filling, or converting of most wetlands, Congress took a small step by including a section in the 1985 farm bill referred to as the "Swampbuster Provision," aimed at discouraging draining of wetlands for agriculture by stating that farmers who do so will lose their farm program benefits. The Conservation Reserve Program, enacted under that same legislation, provided farmers with financial incentives to protect lands taken out of cultivation and thereby fostered the restoration of critical wetlands habitat. In 1989 federal legislation created one of the most significant conservation programs in U.S. history. The North American Wetlands Conservation Act (NAWCA) provides matching grants for wetlands conservation programs throughout North America and since 1989 has helped finance projects in all 50 states, Canada, and Mexico.

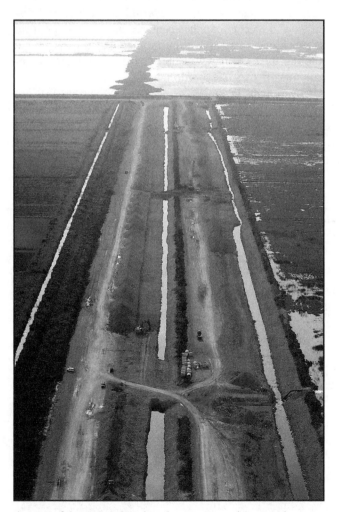

As part of the comprehensive plan to restore the natural water flow patterns in the Florida Everglades (the world's largest freshwater marsh), more than 30 million tons of earth will be moved to build a massive reservoir capable of holding 62 billion gallons of water. [*AP Photo/J. Pat Carter*]

With private groups such as Ducks Unlimited and the Nature Conservancy matching federal money dollar for dollar, over the last 20 years approximately 25 million acres of wetlands and associated uplands have been restored and protected, thanks to NAWCA.

Since almost three-fourths of all wetlands acreage in the United States is privately owned, the ultimate success of wetlands preservation attempts hinge on efforts by both government and environmental organizations to educate landowners on the intrinsic value of wetlands, to encourage wetlands conservation and restoration, and to provide the technical assistance and financial incentives that will persuade property owners to protect this precious resource.

LOSS OF BIODIVERSITY

Extinction of a species, like the death of an individual, is a natural process. As fossil evidence clearly indicates, many groups of plants and animals that dominated life on earth in past millennia have died out, only to be replaced by newly evolving organisms. The rise and fall of species throughout the course of earth's history was determined largely by a population's ability to adapt to changing environmental conditions or to become increasingly specialized for life in a particular ecological niche. As evolution proceeded, the number of plant and animal species proliferated as populations dispersed into far-flung geographic regions and adapted to life in a seemingly endless variety of ecological niches. Today biologists have described 1.8 million species, but estimate that the actual number currently in existence, many yet undiscovered, ranges from 5 to 30 million, the largest number being small creatures living in tropical forests and in the deep oceans. Unfortunately, it is widely feared that many of these species will vanish before their existence is ever noted or recorded.

The sad truth of the present situation is that human actions have greatly accelerated the rate at which species are becoming extinct; indeed, for the first time since the last great die-off at the end of the Cretaceous Period 65 million years ago, species are vanishing more rapidly than new ones are evolving, resulting in a diminishing diversity of life forms. The first recorded animal extinction—that of the European lion—was documented in AD 80; more than half of the animal species that have disappeared since that time have become extinct since 1900. Just as human populations have been increasing at an ever-faster pace in recent centuries, so has the rate of species loss. While estimates indicate that over the vast span of geologic time one mammalian species suffers extinction every 400 years and one bird species every 200, the record for the past 400 years shows a dramatic acceleration in the rate of extinction: 58 mammalian species and 128 bird species. Even these numbers don't accurately represent the true toll, especially for recent decades, since, by international agreement, a species isn't classified as extinct until 50 years after its last sighting. In addition, with millions of species still undiscovered and unnamed, it is quite likely that large numbers are quietly disappearing, unnoticed and unmourned (Wilcove, McMillan, and Winston, 1993). In 2008, the World Conservation Union (IUCN) evaluated 44,838 species, of which it placed 38% on its *Red List of Threatened Species;* included were 22% of mammalian species and 14% of birds. The IUCN *Red List* also includes 869 species (2% of those evaluated) that it identifies as already extinct or "extinct in the wild," though it acknowledges that this number could exceed 1,100 if those species within the "critically endangered" group categorized as "possibly extinct" are, in fact, no longer in existence.

When *all* types of organisms are considered—not just the feathered or furry creatures that appeal to human emotions, but the myriads of insects, mollusks, fish, fungi, plants, and other organisms that greatly enrich the diversity of life—then current rates of extinction are even more alarming. Harvard biologist E. O. Wilson estimates that in tropical forest areas alone, home to a conservatively estimated 10 million species, the world is currently losing 3 species every hour, 74 per day, 27,000 each year. If present trends of rain forest destruction are not reversed, 10–20% of all rain forest species will be extinct within 30 years—a number equivalent to at least 5–10% of all species on earth (Wilson, 1992).

The magnitude of such a loss is staggering. Species diversity is generally considered a prime determinant of ecological stability; extinction of key species, particularly plant species, may lead to the collapse of whole ecosystems. Less spectacular but equally distressing from a human viewpoint is the prospect of many potentially useful plant species being lost before their food or medicinal value is discovered. Even today, one-fourth of all pharmaceutical products bought by Americans contain active ingredients derived from plant products. The discovery of taxol, a potent anticancer drug derived from the bark of the Pacific yew (formerly regarded as a weed tree in old-growth forests of the Pacific Northwest) is but one of the more recent additions to a long list of valuable medicinal products extracted from forest plants. From a philosophical viewpoint also, the implications of the wholesale destruction of nonhuman life is profoundly disturbing. Over a century ago Thoreau proclaimed that "in wildness is the preservation of the world." Much ethical discussion in recent years has centered around the question of whether humans have the moral right to exterminate another form of life, to abruptly terminate the product of millions of years of evolution.

Although the causes of accelerating species loss are by now fairly well understood, reversing these trends will be extremely difficult, particularly in regions where rapidly growing human populations are in direct competition with wildlife. Human pressures on other species can assume a variety of forms, as detailed next.

Table 5-3   Representative Examples of Threatened Species by Major Groups of Organisms (1996–2010)

	Number of described species	Number of threatened species in 2010	Number threatened in 2010, as % of species described
Vertebrates			
Mammals	5,490	1,130	21%
Birds	10,027	1,240	12%
Reptiles	9,084	467	5%
Amphibians	6,638	1,895	29%
Fishes	31,600	1,771	6%
Invertebrates			
Insects	1,000,000	733	0.1%
Mollusks	85,000	1,114	1%
Crustaceans	47,000	596	1%
Corals	2,175	235	11%
Others	68,658	24	0.03%
Plants			
Mosses	16,236	80	0%
Ferns and allies	12,000	148	1%
Gymnosperms	1,052	371	35%
Flowering Plants	268,000	8,084	3%

Source: Excerpted from *2010 IUCN Red List of Threatened Species*. Version 2010.2. www.iucnredlist.org.

Direct Killing or Collecting of Wildlife for Food, Pleasure, or Profit

From the Paleolithic hunters who decimated the woolly mammoths and mastodons with primitive weapons to the modern Russian and Japanese fishing fleets that have brought several species of whale to the brink of extinction, predatory humans have totally eliminated a number of bird and mammalian species. Of all the animal extinctions known to have occurred within the past 400 years, the World Conservation Union estimates that nearly one-fourth (23%) were caused by overhunting. Collectors who dynamite reefs to obtain chunks of coral or capture rare tropical fish for sale to aquarium hobbyists; cactus "rustlers" who steal plants from nature preserves to satisfy the growing demand for rare houseplants; African poachers who shoot the endangered rhinoceros for the high profits its horn will bring in the markets of the Orient (powdered rhinoceros horn has long been considered an aphrodisiac in China and the Far East)—all contribute to the demise of species, as do the consumers who provide the incentive for such actions.

In recent years commercial hunting of wild animals for their meat has emerged as the most serious threat to wildlife in Africa, as well as in many other parts of the world (see box 5-2). Local extinctions of some species in West Africa and Asia have already been documented by groups such as the Bushmeat Crisis Task Force, who warn that the slaughter is rapidly expanding into formerly unaffected areas and decimating animal populations previously not at risk. Closer to home, commercial hunting has placed the Cuban crocodile in the "critically endangered" category due to illegal killing of the reptile for its meat and skin.

In an effort to remove the financial incentives for exploitation of wildlife, conservation groups mustered enough support to secure passage of the 1973 **Convention on International Trade in Endangered Species of Flora and Fauna (CITES)**. Meeting twice a year, CITES' governing body regulates international trade in specified animal and plant products and flatly prohibits trade in products from endangered species. CITES initially received praise for stemming the slaughter of African elephants after issuing a ban in 1989 on ivory trading (the ban exempted domestic sales on ivory harvested prior to 1989). Although poaching appeared to be on the decline during the 1990s, a quadrupling in the value of illegal ivory since 2004 has reversed previous gains. Prior to the 1989 ban, approximately 7.4% of the world's elephants were being killed each year for their tusks and other body parts; today, in spite of the ban, the annual toll is estimated at 8% and elephant herds continue to shrink (Block, 2008).

CITES has been even less effective in curbing the illicit trade in tiger parts, which has resulted in such a precipitous decline in populations of the big cats that many wildlife biologists hold out little hope for the survival of tigers outside of zoos. Whereas the world's tiger population numbered approximately 100,000 a century ago, experts estimate that today there are fewer than 4,000 tigers in the wild, inhabiting only 7% of their original range. In countries such as China and Taiwan, virtually every part of the animal's body brings premium prices due to their supposed medicinal benefits: tiger

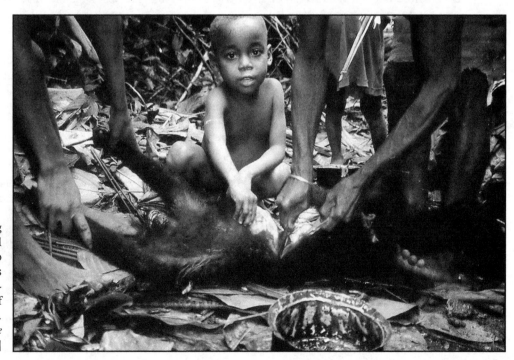

The indiscriminate hunting of "bushmeat" for both local consumption and for sale to large commercial markets has become the most immediate threat to the future of wildlife in the Congo basin. [*Heidi Verhoef, courtesy of the Bushmeat Crisis Task Force*]

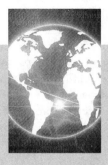

· · · · · · · 5-2 · · · · · · ·

Slaughter in the Jungle: Bushmeat's Tragic Toll

"Bushmeat," a common term for the flesh of wildlife living in the jungles and shrub-land ("bush") of Africa, has always been a dietary staple for people inhabiting the vast forests of that continent. From time immemorial, subsistence hunters armed with bows and arrows, nets, and other traditional weapons have stalked, killed, and eaten a wide array of the native animals and birds whose habitat they shared. So long as human populations were relatively small and weapons primitive, when the hunters' goal was simply to secure enough meat to feed their own families or village, such predation had only a localized impact and was sustainable in terms of preserving stable wildlife populations.

That situation has now changed dramatically with the commercialization of hunting throughout the forests of western and central Africa. Horrified conservationists are now warning that nothing—not even habitat loss—poses a greater threat to biodiversity throughout this vast region than does the relentless slaughter of wildlife for human consumption.

Each year the 30 million people living in the countries of the Congo River basin eat an estimated 5 million metric tons of forest antelopes, bush pigs, monkeys, gorillas, chimpanzees, elephants, monitor lizards, guinea fowl, and cane rats—among others. The demand for bushmeat is enormous and growing. Central Africans eat as much or more meat on a daily basis per person as do Americans or Europeans, but most of the meat they consume—about 80%—comes from wildlife rather than domestic animals. The lack of available grasslands for cattle grazing, the density of forests, and the prevalence of tropical diseases and insects lethal to temperate-zone livestock have made beef, mutton, and poultry rare items on Central African dinner tables; it's always been much easier and cheaper to look to the forest for the daily supply of meat. Rapidly growing urban populations in the region are increasing the demand for bushmeat; unlike the situation in rural areas where bushmeat is the cheapest source of animal protein, in the cities it is more expensive than shipped-in domestic meats. Many affluent Africans, however, are happy to pay premium prices for gorilla, chimpanzee, or other bushmeat, regarding it as a status symbol and a way to maintain cultural ties and ethnic identity with their rural roots.

It is economics, however, that is driving the bushmeat business. Throughout central Africa, collapsing commodity prices for cash crops such as cocoa and coffee have caused widespread unemployment; to men desperate to support their families, the burgeoning bushmeat trade offers lucrative opportunities. As long as the supply of wildlife is abundant, hunters can earn from $400–1,100 per year, a sum higher than the average yearly income in the region (and greater than the salary paid to guards hired to prevent hunting). Resources needed to become a hunter are few and relatively inexpensive; a rifle, often borrowed, some cartridges, and perhaps some wire snares. Add to this the fact that few Africans see anything wrong with killing wildlife and it's not surprising that economic incentive coupled with cultural values gives the bushmeat trade widespread public acceptance.

Commercial hunting has been greatly facilitated and the demand for bushmeat substantially boosted by industrial logging operations in the Congo basin. Dozens of foreign timber companies have been granted logging concessions to extract timber from vast expanses of pristine tropical forests. The forest fragmentation caused by such operations and the network of access roads built to transport the logs to market have made native wildlife easy prey for hunters. By affording easy access to formerly impenetrable jungle and by allowing hunters to hitch rides on logging trucks, timber companies have, intentionally or not, greatly increased the supply of bushmeat and the profitability of the trade. Logging operations have also boosted demand; with thousands of itinerant loggers and their families moving into once sparsely settled areas, a market for bushmeat has arrived at the source of supply. Needing meat for their workers, some logging companies hire professional hunters directly or may provide them with guns and wire snares in return for a portion of the kill. Even without direct subsidies, bushmeat hunters ply a profitable trade among loggers who have money to spend, big appetites, and no other readily available source of meat. Elsewhere in the region, notably in the eastern section of the Democratic Republic of the Congo, wildlife has been decimated by the bushmeat demands of thousands of peasant farmers-turned coltan miners (coltan, a tantalum-containing ore, is a key component for circuitry in cell phones, video games, laptop computers, and other electronic devices). In the late 1990s, coltan prospectors began digging in Kahuzi-Biega National Park, supposedly a protected World Heritage Site. The hunters who arrived to supply them with food successively killed off the elephants, gorillas, chimpanzees, buffaloes, and antelopes. As the larger species were wiped out, hunters moved on to smaller prey; within a few years there was little left to shoot other than some small antelopes, birds, monkeys, and tortoises.

The scope of the ongoing massacre is immense. In some areas observers now refer to the "Empty Forest Syndrome"—regions where the jungle is relatively intact but devoid of all large animals. While the loss of any species is tragic, the plight of the region's great apes—gorillas, chimpanzees, and bonobos—is of special concern. Although these large primates comprise but a small percentage of bushmeat in the marketplace, perhaps just 1%, they are likely to be the first species hunted to extinction for their tasty flesh. Already rare, apes are exceptionally vulnerable to hunting pressures because of very low fertility rates. The fact that they are large, noisy, and gregarious makes it very easy for hunters to locate and shoot them and cultural values place a high premium on their meat, especially gorilla hands, which are considered a delicacy and fetch a high price. Since all great apes are classified as "endangered" or "highly endangered," it is illegal in every African country to kill them or to sell their flesh. Such laws are largely ignored, however, and seldom enforced. Recently, public health authorities have been raising an additional concern related to the bushmeat trade in chimpanzee and gorilla flesh, citing the potential for disease transmission. Evidence has been emerging of a possible link between exposure to dead apes and human outbreaks of HIV, Ebola, and Marburg virus. It is well-known that disease organisms can spread from one species to another and health officials fear that butchering and eating bushmeat places humans at increased risk of contracting deadly animal-borne diseases.

Unfortunately, prospects for any substantial curtailing of the bushmeat trade appear grim. With regional economies in a free-fall and government officials easy to bribe, the will and ability to monitor hunting and logging practices is largely nonexistent. Since the late 1990s international conservation groups have entered into cooperative agreements with some of the large logging companies, trying to enlist the industry's support for curbing the worst abuses of bushmeat trafficking while conceding that the timber industry has an important role to play in African development. Critics charge such associations give "green cover" to loggers who have been among the worst offenders in sanctioning the bushmeat business, adding that the agreements signed leave most of the costs for ameliorating problems with the "feel-good" environmental groups rather than with the highly profitable exploitive industries.

Barring a total moratorium on commercial hunting of bushmeat, extinction within the foreseeable future is a likely prognosis for many species in the Congo basin. With Central African populations doubling in size roughly every 25 years, bushmeat consumption is expected to increase by about 3% a year. With the current annual take already at an unsustainably high level, human demographic trends leave little room for optimism about Africa's large animals. While some might argue that well-fed Westerners have little right to criticize Africans' exploitation of their own natural resources—especially when so many of them are poor and have no other source of affordable protein—the fact remains that once the animals are eaten to extinction they are gone forever. African cooking pots will be empty and all of humankind will be the poorer for the demise of magnificent species, among them several of our closest relatives. How do we explain *that* to future generations? (Bushmeat Crisis Task Force [BCTF], 2003; Peterson, 2003.)

bones for potions to cure rheumatism, tiger whiskers to provide strength, tiger eyes to calm convulsions, and tiger penis, simmered in a soup, to rekindle male sexual prowess among senior citizens (only wealthy senior citizens need apply, however—a bowl of tiger penis soup may cost over $300!).

In 1993 China enacted a law prohibiting domestic sales of tiger products, but due to continuing demand, a brisk illicit market in such items quickly sprang up and continues to the present day. Organized crime rings are intimately involved with the trade in tiger parts; law enforcement authorities estimate that, worldwide, criminal trafficking in wildlife and forest products (more than half from Asia) has become a $10 billion/year business, second only to the illegal trade in drugs and weapons. Demand for such products among the growing numbers of affluent Chinese consumers, as well as by those in Europe and the United States, continue to drive this illicit trade (O'Neill, 2008). Since CITES has no enforcement powers of its own, protection of endangered species from the ongoing indiscriminate slaughter will depend on the political determination of national governments to protect and preserve their own threatened wildlife—and on the general public's willingness to place a higher value on the continued existence of creatures in the wild than on personal possession of pricey animal pelts, aphrodisiacs, and culinary treats.

Introduction of Invasive Species

The deliberate or accidental introduction of nonnative plants, animals, or microbes into new environments has, until relatively recently, been the single most important factor accounting for species loss. Though now outranked by habitat destruction as the most critical threat to biodiversity, the growing number of "bioinvasions" has assumed such alarming proportions that in 1997 the United Nations established its Global Invasive Species Programme to focus international attention on the problem. In 1999, President Bill Clinton issued an executive order creating the National Invasive Species Council which, two years later, released a management plan to enhance the United States' ability to minimize the impact of bioinvasions and to prevent their spread. The concern is economic as well as environmental; Dr. David Pimentel, an ecologist at Cornell University, estimates that in the U.S. alone, damages caused by invasive species and expenditures for their control add up to $137 billion annually. Biologists estimate that more than 6,000 exotic plant and animal species have now become permanent residents of the United States. While not all bioinvaders cause problems, many are now numbered among our most troublesome pests. Proliferating uncontrollably, threatening native ecosystems, or causing economic damage, these unwelcome newcomers are termed **invasive alien species**. Lacking natural enemies to curb their rampant spread, these aggressive invaders have overwhelmed and decimated many indigenous species—eating them, outcompeting them for available resources, spreading disease, or in various ways altering ecosystems to the detriment of native flora and fauna.

Examples are legion: European starlings, forty pairs of which were deliberately released by a bird-lover in New York's Central Park in 1890, within 50 years had spread coast-to-coast, driving many less-aggressive songbirds from their original range; Eurasian cheatgrass, introduced when weed-infested seed grain carried by westward-bound immigrants fell alongside late-19th-century wagon trails, subsequently spread over millions of acres of rangeland and even today greatly enhances the frequency of wildfires on the western plains; zebra mussels, first observed in Lake St. Clair near Detroit in 1988, have now spread throughout inland waterways in much of the eastern and central U.S., causing billions of dollars in damage to water intake pipes and overwhelming native mussel species.

A recent newcomer is the Asian longhorned beetle, native to China, Korea, and Japan. Discovered in 1996 on Long Island, in 1998 in Chicago, in 2002 in northeastern New Jersey, and in 2003 near Toronto, the large, shiny black-and-white beetle poses a serious threat to many species of hardwood trees, especially maples, into which it tunnels and feeds. Aggressive eradication efforts were launched in the localized areas where infestations have been identified (these efforts seem to have been effective in the Chicago area, where the Asian longhorned beetle was officially declared "eradicated" in 2008) and regulations have been imposed requiring that wooden shipping crates from China be heated and chemically treated to kill any beetles they might be harboring. Such precautions, unfortunately, didn't prevent the arrival of yet another uninvited guest from northeast Asia. In the summer of 2002, the emerald ash borer—a small, tree-infesting insect—was discovered in both Michigan and Ontario. By 2009 the borer had spread throughout the state of Michigan, to additional locations in Ontario, and had also been found in Quebec, across most of Ohio, and in parts of Indiana, Illinois, Wisconsin, Missouri, Pennsylvania, West Virginia, Virginia, and Maryland. Since the insect is usually established for several years prior to its detection, it's likely that additional states will soon discover that they, too, are unwilling hosts to this new invader. Entomologists gloomily predict it will eventually spread throughout North America, killing untold millions of ash trees and causing enormous economic losses.

In addition to such accidental arrivals, numerous fish-stocking programs since the 1950s have quite intentionally introduced nonnative brown and rainbow trout, as well as other game fish, into waterways where they previously didn't exist, pleasing sports fishermen but decimating populations of indigenous fish and amphibians. It's estimated that half the fish now on the "endangered" list are thus imperiled because of introduced exotics (Baskin, 2002). Another deliberately introduced fish species that has already created ecological havoc in the Mississippi/Illinois River basin and poses a serious threat to the Great Lakes ecosystem is the Asian carp, imported by southern catfish farmers in the early 1970s to keep their ponds free of algae and suspended solids. So long as they were confined to aquaculture ponds, the carp posed no problems, but major flooding in the Mississippi River Valley during the summer of 1993 caused catfish farm ponds to overflow, releasing the carp into local waterways, from which they made their way up the Mississippi River. Due to their large size and rapid rate of reproduction, Asian carp have become the dominant fish species in some parts of the river basin, outcompeting native species and decimating local fisheries.

Concerned that these invaders might gain access to Lake Michigan, the federal government and the State of Illinois have funded construction of a multi-million dollar electric barrier across the Chicago Sanitary and Ship Canal near Romeoville, Illinois, to block further advance of the carp. In July 2010, the states of Michigan, Wisconsin, Ohio, Minnesota, and Pennsylvania filed a federal lawsuit seeking to force the Metropolitan Water Reclamation District of Greater Chicago and the U.S. Army Corps of Engineers to close two Chicago-area shipping locks and to conduct poisoning and netting programs for Asian carp that may already have breached the electric barrier near Romeoville. At stake is the $7 billion-a-year Great Lakes fishing industry, which some experts fear would be decimated by the ravenous carp. The city of Chicago and regional shipping interests opposed the closing of the locks. A U.S. District Court judge ruled in December 2010 that the locks will remain open.

The impact of nonnative species can be seen most dramatically in island ecosystems such as Hawaii, site of fully three-fourths of all known bird and plant extinctions in the United States. The goats, pigs, sheep, rats, and mongooses that came ashore with European settlers in the years after Captain Cook's voyage to the islands in 1778 are the most notorious of approximately 3,900 plant and animal species arriving in Hawaii over the past two centuries. Today, of the remaining native Hawaiian plants, one-fifth are endangered; for native bird species, nearly half are at risk, primarily due to the impact of exotic newcomers. On the Pacific island of Guam, the brown tree snake has virtually wiped out native bird populations since it was first introduced in the mid-1940s.

Nowhere, however, has the impact of alien species been more devastating than in Africa's Lake Victoria, a waterway once renowned for its amazing diversity of

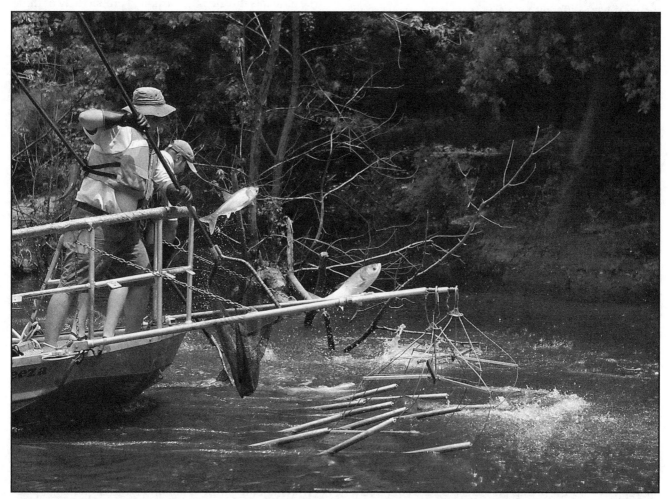

Asian carp loom as a threat to the Great Lakes ecosystem after having made their way from flooded catfish ponds in the South up the Mississippi and Illinois rivers. [*U.S. Fish and Wildlife Service*]

cichlid fishes—more than 300 species found nowhere else in the world. In 1959 Nile perch, a type of carnivorous fish growing up to six feet in length, were introduced into the lake by British settlers who thought they would enhance sports-fishing opportunities. Within 25 years the invaders had gobbled up so many of the native cichlids that several species disappeared completely; it is expected that eventually over half the native species will become extinct. The demise of the plant-eating cichlids has had far-reaching effects on the Lake Victoria ecosystem, leading to algal blooms, oxygen depletion, and the decline of many other lake species. While the decision to introduce the perch had no malicious intent, the catastrophic results of this act led a team of biologists to observe: "Never before has man in a single ill-advised step placed so many vertebrate species simultaneously at risk of extinction and also, in doing so, threatened a food resource and traditional way of life of riparian dwellers" (Wilson, 1992).

Problems due to invasive species are nothing new; for millennia as human populations moved about the globe they carried other species with them into new territories. What's different today is the quantum increase in numbers of species on the move, facilitated by more rapid transportation (permitting stowaways to survive long journeys), globalization of trade, and record numbers of people traveling to distant lands for business or pleasure. While some of the species introductions in recent years have been a deliberate result of commercial transactions, most are accidental consequences of the global distribution networks that facilitate international commerce. Exotic species frequently invade new territory attached to the hulls of ships; as stowaways in wooden crates or packing materials; hidden inside unprocessed logs, fruits, or seeds; as unticketed passengers on aircraft; or, most common of all, swimming in the ballast water discharged by ships entering ports (the zebra mussel's presumed route of entry). The impact of exotics has been particularly severe on coastal ecosystems. In San Francisco Bay alone, according to a spokeswoman at the Center of Marine Conservation, a new species is discovered entering the bay, on average, every 14 days.

At the level of international policy making, stemming bioinvasions is more difficult and complex than curbing trade in endangered species. With the exception of various protocols that categorically exclude exotic organisms from Antarctica, there are no treaties specifically enacted to prevent bioinvasions. The 1992 Convention of Biological Diversity, which emerged from the UN-sponsored Earth Summit that year, requires signatory nations to prevent the introduction of alien species that pose a threat to ecosystem stability but to do so "as far as possible and appropriate"—a qualifying phrase that makes the treaty little more than a weak statement of noble intentions. For the foreseeable future, efforts at mitigating the impact of exotic species will likely remain a combination of port-of-entry inspections, prohibitions or controls of listed problematic species or items (e.g., potentially insect-infested logs from Siberia, nontreated wooden crates from China), and eradication or control programs targeting already established exotic pests. The task is daunting, but biologists are convinced that over the long term controlling exotic species will be just as important for protecting biodiversity as are efforts to save those that are threatened and endangered; indeed, the two activities may be but opposite sides of the same coin (Bright, 1998).

Pollution of Air and Water with Toxic Chemicals

The death of entire aquatic ecosystems due to acid rainfall is but one example of the effect toxic pollutants are having on other forms of life. Particularly since the introduction of the synthetic organic pesticides after World War II, numerous wildlife species, especially carnivorous birds, have suffered sharp population declines. Contamination of rivers, lakes, and estuaries with industrial effluents threaten the sustained productivity of those ecosystems. The problem is even more acute in the developing nations, where environmental laws regulating toxic discharges are either weak or nonexistent and where many of the hazardous pesticides now banned in most industrialized countries are still widely and indiscriminately used (Tuxill, 1998).

Among the more noted casualties have been the beluga whales inhabiting the St. Lawrence River. Once numbering in the thousands, the belugas have dwindled to an estimated population of 700 animals, large numbers of which are afflicted with various types of tumors, ulcers, lesions, cysts, pneumonia, and reproductive problems. Scientists attribute the whales' plight to chemical contamination of the river with mercury, lead, PCBs, and various organochlorine pesticides. Analyses of tissue samples from dead belugas show concentrations of all these chemicals at levels far above those in whales from Arctic waters. While marine mammals and fish are particularly hard hit because of the toxic soup that constantly surrounds them in many waterways, polluted air also is taking its toll on sensitive species. In western Europe fungi appear to be dying off *en masse*, with a 40–50% loss of species in certain areas of Germany, Austria, and the Netherlands. Among those adversely affected are the mycorrhizal fungi that live in symbiotic association with plant roots, promoting the uptake of dissolved nutrients. The fact that these inconspicuous organisms play an important role in the normal functioning of many plant species gives their demise far-reaching significance (Wilson, 1992).

Yet another form of pollution, certain mining operations pose a serious hazard to migratory waterfowl species. The Natural Resources Defense Council (NRDC) estimates that as many as 100,000 birds die each year from swimming in ponds contaminated with toxic mining wastes. NRDC is particularly concerned about the threat to millions of birds posed by Canada's massive tar sands mining and drilling operations in Alberta's boreal forest, where critical habitat is being destroyed and toxic holding ponds created. Efforts to curb pollution will have a beneficial impact on the health of both humans and ecosystems.

Habitat Destruction

By far the greatest threat to biodiversity today—and the most difficult to control—is the destruction of those natural areas that wildlife require for breeding, feeding, or migrating. As the pressures of expanding populations and economies increase, forests are chopped down, swamps are drained, prairies are put to the plow, rivers are dammed. Some wildlife species can thrive in close proximity to humans; most cannot and perish when their natural habitat is destroyed or reduced in size below a critical minimum.

While there is little disagreement that preservation of biodiversity is a lost cause without a significantly greater commitment to conserving natural habitats, the question of how to maintain the integrity of dwindling expanses of forest, savannah, and grasslands at a time of exponentially increasing human needs is a vexing one for policy makers everywhere. Since 1872 when Yellowstone was established as the world's first national park, the conventional approach to preserving wild areas of great beauty or biological richness has been to set aside **protected areas** as wildlife refuges, national parks, or wilderness areas. Extending this concept to the ocean environment, some fisheries experts are now advocating marine reserves as the only effective way to save endangered fish stocks. Currently a few small, widely scattered "no-take zones" exist and have been very effective in boosting catches in nearby waters, but these collectively encompass only 0.01% of the ocean surface. In one of his last acts as President, George W. Bush in January 2009 designated a vast expanse of U.S.-controlled Pacific Ocean reefs, surface waters, sea floor, and islands as marine national monuments. This action limits fishing, mining, oil exploration, and other commercial activity in an area larger than Oregon and Washington combined and provides long-term protection of habitat critical to the survival of hundreds of species of rare birds and fish (Broder, 2009). Some biologists are calling for 20% of the oceans to be set aside as protected zones, though many concede that it would be virtually impossible to police such vast areas (Pauly and Watson, 2003).

Today 4% of the earth's total land surface has been set aside in approximately 8,000 protected areas worldwide, their natural wealth safeguarded by limiting human access to such areas. A modification of this approach is now being proposed by a number of promi-

nent biologists who fear the number of endangered species far outstrips current resources to protect them. They advocate a scheme to prioritize preservation efforts by identifying **biodiversity "hot spots"**—areas characterized by exceptionally high numbers of native species facing likely extinction due to extensive loss of habitat. By focusing available financial resources on these critical areas, society could reap the most benefit in terms of protecting species. These scientists have identified 25 such "hot spots" they deem worthy of special conservation efforts and are trying to attract funding to implement their proposals (Myers et al., 2000).

While the protected areas approach has been relatively successful, particularly in regions such as North America where population pressures are modest, trends suggest that in the years ahead preservation of critical habitat through reliance on government-established exclusion zones cannot adequately protect biodiversity and is ultimately doomed to failure. This is true for a number of reasons: (1) in most cases, the protected areas are too scattered, small, and fragmented to sustain the long-term stability of their biotic communities; ecologists have documented the adverse impact of crowding species into isolated "islands" of woodland or tropical forest, surrounded by a "sea" of farmlands or urban development. The "edge effect" experienced around the periphery of these fragmented habitats (i.e., increased exposure to wind, sunlight, decreased humidity, vulnerability to new predators) may result in the loss of many species highly adapted to life within a narrow range of environmental conditions; (2) many so-called protected areas, particularly those in developing countries, are protected in name only, since governments frequently lack the financial resources, the technical expertise, or the will to enforce their borders. The wide-scale poaching of endangered rhinos in East Africa or of tigers in India—both legally protected animals—is indicative of the difficulty many poor countries face in trying to safeguard their natural heritage; (3) finally, and perhaps most importantly, the protected area strategy doesn't take into account the fact that humans are an integral part of ecosystems also. Most of the areas set aside for wildlife once sustained the needs of local people who are now forbidden to hunt, fish, or grow crops on lands they once considered theirs to use. As growing human populations press against park boundaries, it will be impossible and, indeed, unjust, to forbid them the use of their own surroundings without providing viable alternatives for survival.

Accordingly, a radically different approach to habitat conservation has gradually been gaining adherents, an approach that attempts to make local communities both the beneficiaries and the custodians of efforts to safeguard biodiversity. Called **community-based conservation**, this concept recognizes that the exclusionary policies of the past, as embodied in the wildlife reserves, cannot be sustained in the face of mounting human poverty and hostility to programs that seem to place greater value on elephants or pandas than on people. Community-based conservation relies on positive grassroots participation, relinquishing the traditional top-down planning by central government officials in favor of involving local people in the planning, design, and implementation of conservation efforts which will benefit them directly and give them a personal stake in the successful outcome of such ventures. Community-based conservation efforts are quietly underway in a number of areas around the world and involve situations as diverse as the "extractive reserves" in Brazilian Amazonia, subsistence farming combined with ecotourism in Papua New Guinea, forest management by community councils in India, or incentive payments to private landowners for fostering biodiversity in England (Wright, 1993).

Another interesting approach to involve local people in wildlife conservation efforts is that of **biodiversity prospecting**—enlisting residents of species-rich tropical countries to assist in the search for plants or animals of potential medicinal, pesticidal, or agricultural value. Several bioprospecting agreements have been signed since the early 1990s between drug companies and national governments or institutes in the developing world (the U.S. National Parks Service has also indicated an interest in similar arrangements involving bioprospecting in such unique ecosystems as the hot springs at Yellowstone National Park). Merck & Co., the world's largest pharmaceutical corporation, now pays a private nonprofit organi-

zation in Costa Rica to send the company a steady supply of plant, animal, and microbial specimens to be analyzed for possible medicinal properties. Merck has agreed to pay royalties to its Costa Rican partner, the Instituto Nacional de Biodiversidad (INBIO), for any commercial products developed from Costa Rican specimens. It is assumed that once the biochemically active ingredient of a newly discovered species is identified, it will be possible to mass-produce an identical synthetic compound, thereby avoiding further exploitation of the species in its native habitat. By intimately involving local people in cataloging their country's biodiversity, INBIO gives Costa Ricans an in-depth understanding of their natural heritage and a personal stake in protecting it. Similar arrangements involving other pharmaceutical firms are now in effect in Ghana, Nigeria, and Surinam (Tuxill, 1998).

The shift in focus from preserving wildlife to acknowledging the need to factor human needs into the equation may be the only practical approach to saving as much biodiversity as possible, particularly at a time when human-modified landscapes are relentlessly expanding. Convincing local people that their own well-being can best be ensured by conserving and sustainably using the biological wealth of their surroundings may ultimately be the key to species preservation.

Climate Change

Although habitat loss is currently the greatest threat to biodiversity, climate change may become an equally important cause of species loss in future decades. An

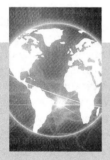

· · · · · · · *5-3* · · · · · · ·

Endangered "Rain Forests of the Sea"

Coral reefs constitute far more than a profitable tourist attraction. Sometimes dubbed "rain forests of the sea," coral reefs, especially those in warm shallow waters, harbor incredible biodiversity, providing habitat for an estimated 9 million species, including 4,000 species of fish. Offshore barrier reefs protect low-lying coastlands from the fury of tropical storms and provide a livelihood for 100 million people in developing countries who depend on reefs for subsistence fishing and tourism (Normile, 2009). Their enormous ecological and economic value make it especially worrisome that coral reefs today face unprecedented threats, both from natural disasters and human activities; moreover, climate change, if not averted, could doom them to extinction.

For decades marine biologists have documented reef degradation in various parts of the world, caused by factors such as urban development along coastlines, sedimentation from poor land-use practices, and pollution due to runoff of farm chemicals or untreated sewage discharges. Bottom-trawling fisheries, careless navigation practices by cruise ships, and scuba-divers or snorkelers collecting reef "souvenirs" have all taken their toll on these easily damaged underwater habitats. Over-harvesting of reef-dwelling fish and other marine creatures has been especially problematic, especially in recent years as fishers attempt to facilitate their efforts by using explosives to blast chunks of coral off reefs or pour cyanide into the water to stun fish that will subsequently be collected and sold to upscale restaurants. A flourishing trade in living red and pink corals, used both for jewelry and for aquarium decorations, also despoils reef ecosystems. By 2008, according to the Global Coral Reef Monitoring Network, 19% of the world's coral reef areas had been destroyed and another 15% could be lost by 2030 if no remedial actions are taken.

The actual toll could be far worse if predictions regarding climate change prove accurate—and a growing body of evidence suggests that global warming is already having a deleterious effect on some reef communities. The impacts of climate change on coral reefs are two-fold, causing (1) a rise in ocean temperature and (2) an increase in the acidity of seawater. The former is deleterious to the health of corals because it causes them to "bleach"—a process whereby the heat-stressed corals expel the symbiotic algae that provide them with nutrients and give them their distinctive color. "Bleached" corals appear unnaturally white and unless the algae return to their hosts within a few weeks, the coral will starve to death. Most corals require water temperatures in the range of 74–84°F (23–29°C) for optimal growth and even a slight increase in water temperature can cause some species to bleach, especially if the warming is prolonged. In 1998, unusually warm waters in the eastern Pacific resulted in the death of 16% of corals worldwide, with mortality rates reaching 70–80% of all shallow-water corals on many reefs in the Indo-Pacific region. Eventually many of the reefs affected were re-colonized and are gradually recovering, but others seem to have been irreversibly destroyed. In some of the affected regions, the 1998 bleaching event was followed by two subsequent bleachings, further undermining the reefs' ecological stability. Stresses imposed on coral colonies by warming sea waters or by pollution can also render reefs more susceptible to disease outbreaks, the rate of which seem to be increasing and affecting more reef species. Human activities contributing to reef degradation make recovery from bleaching even more difficult and have led some researchers to conclude that the risk of extinction for a number of coral species has increased significantly since 1998 (Carpenter et al., 2008). Scientists with the World Conservation Union's Species Survival Commission have assessed the potential susceptibility of 799 species of warm-water reef-forming corals to climate change-induced warming of the oceans. They concluded that 71% are at risk due to their sensitivity to temperature increases, both as adult polyps and free-living larvae, and warn that more than three-fourths of the species assessed could vanish if global temperatures continue to climb (Foden et al., 2008).

Equally problematic, though not yet quantified, is increasing acidification of the oceans due to increasing atmospheric concentrations of CO_2. Approximately 30% of the carbon dioxide released by fossil fuel combustion and other human activities has been absorbed by the world's oceans—the main reason that climate change to date has been relatively modest. However, the CO_2 absorbed by ocean waters reacts with dissolved carbonate ions to form carbonic acid, lowering seawater pH. Today the oceans are 30% more acidic than they were in the pre-industrial era—and that fact constitutes another threat to the survival of coral species. As soft-bodied larvae, young corals settle on a hard surface, acquire algal partners, and begin to secrete a hard skeleton by extracting calcium compounds from the water. The more acid the water becomes, the more difficult it becomes for the coral polyps to obtain the calcium they require. Research conducted on Australia's Great Barrier Reef showed that the rate at which corals absorbed calcium from seawater has dropped dramatically since 1990, resulting in slower growth of coral colonies. Since coral reefs are constantly eroding due to wave action, inability of the corals to calcify their skeletons quickly enough to keep pace with natural losses could have serious consequences for their long-term survival (Pennisi, 2009).

Ambitious but small-scale efforts to restore damaged or ailing reefs have been launched in Japan, the Philippines, Israel, and several other countries where researchers are experimenting with various methods—both high-tech and low-tech, including coral nurseries and coral transplants—in an effort to restore at least the functionality of reefs, if not their original biodiversity and beauty. Some experts doubt that these efforts, even if greatly expanded in scope, will make much difference, arguing that the only way to save reefs is to eliminate the stresses causing their degradation (Normile, 2009). Restoration tasks will be much more difficult if action to combat climate change is delayed and ocean temperatures continue to rise. If bleaching events become more frequent, and especially if other human-generated pressures persist, corals may be unable to maintain breeding populations and could experience irreversible declines. If that happens, large-scale loss of biodiversity is inevitable.

international group of researchers based in the United Kingdom warns that anticipated increases in average global temperatures caused by human-generated greenhouse gas emissions may become a significant cause of species extinctions by the mid-21st century. As temperatures rise, provoking habitat change, many species living in those areas will either die out or move elsewhere. However, fragmentation of habitat could make such migration impossible and even if species succeed in reaching a new area of suitable climate, inappropriate soils or lack of food resources may prevent establishment of a viable population. For those species remaining in the original climate-altered habitat, the encroachment of invasive species moving in from disturbed ecosystems elsewhere may be the "straw that breaks the camel's back," precipitating their descent to oblivion. Estimates of the number of species "committed to extinction" vary in direct proportion to the amount of warming realized, with higher temperatures producing the greatest impact on species loss. Accordingly, concerned scientists are urging governments to implement policies for reducing greenhouse gas emissions as rapidly as possible in order to minimize the ultimate extent of climate change and thereby save a substantial percentage of species from extinction (Thomas et al., 2004).

Protecting Biodiversity: The Endangered Species Act

Since its enactment in 1973, the **Endangered Species Act (ESA)** has constituted the nation's most effective weapon for ensuring the survival of native plants and animals. Probably the toughest wildlife protection law anywhere in the world, the ESA prohibits the killing, collecting, harassment, or capture of any species listed by the U.S. Fish and Wildlife Service (FWS) as "endangered" or "threatened." It also provides strict protection for the critical habitat of endangered species and requires FWS to develop recovery programs for each species listed. By mid-2010, FWS had officially designated 1,371 U.S. species as endangered or threatened (576 animals and 795 plants), up from just 78 in 1967 when the original endangered species list was compiled.

While environmentalists hail the ESA for noticeably slowing the pace of wildlife extinction in the United States, citing as evidence the fact that 60 endangered species have increased their numbers or expanded their range since being listed, opponents strive to weaken the law whenever it comes up for reauthorization. Charging that the act has excessive power to supersede individual property rights, hinder economic progress, and threaten jobs, such disparate constituencies as land developers, Gulf Coast shrimpers, and loggers in the Pacific Northwest would like to see the act significantly weakened.

These groups raise the question of how much biological diversity can or should be preserved, especially when the species in question isn't particularly cute or fuzzy. Some people find it hard to get emotional about the Colorado squawfish or the scrub plum!

ESA defenders point out that, for the vast majority of protected species, recovery plans seldom provoke conflict. Perhaps one explanation for increasing antagonism toward ESA is the fact that in recent years it has begun to affect entire regions rather than just isolated projects, as was generally the case in the past. For example, in the early 1990s attempts to save the northern spotted owl by declaring large areas of the Northwest's old-growth forest off-limits for timber harvesting prompted vociferous complaints that the ESA favors wildlife over people.

In fact, contrary to detractors' claims, the ESA *does* make an effort to accommodate societal concerns. Economic considerations are taken into account to some degree when designations of critical habitat are made; in situations where proposed projects threaten endangered species, the act requires that an effort be made to find alternative means of carrying out the activity without endangering survival of the species in question. In those rare cases where the conflict is irreconcilable, an official panel (the "God Squad") can give the green light to projects deemed of sufficient importance, even if this action constitutes a death sentence for an endangered species.

Even supporters admit, however, that implementation of ESA is in need of improvement. To some extent, problems center around insufficient money and personnel to carry out the intent of the act. Even more problematic is the cumbersome process of officially listing rare species as threatened or endangered. Frequently the official designation comes so late that populations of the species in question may already be too low to halt the slide into oblivion. In other cases, only costly rescue missions such as captive breeding programs can guarantee long-term survival, when earlier action could have achieved success through less extreme measures. Although studies suggest that a minimum population in the low thousands is a prerequisite for viable vertebrate populations, the average number of individuals remaining in vertebrate groups listed as endangered was just 1,075; for invertebrates it was even lower—999. For plants, the average number of remaining specimens in at-risk populations at the time of official listing is a mere 120, making recovery of such species extremely difficult. Biologists suggest that the minuscule number of species that have rebounded and been removed from the endangered list can be explained by the fact that official designation often comes too late to implement effective recovery plans.

In spite of its limitations, the Endangered Species Act can claim its share of notable success stories. Although only 21 species have been delisted as "recovered," a number of others have made a remarkable comeback from near-extinction. These include the bald eagle, the American alligator, the whooping crane, peregrine falcon, California sea otter, grizzly bear, black-footed ferret, and the red wolf. All now have a new lease on life, thanks to the Endangered Species Act.

While ESA historically has focused on protecting individual species on a case-by-case basis, a 1982 amendment established an alternative approach to preserving biodiversity known as **habitat conservation planning (HCP).** Devised as a way of striking a balance between pressures for economic growth and habitat preservation, HCP allows landowners to develop property occupied by endangered species if they agree to minimize the loss of critical habitat or offset that loss by providing additional land nearby. While this approach implicitly permits the loss of some members of the endangered species in question, it guarantees that enough critical habitat will be preserved to sustain the remainder of that population indefinitely. Drawing up an acceptable plan may involve years of negotiations among developers, environmentalists, local governments, and Fish and Wildlife Service personnel who supervise the process and must ultimately approve the plan. Nevertheless, both environmentalists and property rights advocates are supportive of the HCP concept, the former seeing it as a way of winning concessions from landowners who might otherwise ignore the law, the latter preferring negotiated plans rather than blanket restrictions on land use.

By 2009, 660 habitat conservation plans had been approved, protecting more than 544 species. The HCP process has been particularly important in southern California, where intense development pressures on biologically rich natural areas have pitted preservationists against developers for years. In 1993 Interior Secretary Bruce Babbitt worked out an agreement between environmentalists and developers who had been at loggerheads for years over the fate of a diminutive songbird, the California gnatcatcher. Since fewer than 3,000 nesting pairs remained in the 250,000 acres of sage scrub stretching along the Pacific Coast from Los Angeles to San Diego, environmentalists had been demanding that the Fish and Wildlife Service list the gnatcatcher as endangered; developers were adamant that such action, automatically triggering prohibitions on the use of valuable real estate, would impose serious economic hardships. Under the HCP brokered by Babbitt, the gnatcatcher was listed as merely "threatened" rather than "endangered," thus permitting a more flexible recovery plan; in return, development interests agreed to protect critical habitat by setting aside up to 12 reserves, an act that benefited not only the gnatcatcher, but as many as 40 other species as well. Habitat conservation planning has continued to win proponents throughout southern California, particularly in the San Diego area where what has been billed as a model HCP was approved by the city council in 1997. Under the agreed-upon arrangement, specified natural areas adjacent to the city will be acquired and permanently set aside for habitat preservation while other still-open lands will be available for unrestricted development.

While experience with habitat conservation planning is not yet extensive enough to render a verdict on its ability to save species, hopes are high that it provides a means for avoiding bitter confrontations and halting the decline of species long before their situation deteriorates beyond redemption.

We have met the enemy, and it is us.
—Walt Kelly

······· Part 2 ·······

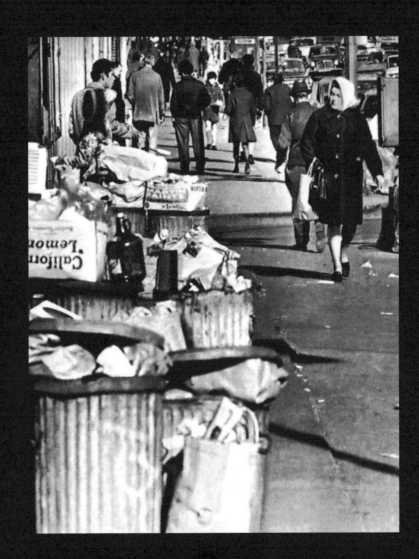

Our Toxic Environment

Does Everything Cause Cancer?

Newspaper headlines screaming "Ozone Alert!"; a $1 million damage settlement to an asbestos worker's widow; public protests over a leaking hazardous waste dump; migrant workers hospitalized for pesticide poisoning; accidental sewage discharge forcing closure of public beaches—such situations represent but a handful of the issues daily facing modern society in which some aspect of environmental quality has a direct impact on human health.

From primitive times up until the mid-19th century, the idea that health and disease were determined, at least in part, by environmental factors was widely accepted (witness the belief that night air precipitated fever and chills). The mid-1800s, however, marked a period of rapid progress in research relating to disease causation. The discovery of the anthrax bacterium by the German microbiologist Robert Koch and his demonstration in 1877 that this organism was responsible for an important human disease revolutionized society's view of health. For the next 70 years virtually all human ailments were blamed on pathogenic organisms such as bacteria, viruses, and protozoans. It was widely assumed that the development of preventative vaccines or curative antibiotics should be our main focus in protecting public health.

More recently, however, recognition of the role that deprivation or stress can play in initiating serious health problems, as well as the sharp increase of the so-called "degenerative diseases" (cardiovascular disease, cancer, hypertension) have led to the realization that good health depends on more than just the absence of disease-causing microorganisms. Some of today's most prevalent ills are increasingly blamed on toxic environmental contaminants—synthetic chemical wastes carelessly dumped in waterways or landfills, products of combustion spewed into the air, pesticide residues in the food we eat. Other illnesses are associated with personal habits that in the broad sense can be considered aspects of environmental quality—smoking, drinking, high-fat diets, lack of regular exercise. Perception of the threat that such factors pose to human well-being provided the main thrust behind the modern environmental movement. Preservation—or restoration—of environmental quality means far more than protecting bald eagles or ensuring that the last coastal redwood isn't converted into a picnic table; the prime emphasis among environmental advocates has always been the protection of human health, with the implicit recognition that human well-being is inextricably intertwined with the health and stability of the natural ecosystems of which we form an integral part.

While not a perfect standard, the health status of societies is often measured in terms of life expectancy—the number of years an average individual in that society can expect to live. In terms of longevity, health conditions in the Western world have improved markedly in recent centuries. Whereas in the days of Roman emperors the average life expectancy at birth was about 30 years, today in most industrialized countries it has reached 77 years, up from 50 years at the turn of the century (Japanese are currently the world's longest-lived people, with an average life expectancy of 83, compared to 78 in the United States and 81 in Canada). Among the developing nations average longevity is more variable, ranging from a low of 41 in Lesotho (due largely to the AIDS epidemic) to the mid-40s in Afghanistan and some African countries to the mid-70s in parts of Latin America and the Caribbean. Many people, looking at such statistics, assume that the major factor accounting for

124

increased longevity worldwide was the introduction of modern medicines and pesticides that provided the first really effective weapons against many of the infectious epidemic diseases. While medical science undoubtedly played a part in reducing mortality rates, many observers feel that a more fundamental factor was a general improvement in living conditions: better nutritional levels made possible by increased agricultural productivity; improved sanitary conditions as a result of sewer system construction; the provision of safe drinking water supplies; refuse collection; sewage treatment; the enforcement of housing codes, and so forth. Rising incomes, increasing levels of education, mass communications, and improved standards of personal hygiene also have been extremely important determinants in furthering the health advances observed in most parts of the world.

However, we seem to have now reached a longevity plateau and are no longer observing a continued rapid drop in death rates such as characterized the years between 1950–1960. Indeed, longevity is actually declining in Russia, where high levels of pollution, added to the ravages of alcoholism and substandard health care, have caused male life expectancy to fall to 62 years, the lowest for any industrialized country (female life expectancy has remained stable at 74 years). There appears to be general agreement that future gains will come, not so much through new medical discoveries, but when—and only when—essential preconditions of better health are everywhere available. These essential preconditions relate largely to environmental considerations: sufficient quantities of uncontaminated water, elimination of malnutrition, proper handling and disposal of human wastes, control of toxic pollutants, adoption of healthier personal lifestyles. The environmentally induced diseases currently plaguing much of humanity can best be controlled through a strategy of prevention, rather than cure, requiring not only application of technology but also social, political, and behavioral changes. Adopting such a strategy and enlisting the public support necessary to attain the goal of a healthful society require a thorough understanding of the issues and dilemmas involved. The following chapters will delineate the major concerns regarding our increasingly toxic environment and the health implications inherent in our present lifestyle; they also attempt to show that improving human health and enhancing environmental quality are but two sides of the same coin.

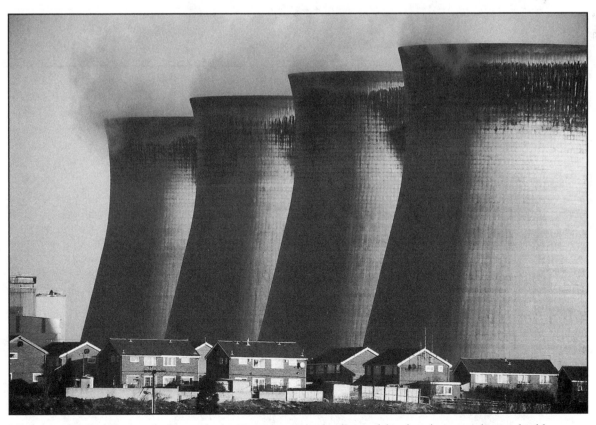

Modern society is daily assaulted by toxics in our environment that have a deleterious impact on human health.

········ 6 ········

Environmental illness is simply an incurable disease.
There is no cure. It can only be prevented.
—Barry Commoner, 1990

Environmental Disease

Polluted air and water, excessive levels of noise, sunshine, nuclear weapons fall-out, overcrowded slums, toxic waste dumps, inadequate or overly adequate diet, stress, food contaminants, medical X-rays, drugs, cigarettes, unsafe working conditions—these comprise but a partial listing of the many environmental factors which, through their adverse impact on human health, can be regarded as causative agents of environmental disease. In recent decades public concern about rising levels of pollution and environmental degradation has increasingly focused on the question of whether such trends may be influencing disease rates, particularly ailments such as heart disease, cancer, and stroke. If such a connection exists, as virtually all authorities agree it does, then society's response should be clear: most environmentally induced diseases, unlike those caused by bacteria or other pathogens, are difficult to cure but theoretically simple to prevent; remove the adverse environmental influence and the ailment will disappear. In other words, by preventing the discharge of poisons into our air, water, and food, by avoiding exposure to radiation, by refusing to fill our lungs with cigarette smoke or our stomachs with saturated fats, we can protect our health far more effectively and cheaply than we can by desperately searching for a cure after our bodies succumb to a malignancy or degeneration of vital organs or when our children are born deformed. The old adage, "Prevention is the best cure," has never been more true than when applied to environmentally induced disease.

In spite of the fact that environmental factors can affect human health in many ways, the focus of most concern today in this age of toxic pollutants is on those substances that, in ways not yet completely understood, act at the cellular level to initiate often irreversible changes that can kill or damage the cell. Although health damage due to environmental pollutants may be manifested by outward symptoms, research has shown that such contaminants in fact act at the level of an individual cell or cells. In spite of its small size, the cell is an exceptionally complex structure—the end product of billions of years of evolution and natural selection in response to existing environmental conditions. Thus it should not be surprising to find that a sudden change in the environment (e.g., exposure to X-rays, synthetic organic chemicals, heavy metals, etc.) to which a cell has become so finely adapted can kill or injure the cell. Cell death, in many respects, is a lesser concern than cell injury because it has no further implications. Cell damage, on the other hand, has more ominous implications. The subject of extensive scientific and medical research for the past half century, cell damage can be manifested as mutations, birth defects, or cancer.

MUTATION

Mutation, defined as any change in the genetic material, is perhaps the most worrisome type of cell damage because of its potential for harming not only the person or organism with the mutant cell but, if the mutation occurs in an egg or sperm, unborn generations as well. To understand the impact of mutation, it is necessary to examine the nature of the hereditary material itself.

The most conspicuous organelle in most cells is the nucleus, readily visible under an ordinary light microscope. The nucleus contains threadlike structures called **chromosomes**; each species of plant or animal has its own characteristic number of chromosomes per cell. In humans the normal chromosome number is 46. When cells undergo **mitosis** (cell division), each chromosome splits longitudinally into two daughter **chromatids**, one of which goes into each of the two newly forming cells. Thus the number of chromosomes per nucleus remains constant and the hereditary material contained within the chromosomes is equally shared.

Chemically, each chromosome consists of a single giant molecule of DNA (deoxyribonucleic acid) and associated histone and nonhistone proteins. The DNA molecule itself is composed of two antiparallel strands of alternating units of a five-carbon sugar and phosphate molecules, cross-linked by one of four different nitrogenous bases (adenine, guanine, thymine, and cytosine), and twisted into a helical configuration (see figure 6-2). The pairing of the nitrogenous bases is quite specific: adenine can pair only with thymine and guanine with cytosine. Along any one strand bases can occur in any sequence, but once the order on one strand is given, the sequence on the antiparallel strand is automatically determined. The adenine-thymine (A-T) or guanine-cytosine (G-C) combination making up each cross-connection is referred to as a **base pair**.

DNA is vitally important to cellular function and is often referred to as the "Master Molecule" because (1) it passes genetic information from one generation to the next and (2) it controls cellular metabolism by giving the instructions for protein synthesis. The hereditary charac-

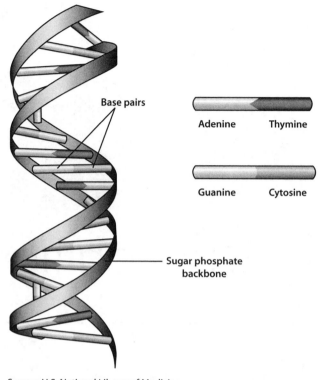

Source: U.S. National Library of Medicine.

Figure 6-2   DNA Double Helix

teristics are controlled by **genes** along the length of the chromosome. In essence, a gene is a section of chromosome consisting of thousands of base pairs. Genes are responsible for the production of proteins necessary for proper cell function. It is absolutely essential that the integrity of the DNA molecule be maintained if the correct information for protein synthesis is to be passed from one generation to the next. Any change within the gene constitutes a mutation.

Types of Mutations

There are two basic types of mutations recognized.

"Point" Mutation (Single Gene Mutation)

By far the most common type of mutation, point mutations involve a change at the molecular level within a gene. Such a change could consist of the deletion, addition, or substitution of a single base pair or could involve a small portion of a single gene (e.g., a so-called "jumping gene," more properly referred to as a **transposable**

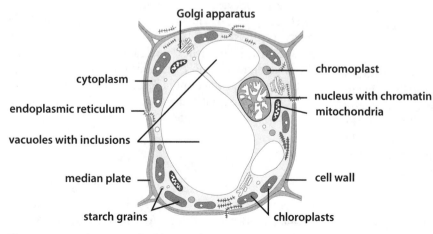

Figure 6-1   Diagram of a Plant Cell

element). Any of these changes would result in the "misreading" of the genetic code (the sequence of bases along a DNA strand is all-important; any change can result in the wrong protein being formed). The severity of a point mutation depends on precisely where within a gene the change occurs; it can range from being lethal to causing an almost imperceptible loss of vigor. Point mutations are now known to be responsible for several serious human ailments, including sickle-cell anemia, hemophilia, diabetes, and achondroplastic dwarfism. Though such ailments are tragic for the victim (prior to modern forms of treatment, which are only partially effective, these diseases invariably resulted in death at a fairly early age), many geneticists are more concerned about the accumulation of sub-lethal mutations in populations. Such sub-lethal mutations don't kill their victims outright, but render them less fit than they would otherwise be. Examples of the types of impairment that could result from a sub-lethal mutation include reduced physical or mental vigor, shortened life span, increased susceptibility to disease, or varying degrees of malformation of some organ. Such changes, though possibly debilitating, nevertheless permit afflicted individuals to survive, reproduce, and pass altered genes on to succeeding generations.

Chromosome Abnormalities

Chromosome abnormalities are thought to be the leading cause of fetal loss, responsible for half of all first trimester miscarriages and 20% of spontaneous abortions during the second trimester. They also are regarded as the primary cause of intellectual disability. Chromosome abnormalities can include the loss or addition of sizeable pieces of a chromosome or the reversal of parts of the same chromosome—events that most commonly occur during a stage of meiosis (reduction division) when the homologous chromosomes are in synapsis and crossing-over takes place. Although some of these rearrangements seem to have little outward effect, others can have serious consequences. In humans, the reciprocal translocation of sections of chromosomes 9 and 22 represents a specific chromosomal abnormality (the "Philadelphia chromosome") that results in the development of chronic myelogenous leukemia, a form of cancer. Rearrangements of chromosomal material have now been observed in more than 40 different kinds of cancer (Jorde et al., 1999).

A second type of chromosome abnormality involves a change in the number of chromosomes within the nucleus of a cell. This situation occurs when paired homologous chromosomes fail to separate (nondisjunction) during meiosis, resulting in some cells with more than the normal chromosome number, others with less. In some cases, a change in chromosome number can be lethal. Having three copies (**trisomy**) of chromosome 16 is relatively common in the very early stages of human development; however, none of the fetuses characterized by this condition ever survives to birth. Trisomy of chromosomes 13 and 18 also is seen relatively often in fetuses miscarried during the first few months of pregnancy, but the condition is extremely rare among liveborn infants and almost all of them die soon after birth (Sack, 1999).

The best known human ailment resulting from a change in chromosome number is Down syndrome. Afflicting about one baby out of every 800 live births, Down syndrome, in most cases, results in intellectual disability (IQ seldom exceeds 70) as well as below-average physical and psychomotor skills. Victims often exhibit heart malformations and respiratory problems; few live beyond the age of 50. Down syndrome occurs due to the presence in the person's cells of 47 chromosomes instead of the normal 46 (to be more precise, three copies of chromosome 21 rather than two). Interestingly, the likelihood of a woman's giving birth to a Down syndrome child increases as the mother gets older. While the likelihood of a 30-year-old woman giving birth to a Down syndrome child is one in 1,000, the risk at age 35 rises to one in 400; at age 40 it increases tenfold, to one in 100; at 45, it is still higher—one out of every 50 infants is likely to be a Down syndrome baby. Although the reason for

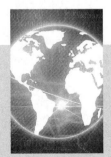

········ 6-1 ········

Microbial Killers

Toxic chemical pollutants may be the current "hot button" issue among many environmentalists today, but historically the primary focus of environmental health practitioners has been reducing the incidence of infectious epidemic disease. Fostered by poor living conditions and spread through contaminated food and water, bacterial, viral, and parasitic pathogens have been responsible for the vast majority of human deaths from time immemorial until the early 20th century. Even today throughout much of the developing world, infectious killers such as tuberculosis, malaria, and diarrheal diseases remain leading causes of mortality.

In North America and Europe, however, deaths caused by infectious microbes began to decline noticeably about 100 years ago, thanks in large part to drinking water purification, sewage treatment, and vector control. In the United States, infectious disease mortality rates dropped by approximately 2.8% annually between 1900 and 1937 (with the exception of 1918 when a worldwide outbreak of "Spanish flu" sent death rates soaring everywhere). From 1937 until 1952, mortality rates due to infectious diseases dropped even more precipitously—8.2% per year—as cases of pneumonia, influenza, and tuberculosis plummeted (Armstrong et al., 1999). These years witnessed the introduction of powerful new antibacterial drugs—sulfonamides, penicillin, streptomycin, isoniazid—but it's likely that a number of factors in addition to improved medications account for mortality declines. From the mid-1950s until 1980 infectious disease death rates continued to drop, albeit more slowly than during the preceding 15 years. By this time it had become an article of faith that humankind (or at least those fortunate enough to live in affluent, sanitized, well-fed nations) had forever left behind the "age of pestilence and famine"—characterized by high rates of infectious disease mortality, especially among children and young adults. We had transitioned, so it was believed, into the modern age of degenerative diseases where most deaths occur among the elderly and are due to chronic ills such as cardiovascular disease or cancer.

Dismissal of microbial threats as a thing of the past proved premature, however. In 1981 medical recognition of Acquired Immune Deficiency Syndrome (AIDS) reminded the world that pathogens still lurk among human populations. From 1981–1996 the U.S. witnessed a steady rise in mortality rates due to infectious diseases, primarily AIDS and tuberculosis. Unfortunately, AIDS was only the first of several frightening diseases to make headlines over the past several decades. Medical researchers now speak of "newly emerging pathogens" to describe outbreaks of previously unknown ailments such as Lassa fever, Legionnaires' Disease, toxic shock syndrome, Ebola virus, hantavirus, E. coli 0157:H7 food poisoning, and SARS (Severe Acute Respiratory Syndrome). In addition, old microbial diseases are now showing up in new places, South America's cholera epidemic of the mid-1990s being a case in point (Armstrong et al., 1999).

Other killers of yesteryear are surfacing in new forms; in late 1997, "bird flu"—a strain of influenza previously documented only among avian species—broke out in Hong Kong, killing four of the 16 people infected. A new and even more ominous strain of avian influenza, H5N1, surfaced in late 2003 in several southeast Asian countries. The causative virus, continually mutating to more dangerous forms, jumped from birds to people, sickening 250, terrifying millions, and resulting in more than 100 deaths worldwide before the outbreak subsided. Global health experts are extremely worried that if this highly lethal pathogen develops the ability to spread person-to-person, a global pandemic will result, ravaging populations worldwide, since no baseline immunity currently exists against this new disease. In 2009 another flu variant, termed H1N1 or "swine flu," emerged in Mexico and quickly spread worldwide. By the end of that year it had affected more than 200 countries and overseas territories and resulted in an estimated 12,200 deaths, according to WHO data. Fortunately, the virus proved to be much less deadly than originally feared; humanity seemed to have "dodged the bullet" so far at H1N1 was concerned, but health authorities worry that the world may not be so lucky next time—and they're certain there *will* be a next time.

AIDS may be the first large-scale modern epidemic of infectious disease, but almost certainly it won't be the last. The world today is more vulnerable than ever before to the global spread of infections. As ever-more crowded human populations invade previously undisturbed ecosystems, especially in the tropics, opportunities for contact with animal pathogens proliferate. The rapid expansion of global commerce and tourism provide easy access for microbes on one continent to travel quickly to distant locations, either riding along with cargo, harbored by stowaway insects, or incubating in the bodies of travelers. Unfortunately, the Western world's single-minded preoccupation with finding a cure for cancer and other degenerative diseases has caused us largely to ignore the microbial pathogens that remain an ever-present threat. The nations of the world still lack an "early warning system" to ensure the quick detection of new diseases when they first appear or to identify old diseases when they show up in unexpected places or in clever disguises. Continued delay in confronting this challenge due to a misplaced faith in humanity's supposed conquest of infectious disease is a risky tactic. As Dr. Richard Krause of the U.S. National Institutes of Health commented more than 25 years ago, "Plagues are as certain as death and taxes" (Garrett, 1994).

the increased frequency of this birth defect among older mothers is not known with certainty, the prevailing theory is that the rate of nondisjunction is considerably higher among older women, possibly due to impairment of aging egg cells (since each female child is born with all the egg cells she will ever have, by the time the mother is 45 years old, her eggs are 45 years old also). Given the enhanced risk, it is now common practice for pregnant women 35 or older to undergo a prenatal diagnostic procedure such as **amniocentesis** or **chorionic villus sampling**. By removing and culturing fetal cells, medical personnel can determine whether the developing child has Down syndrome or any of approximately 100 other genetic diseases. If test results are positive, the parents then have the option of terminating the pregnancy.

It is widely recognized that congenital abnormalities occur with greater frequency among babies of older mothers, but less commonly known is that older fathers also have a greater chance of passing on defective genes to their offspring. Approximately 20 different genetic disorders have been correlated with increasing paternal age, including achondroplastic dwarfism, Apert syndrome (characterized by head, facial, and limb abnormalities), and schizophrenia. Since the number of mutations present in sperm cells increases as men grow older, some European countries now prohibit men from becoming sperm donors once they pass a certain age (Thacker, 2004).

Two other human abnormalities resulting from a change in chromosome number are Klinefelter's syndrome, found only in males, and Turner's syndrome, restricted to females. Whereas a normal man has an X and a Y sex chromosome, victims of Klinefelter's syndrome have an extra X, or 47 chromosomes altogether. This condition, one of the most common of all genetic abnormalities, can cause a variety of problems, ranging from learning disabilities, language difficulties, behavioral problems, infertility, and, in about one-third of cases, enlargement of the breasts following puberty. Many of these symptoms respond to therapy, enabling Klinefelter males to lead normal, productive lives even though they will never be able to father children (nevertheless, many marry and are sexually active). The frequency of Klinefelter's births is relatively high—about one out of every 1,000 male births—and is more prevalent among children of older mothers. Turner's syndrome, by contrast, occurs when one X chromosome is missing; i.e., the victim has only one sex chromosome, for a total of 45 instead of the normal 46. This malady is outwardly expressed by retarded sexual development (no breast development, failure to menstruate or ovulate), unusually short stature (generally under 5 feet), a webbed neck, and broad chest. Treatment methods developed within recent years have made it possible for an increasing number of Turner's syndrome women to live near-normal lives. Interestingly, the incidence of Turner's syndrome is far lower than that of Klinefelter's—about one in 3,000 female births. This discrepancy appears to be due to a very high rate of intrauterine deaths among fetuses with only one sex chromosome (Jorde et al., 1999).

Cause of Mutations

That mutations occur is not in question; their underlying cause is less well understood. A great many mutations occur spontaneously due to natural causes. Some of these spontaneous mutations have been attributed to radiation exposure from cosmic rays and radioactive minerals in the earth's crust. However, it is thought that such relatively low levels of background radiation are insufficient to account for the majority of spontaneous mutations, the cause of which remains a mystery.

Since the early 1900s, several substances identified as capable of inducing mutations have been introduced into the human environment and have raised serious concerns within the scientific community regarding their potential for increasing mutation rates. Such substances are known as **mutagens**. X-rays were the first mutagens to be recognized, their mutagenic effect on fruit flies being described in 1927 by the great geneticist H. J. Muller at Indiana University. Subsequently a number of chemical compounds have been found to possess mutagenic properties, among them formaldehyde, mustard gas, nitrous acid, colchicine, and vinyl chloride. Many other candidates are now under suspicion as being possible mutagens.

Mutation Rates

Although the probability of any given human gene in an egg or sperm cell undergoing a spontaneous mutation is difficult to estimate accurately, it is generally regarded as low. However, one must keep in mind that each person has about 20,000–25,000 genes (Human Genome Sequencing Consortium, 2004). The chances of a mutation occurring in at least one of those genes are thus quite large. In fact, the English geneticist Harry Harris asserts that, on the average, every newborn child may be "expected, as the result of a new mutation in either of its parents, to synthesize at least one structurally variant enzyme or protein." Since only those mutations that occur in an egg or sperm have the potential to be passed on to subsequent generations, studies of mutation frequency have focused on these so-called genetic mutations. Typically, mutations occurring in a person's sex cells have no effect upon him or her but present a risk to succeeding generations of offspring. On the other hand, a mutation occurring in any cell other than an egg or sperm (somatic mutation) can adversely affect the person who sustained the mutation, but such injury will not be inherited by his or her children and thus represents no threat to the human gene pool.

In this context, it is of interest to note that about a third of pregnancies spontaneously abort after implantation of the fertilized egg (it's unknown how many are lost prior to implantation). Geneticists estimate that at least 10–15% of conceptions exhibit some chromosome abnormality and that a significant portion of fetal loss can be attributed to these mutations (Jorde et al., 1999).

The great concern among geneticists today is that exposure of populations to the artificial mutagens so common in the modern environment could further increase mutation rates. Since most mutations are harmful to some degree, it is in humanity's long-term interest to keep mutation rates as low as possible.

BIRTH DEFECTS

As we have seen in the previous section, mutations in parents' sex cells can result in their children being born with structural or functional abnormalities, but by no means are all birth defects due to mutations. The CDC (Centers for Disease Control and Prevention) estimates that major birth defects affect approximately 3% of all births in the United States each year (CDC, 2008e); mutations are believed to account for approximately 25% of the total. Since birth defects constitute the leading cause of infant mortality in the United States and are responsible for billions of dollars spent for medical care, efforts to understand why fetal malformation occurs and how to prevent such a tragic course of events assume added urgency.

Living things are far more sensitive to adverse environmental influences during their early stages of development than they are at any other time. Embryos that are perfectly normal genetically can be seriously or fatally damaged if exposed to extraneous hazards. Investigations over the past several decades have revealed the sad truth that the womb is not the safe haven it was once assumed to be.

The likelihood that all abnormal development is triggered by some aspect of the environment (even hereditary disorders were at some point initiated by a mutation) has given rise to the science of **teratology**—the study of abnormal formations in animals or plants—and to the search for **teratogens,** substances that cause birth defects.

Interest in birth abnormalities is undoubtedly as old as humanity itself, although prior to the 20th century most ideas regarding birth defects involved considerably more fantasy than fact. From ancient times until fairly recently, some societies believed that the emotional state and visual impressions of an expectant mother could influence the physical development of her child. For this reason women in ancient Greece were encouraged to gaze at statuary representing the ideal human form, while Norwegian mothers-to-be were cautioned against looking at rabbits, for fear their babies would be born with harelip! The Babylonians and Sumerians regarded certain types of malformations as portents of coming events; medieval Europeans regarded them as evidence that the mother had indulged in intercourse with Satan or other demons and occasionally used this as an excuse to execute the mother and child. The so-called "Theory of Divine Retribution," also prevalent in Europe during the Middle Ages, viewed the birth of a defective child as God's punishment on the parents for past sins.

With the rebirth of scientific inquiry in the Western world following the Renaissance, less mythical interpretations of teratogenesis were sought. In the 17th century birth defects were attributed to such factors as the narrowness of the mother's uterus, poor posture of the pregnant woman, or to a fall or blow on the abdomen during pregnancy. Though inaccurate, these explanations at least were an attempt to find a rational explanation for what remained a mysterious phenomenon. Gregor Mendel's discovery of the laws of genetics, followed by an explosion of research into the mechanism of heredity, led in the early 20th century to acceptance of the idea that all developmental errors could be attributed to faulty genes. This view prevailed until the mid-20th century, but a series of significant discoveries and observations since that time has once again altered our perception regarding teratogenesis and has given new impetus and urgency to the field of teratology.

The first key discovery to contradict the prevailing view that heredity is all-important emerged from animal studies investigating the influence of maternal diet on the outcome of pregnancy. In 1940 a report was published showing that specific types of nutritional deficiencies in pregnant rats caused predictable types and percentages of malformations in their offspring (Warkany, 1972). This finding effectively shattered old ideas about the overriding importance of genes and the conviction that the fetus could parasitize the mother if necessary to ensure normal development. Continued research into the influence of maternal diet on fetal development has confirmed and broadened these original findings. It is now known that a wide range of nutrients, from proteins to trace minerals to specific amino acids, are essential for normal development. Conversely, an excess of some of these necessary substances (e.g., phenylalanine, vitamin A) can exert teratogenic effects. Among the birth abnormalities associated with a specific nutritional deficiency are neural tube defects such as spina bifida and anencephaly. Recognition that up to 75% of these devastating birth abnormalities could be prevented simply by increasing a pregnant woman's dietary intake of **folic acid,** one of the B vitamins, led the FDA to mandate the fortification of flour, corn meal, pasta, and rice with this micronutrient. The FDA action, which took

Table 6-1   Some Known Human Teratogens

Teratogen	Effect
Ionizing Radiation	
X-rays	central nervous system disorders, micro-
Nuclear fallout	cephaly, eye problems, mental retardation
Pathogenic Infections	
German measles	congenital heart defect, deafness, cataracts
Syphilis and herpes simplex type 2	mental retardation, microcephaly
Cytomegalovirus	kidney and liver disorders, pneumonia, brain damage
Toxoplasmosis	fatal lesions in the central nervous system
Drugs and Chemicals	
Thalidomide	phocomelia
Methyl mercury	mental retardation, sensory and motor problems
DES	vaginal cancer in girls, genital abnormalities in boys
Dioxin	structural deformities, miscarriages
Anesthesia	miscarriages, structural deformities
Alcohol	mental retardation, growth deficiencies, microcephaly, facial irregularities
Cigarette smoke	low birth weight, miscarriage, stillbirth
Dilantin	heart malformations, cleft palate, harelip, mental retardation, microcephaly
Valproic acid	spina bifida
Accutane	cardiovascular abnormalities, deformation of the ear, hydrocephaly, microcephaly
Tegison	same effect as for Accutane

effect on January 1, 1998, marks the first time the federal agency has required fortification of a food for the express purpose of preventing a birth defect.

In 1941 an unusually large number of babies in both the United States and Australia were born suffering from congenital cataracts, heart defects, or deafness. Epidemiological studies launched to try to determine the cause for such an outbreak found that the only common thread linking all the victims was the fact that during the first trimester of pregnancy, their mothers had contracted German measles (*Rubella*), which had reached epidemic proportions that year. The fact that a virus could cross the placental barrier and damage the fetus was thus established.

While these two developments demonstrated that mammalian embryos are vulnerable to such commonplace environmental influences as inadequate diet and infections, the most dramatic confirmation that certain environmental factors (in this case an artificially synthesized drug) must be regarded as a potential risk to the unborn came in the early 1960s with revelation of what has since become known as the "Thalidomide Tragedy."

Thalidomide was a drug first synthesized by a pharmaceutical company in Germany in 1953 and subsequently developed and widely marketed in western Europe as a mild sedative and as a treatment for morning sickness. Preliminary testing on laboratory animals indicated that thalidomide had little injurious effect even when taken in quantity (in fact, humans who attempted to commit suicide using the drug survived extremely large doses). With evidence of its safety regarding overdosing, but with virtually no testing for other side effects, the German manufacturer put thalidomide on the market as a nonprescription sleeping pill. Thanks to an aggressive advertising campaign stressing its safety, thalidomide (sold under the trade name *Cantergan*) became the most widely used sedative in Germany and was extensively sold in the United Kingdom; altogether, the drug was marketed in 48 countries during the early 1960s. Two American drug companies initially showed interest in acquiring thalidomide but concluded from their own tests that the drug was less effective than the brands they were already marketing. Somewhat later another American firm, impressed by the growing popularity of thalidomide in Europe, began another series of tests and released the drug for prescription use in Canada. In the United States, however, a doctor with the Food and Drug Administration had nagging doubts about some unexplained neurological results among long-term thalidomide users and restricted use of the drug in this country to a small clinical human trial.

At about this time (1960) the European medical community was becoming increasingly puzzled by the sudden increase in what had formerly been an extremely rare type of birth abnormality. In near-epidemic proportions children were being born with a condition known as **phocomelia** (seal-limb), in which there is typically a hand or foot attached directly to the torso without an arm or leg. In some cases, however, even the hands and feet were absent, the babies being born with only a head and torso. The presence of large numbers of babies with such an obvious deformity couldn't be overlooked, but intense questioning of the parents regarding their hereditary background, blood type, radiation exposure, or chromosomal aberrations in other children failed to reveal a common link. Finally two alert physicians made the connection between thalidomide use early in pregnancy to the birth of limbless babies. Subsequent studies revealed that 40% of the women who had taken thalidomide during their

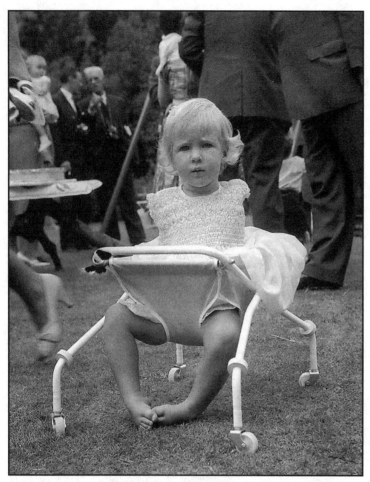

This young British girl is one of the approximately 12,000 children born with missing arms or legs as a result of fetal exposure to thalidomide—a nonprescription sedative widely used in Europe in the early 1960s. [*Press Association via AP Images*]

first trimester of pregnancy delivered babies afflicted with phocomelia. As proof of thalidomide's teratogenic properties gained acceptance, use of the drug was gradually discontinued in country after country, but not before nearly 12,000 children had been permanently disabled.

Ironically, thalidomide's unsavory reputation may yet be redeemed. Research demonstrating that thalidomide acts by inhibiting blood vessel growth has suggested its potential for combating a number of serious human ailments, including brain cancer, AIDS, and lupus. The drug also offers hope for treating diabetic retinopathy and macular degeneration, the two leading causes of blindness in the United States. In July 1998, the FDA approved the use of thalidomide for treating a serious inflammatory skin condition in patients with leprosy (*erythema nodosum leprosum*), and by October of that year thalidomide became commercially available in the U.S. for the first time. In May 2006, the FDA approved thalidomide (in conjunction with another drug) for treating

newly diagnosed multiple myeloma, a blood and bone marrow cancer. Produced exclusively by Celgene Corporation under the trade name "Thalidomid," thalidomide is now being prescribed for hundreds of critically ill cancer patients as tests of its safety and efficacy are ongoing (Henderson, 1999; FDA, 1998; Mayo Clinic, 2008).

In the early 1970s, not long after the heartbreaking photos of thalidomide babies had receded from media attention, another teratogenic chemical made headline news. Diethylstilbestrol, or **DES,** was first synthesized in 1938 and widely prescribed to pregnant women in the United States and Latin America for several decades thereafter. Because its biological action resembles that of natural estrogen, doctors began administering it to women experiencing problem pregnancies in the mistaken belief that it would prevent miscarriages. In the late 1950s one drug company, touting the miraculous properties of DES, even urged that *all* pregnant women use the drug to produce "bigger and stronger babies!" Eventually it was demonstrated that DES had no beneficial health effects; in fact, when given in high doses before the 20th week of pregnancy, DES actually *increased* the risk of miscarriage. Gradually the popularity of the drug began to wane, but not before an estimated 5 million pregnant women had used it.

Little more was heard about DES until the late 1960s when doctors at Massachusetts General Hospital in Boston made the connection between a rare form of vaginal cancer (clear-cell adenocarcinoma) in young female patients and the use of DES by their mothers during pregnancy. The fact that teratogenic effects could lie hidden for years, only to manifest themselves when the affected child became an adult hit the medical world like a bombshell—obviously birth defects don't have to be immediately visible to be important. Over the years that followed, several hundred cases of vaginal cancer were diagnosed among "DES daughters." While DES-related troubles initially focused on the daughters of women who had taken the drug, it gradually became apparent that girls were not the only victims nor was vaginal cancer the only problem. Many DES sons exhibit congenital deformities of the reproductive system and reduced fertility—problems experienced by DES daughters as well. DES daughters are at heightened risk of tubal pregnancies, miscarriages, and premature deliveries—if they are able to become pregnant in the first place. Perhaps most ominous of all are research results suggesting that DES exposure *in utero* causes genetic changes in a female embryo's egg cells that may pose a cancer threat to yet a third generation—the DES *granddaughters.* Unfortunately, hopes that the sad saga of DES would be confined to the generation exposed in the womb may prove too optimistic (Colborn, Dumanoski, and Myers, 1996; Newbold et al., 1998).

The thalidomide and DES episodes not only emphasized the importance of testing new drugs for their teratogenic effects, but also raised the profoundly disturbing question of what other drugs and medicines widely used by pregnant women might be doing to their unborn babies. That harmful effects could indeed result from medications used by pregnant women was confirmed again in the early 1980s when a French physician linked numerous cases of spina bifida to maternal use of valproic acid to control epileptic seizures (Harris and Wynne, 1994). A very beneficial medication for the mother's health problems, valproic acid proved devastating for unborn children exposed to the medication *in utero.* Valproic acid and thalidomide produced such distinctive types of abnormalities that they could scarcely go unnoticed. Conceivably, however, other teratogens that result in slight impairment of mental abilities, slight physical abnormalities, or diminished vigor might never be suspected as harmful.

These tragic episodes stimulated research, still ongoing, into what other substances present a threat to the unborn. Though much remains to be learned, investigations over the past several decades have implicated an increasing number of drugs and chemicals as proven or suspected teratogens. Among them, in addition to thalidomide and DES: dioxin, organic mercury, lead, cadmium, anesthetic gases, alcohol (see box 6-2), and cigarette smoke. While nonsmokers of any age can suffer health problems when exposed either to mainstream smoke exhaled by a smoker or from the sidestream smoke emanating from the end of a burning cigarette, infants in the womb are the most vulnerable. When a pregnant woman smokes—and nearly 20% of expectant mothers in the U.S. *do* smoke—she is exposing her fetus to nicotine, carbon monoxide, radioactive polonium, and numerous other toxic chemicals. Carbon monoxide appears to be the most fetotoxic of these, causing a rise in carboxyhemoglobin in the blood of both mother and child and resulting in retarded fetal growth rates. Pregnant women who smoke 20 or more cigarettes daily are at heightened risk of bearing an infant with cleft lip and palate; maternal smoking during pregnancy also is associated with a significantly higher chance of giving birth to a child with intellectual disabilities. Medical experts estimate that 30% of all low-weight births can be directly attributed to maternal smoking during pregnancy. Infants born to smoking mothers weigh on the average about 10% less at birth than do babies of nonsmokers. Since low birth weight is a major risk factor for infant mortal-

ity, it is not surprising that approximately 5% of all U.S. neonatal deaths each year are blamed on maternal smoking. Smoking during pregnancy also is blamed for an estimated 50,000 miscarriages annually and for 10% of all premature births. In addition, the incidence of Sudden Infant Death Syndrome (SIDS) is 1.4–3 times higher among babies whose mothers smoked during pregnancy (Tong et al., 2009; CDC, 2009f). In spite of the gruesome lessons of past tragedies, pregnant women continue using various drugs (e.g., aspirin, antacids, barbiturates, tranquilizers, cough medicines), drinking, and smoking, even though it is generally accepted that excess use of any of the above substances carries some risk of fetal damage.

Self-administered drugs or medications are not the only source of teratogenic exposure, of course. Hundreds of thousands of American workers currently are employed in occupations that expose them to reproductive hazards—lead, anesthetic gases, ethylene oxide (used as a sterilant for many hospital supplies), and certain pesticides. While few well-documented associations between specific workplace chemicals and reproductive problems (i.e., miscarriage, reduced fertility, neonatal death, birth defects) exist at present, this doesn't mean such a linkage is nonexistent. Very few well-designed clinical or epidemiologic studies on the issue have been conducted, making it impossible to draw definitive conclusions. Nevertheless, a 1985 review of 2,800 chemicals evaluated for their ability to induce birth defects in animals indicated that more than a third exhibited some teratogenic potential (Chivian et al., 1993). Unfortunately, most workplace teratogens are identified only after significant numbers of employees experience personal tragedies. Among the more recent reproductive hazards to make headlines are two glycol ethers, widely used as solvents in the manufacture of computer chips. Studies conducted during the early 1990s on female workers exposed to the chemicals during the chip-making process found that the women suffered miscarriages 20–40% more frequently than did nonexposed women in the industry and experienced 30% fewer pregnancies. As a result of these findings, several of the corporate giants in the semiconductor industry assigned pregnant female employees to work outside the chip fabrication area of the plant and in 1994 began phasing ethylene-based glycol ethers out of the production process altogether (Pellow and Park, 2002).

The widespread assumption that such workplace precautions need apply only to female workers is now being challenged by provocative, though inconclusive, evidence that a father's exposure to environmental hazards may also lead to defective offspring. It has long been observed that men working as painters, farmers, or mechanics—jobs involving exposure to certain solvents and pesticides—tend to be at higher risk of fathering children with birth defects than do men in other occupations.

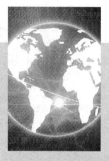

········ 6-2 ········

A Totally Preventable Tragedy

Fetal Alcohol Syndrome (FAS) afflicts 1–3 of every 1,000 babies born in the world today and is the leading known cause of intellectual disability. In the United States, an estimated 6–22 FAS-afflicted infants are born every day and the lifetime cost to care for each of them will exceed $1.5 million. Fetal Alcohol Syndrome is a lifelong, permanently disabling condition that cannot be reversed by providing prenatally damaged children with a high-quality, stable home environment after birth. Because it forever deprives its victims of a normal, productive life, FAS can justifiably be regarded as an extreme form of maternal child abuse.

As the name suggests, Fetal Alcohol Syndrome is a birth defect resulting from alcohol consumption during pregnancy. More toxic than any other abused drug, alcohol rapidly crosses the placental barrier from mother to fetus; within a few minutes after a pregnant woman drinks, blood alcohol levels in her fetus approximate her own.

Although surveys indicate most women are aware that drinking during pregnancy poses risks to a developing fetus, many choose to indulge regardless. Survey statistics published in 2004 revealed that each year approximately half a million pregnant women in the U.S.—about one in eight—report some degree of alcohol use, with 80,000 admitting to binge drinking.

Admittedly, not all babies born to heavily drinking mothers have FAS—perhaps as few as 4 out of 100 have the full complement of symptoms. Why this is the case remains a subject of research, with individual genetic factors assumed to be the most likely explanation. However, the fact that all babies born with FAS have mothers who drank heavily during pregnancy supports a direct cause-and-effect relationship.

Fetal Alcohol Syndrome was first described in the early 1970s as a complex of physical and neurobehavioral defects resulting from prenatal alcohol exposure. (Note: More recently the term Fetal Alcohol Spectrum Disorders [FASDs] has been introduced to describe the full range of conditions that can afflict a person whose mother consumed alcohol during pregnancy. A designation of FAS is applied to cases with the most extreme symptoms.) Some of the more common physical features associated with FAS babies include:

1. smaller than average body size and weight—a characteristic that persists throughout childhood

2. facial abnormalities, the most apparent of which are small eye openings, skin webbing between the eyes and base of the nose, thin upper lip, indistinct or absent groove between the nose and upper lip, low nasal bridge, short nose, small jaw, and low-set ears.

FAS children often exhibit congenital heart defects, cleft lip and palate, kidney and urinary tract defects, and/or malformed genitals. Skeletal defects such as a small head, deformed ribs and breastbone, hip dislocations, curved spine, and fused, webbed, or missing fingers or toes may also be manifest. Some of these physical characteristics become less obvious as the child grows older, but the same cannot be said of the neurobehavioral traits that are a result of alcohol's devastating effects on the central nervous system (CNS) and which frequently become even more noticeable after puberty. Because prenatal alcohol exposure damages the developing brain, FAS children often, though not always, experience some degree of mental retardation and low I.Q. Learning disabilities—particularly difficulty with arithmetic—are common, as is short attention span, hyperactivity, and poor body, hand, and finger coordination. As they get older, outbursts of aggression and lack of impulse control become an issue, schooling is frequently disrupted, and the children have difficulty maintaining friendships. As adults, FAS victims often experience mental health problems, find it difficult to hold a regular job, and not infrequently find themselves in trouble with the law. They typically exercise poor judgment in making decisions, have little understanding of danger, and find it difficult to use past experience in planning and organizing future actions. As a result, many are unable to care for themselves adequately, with homelessness often a result.

Combating FAS requires a thorough understanding of causation and although three decades of research have revealed a great deal of information, a number of questions remain unresolved. Confounding easy answers is the fact that, as a teratogen, alcohol produces a continuum of effects, making diagnosis problematic. While some children show the classic symptoms of FAS, nearly twice as many more display only a few or no facial abnormalities, yet still exhibit the behavioral dysfunction characteristic of alcohol-induced central nervous system damage. These children are designated as suffering from either Alcohol-Related Neurodevelopmental Disorder (ARND) or Alcohol-Related Birth Defects (ARBD), a continuum of symptoms that, along with FAS, includes the various conditions comprising FASDs. The range of symptoms manifested appears to be dependent on dose; children whose mothers are confirmed alcoholics suffer more severe effects than those whose mothers drank only moderate amounts during pregnancy. However, the question of "how much is too much?" has proven difficult to answer. Until relatively recently, medical researchers believed that a pregnant woman could safely consume one drink per day (one drink is defined as 12 ounces of beer, 5 ounces of wine, or 1.5 ounces of hard liquor) without incurring any greater risk of harm to her baby than that of women who abstained completely. A study published in 2002, however, showed that mothers who had only 1½ drinks per week gave birth to babies who were shorter, weighed less, and had smaller heads than infants whose mothers never drank during pregnancy.

Regardless of the total amount of alcohol consumed, studies have conclusively shown that consuming a large number of drinks within a short time period (so-called binge drinking) is significantly more harmful to the fetus than drinking the same total quantity in smaller amounts over a period of several days. The stage of fetal development at the time of alcohol exposure is an important determinant of the specific type of damage inflicted on the fetus. During the first trimester, when the basic organs of the body are forming, maternal drinking results in the facial abnormalities typically associated with FAS; at this time exposure can also result in skeletal deformities and, if occurring during the 3rd–4th week of gestation, in malformation of the heart. During the second trimester, alcohol disrupts nerve formation in the brain, while in the third trimester it interferes with nervous system development. Both the second and third trimesters are critical periods for fetal growth, so alcohol exposure during these periods has a pronounced dose-dependent effect in terms of reduced body weight, length, and head size. As one might expect, the most severely damaged children are those whose mothers drank heavily throughout their pregnancy.

Health care professionals are now striving to develop effective ways of identifying and helping alcohol-dependent pregnant women. The need to reach and educate sexually active teenagers is considered especially urgent, since many become pregnant and continue using alcohol, often with little or no understanding of the risks or consequences of FASDs. Doctors and staff at prenatal clinics could be effective educators by asking these young women about their drinking habits and encouraging them to cease using alcohol while pregnant. Altering behavior of chronically alcoholic women is much more difficult than dealing with binge-drinking teenagers, since even when they understand the risk, many are unable to break their addiction. Warning labels regarding the dangers of drinking while pregnant, now required on all alcoholic beverages, have raised awareness of the problem but have had minimal impact in changing the behavior of long-time heavy drinkers who tend to have numerous other problems, including drug abuse, smoking, and malnutrition.

For the majority of expectant mothers who are not alcohol-addicted but may be social drinkers, constant reminders by friends, relatives, and health care providers about the hazards of drinking while pregnant are appropriate. Since science has yet to identify a foolproof method for determining which infants are genetically predisposed to harm from even very low exposure to alcohol in the womb, it is only prudent for every pregnant woman to assume that her fetus is in this extra-vulnerable category and act accordingly. Although the global incidence of FASDs continues to climb, the strategy for eliminating this cruel but completely avoidable birth defect is utterly straightforward: while pregnant, women should not drink any amount of alcohol—period. It's that simple (Eustace et al., 2003; Floyd and Sidhu, 2004; CDC, 2010a).

These observations have stimulated a new look at the impact that mutagenic or teratogenic substances might have on sperm production or on the chemical composition of semen, and thereby on the development of a fertilized egg (Stone, 1992).

While some progress in elucidating the mechanism of teratogenesis has been made in recent years, much

more research is needed. Nevertheless, some broad generalizations about the causation of birth defects can be made. Perhaps most critical is the finding that fetal vulnerability to teratogens depends on the stage of development at the time of exposure. By far the most sensitive period is the time of tissue and organ formation (organogenesis), a period lasting from about the 18th day after

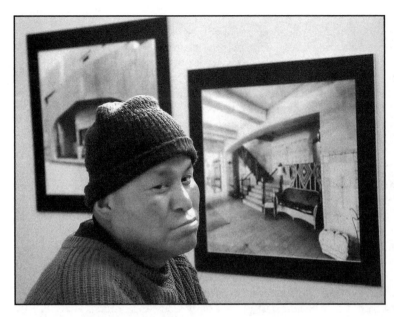

Maternal consumption of alcohol during pregnancy can result in a birth defect characterized by physical and neurobehavioral defects known as Fetal Alcohol Syndrome (FAS). As adults, FAS victims often experience mental health problems, find it difficult to hold a regular job, and may find themselves in trouble with the law. [*AP Photo/Albuquerque Journal, Richard Pipes*]

conception to approximately the 60th day, with the peak of sensitivity around the 30th day. During this time, interference with development can result in gross structural defects. In the case of the thalidomide episode, it was found that virtually all of the thalidomide mothers had taken the drug precisely during those few days when the limb buds were forming. Those women who used thalidomide before or after this critical time gave birth to normal babies. Similarly, DES exposure after the 20th week of pregnancy did not result in reproductive tract deformities, while exposure before the tenth week increased the risk of cancer in DES daughters. During the first week after conception, when the embryo is a relatively undifferentiated mass of cells, any damage caused by teratogenic exposure will be lethal to the developing embryo. After the 8th week, though the fetus is barely an inch long, its organs are already basically formed. Exposure to teratogens after this time can cause such harm as intellectual disability, blindness, or damage to the external sex organs, but the time for major structural deformation has passed. It must be recognized, however, that individual genetic differences in both mother and child will determine the extent of damage caused by teratogenic exposure. No teratogen causes birth defects in 100% of those exposed; if a group of women, all at the same stage of pregnancy, were exposed to equal concentrations of the same teratogen, some would give birth to babies with serious abnormalities, others with only moderate damage, and some would deliver infants who were perfectly normal (Harris and Wynne, 1994).

A second widely accepted generalization about teratogenesis is that as the dosage of a teratogen increases, the degree of damage increases. Basing their assumptions on the results of animal studies, teratologists thus presume the existence of a threshold below which no injury of any kind can be demonstrated. Determining exactly where that threshold is for any particular substance is, however, uncertain at best, and expectant mothers are well advised to limit their exposure to potential teratogens to the greatest extent possible.

CANCER

Few words arouse such emotions of sheer terror and hopelessness today as does the term "cancer." As the second leading cause of death in the United States (heart disease ranks first), and with over 1.5 million new cases diagnosed annually, cancer appears to have assumed epidemic proportions. Throughout the industrialized nations, cancer now accounts for 20–25% of all deaths each year; worldwide, according to the World Health Organization, cancer claims almost 6.5 million victims annually. In the United States, over 1,500 people die of cancer every day, with a yearly toll exceeding 560,000. Cancer is not an age-specific disease; although incidence rates are considerably higher among the elderly, cancer is the second-leading cause of death, after accidents, among children aged 1–14. In general, cancer death rates are considerably higher in developed countries than in the developing world, but the *types* of cancer that are most prevalent in various parts of the world differ sharply. Malignancies associated with cigarette smoking, asbestos exposure, or high-fat diets are far more common among populations in industrialized countries, while cancers linked to certain food preservatives, viral infections, or fungal toxins in food are more prevalent in the developing world.

In the United States, the *incidence* rate for all cancers as a group climbed steadily from 1973 to 1992, the peak year for new cancer cases, but has been gradually declining since then (cancer incidence for certain sites continues to increase however, most notably for breast cancer among women over the age of 50). The same trend holds true for cancer *mortality* rates. Since cancer record-keeping began in 1930, cancer death rates increased inexorably, year after year, reaching a peak in 1990. In 1991, however, overall U.S. cancer mortality rates began a slow but steady decline; over the next 15 years, from 1991–2006, cancer death rates for men dropped by 21%, while the decline for women was 12.3%. By 2003–2004, the actual *number* of annual cancer deaths, not only death rates, began to fall as well, though the decline was quite modest in comparison with overall cancer mortality figures. A slight drop in the number of new cancer cases has also become evident in recent years, with the incidence of malignancies among men falling 1.3% annually from 2000–2006 and among women by 0.5% per year from 1998–2006 (Jemal et al., 2010; Cole and Rodu, 1996).

The welcome reversal is attributed to a variety of factors: decades of anti-smoking campaigns and other preventive efforts, as well as to improvements in early detection and treatment of colorectal, breast, and prostate malignancies (Cole and Rodu, 1996). For some types of cancer, the turnaround in mortality rates was achieved long before the 1990s. For over a half-century, deaths due to cancer of the uterus, cervix, and stomach have fallen by more than 70% in the United States. In the case of uterine and cervical cancers, credit for the decline in death rates is attributed to widespread use of the Pap smear test, which provides early diagnosis when the disease is still treatable. Experts estimate that a further 90% reduction in the current annual number of U.S. cervical cancer deaths could be achieved if all American women would take advantage of this simple procedure. Regarding stomach cancer mortality, which is lower today in the

Estimated New Cases*		Estimated Deaths	
Male	**Female**	**Male**	**Female**
Prostate 217,730 (28%)	Breast 207,090 (28%)	Lung & bronchus 86,220 (29%)	Lung & bronchus 71,080 (26%)
Lung & bronchus 116,750 (15%)	Lung & bronchus 105,770 (14%)	Prostate 32,050 (11%)	Breast 39,840 (15%)
Colon & rectum 72,090 (9%)	Colon & rectum 70,480 (10%)	Colon & rectum 26,580 (9%)	Colon & rectum 24,790 (9%)
Urinary bladder 52,760 (7%)	Uterine corpus 43,470 (6%)	Pancreas 18,770 (6%)	Pancreas 18,030 (7%)
Melanoma of the skin 38,870 (5%)	Thyroid 33,930 (5%)	Liver & intrahepatic bile duct 12,720 (4%)	Ovary 13,850 (5%)
Non-Hodgkin lymphoma 35,380 (4%)	Non-Hodgkin lymphoma 30,160 (4%)	Leukemia 12,660 (4%)	Non-Hodgkin lymphoma 9,500 (4%)
Kidney & renal pelvis 35,370 (4%)	Melanoma of the skin 29,260 (4%)	Esophagus 11,650 (4%)	Leukemia 9,180 (3%)
Oral cavity & pharynx 25,420 (3%)	Kidney & renal pelvis 22,870 (3%)	Non-Hodgkin lymphoma 10,710 (4%)	Uterine 7,950 (3%)
Leukemia 24,690 (3%)	Ovary 21,880 (3%)	Urinary bladder 10,410 (3%)	Liver & intrahepatic bile duct 6,190 (2%)
Pancreas 21,370 (3%)	Pancreas 21,770 (3%)	Kidney & renal pelvis 8,210 (3%)	Brain & other nervous system 5,720 (2%)
All sites 789,620 (100%)	All sites 739,940 (100%)	All sites 299,200 (100%)	All sites 270,290 (100%)

*Excludes basal and squamous cell skin cancers and in situ carcinoma except urinary bladder

©2010, American Cancer Society, Inc., Surveillance and Health Policy Research

Source: *Cancer Facts & Figures—2010.* Reprinted with permission of the American Cancer Society, Inc., Atlanta.

Figure 6-3   Leading Sites of New Cancer Cases and Deaths—2010 Estimates

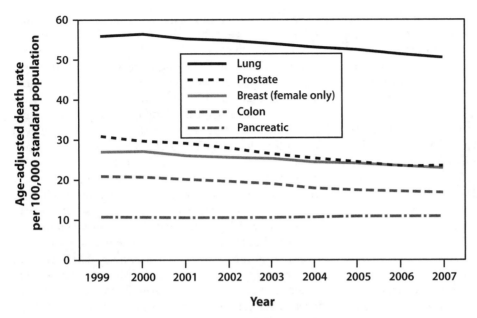

Source: CDC, *Morbidity and Mortality Weekly Report* 59(39), October 2010.

Figure 6-4   Death Rates for Five Leading Types of Cancer, U.S., 1999–2007

United States than anywhere else in the world (at present the East Asian countries and several of the former Soviet republics, including Russia, have the highest incidence of stomach cancer mortality), favorable trends are probably due to improved methods of transport and to refrigeration, which have made fresh produce available year-round. These advantages of modern life are significant in terms of cancer prevention because they have led to increased consumption of fresh fruits and vegetables (known to contain anticarcinogenic compounds), thereby lessening dependence on the salted, pickled, or smoke-preserved foods that are thought to pose a cancer risk.

More recently, colorectal cancers have declined dramatically in both North America and western Europe; breast cancer, prostate cancer, and childhood leukemia mortality rates exhibit similar downward trends. Most encouraging, however, is the long-awaited reversal in the lung cancer death rate. Although lung cancer remains by far the leading cancer killer among Americans of both sexes, death rates for this disease are finally beginning to drop sharply for U.S. men and have begun to plateau for U.S. women. The only significant increase in cancer death rates since the early 1990s is for non-Hodgkin's lymphoma.

Cancer, of course, is not a new disease; ancient societies were familiar with the ravages of cancer. Indeed, all multicellular organisms, plant and animal, are subject to the occasional development of malignancies. However, cancer's rapid rise to prominence as a leading cause of illness and death over the past century has imbued it with an aura of dread and fatalism. Until recently, progress achieved in the so-called war against cancer remained disappointingly limited after decades of intensive medical research and the expenditure of billions of dollars. Major gains were achieved in prolonging a cancer patient's survival time after the initial diagnosis, and notable successes were scored in reducing deaths from childhood leukemia and Hodgkin's lymphoma; nevertheless, the "magic bullet" that would provide a cure for cancer was nowhere in sight. Research and observation strongly suggested that a majority of cancers were associated with environmental causes (using the term "environment" in its broadest sense to include diet, smoking, sun exposure, chemical pollutants, and so forth), yet the mechanism for such interaction remained unknown. During the past several decades, however, a number of major breakthroughs in cancer research have revolutionized our understanding of carcinogenesis. While a great deal more remains to be learned, these findings have provided important information on how once-healthy cells become malignant and offer new hope for both prevention and treatment of this formidable killer.

What Causes Cancer?

"Cancer" is a collective term used to describe a number of diseases that differ in origin, prognosis, and treatment. It is essentially a condition in which the regulating forces that govern normal cell processes no longer function correctly, leading to uncontrolled cell proliferation. Cancerous cells, unlike normal ones, continue to divide and spread, invading other tissues where they interfere with vital bodily functions and eventually lead to death of the organism. The search for agents responsible for initiating this chain of events has been ongoing for years and has focused on a number of possibilities including pathogens, hereditary factors, oxidation damage within cells due to normal metabolic processes, and exposure to a wide range of environmental **carcinogens** (substances that can cause cancer) such as toxic chemicals and radiation.

Viruses have long been known to cause some forms of cancer in animals (e.g. viral leukemia in cats, Rous sarcoma in chickens). It is now recognized that at least seven viruses cause cancer in humans as well. Among the most significant are the hepatitis B and C viruses that predispose infected individuals to liver cancer, one of the most common and deadly forms of cancer worldwide; about 70% of all liver cancers are a result of hepatitis infections. Another prominent carcinogenic virus is the herpes papillomavirus, associated with approximately 90% of all cervical cancers (Parkin et al., 1999). For decades it had been assumed that **bacteria** had no part to play in the cancer drama, but in the early 1990s researchers found that both gastric cancer and non-Hodgkin's lymphoma of the stomach are markedly higher among people infected with the bacterium *Helicobacter pylori*, the common microbe recognized as the leading cause of stomach ulcers. Interestingly, while non-Hodgkin's lymphoma of the stomach is extremely rare in the United States, it is relatively common in the Veneto region of Italy where 90% of the population is infected with *H. pylori* (Parsonnet et al., 1994; Isaacson, 1994). Together, viruses and bacteria are now viewed as causative agents for almost 15% of all human cancers—over a million new cases annually—with viruses responsible for the large majority of these (Parkin et al., 1999).

Since the rediscovery of Mendelian principles of genetics in the early 1900s, **heredity** has been a prime suspect for cancer causation, particularly because certain kinds of malignancies are more common in some families than in others. It is well established that a few types of cancer are hereditary; among the best known inherited cancers are retinoblastoma, a cancer of the eye, and familial polyposis, a rare type of colon cancer. For the most part, however, studies carried out decades ago discounted heredity as a significant factor in cancer causation. These studies compared the incidence of specific types of cancer among descendants of immigrants to the United States and members of the same ethnic group remaining in the homeland. For example, a 1944 study of the incidence of liver cancer showed that African-Americans have much lower rates of this disease than do native African populations; similarly, Japanese-Americans exhibit low rates of stomach cancer—comparable to those of the general American population—while stomach cancer remains very common in Japan. By contrast, these Japanese-Americans, like other U.S. residents, experience typically high rates of colon cancer, a disease quite rare in Japan.

A subsequent study of immigrants to Australia and Canada found that a woman's risk of breast cancer shifted from the rate prevailing in her country of origin toward the rate observed among native-born women in the country to which she moved. Thus women who emigrated from England, where breast cancer rates are relatively high, experienced a lowering of risk in their new country of destination; conversely, female emigrants from Asian countries, where breast cancer rates are lower than those prevailing in Canada and Australia, were

more likely to develop breast cancer in their adopted countries than were women in their homelands. Study results strongly suggest that risk of breast cancer has little to do with heredity, but rather is associated with as-yet unidentified environmental and lifestyle factors. Since most of the women emigrated as adults, it also suggests that one's risk of breast cancer can be altered later in life (Kliewer and Smith, 1995).

However, while most breast cancers are not hereditary, within some population subgroups, particularly those with an Eastern European Jewish background, genetics does play a role in cancer causation. Medical research has revealed the existence of two tumor-suppressing genes known as BRCA 1 and BRCA 2 (shorthand for breast cancer susceptibility gene); if a mutation "turns off" one or both of these genes, uncontrolled cell growth (i.e., a malignancy) may result. A woman's lifetime risk of developing breast or ovarian cancer is greatly increased if she inherits a defective BRCA 1 or BRCA 2 gene—about five times higher than that of a woman with normal BRCA genes. Similarly, her chances of developing such cancers at an early age, prior to menopause, are also enhanced if she harbors a mutant BRCA gene. Since such genes are passed from generation to generation, it's not uncommon for many women in the same family to be diagnosed with breast and ovarian cancers, as well as a number of other malignancies whose incidence has been linked to defective BRCA 1 or BRCA 2 genes. Even male relatives can be affected, since harmful BRCA 2 mutations have been shown to increase the risk of male breast cancer, prostate cancer, and pancreatic cancer. For those whose family history suggests they should be concerned about possible BRCA gene mutations, genetic testing of blood samples can reveal whether a defective gene is present; if so, various risk management options can then be pursued (National Cancer Institute, 2010).

Although few types of cancers are directly associated with "cancer genes," a tidal wave of new discoveries during the past two decades has demonstrated the existence of an inherited *predisposition* to cancer that explains the prevalence of specific types of malignancies within certain families. These findings not only help to explain why some people exposed to known carcinogens remain hale and hearty while others sicken and die, but also offer promising therapeutic approaches for reducing cancer mortality among those likely to develop the disease. A classic example of genetic predisposition to cancer is that of hereditary non-polyposis colon cancer, a common type of colorectal malignancy. Victims of the disease carry an inherited defective gene which, in its normal state, produces a DNA repair protein that acts as a cellular "spell checker," correcting errors in the order of nucleotide base pairs during DNA replication. In mutated form, the gene is no longer able to produce its key protein, so mistakes occurring after replication rapidly accumulate throughout the genetic material, creating a situation that may eventually result in cancer (Leach et al., 1993; Fishel et al., 1993). For individuals with a predisposition for hereditary non-polyposis colon cancer (about 10% of all colon malignancies), the chances of eventually developing colon cancer range between 70–90%, with many victims developing tumors before the age of 50. The practical significance of these recent findings is therefore immense: if carriers could be identified through genetic screening programs, they could begin having regular colonoscopic examinations at an early age in order to detect precancerous polyps when they can be easily removed. Similarly, identified bearers of the defective gene could be strongly advised to adopt the low-fat, high-fiber diet that is known to reduce the risk of colorectal cancer (Weinberg, 1998; Papadopoulos et al., 1994; Bronner et al., 1994).

A great many **environmental agents** such as cigarette smoke, radon gas, sunlight, heavy metals, X-rays, chemical pesticides, some air pollutants, and high-fat diets are known to be carcinogenic. These environmental factors, acting in conjunction with an individual's inherited predisposition to cancer and with acquired susceptibility, are believed to be responsible for an estimated 80% of all human cancers. The exact mechanism by which such agents induce a malignancy is still not completely understood, but recent progress in unraveling cancer's mysteries has brought us tantalizingly closer to that goal (Perera, 1997).

How Does Cancer Develop?

The exact mechanism of carcinogenesis is still being unraveled, with various theories being proposed as new findings emerge from medical research. The currently prevailing hypothesis is that cancer develops as a multistep process that begins when a single cell undergoes a mutation. The mutant cell then slowly proliferates to form a small group of genetically identical precancerous cells. This first step, termed **initiation,** is possibly provoked by a brief interaction between the target cell and a carcinogenic agent. It has been demonstrated that many environmental carcinogens (e.g., ultraviolet light, aflatoxin, vinyl chloride, certain components of tobacco smoke, etc.) bond tightly with DNA to form DNA-carcinogen **adducts,** causing genetic damage that can eventually lead to cancer. Researchers can utilize the unique "biomarkers" left at characteristic locations along certain genes to identify the causative agent of a specific cancer (Semenza and Weasel, 1997).

Cells that have undergone initiation do not inevitably give rise to malignancies, however. Tumor progression is dependent on the **promotion** of initiated cells by long-term exposure to nonmutagenic agents that stimulate cell proliferation, thereby expanding the number of initiated cells and increasing the likelihood that additional mutations will occur within this population. Unlike initiation, which is an irreversible event, promotion can be reversed if the promoting agent is removed (Pitot, 2002). It has long been observed that onset of malignant disease almost always occurs many years after initial exposure to a cancer-causing agent. This characteristically long **latency period** can be explained by the fact that **progression** of cancer requires considerable time (10–30 years or more, depending on the type of cancer) for a precancerous tumor to accumulate the three to seven additional independent, random mutations generally needed to cause malignant growth—a fact which may explain why the chances of developing cancer increase exponentially after the age of 55 (Levine, 2002).

During the 1990s, a number of significant findings by cancer researchers further clarified the nature of the molecular changes within genes that lead to the outward manifestation of cancer. It is now known that two major types of genes are of fundamental importance in cancer causation: **proto-oncogenes** and **tumor-suppressor genes,** both of which play an essential role in regulating the cell cycle. Proto-oncogenes tell the cell when to begin dividing; in so doing, they orchestrate orderly fetal development, the routine replacement of worn-out cells, healing of wounds, and so forth. Mutant versions of these genes, called **oncogenes** (from the Greek word *onkos*, meaning "lump" or "mass"), cause cells to divide endlessly when they should not. By contrast, normal tumor-suppressor genes halt uncontrolled multiplication of cells, acting in a manner analogous to the brakes on an automobile. In mutant form, normal gene function is inactivated, resulting in runaway cell proliferation. Approximately 100 oncogenes and 25 tumor-suppressor genes have now been identified as key contributors to the development of many cancers. The *ras* oncogene is known to occur in 50% of colon cancers and 90% of pancreatic cancers. Even more ubiquitous is the tumor-suppressor gene, *p53*, found in altered form in the tumors of more than half of all cancer patients, regardless of the type of cancer involved. Normal functioning of *p53* is especially important because, in addition to preventing uncontrolled cell division, the gene gives instructions for a cell to self-destruct when it detects irreparable damage to DNA during cell division. Because of its role in preventing the dangerous proliferation of mutant cells, *p53* is sometimes referred to as the "guardian of the genome."

Research has shown that the progression of a precancerous tumor to a full-blown malignancy requires a series of mutations that both activate specific oncogenes and inactivate specific tumor-suppressor genes. This sequence of events can be, and usually is, blocked by a number of

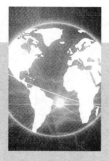

········ 6-3 ········

Lab Tests for Carcinogenicity—Are They Valid?

In 1977 a Canadian study documenting an excess incidence of bladder cancer among male rats fed a 5% diet of saccharin created a furor among an American public unconvinced that the food additive posed a real health threat and dismayed at the possible banning of the only noncaloric sweetener on the market at that time. Intelligent assessment of the implications of the saccharin research was not helped by the statement by a top FDA official that humans would have to drink 800 cans of diet soda daily to consume an amount of saccharin equivalent to that fed the experimental rats. The issue was widely aired in outraged letters to Congress and newspaper opinion pages, laughed about on late-night talk shows, and used as the butt of cartoonist's jokes. The public was given the impression that the tests were meaningless as far as human health was concerned, an attitude aptly expressed by Congressman Andrew Jacobs of Indiana who proposed passage of a bill requiring that products containing saccharin bear the label: "Warning: the Canadians have determined that saccharin is dangerous to your rat's health."

Unfortunately, the congressman's remarks revealed a profound lack of understanding regarding the methods routinely used for determining the safety of new chemicals. The objections raised to the Canadian saccharin tests—and to animal testing procedures in general—focus primarily on two points:

1. The question of dosage. Does *everything* cause cancer when present in excess? Contrary to popular belief, only carcinogens cause cancer. A test animal might be fed a mountain of sugar or salt and die of toxemia, but it will not develop a malignancy because neither substance is a carcinogen. Some would qualify this statement by pointing out that because hyper-obesity is a risk factor for certain types of cancer, excessive consumption of chocolate fudge sundaes could lead to cancer; nevertheless, it would be difficult to argue that ice cream is an environmental carcinogen in the same sense that aflatoxins or nitrosamines are known to be. Feeding or exposing test animals to extremely high doses of a suspected chemical is a widely accepted procedure necessary for obtaining meaningful results within a reasonable period of time, given the constraints of such experiments. In a typical study, for reasons of expense and space considerations, only 50 to 100 experimental animals are used in each test group. Such animals have a relatively short life span in comparison with humans, so in order to compensate for the long latency period involved in cancer initiation and to increase the chances for a weak carcinogen to be revealed in the small study population, massive doses are used. This method simply facilitates the collection of data within a reasonable time and at considerably less expense than would be possible using larger test populations and lower dosages.

That such tests are valid and that administration of large doses, per se, does not lead to carcinogenesis are supported by the results of past experimentation. A researcher at the National Cancer Institute some years ago reported that of 3,500 suspected carcinogens tested in the routine manner, only 750 proved, in fact, to be carcinogenic—hardly support for the thesis that large doses in themselves are cancer-causing.

2. Animals aren't humans. Do the substances that cause cancer in mice, monkeys, or rats predict cancer causation in humans? The prevailing assumption among researchers is that the basic biological processes in all mammals are fundamentally the same. For ethical reasons it is impossible to prove the thesis that any chemical that causes cancer in animals also causes the disease in humans—to do so would require deliberately exposing humans to a known animal carcinogen and waiting to see if cancer develops! However, numerous tests have been successfully carried out to prove the reverse: every substance known to induce human cancer causes cancer in animals as well (with the sole exception of arsenic, a heavy metal that is a human carcinogen, is mutagenic to bacteria and to cells grown in tissue culture, yet has never been shown to have carcinogenic potential in animals). Thus it seems logical to assume that the opposite is true also and that animal testing is a valid method for determining which chemicals are carcinogenic. What animal testing cannot tell us, however, is how strong or weak a given carcinogen will be in humans. This is because different species show varying degrees of sensitivity to the same substance, some developing cancer only at high levels of exposure while others are vulnerable to relatively low doses. Unfortunately, it is not possible to calculate the level of human risk based on the risk level in animals. We may be more or less vulnerable; the tests indicate only which substance can be expected to result in a given number of human cancer cases.

Animal models, of course, provide but one of several methods for studying the mechanism of carcinogenesis. Other approaches for advancing our understanding of cancer include: **mutagenesis studies using bacteria** which, due to their very large population size and short generation time, allow rapid screening of numerous potential carcinogens; **tissue culture research,** which permits examination of DNA damage and mutagenesis in eukaryotic cells (as opposed to prokaryotic bacterial cells); and **epidemiologic studies** of cancer incidence among human populations. Each of these lines of investigation has inherent limitations, and results yielded by one type of study may not always correspond with conclusions drawn from an alternative mode of inquiry. For example, nickel compounds are potent carcinogens in both humans and animals but are not mutagenic to bacteria. Conversely, organic mercury compounds damage DNA in bacterial cells and are mutagenic to cells in tissue culture, but have not been shown to induce cancer either in humans or animals. Cadmium and chromium, however, show carcinogenic potential in all four systems.

The disturbing lack of consistency in results among these various test models has led some observers to question the validity of current testing procedures and to challenge government regulations based on the results of carcinogenicity studies on animals. Most investigators would argue, however, that in an admittedly imperfect world, we must continue to use the only tools currently available, always bearing in mind their limitations and exercising due caution when interpreting data or extrapolating results from such experiments.

different bodily defense mechanisms that limit the number of times a cell can divide before dying (cell mortality) or that cause defective cells to self-destruct (apoptosis). Only when all such obstacles are surmounted does cancerous growth commence (Weinberg, 1998).

Undoubtedly, coming years will witness unprecedented expansion of our knowledge regarding cancer causation—knowledge that will provide an increasing number of weapons for fighting and eventually controlling this dreaded disease. In the meantime, however, society must continue ongoing efforts to prevent exposure to the myriad of environmental agents that are believed responsible for the majority of cancers. While new evidence of inherited predisposition to specific cancers explains why some people are more likely to develop cancer than others, it holds true nevertheless that with most cancers even susceptible individuals are unlikely to develop a malignancy in the absence of adverse environmental exposure. Conversely, even individuals who are not genetically predisposed can experience the DNA damage leading to carcinogenesis if exposure to cancer-causing agents is excessive. By eliminating contact with known carcinogens, one can drastically reduce the incidence of a malignancy—as in so many other realms of life, prevention is the best cure for cancer.

Environmental Carcinogens

The fact that an environmental agent can cause cancer was first reported more than two centuries ago when, in 1775, an English physician, Sir Percival Pott, recognized an association between cancer of the scrotum and exposure to soot. Every patient he examined with this relatively rare ailment had, as a child, worked as a chimney sweep, being lowered naked into chimneys to clean out the soot that accumulated there. In the process, the boys were covered with soot and grime themselves and with the low standards of personal hygiene that characterized those times, some of this soot remained in the folds of the scrotum for long periods, eventually resulting in the development of scrotal cancer years later (more recently the active ingredient in this soot was identified as benzopyrene, known as a very potent carcinogen). Not until the 20th century, however, was much research directed toward detecting environmental carcinogens. Work during the early 1900s revealed the cancer-causing properties of a number of coal tar products and of X-rays, but not until mid-century as age-adjusted cancer rates began to soar did the search for cancer causation acquire new urgency. Since that time the public has been bombarded with so many dire warnings that the average citizen may be excused for thinking that indeed *everything* causes cancer. This of course is untrue, but the very large number of new chemicals and products that are introduced each year, many without adequate testing for harmful side effects, justifies concern. Epidemiologic surveys carried out on the "geography of cancer" indicate that the incidence of certain types of cancer is elevated in heavily industrialized areas.

Researchers and environmentalists alike continue to debate the extent to which present cancer rates reflect exposure to chemical pollutants as opposed to personal habits such as smoking or diet. The outcome of this controversy is obviously of political and economic importance, since extensive regulation would be required to control the former, while education and persuasion represent the practical limits to modifying the latter. Several of the most prominent public concerns in relation to cancer causation include the following.

Smoking

Tobacco use, particularly cigarette smoking, is now recognized as far and away the leading contributor to cancer mortality. Rates of lung cancer are most reflective of the impact of smoking on health, and the drastic rise in this disease in the United States neatly parallels the increase in the smoking habit in American society. Today almost one-third of all U.S. cancer deaths are due to lung cancer, and of the more than 220,000 new lung cancer victims diagnosed annually in recent years, 87% are cigarette smokers (most of the others are individuals industrially exposed to carcinogens such as asbestos fibers or those exposed to radon gas inside their homes). Death rates among lung cancer victims, as opposed to victims of some other types of cancer, are quite high largely because

lung malignancies are seldom diagnosed before the mass has reached a size of about 1 cm in diameter. By that time it has been growing for about 10 years and has usually spread to other parts of the body.

Lung cancer rates began their steady rise in the mid-1930s, approximately 20 years or so after cigarette smoking became popular. Interestingly, until the mid-1950s it was widely assumed that women were resistant to the disease because the incidence of lung cancer among females was negligible compared to that among men. However, over the past 50 years, the incidence of lung cancer among women has soared by 600%, reflecting the growing social acceptance of women's smoking following the "female emancipation" of the 1920s and 1930s. In 1987 lung cancer surpassed breast cancer as the leading cause of cancer mortality among women, making it for the first time the number one cancer killer among both sexes. As the advertisement for Virginia Slims puts it, "You've come a long way, Baby"—all the way from virtually no lung cancer prior to the 1950s to the current situation where more than 100,000 American women are diagnosed with lung cancer each year (American Cancer

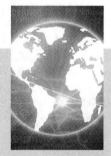

· · · · · · · 6-4 · · · · · · ·

Synergism: 1 + 1 = 5

Virtually all laboratory tests to determine carcinogenicity of suspected substances are based on responses to single-source exposures. Results of such testing methods may significantly underestimate risks in the real world because it is now well known that certain substances in combination are far more hazardous than either one would be if acting independently. For example, people who smoke cigarettes are 10 times more likely to develop lung cancer than are nonsmokers; asbestos workers incur significantly higher risk of lung cancer than do people not exposed to asbestos. However, a person who both smokes cigarettes and works with asbestos is 60 times more likely to get lung cancer than is a person exposed neither to cigarette smoke nor to asbestos—far higher than the risk factor for either type of exposure separately. This phenomenon, where the interaction of two or more substances produces an impact greater than the sum of their independent effects, is known as **synergism** and can perhaps be most easily thought of as a situation where 1 + 1 = 5.

Synergistic effects are well documented in relation to interactions between various air pollutants, water pollutants, and so forth and will be mentioned again in the chapters dealing with those topics. Synergism has been most studied, however, in the context of cancer and smoking in an effort to demonstrate the degree of risk inherent in various types of smokers' lifestyles. In addition to the smoking-asbestos connection, other synergistic associations with smoking include:

1. Smoking and alcohol consumption—as much as a thirtyfold increase in the risk of mouth and throat cancer.

2. Smoking and living in areas of high air pollution—elevated risk of lung cancer.

3. Smoking and working with chemicals or in uranium mines—high lung cancer risk.

Society, 2010). Thanks to increasing public awareness of the many adverse health impacts of tobacco use following the 1964 Surgeon General's report, the incidence of cigarette smoking among adults in the United States steadily declined from a national average of 42% in 1965 to 20.6% in 2008, holding relatively steady for the last several years. The percentage varies widely among states, with a high of 28.3% in Kentucky and a low of 11.7% in Utah (the U.S. Virgin Islands does even better, with smokers constituting only 8.7% of the adult population). Smoking prevalence is higher for men (23.1%) than for women (18.3%) and is highest among Native Americans (32.4%) as compared with other ethnic groups. Smoking prevalence is inversely associated with educational level, reaching its peak among adults with a GED diploma (41.3%) and lowest (5.7%) among those people with master's, doctoral, or professional degrees (CDC, 2009c; 2009f).

Since most smokers acquired their habit as teenagers, health officials have been closely watching trends in tobacco use among young people. They were heartened to note that between 1997–2003, cigarette smoking among high school students declined from 36.4% to 21.9%; however, since 2003 teen-age smoking rates have remained relatively stable overall—except among black students, whose tobacco use has been steadily declining, with just 11.6% of males and 8.4% of females now smoking, compared with corresponding male/female rates of 23.2% and 22.5% for non-Hispanic white students. Smoking rates among Hispanic students were in between these two extremes, at 18.7% for males and 14.6% for females. Disappointingly, surveys show that smoking frequency tends to rise with grade level: 14.3% of 9th graders, 19.6% of 10th graders, 21.6% of 11th graders, and 26.5% of 12th graders reported being current smokers (CDC, 2008c).

Elsewhere in the world, the toll of tobacco-related disease mirrors that in the United States. Smoking prevalence in other industrialized countries has equaled or exceeded that in the U.S. for many years and in recent decades many newly affluent developing nations also witnessed an explosive increase in cigarette sales and per-capita cigarette consumption. Some representative examples of adult male smoking prevalence elsewhere in the world include: Greece, 45%; India, 50%; Egypt, 50%; Russia, 60%; and Turkey, 66%. As a result, throughout the world lung cancer is the leading cause of cancer mortality. There are currently an estimated 1.3 billion smokers worldwide and the consequences of their addiction are evident in the nearly 6 million deaths globally caused by smoking-related illnesses each year. The number of victims today is almost evenly divided between those living in developed vs. developing nations—evidence that tobacco is an equal-opportunity killer (Ezzati and Lopez, 2003).

Such trends cause dismay to those who realize that cigarette smoke contains more than 4,700 chemical compounds, of which at least 43 are known carcinogens, including benzo(a)pyrene, arsenic, cadmium, benzene, and radioactive polonium. Since these substances are inhaled, it is not surprising that the lungs are the tissue most directly affected. However, smoking also has been documented as the single most important cause of bladder cancer, accounting for an estimated 40-70% of all cases; smokers run 2–3 times the risk of developing bladder cancer as nonsmokers. Cancers of the mouth, throat, and esophagus are also highly correlated with tobacco use. Smoking contributes to the development of kidney, pancreatic, and colon cancer and also significantly increases the risk of breast cancer for women who began using tobacco at an early age. Research has shown that girls who start smoking within five years of their first men-

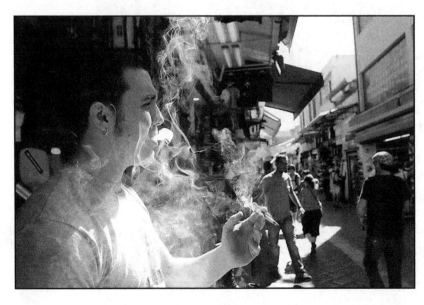

A Greek shopkeeper steps outside for a cigarette after a comprehensive ban on smoking in indoor public places went into effect in Greece on September 1, 2010. Greek males have one of the highest smoking rates in the world. [*AP Photo/ Petros Giannakouris*]

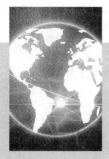

········ *6-5* ········

International Initiative to Fight Tobacco: The Framework Convention on Tobacco Control

As the number of smokers in the United States, Canada, and many Western countries continues to fall, tobacco companies seeking to maintain sales and profits are looking to the nations of Asia, Africa, and eastern Europe, where millions of new smokers are taking up the habit. Of the estimated 1.3 billion smokers in the world today (47.5% of all men and 10.3% of women currently use tobacco, according to WHO statistics), 84% live in low or middle-income countries. The global tobacco epidemic, which began in North America and western Europe, is now taking a heavy toll in the developing nations where nearly half of the 5.4 million smoking-related annual deaths occur. Unless action is taken to reverse present trends, experts fear annual global mortality caused by tobacco could rise to 6.5 million by 2015, 8.3 million by 2030, with smokers in poor and middle-income countries accounting for over 80% of these fatalities. In China, where approximately 60–65% of males smoke, researchers warn that more than a million men per year are likely to die of tobacco-related diseases during the first few decades of the 21st century—a number predicted to rise to 3 million annually by 2050 (until quite recently, only 1% of Chinese women smoked, hence the restriction of tobacco-related mortality to men in that country). Russia and the eastern European nations constitute several of the most rapidly growing markets for tobacco sales; Russians now lead the world in per capita cigarette consumption, a fact with ominous implications for Russia's health statistics in the years ahead (Ezzati and Lopez, 2003).

As tobacco-related deaths and disease continue to climb throughout the world, many governments—particularly those in developing countries whose health-care budgets are already stretched thin trying to deal with infectious diseases—are beginning to implement antismoking initiatives similar to those already widespread in the United States and some European countries. The international community as a whole became actively involved in fighting the scourge of tobacco-related disease in 1999 when Gro Harlem Brundtland, then Director-General of the World Health Organization, decided to make global tobacco control a WHO priority. During the next four years, representatives from around the world negotiated the details of what was to become the **Framework Convention on Tobacco Control (FCTC),** an international treaty unanimously approved by delegates from 192 countries in March 2003. Despite efforts by "Big Tobacco" to undermine FCTC and to exert pressure on governments to spurn the agreement, the treaty entered into force and became legally binding on Feb. 27, 2005, 90 days after ratification by the requisite 40 signatory nations. By the end of 2009, 168 countries had ratified the FCTC; the U.S. signed the treaty in 2004 but has not yet ratified it. Stating that FCTC's goal is "to protect present and future generations from the devastating health, social, environmental, and economic consequences of tobacco consumption and exposure to tobacco smoke," framers of the Convention incorporated numerous provisions to achieve this objective, the most significant of which include:

- **Encouragement of higher cigarette taxes.** Experience in several countries has shown that increasing the cost of tobacco products via higher taxes is the most effective means of discouraging smoking, particularly among adolescents. All but four U.S. states have increased their cigarette tax rates since 1999, in part to enhance state revenues but usually with the justification that doing so served as a deterrent to teenage smoking. In 2009 President Obama signed legislation raising the federal tax on cigarettes from 39¢ to $1.01 per pack and increasing the tax on chewing tobacco from 19.5¢ to 50¢ per pound. Many western European countries have taken similar action; Norway, the first nation to ratify the FCTC, promptly imposed a whopping cigarette tax of $5.99 per pack. Governments that ratify FCTC are urged to consider national health objectives when deciding how to tax tobacco products and are also encouraged to restrict or prohibit their duty-free sale.

- **A comprehensive ban on tobacco advertising and promotion** within 5 years of ratification. Sponsorship of sporting events by tobacco companies—a more recent tactic by tobacco companies to evade advertising bans—would also be prohibited, as would cross-border advertising (e.g., TV or Internet ads that could be seen by viewers in another country) originating within nations that ratified the treaty.

- **Requirement for prominent warning labels.** FCTC calls for health warning labels to cover at least 50% of the principle display area of the packet and stipulates that these warnings be printed in the language of the country where the product is sold. Although by late 2009 the U.S. had still not ratified the treaty, Congress that year enacted legislation giving the FDA authority to regulate tobacco products. Among the law's requirements is a provision that by 2012 each package of cigarettes must bear a large FDA-approved warning label containing graphic color pictures that depict smoking's negative health consequences. Within three years of ratification, parties to the agreement must also prohibit misleading terms. The 2009 U.S. law regulating tobacco use also conforms with this FCTC mandate by prohibiting the industry from claiming its products are "light," "mild," or "low-tar"—terms that give consumers a false impression that those brands are safer.

- **Protection of nonsmokers.** Legislating smoke-free workplaces, public transport, and other indoor public spaces was a concept pioneered in the U.S. and constitutes another requirement of FCTC. Supported by scientific research proving that secondhand smoke can cause death and illness among exposed nonsmokers, mandatory smoking restrictions have been adopted by numerous U.S. cities and most states; more recently, other countries have followed suit, recognizing that only a complete ban on public smoking can effectively protect nonsmokers.

The trend toward smoke-free areas seems to be spreading and, in some countries, restrictions are even more comprehensive than the antismoking laws in the United States. By 2005, Ireland, Norway, and the Netherlands, despite considerable controversy, had imposed nationwide bans on smoking in restaurants and bars (immediately after Ireland's prohibition on smoking in pubs went into effect in March 2004, sales of outdoor heaters and awnings for installation outside pubs soared). Most far-reaching of all are the actions of the small Himalayan kingdom of Bhutan which, on the last day of 2004, banned cigarettes completely, making the sale of tobacco products illegal and imposing fines on anyone caught smoking in public.

Additional issues addressed by FCTC provisions include requirements to eliminate tobacco smuggling, to include in national health programs services to help smokers break the habit, to prohibit the sale of tobacco products to minors, and to encourage litigation against tobacco interests as an antismoking strategy.

Even before the treaty became legally binding on the countries that had ratified it, FCTC motivated many governments to strengthen their own national antismoking programs. Examples include Thailand's crackdown on cigarette smuggling; Tanzania's prohibition on smoking in public places; and North Korea's doubling of cigarette prices. In Taiwan, where a smoking ban for public indoor areas took effect early in 2009, the government may impose a further requirement that if smokers go outside to indulge their habit, they must carry personal ashtrays! In Europe, where the percentage of adults who smoke remains considerably higher than in the U.S., large black-and-white warning labels bearing such blunt admonitions as "Smoking May Cause a Slow and Painful Death" are now mandatory under European Union law. By mid-2005, tobacco advertising on television, radio, and the print media had become illegal throughout the EU; tobacco sponsorship of sporting events had been banned as well (ASH, 2004).

Of course laws are one thing, enforcement another matter entirely. Antismoking advocates acknowledge that achieving a smoke-free environment, regardless of legal victories, will not be easy. Even in countries like France and Germany where laws already call for restaurants to provide nonsmoking sections, few establishments comply. In some countries, especially in southern Europe, it's commonplace to see smokers puffing away while leaning against a "NO SMOKING" sign!

Nevertheless, bit by bit, attitudes are changing as the public and policy makers alike contemplate the devastating health and financial impact wrought by smoking-related disease and acknowledge the validity of the WHO's declaration that:

"A cigarette is the only legally available consumer product that kills through normal use."

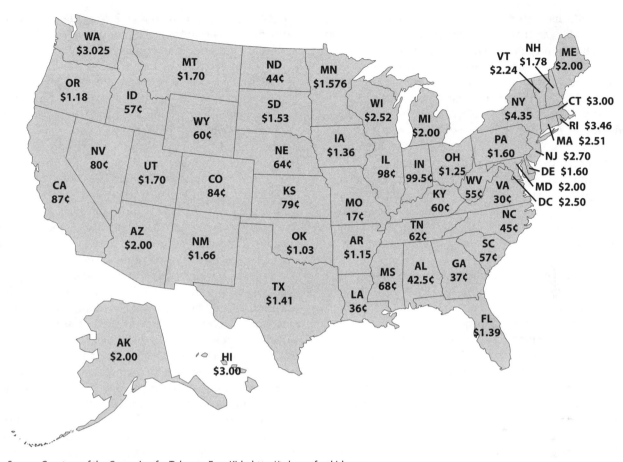

Source: Courtesy of the Campaign for Tobacco-Free Kids, http://tobaccofreekids.org

Figure 6-5   Map of State Cigarette Tax Rates (as of mid-2010)

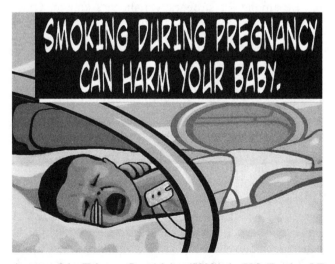

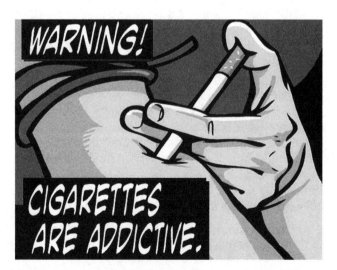

As part of the Tobacco Control Act (2009), the U.S. Food and Drug Administration has unveiled dozens of larger, more graphic proposed cigarette warning labels, two of which are shown here. After a period of public comment, the FDA will select nine of the new labels by mid-2011; they will appear on all U.S.-sold cigarettes by October 22, 2012. [*www.fda.gov/TobaccoProducts/Labeling*]

strual period have sharply higher rates of breast cancer during middle age than do women who began smoking after a full-term pregnancy. The presumed explanation for this observed fact is that cells within the breasts of adolescent girls are not yet fully differentiated and are thus quite susceptible to the effects of environmental carcinogens like cigarette smoke; breast cells become fully differentiated only after a first pregnancy, after which they are much less sensitive to carcinogenic chemicals. Such findings make it especially important to intensify public health efforts aimed at discouraging cigarette smoking among young teenage girls. Interestingly, older women who have never been pregnant and who have been heavy smokers (20 or more cigarettes daily) for at least twenty years are also at increased risk of developing breast cancer (Band et al., 2002).

Whatever their age, smokers who quit live longer than those who continue to smoke. However, they continue to have a higher risk for certain types of cancer than do people who never used tobacco. During the past few years, a growing number of smokers report cutting back on the frequency of smoking, using cigarettes some days but not on others. Whether this trend is due to higher taxes on tobacco products, to smoking restrictions, or to personal health concerns is not clear, but research has shown that individuals who reduce their tobacco use, even by 50%, as opposed to quitting entirely are just as likely to die of smoking-related diseases as those who are heavy smokers. Risk begins to decline only with complete cessation of smoking (CDC, 2003b).

Most troubling are research findings that smoking during childhood or adolescence, when lung tissue is particularly sensitive, confers a heightened lifelong risk of cancer even when the individual involved subsequently kicked the habit. Such results are especially disturbing in light of the growing numbers of very young smokers. As one cancer researcher remarked, "We have a generation of people who smoked as teenagers, quit, changed their lifestyles, and now are just walking time bombs for cancer to develop" (Wiencke et al., 1999).

Altogether, it is estimated that smoking is responsible for fully 30% of all cancer-related deaths. In light of these realities, those who look forward to a long and healthy life would do well to consider the categorical advice offered by a former U.S. Surgeon General:

> There is no single action an individual can take to reduce the risk of cancer more effectively than to stop smoking—particularly smoking cigarettes.

Dietary Factors

Approximately one-third of all U.S. cancer deaths are believed to be due to dietary factors, but judging from media accounts, most of us misidentify the main culprits. Recent scares about everything from coffee to charcoal-broiled meat to peanut butter having the potential to cause cancer have prompted consumers to fear that many food additives and contaminants are potential carcinogens—a concern that is reflected in the growing popularity of so-called natural or organic foods. This topic will be discussed at greater length in chapter 9. Suffice it to say here that although some food additives—particularly the coal tar dyes used for artificial coloring and sodium nitrite in hot dogs—are known to be carcinogenic in tests on laboratory animals, no solid evidence yet exists to indicate that human cancer rates are rising because of these substances in food. However, bearing in mind the long latency period of many forms of cancer and the fact that many additives have been widely used for only a few decades, it may yet be too early to state categorically that such chemicals won't cause future problems.

Ironically, while many people worry, perhaps unjustifiably, about synthetic food additives, they pay little attention to findings regarding naturally occurring carcinogens in food. Substances called **aflatoxins,** potent carcinogens produced by the fungus *Aspergillus flavus*, cause liver cancer in both humans and animals and are suspected of contributing to the high rates of that disease observed in parts of Africa and Southeast Asia. Aflatoxins are known to act synergistically with the hepatitis B virus and with chronic alcohol consumption (National Research Council, 1996). The toxin-producing mold grows on peanuts, pistachios, corn, rice, and certain other grains and nuts when temperatures and humidity are high. If large quantities of aflatoxin are present in the food, liver damage and death may occur very quickly; in small amounts, consumed over a period of time, aflatoxins are among the strongest carcinogens known. Other natural carcinogens in food include safrole, an extract of sassafras long used to flavor root beer until banned by the FDA in 1960, and oil of calamus, used until 1968 to flavor vermouth. On a more cheerful note, it also has been demonstrated that many foods contain anticarcinogenic compounds whose regular inclusion in one's diet can be protective against many types of cancer. Most notable in this regard are members of the cabbage family—broccoli, cauliflower, cabbage, kale, and brussels sprouts—whose cells contain **sulforaphane,** one of the most potent anticarcinogens yet discovered. Cooked tomato products rich in **lycopene**—especially tomato sauce, tomato juice, and pizza—have long been associated with a reduced risk of prostate cancer. Other tasty sources of protection against cancer include yellow and green vegetables, citrus fruits, apricots, cantaloupe, brown rice, wheat germ, soy products, onions, and garlic (Davis, 1990; Giovanucci et al., 1995; Kliewer and Smith, 1995).

Alcohol is another dietary factor recognized as increasing one's risk for cancer, although the mechanism of causation is still not well understood. Research has shown that men who consume two or more alcoholic drinks a day, and women who have just one, enhance their chances of developing certain types of cancer. One of the strongest alcohol-cancer links concerns liver cancer; heavy alcohol consumption can cause cirrhosis of the liver, especially when combined with a hepatitis C infection. Other cancers showing a strong association with alcohol use are those of the mouth, esophagus, and pharynx; according to the American Cancer Society, 75–80% of people who develop oral cancers are heavy drinkers. The risk is even greater if alcohol consumption is accompanied, as it often is, with tobacco use, since alcohol and cigarette smoke interact synergistically.

Perhaps most important of all in reference to food and cancer is the conviction among many researchers that there is a direct correlation between high fat intake and rates of colon and prostate cancer, as well as a relationship between stomach cancer and consumption of smoked, salt-pickled, and salt-cured foods. In addition, being excessively overweight seems to favor development of cancer of the endometrium, esophagus, and gall bladder (Doll, 1996; Willett, 1994). Women who are more than 50 pounds overweight are also at significantly enhanced risk of breast cancer, particularly after menopause (Rose, 1996). However, the widespread suspicion among health experts that breast cancer incidence is closely associated with high-fat diets was dispelled by results of a 14-year study of almost 89,000 women, which demonstrated that those who consume large amounts of fat have no higher risk of developing breast cancer than women whose diet is low in fat. Reducing dietary fat intake confers significant benefits in preventing heart disease, but apparently has no impact one way or the other in reducing breast cancer risk (Holmes et al., 1999). Although much remains to be learned concerning the relationship between dietary factors and cancer, current scientific evidence strongly suggests that a diet rich in a wide variety of fruits, vegetables, beans, and grain products and low in meat, dairy products, and other high-fat foods can significantly reduce overall cancer risk.

Air Pollution

It has long been known that urban air contains a number of carcinogenic substances, benzo(a)pyrene among the most potent. Obtaining conclusive proof that breathing polluted air, by itself, induces cancer has been complicated by the fact that many cancer victims living in regions of poor air quality are also smokers. However, a number of well-designed epidemiologic studies, along with research utilizing techniques from molecular genetics, have yielded results demonstrating a clear association between polluted air and increased incidence of lung cancer. In southern California, a study of more than 6,000 nonsmoking Seventh-Day Adventists who had lived in areas with elevated levels of particulate matter, sulfur dioxide, and ozone found an excess rate of lung cancer among both men and women within this population (Beeson, Abbey, and Knutson, 1998). Halfway around the world, in a heavily industrialized region of Poland where coal combustion for industry and home heating has fouled the air for decades, studies have shown a close correlation between lung cancer incidence and residence in highly polluted neighborhoods. Scientists working in Krakow have demonstrated how air contaminants can damage the molecular structure of genes. Examining DNA from white blood cells of Polish central-city residents, researchers found that certain polycyclic aromatic hydrocarbons (PAHs) produced from burning coal bond to the DNA molecule to form PAH-DNA adducts. Since adducts at that location on the gene had previously been linked to elevated lung cancer risk, this finding provides additional evidence that certain air pollutants damage the genetic material and hence play a direct role in cancer causation (Whyatt et al., 1998).

Occupational Exposure

It has long been recognized that certain occupations entail heightened risk of specific diseases. In recent decades the proliferation of new synthetic chemicals in industry, as well as the continued use of older substances only recently recognized as hazardous, has been reflected in cancer rates far higher among certain segments of the workforce than among the general public. Estimates of the number of American workers potentially exposed to chemicals considered by the National Institute of Occupational Safety and Health (NIOSH) to be proven or likely carcinogens range from 3–9 million; many others work with materials suspected to be carcinogens but on which the necessary testing has not yet been done. NIOSH estimates that less than 2% of all workplace chemicals have been tested for carcinogenicity. Occupational exposure is believed responsible for 12,000–26,000 U.S. cancer deaths each year, with estimates of 152,000 for the worldwide toll. In addition, 40,000 new cases of cancer in the U.S. each year are blamed on workplace exposure (NIOSH, 2009).

Until passage of the Toxic Substances Control Act in 1976, giving the federal government the power to require testing of potentially hazardous substances before they go on the market, hundreds of new chemicals with unknown side effects came into industrial use each year. Unfortunately, the carcinogenicity of many substances was recognized only after exposed workers, like human "guinea pigs," fell sick or died. Some of the most significant industrial carcinogens thus discovered include:

- **asbestos,** one of the best-known occupational hazards, which is expected to cause the death of 30–40% of all asbestos workers

- **vinyl chloride,** a basic ingredient in the manufacture of plastics, found in 1974 to induce a rare form of liver cancer among exposed workers

- **anesthetic gases** used in operating rooms have been identified as the reason nurse anesthetists develop leukemia and lymphoma at three times the normal rate and also experience higher rates of miscarriage and birth defects among their children

- **benzene,** long known to be a powerful bone marrow poison capable of causing aplastic anemia, has now been shown to cause leukemia as well

- **coke oven emissions** have been linked with cancers of the lung, trachea, bronchus, and kidneys and are now regulated as hazardous air pollutants when vented to the outdoor air

- **benzidine, naphythylamine,** and several other chemicals associated with rubber and dye manufacturing pose an excess risk of bladder cancer to exposed workers in those industries

- **hardwood dust** inhaled by cabinet and furniture makers can lead to malignant nasal tumors

- **radioactive mine dusts** have been a particular problem in uranium mines, resulting in lung cancer rates among miners four times higher than the national average

Although pressure from labor unions and adoption of protective government legislation have resulted in some improvements in reducing occupational hazards, standards set for protecting workers are far less stringent than those set for protecting society at large. In addition, workers years ago often lacked basic information about the nature of the materials with which they worked and were thus unable to take precautions even if they desired to do so. A major step forward in this regard was promulgation by the Occupational Safety and Health Administration (OSHA) in 1983 of its Hazard Communication Standard, intended to provide employees in manufacturing industries access to information concerning the hazards of chemicals that they encounter in the workplace. Essentially a federal "Employee Right-to-Know" law, this ruling requires that U.S. manufacturers inform their employees of any workplace hazards and how they can minimize risk of harm. Manufacturers must also ensure that all chemicals are properly labeled and that Material Safety Data Sheets for each chemical are available for any employee who requests them.

Reproductive/Sexual Behavior

The National Cancer Institute estimates that 7% of all cancer deaths can be linked with reproductive factors or sexual practices. For reasons thought to relate to hormone levels, breast cancer incidence is significantly higher among women who experienced early onset of menstruation, childless women or women who first gave birth at a late age, and women who were older than average at the time of menopause. Conversely, research suggests that mothers who breast-feed, especially *teenage mothers* who nurse their babies for at least six months, cut their risk of developing breast cancer before menopause nearly in half. For women in their 20s and 30s, prolonged breast-feeding reduces cancer risk by approximately 22%. Although such risk factors are largely beyond the control of the women involved, those who fall into one or more of these categories should be especially conscientious about having regular mammograms once they reach age 40.

Risk factors for cervical cancer are more subject to self-control: early age at the time of first intercourse and multiple sex partners predispose a woman to subsequent development of this type of cancer. Chances of contracting uterine cancer are enhanced by early onset of menstruation, late menopause, a failure to ovulate, a history of infertility, or by excessive obesity (Pitot, 2002).

Preventing Cancer

The preceding discussion should make it apparent that while we still have much to learn about the nature of carcinogenesis, we have already discovered enough to suggest a variety of personal actions that individuals can take to substantially reduce their own risk of developing cancer. Malignancies caused by tobacco use, responsible for more than 170,000 U.S. cancer deaths every year, could be prevented entirely. Eating generous amounts of fruits and green and yellow vegetables daily, while cutting down on meat and total calories could, along with regular exercise, significantly reduce the estimated one-third of fatal cancers attributed to dietary factors. Avoiding excessive sun exposure and using a high-SPF sunscreen when such exposure is unavoidable could have a major impact on reducing new cases of skin cancer, currently totaling over one million annually in the United States. More widespread use of vaccines and antibiotics to prevent or treat infections known to cause several major types of cancer could have a significant impact on lowering cancer incidence, particularly in developing countries where such infections are rampant. Although medical science continues its aggressive search for a cancer cure, even the most optimistic researchers affirm that preventing cancer from ever developing is the most effective way of combating this dreaded, but certainly not inevitable, disease.

⋯⋯⋯ 7 ⋯⋯⋯

What is it that is not poison?
All things are poison and nothing is without poison.
It is the dose only that makes a thing not a poison.
—Paracelsus (16th Century)

Toxic Substances

Human illness or death due to contact with toxic materials in the environment is certainly not unique to the modern age. Hippocrates described the symptoms of lead poisoning as early as 370 BC; mercury fumes in Roman mines in Spain made work there the equivalent of a death sentence to the unfortunate slaves receiving such an assignment; for centuries Turkish villagers in central Anatolia who live in homes built of asbestos-containing volcanic rock have been dying of lung disease. Yet for the most part, such examples of illness caused by direct contact with toxic substances have been confined to certain occupational groups or to people who, by chance, happened to be living in an area where there was an unnaturally high concentration of some toxic material. In the past, large populations seldom, if ever, were exposed to significant amounts of toxicants on a sustained basis. Since the early 20th century, however, that situation has changed, thanks in part to the tremendous increase in industrial production, as well as to the "chemical revolution" that has introduced thousands of new synthetic compounds into widespread use in recent decades. Some of these substances, several of which were briefly mentioned in the preceding chapter, are largely confined to an occupational setting and pose little threat to the general public. Others, however, are now virtually omnipresent throughout the human environment and are generating considerable controversy as to the degree of public health threat they present.

In this chapter we will describe the process by which chemicals are tested for toxicity and their health risks assessed. We will then take a closer look at several of these substances—some naturally occurring, others artificially produced—to which human exposure is nearly universal and which are known to cause serious health damage.

TESTING FOR TOXICITY

"Toxic" or "toxicant" are terms scientists use to describe a chemical that provokes an adverse systemic effect on living organisms. That is, **toxicants** have the ability to cause harm to organs or biochemical processes away from the site on the body where exposure occurred. In this sense they differ from other harmful chemicals such as corrosives or irritants, which damage only the tissues they contact. For example, spilling concentrated acid on one's hand will result in a painful chemical burn, followed by loss of skin, but damage is localized to that area. By contrast, ingesting small amounts of arsenic over an extended time period can result in cirrhosis of the liver, skin discoloration, and peripheral nerve damage, among other problems. **Poison,** a word many people use as a synonym for toxic, actually has a much narrower meaning, referring to a chemical that can cause illness or death at a very low dose of exposure—approximately 3/4 of a teaspoon for an adult or 1/8 of a teaspoon for a toddler.

Very few chemicals are capable of causing death in such low amounts, hence the list of true poisons is much shorter than commonly believed. Another term frequently equated with "toxic" is **hazardous,** whose actual meaning is more complex. The hazardous nature of a substance is dependent both on its inherent capacity to do harm (e.g., its degree of toxicity, corrosiveness, flammability, etc.) and, equally important, on the likelihood of that substance coming into contact with people. Methyl parathion, one of the most toxic insecticides, presents an extreme hazard to migrant farm workers entering a just-sprayed field without protective clothing; the very same chemical presents virtually no hazard when stored in its original container inside a securely locked storeroom.

The study of toxic substances, or **toxicology,** in an informal sense is probably as old as the human species. Long before written records were kept, ancient peoples learned through trial and error which plants and animals should be avoided because of their toxic properties. Among classical civilizations, knowledge of mineral toxicants was well established and was extensively applied to the art of poisoning one's enemies! Modern toxicology is a relatively recent offshoot of pharmacological science, its origin as an independent field of inquiry prompted initially by the needs of occupational medicine. Toxicology has gained added importance in recent decades due to the rapid growth of the chemical industry and associated public concerns regarding health effects of toxic chemicals.

Whether a chemical provokes a toxic effect—or any effect at all—is dependent on a number of variables, the most important of which is the **dose-time** relationship, that is, the amount of the chemical in question (dose) and the duration of exposure (time). Depending on the nature of the dose-time relationship, toxicity can be categorized as either acute or chronic. A chemical's **acute toxicity** refers to its ability to cause harm as a result of one-time exposure to a relatively large amount of the substance. Most accidental childhood poisonings (e.g., drinking a liquid pesticide stored in a cola bottle) represent harm caused by acutely toxic chemicals. **Chronic toxicity,** by contrast, refers to a chemical's ability to impair health when repeated low-dose exposure to the chemical occurs over a long time period. Interestingly, the effects of acute vs. chronic toxicity for the same chemical are often quite different in terms of symptoms and bodily organs involved. As an example, with acute exposure lead poisoning manifests itself as severe abdominal pains, while chronic lead toxicity provokes anemia and nervous system damage. Not only is there no correlation between acute and chronic toxicity symptoms, there also is no connection between their relative potency. A chemical that is very toxic in acute exposure situations may be nontoxic chronically. Similarly, a chemical with minimal acute toxicity may present a greater danger when exposure is chronic.

Another parameter influencing toxicity is the chemical's route of exposure. Toxic substances can enter the body through the mouth when a person eats, drinks, or smokes (**oral**); through the skin (**dermal**); or via the lungs if the substance is inhaled (**respiratory**). Depending on the chemical in question, toxicity will vary, depending on the route of exposure—very few chemicals are equally toxic by all three routes.

Toxicity is also profoundly affected by species, a fact that troubles those questioning the validity of animal testing procedures. Chemicals that are very toxic to some animal species may be only slightly toxic or nontoxic to others, including humans. Close taxonomic relationship is no predictor of how a particular species will react in a toxicity test. For some chemicals, toxicity in both humans and monkeys is very similar, while for other substances humans may join cats and dogs in being highly sensitive while monkeys suffer no adverse effects. Just as genetic variability among species influences toxicity, so do genetic differences *within* a population. Individual susceptibility, based on each person's (or each guinea pig's) biochemical makeup, explains the range of effects among members of a group exposed to exactly the same dose of any substance.

Determining the acute, subchronic, and chronic toxicity of a chemical is necessary in order to establish protective regulations. Acute toxicity is generally described using the technical term **LD_{50}** (LD = lethal dose), which refers to the amount of the chemical, administered in one dose, that is required to kill 50% of a population of test animals within a 14-day period. LD_{50} is expressed as the number of milligrams of chemical per kilogram of body weight. Thus the lower the LD_{50}, the smaller the dose required to kill; in other words, the lower the LD_{50}, the more acutely toxic the chemical is (substances legally termed "poisons" are those with an LD_{50} of 50 or less). For obvious reasons, acute toxicity testing is restricted to populations of laboratory animals; thus when results are used to estimate lethal doses for humans, considerable judgment must be exercised, recognizing that humans may be more or less sensitive than the test species. For some chemicals, unfortunately, direct human results may supplement animal data. When known quantities of a toxicant are involved in accidental poisonings, suicides, murders, or industrial accidents, these quantities can be related to the severity and type of symptoms and then compared with animal test results. If such data indicate the chemical is more or less toxic to humans than to animals, the human results supersede the animal data.

Testing for subchronic and chronic toxicity is more difficult, time-consuming, and expensive than acute toxicity testing and considerably less is known about the long-term effects of a chemical than about its acute effects. Symptoms of chronic toxicity may take months or years to manifest themselves, and because such symptoms are often similar to other common health complaints they may be misdiagnosed.

Testing for subchronic and chronic toxicity involves animal-feeding experiments, most commonly using rats or dogs. After determining the daily dose of chemical the animals are likely to be able to tolerate for long periods (a determination based on the chemical's LD_{50}), the animals are divided into three or more test groups, plus a control group. Each group will have the same number of animals and a balanced male/female ratio. Beginning at the time the animals are weaned, each group of test animals is fed a specified level of the toxicant mixed with its feed. One group receives a dose expected to have significant sublethal chronic effects; one group receives an amount of the toxicant predicted to have no effect; the third group is fed a level of toxicant intermediate between the other two. The control group is treated in exactly the same manner as the other animals except that no toxicant is added to its food. Subchronic toxicity tests typically are run for 90 days, their main intent being to establish levels of exposure at which no adverse effects can be observed and to identify which organ or organs suffer damage after repeated exposure to the toxicant being tested. Daily records are kept detailing the animals' appearance and behavior. At the end of the three-month test period, the animals are killed and autopsied, being carefully examined for evidence of organ damage or other adverse changes. Tests for chronic toxicity are conducted in the same manner as described for subchronic testing, except that the duration of exposure to the chemical is considerably longer. Chronic toxicity tests are usually carried out for a time period equivalent to the average lifespan of the test animals (generally rats or mice). Since determination of a chemical's carcinogenicity is a prime goal of chronic toxicity tests, autopsies performed at the conclusion of the test period are focused specifically on the incidence and location of tumors.

The data collected from these studies are plotted on a **dose-response curve,** which has three parts. The first portion of the curve, on the far left, is horizontal—an indication that low doses of the toxicant produce no ill effects. The middle portion of the curve begins at a point called the **threshold,** where increasing dosage is beginning to provoke adverse symptoms. The curve continues to climb upward as the dose increases until, in its final portion, it again flattens out after reaching its maximum effect (i.e., death). The dose-response curve describes one of the most basic principles of toxicology—the greater the dose of a toxicant, the greater the effect. If all groups of test animals displayed the same symptoms of harm, or if the group fed the lowest level of toxicant suffered more adverse health effects than the group receiving the highest dose, it could be concluded that something other than

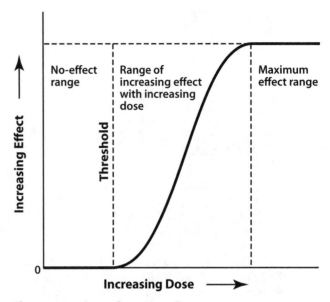

Figure 7-1   Dose-Response Curve

the toxicant caused the observed problems. Demonstration of the existence of thresholds is also of great importance to an understanding of toxicity. Because the threshold of toxicity for a chemical varies among species, as well as within a population of the same species and even in the same individual, depending on age and health status, it will probably never be possible to determine precisely where the threshold of tolerance is for any particular person. Nevertheless, knowing that there is a safe level of exposure facilitates regulation by providing a basis for establishing **margins of safety**—a buffer zone between the highest level of a chemical that produces no adverse effect in an animal species and a level of exposure assumed to be safe for humans. In the United States, a hundredfold margin of safety has traditionally been employed for regulatory control of toxic substances. This number was arbitrarily chosen, based on the assumptions that (1) humans are 10 times more susceptible to the toxic effects of chemicals than are laboratory animals and (2) the more vulnerable members of the population—young children, the elderly, the immunocompromised—are 10 times more sensitive than the average healthy adult. In spite of the uncertainties inherent in such assumptions, the fact that legal exposure limits to toxicants are well below the no-effect level should provide some reassurance (Ottoboni, 1991).

ASSESSING HEALTH RISK

As fears of the potentially harmful health effects of chemical exposure have increased in recent decades, a concerned public has demanded that government act to manage such risks. Doing so effectively requires decision

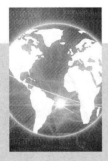

······ 7-1 ·······

Bisphenol A—Should We Worry?

There's no question that humans are widely exposed to bisphenol A (BPA), over 6 billion pounds of which are produced in the U.S. each year for making plastics. Tests conducted by the CDC on more than 2,500 volunteers ages 6 to adult found that 93% of them had detectable traces of BPA in their urine; since BPA is a rapidly metabolized chemical, its presence in such a large proportion of the test population indicates near-constant exposure (BPA has also been found in human blood and breast milk). Such statistics, bolstered by over a thousand animal studies showing adverse health effects in mammalian fetuses and newborns exposed to BPA, have led to serious concern among some scientists, consumer groups, environmentalists, and parents as to whether low-level exposure to this chemical could be insidiously undermining children's health.

Human exposure to bisphenol A is nothing new. The chemical has been used commercially since 1936 when it came into use as a synthetic estrogen, but today BPA is employed primarily in the production of polycarbonate plastics and epoxy resins. The former, identified by the #7 on items made of this material, are used for food and drink containers, baby bottles, sippy cups, and plastic tableware, as well as a number of other products. Epoxy resin lacquers are found as coatings on metal products such as food cans, bottle tops, and water supply pipes. In some cases, dental sealants can also constitute sources of BPA exposure. Unfortu-

nately, bisphenol A can leach from plastic food or beverage containers or from the epoxy coating in food cans, resulting in chemical contamination of the contents. The amount of leaching that occurs depends largely on the surrounding temperature—the hotter it is, the more likely that BPA will leach into foods or liquids. For this reason, an individual's diet constitutes the primary source of exposure to BPA, with infants and children thought to have the highest daily intake among the general population (NIEHS, 2009).

The Food and Drug Administration (FDA) approved the use of bisphenol A in food contact materials in the early 1960s and has set the safe daily exposure level for BPA at 50 µg/

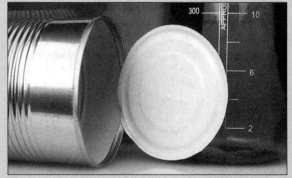

National Institute of Environmental Health Sciences (NIEHS).

kilogram of body weight. For many years its use was largely noncontroversial; when Congress passed the **Toxic Substances Control Act (TSCA)** in 1976, requiring manufacturers to provide EPA with data on the health and environmental effects of new chemicals prior to their introduction, BPA was one of 62,000 chemicals already in use that were "grandfathered" in, not subject to safety testing requirements.

Questions about potential health problems associated with BPA exposure first arose in the 1990s as a result of animal studies showing that rodents exposed to the chemical exhibited a wide range of health effects, including cancers of the mammary and prostate glands, early onset of puberty in females, obesity, and attention-deficit disorder. Knowing that BPA is a hormone-mimic and concerned about the implications of these animal studies for potential human health problems, some of the researchers involved began raising the alarm, arguing that the FDA should act quickly to ban the use of bisphenol A in food contact substances.

Not surprisingly, the chemical industry, as well as a number of scientists, countered with studies of their own showing no evidence of human health damage resulting from exposure to BPA at levels prevailing in the general population. The American Chemistry Council, a trade association representing plastics manufacturers, argues that the toxicology of BPA is well understood and that the chemical is dangerous only when exposure levels are very high. BPA detractors reject such arguments, insisting that because BPA is a hormone-mimic, not a standard toxin, even low-dose exposures can exert harmful effects. In fact, they argue, any exposure at all can cause problems, since when BPA interacts with hormone receptors on cell membranes, even one part per *trillion* can elicit a physiological response (Hinterthuer, 2008). To this, skeptics ask why, with such widespread exposure, don't we see more obvious problems among human populations? Perhaps, they say, BPA is more of a health issue for rodents than it is for people.

In an effort to resolve the debate, the National Toxicology Program (NTP) evaluated the available scientific literature on BPA and issued a report in September 2008, concluding that while considerable uncertainty remains as to whether the effects seen in animal studies are directly applicable to people, the "possibility that BPA may affect human development cannot be dismissed." The NTP report expressed "some concern" regarding bisphenol A's effects on the brain, behavior, and prostate gland of fetuses, infants, and children because animal studies indicated effects occurring at levels of exposure similar to those experienced by humans. By contrast, the report stated there was little reason for concern about most of the other issues raised by BPA opponents, specifically discounting the likelihood of BPA-induced reproductive effects among adults. Nevertheless, the report emphasized the extent of uncertainty in the scientific literature, the conflicting findings, and, especially, the very limited amount of data from human, as opposed to animal, studies. Acknowledging the difficulty in offering advice to the public on this issue, authors of the report conceded the need for more research to understand how these findings relate to human health and development—but added that it's possible that the effects observed with rodents *may* occur in humans as well. They also offered worried parents suggestions on how they can personally reduce exposure. Such precautionary actions include:

- don't microwave any plastic food containers with the #7 on the bottom

- don't wash such containers in the dishwasher

- reduce personal use of canned foods, eating fresh or frozen foods instead

- whenever possible, choose glass, ceramic, or stainless steel food containers, especially for hot foods or liquids

- use only BPA-free baby bottles and choose toys that are labeled BPA-free (NIEHS, 2009)

Although by early 2010 FDA had not yet taken regulatory action regarding BPA, several other governmental bodies have already done so. In 2008, Canada banned the use of BPA in baby bottles, declaring the substance hazardous to humans. Minnesota, Chicago, and Suffolk County, NY, followed suit in 2009, becoming the first state, city, and county, respectively, to ban bisphenol A-containing baby bottles and sippy cups (Chicago's ban became effective in 2010, Minnesota's in 2011). Other states are considering similar bans, and federal legislation to prohibit BPA in all food and beverage containers has been introduced in both the House and Senate. Recognizing the public's misgivings about BPA, several large retailers, including Walmart, CVS, Babies 'R' Us, and Target have phased out selling baby bottles containing BPA. In October 2010, the Canadian government took its opposition to BPA one step further, officially declaring it a toxic substance; this will make it easier to ban in additional consumer products. Canada's move was condemned by the American Chemistry Council as contrary to the

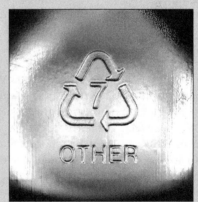

National Institute of Environmental Health Sciences (NIEHS).

weight of scientific evidence. Clearly, the debate among the experts regarding BPA's safety remains unresolved, though there seems to be a mounting groundswell of public opinion to opt for "the precautionary principle" when it comes to bisphenol A.

makers to determine whether a particular substance presents a greater danger than society is willing to accept, to examine the available options for controlling such hazards, and then to adopt policy measures (i.e., regulatory controls, product bans, market-based incentives, educational efforts) that reduce or eliminate unacceptable risk. **Risk management,** however, is dependent on accurate **risk assessment**—determining whether something suspected of presenting a human health threat is in fact dangerous, estimating how much injury or harm is likely to result from a given level of exposure, and determining if those consequences are serious enough to warrant action.

Health risk assessment began to receive serious professional attention early in the 20th century when adverse effects associated with certain types of occupational exposures were described. Investigations into the relationship between levels of exposure and the observed human health effects led to the identification of **no-observed-effect-levels (NOELs)** and the establishment of adequate margins of safety for exposure. By the early 1970s, creation of the U.S. Environmental Protection Agency and the Occupational Safety and Health Administration—agencies charged with writing regulations and implementing the provisions of a number of far-reaching new environmental, health, and safety laws—gave health risk assessment a major boost. By necessity, risk assessment became a prime component of the regulatory decision-making process, and modern quantitative methods of analysis emerged in response to this need. During the past 40 years, health risk assessments have been employed for a wide range of regulatory issues: food additives, pesticide residues, drinking water contaminants, indoor air pollutants, and so forth. Although hazardous substances can adversely affect human health in various ways—immune system dysfunction, reproductive or teratogenic effects, organ damage, nervous system impairment—the potential carcinogenicity of suspect chemicals has been the main focus of health risk assessments in recent years.

Health risk assessment constitutes a four-step process:

1. *Hazard identification.* Aimed at determining whether a particular substance or agent has an adverse effect on human health (e.g., is the substance carcinogenic?). Such a determination is typically made on the basis of animal testing, as described in box 6-3. If these tests indicate no harm from exposure, there is no need for further investigation; on the other hand, if exposure to the substance causes death or injury to some of the test animals, risk assessment proceeds to the next step.

2. *Dose-response assessment.* Since health effects of the same substance can be either harmful, beneficial, or neutral, depending on the amount of exposure received, determining the dose at or below which no effects are detected is important for establishing safety standards. For noncarcinogenic toxic substances this is a relatively straightforward process; empirical evidence has shown that biological effects of exposure to noncarcinogenic chemicals appear only after a threshold level has been exceeded. Exposing laboratory animals to varying doses of the agent in question permits identification of the lowest-observable-effect-level (LOEL), the no-observed-adverse-effect-level (NOAEL)—the dose at or below which no harmful effects are observed, and the no-observed-effect-level (NOEL). This dose-response information facilitates the determination of threshold levels of exposure.

For carcinogens, however, the situation is complicated by a working assumption, adopted by regulatory agencies on the premise it's better to be safe than sorry, that there is no threshold for cancer-causing substances—even one molecule of a carcinogen can initiate cancer. Evidence has been growing that this assumption is incorrect and that, for some carcinogens at least, a threshold does, in fact, exist. Nevertheless, the no-threshold approach to regulating carcinogens still applies. All parties to the controversy agree, however, that the risk of developing cancer is much greater when the exposure dose is high than when it is low.

3. *Exposure assessment.* Attempting to determine the numbers and types of people (age, sex, health status, etc.) who might be exposed to the substance in question, as well as estimating the duration, magnitude, and geographic extent of exposure, constitute the third step in the risk assessment process. In many real-life situations, some of the necessary information is unavailable—particularly actual exposure data—and those performing the analysis frequently must resort to computer modeling based on generalized assumptions about human behavior and how chemicals move in the environment. Generalizations on behavior include guesses on the kinds and quantities of food individuals in the target population eat each day; how much water they drink; how much time they spend indoors vs. outdoors. Assumptions regarding the environmental mobility of a chemical deal with its chemical stability, whether it dissolves in water or animal fat, how quickly it evaporates, or whether it binds to soil. The validity of assumptions about such parameters, in the absence of actual measurements, is questionable, making exposure assessment one of the weaker links in the information chain.

4. *Risk characterization.* Combining the information obtained from the first three steps of the risk assessment process, analysts produce a comprehensive picture of the types of adverse health effects likely to occur in exposed populations and the frequency with

which such effects can be expected to occur. Risk is usually expressed in terms of quantitative probability; for example, one cancer death per 10,000 exposed population or 10^{-4} risk. For noncarcinogens, the risk characterization typically yields **Acceptable Daily Intakes (ADIs)** derived from dividing animal study NOELs by safety factors.

Information gathered through the risk assessment process is of great value to risk managers, but such data are incapable of answering many of the values-based questions with which decision makers wrestle: How safe is "safe enough"? What trade-offs between risks, benefits, and costs of control are justified? Will reducing an existing risk merely replace it with a newer, more dangerous one? Which among competing risks merits the greatest attention and resource allocation for abatement? Societal values and priorities must inevitably be taken into account in resolving these issues. Trade-offs among competing interests, political considerations, legal obligations, and scientific uncertainties are all factors that risk managers weigh as they decide how best to reduce hazards and protect public health. Risk assessment, while not perfect, provides a valuable tool for making appropriate decisions (American Chemical Society, 1998).

POLYCHLORINATED BIPHENYLS (PCBS)

In 1964 Dr. Soren Jensen, a Swedish chemist at the University of Stockholm, began a project to determine DDT levels in human fat and wildlife samples; instead he discovered that the tissues he was examining contained large amounts of synthetic organic chemicals called PCBs. His findings, published in 1966, were greeted with widespread surprise and disbelief because PCBs, unlike DDT and other chlorinated hydrocarbon pesticides, were not being deliberately released into the environment but were restricted to use in industrial settings. Despite the initial skepticism, subsequent studies by researchers in many countries confirmed Dr. Jensen's findings. Virtually every tissue sample tested, from fish to birds to polar bears to animals living in deep sea trenches, contained detectable levels of PCBs. Extensive research during the decades that followed revealed that of all the chemical contaminants known, PCBs are the most widespread throughout the global environment.

How Could This Situation Come About?

Polychlorinated biphenyls were first synthesized in 1929, their production being taken over in 1930 by Monsanto, which sold the chemical under the trade name Arochlor. PCBs, which range in consistency from oily liquids to waxy solids, are extremely stable substances with a high boiling point, high solubility in fat but low solubility in water, low electrical conductivity, and high resistance to heat—all qualities that made them valuable for a wide variety of industrial uses. Primarily employed as cooling liquids in electrical transformers and capacitors, PCBs also have been used in hydraulic fluids, in carbonless carbon paper, insulating tapes, adhesives, paints, caulking compounds, sealants, and as road coverings to control dust.

The chemical stability that made PCBs so attractive to industry, however, is the very characteristic that has made them such an environmental and health hazard. Although designed for industrial use, there are many ways in which PCBs can inadvertently escape and contaminate the environment:

1. Discharge of PCB-laden wastes from factories into waterways have resulted in mammoth pollution problems, the most notorious episodes being Outboard Marine Corporation's dumping of PCBs into Waukegan Harbor (on Lake Michigan) and a similar situation in the Hudson River, traced to two General Electric plants.

2. Vaporization from paints or landfills or burning of PCB-containing material can result in the chemical becoming airborne and then reentering the ecosystem with precipitation. EPA estimates that approximately 89% of PCBs entering Lake Superior are deposited via airborne fallout (EPA, 1994). A classic example of fire causing extensive PCB contamination occurred early in 1981 in Binghamton, New York, where PCB-containing electrical equipment in the basement of the newly built State Office Building caught fire. Although the blaze was quickly extinguished, inspectors subsequently discovered that contaminated soot had been carried through the air conditioning system and deposited throughout the entire building. Air sampling indicated that this soot contained 10–20% PCBs, as well as lesser amounts of dioxin and dibenzofurans formed during the combustion process. The ensuing cleanup operation took seven years to complete and cost New York taxpayers $37 million (Fawcett, 1988).

3. Leaks in industrial equipment have resulted in numerous instances of PCB contamination, such as the case during the summer of 1979 when 200 gallons of PCBs leaked from an electrical transformer at a feed-processing plant in Billings, Montana, contaminating about a million pounds of meal used in chicken feed. Subsequently, $2.7 million worth of chickens and eggs had to be destroyed because the birds had eaten the contaminated meal before the leak was discovered (Regenstein, 1982).

4. Accidental spills or illegal dumping are a source of concern because the high cost of legally disposing of PCB wastes has tempted some haulers to dump such materials along roadsides, in ditches, or other out-of-the-way places. In the summer of 1978 such "midnight dumpers" opened the discharge pipe of their truck while driving along 243 miles of back roads in 14 North Carolina counties, releasing 31,000 gallons of PCB-laden waste oil along the roadside where it remained until a major remediation effort, jointly funded by the EPA and the State of North Carolina, was launched to remove the contaminated soil and bury it in a hazardous waste landfill constructed for that purpose in 1983.

Whatever the route, once PCBs enter the environment they persist there for decades, resisting breakdown. Contamination of living organisms with PCBs generally occurs via the food chain, the concentration of the chemical increasing as it moves from lower to higher trophic levels ("biomagnification," see chapter 8). Within an individual organism, especially among higher-level consumers such as carnivorous birds, fish, and humans, PCBs accumulate in fatty tissues such as liver, kidneys, heart, lungs, brain, and breast milk. By 1976, after more than forty years of PCB production and use, 99% of all breast milk sampled in the United States contained PCBs. A quarter of the samples tested exceeded the legal level of contamination, which would have caused a commercial product to be banned from sale (Steingraber, 1997). With continuing exposure, PCB concentrations in the body increase over a period of time, a process known as **bioaccumulation**.

PCB Threat to Health

Widespread human exposure to PCBs has concerned health and regulatory officials because laboratory testing has shown the chemicals to be toxic to several animal species even at very low concentrations. In experiments with rodents, minks, and Rhesus monkeys, PCB exposure has resulted in the development of a number of adverse health effects: liver disorders, miscarriage, low birth weight, abnormal multiplication of cells, and (in rats only) liver cancer. Researchers presumed that chemicals that could produce such effects in some mammalian species were likely to have similar effects on humans, and the knowledge that virtually everyone on the planet has been exposed to at least trace amounts of PCBs was considered cause for alarm. Evidence that many foods, especially freshwater fish, were contaminated with PCBs prompted the U.S. government to take regulatory action. In 1973 the FDA established tolerance levels for PCBs in food; passage of the Toxic Substances Control Act in 1976 specifically banned the production, sale, distribu-

tion, and use of PCBs in open systems; and in 1977, Monsanto, the sole U.S. manufacturer of the chemicals, terminated PCB production.

In the meantime, research on the human health impact of PCBs continued and today a wealth of scientific data exists on the chemical's toxicological effects. Contrary to popular perception, the acute toxicity of PCBs is quite low. The most frequent complaint provoked by high levels of PCB exposure is the appearance of an acne-like skin disorder referred to as chloracne. Regarded as the most characteristic symptom of PCB poisoning (or poisoning with any of the related group of chemicals known as chlorinated hydrocarbons), chloracne was an occasional occupational health problem among workers during the early years of PCB production and use. Recognition of this hazard led to the establishment in 1942 of recommended maximum allowable concentrations in the workplace. Since then, with the exception of a few cases of chloracne and possibly diminished liver function, scarcely any adverse health effects attributable to PCB exposure have been documented, even among workers who were exposed to PCBs over a period of many years.

For humans, exposure to PCBs could occur via skin absorption if a person happens to touch PCB-containing lubricants or oils leaking from old equipment or if he/she were to swim in PCB-contaminated waters. Dermal exposure, however, poses far less of a health risk than does either inhalation or ingestion of PCBs. People living near hazardous waste sites or landfills where PCBs are present can be exposed to these chemicals by inhaling PCBs evaporating from the soil into the air or by drinking contaminated groundwater. The most common route of entry, affecting the largest number of people, is consumption of sports fish caught in PCB-contaminated lakes and rivers. Meat and dairy products may also constitute dietary sources of PCBs, though to a lesser degree than fish (ATSDR, 2000).

Concerns about PCBs in fish made news in 2004 with the publication of research indicating that farmed salmon, one of America's most popular fish, contains potentially dangerous levels of PCBs, as well as dioxin and several organochlorine pesticides. The presence of these contaminants in farmed salmon is blamed on the fact that these fish are raised on a concentrated feed made of various PCB-tainted fish oils and fish meals (a mixture that is already being modified in response to the adverse market reaction to this news). Interestingly, PCB levels in farmed salmon vary widely, depending on the area where they are raised; those from European salmon farms tested highest for contamination, while those from Chile were lowest, with North American salmon registering levels somewhere in between. The report's authors concluded that because of the high PCB levels, farmed salmon consumption should be limited to one meal per month in order to avoid increased risk of cancer.

Such advice is hotly disputed by other scientists who point out that, although elevated, the PCB levels documented aren't high enough to pose serious danger and don't outweigh the undisputed nutritional benefits of farmed salmon, specifically the protection against heart attacks conferred by their omega-3 polyunsaturated fatty acids. Part of the dispute between scientists relates to the fact that the "safe" level set by the Food and Drug Administration (FDA) for PCBs in fish sold in supermarkets—a level based on nutritional benefits as well as safety considerations—is 40 times higher than EPA's standard for fish caught by sports fishers, for which health is the sole consideration. According to FDA standards, the PCB levels detected in farmed salmon are not excessive, while under EPA guidelines they are. As the experts wrangle over these questions, aquaculturists are hard at work, experimenting with new feed mixtures that will eliminate the PCB problem. One approach would substitute the fish oil component with a variety of transgenic canola oil containing a precursor to omega-3 fatty acids (Hites et al., 2004; Stokstad, 2004).

Since few members of the general public ever receive the relatively high levels of exposure experienced by workers in an occupational setting, the main concern about PCBs' possible health impact has focused on chronic toxicity, specifically their potential to cause cancer. Since animal studies indicate that PCBs are carcinogenic in rodents, it was feared that the same would be true in humans—one of the main reasons advanced to justify banning the chemical. However, after decades of research, no link between chronic PCB exposure and human cancer has been found. In 1999, the largest epidemiologic study to date found no increase in cancer deaths among more than 7,000 workers exposed to PCBs from 1946–1976 (Kimbrough, Doemland, and LeVois, 1999). The evidence thus appears convincing that even among those occupationally exposed to the chemical, PCBs do not cause cancer in humans. PCBs have not yet been acquitted of all charges of adverse human health effects, however. Their role as one of a group of so-called "endocrine disruptors" is now being investigated and may yet vindicate the legal action taken against them some 30 years ago.

Although PCB production in the United States halted in 1977, the chemicals remain very much a part of the American scene. During the years 1929–1977, 1.4 billion pounds of PCBs were produced in the United States. Decades later, millions of pounds remain in use, mainly in closed systems such as high-voltage capacitors (common on ordinary utility poles), electrical transformers, and fluorescent light ballasts. In addition, approximately 500 million pounds of PCBs have been dumped into landfills and waterways where they continue to pose an environmental threat. As existing PCB-containing equipment becomes obsolete and is replaced, safe methods for disposing of this material must be found. Currently, high-temperature (2200°F or above) incineration is the EPA-approved method for destroying wastes containing high concentrations of PCBs.

Many of the locations where PCB wastes were carelessly or illegally dumped years ago have now been targeted for remedial cleanup by state environmental agencies or, in the most serious cases, under the federal Superfund program (see chapter 17). Of the slightly more than 1,500 federal Superfund sites, approximately 500 involve PCB contamination. At present, one of the major projects undergoing Superfund remediation is a 40-mile stretch of the Upper Hudson River where General Electric dumped its toxic wastes decades ago. After years of legal and scientific wrangling over how the problem should be resolved, dredging of the most densely contaminated area of river bottom (94 acres) commenced in the spring of 2009 and concluded several months later. The project's second phase, covering a much more extensive area, is supposed to get underway in 2011, though GE has asked EPA to give the company another year to decide whether to proceed with the cleanup. GE's concerns ostensibly focus on whether the first phase stirred up too much contaminated silt and, if so, what to do about it. New York environmental officials contend that the project has not raised PCB levels in fish or river water to any significant degree and are urging that the EPA not allow any further cleanup delays by GE. The EPA is requiring GE to pay for dredging and removal of approximately 2.65 million cubic yards of PCB-contaminated sediment. The company has built a dewatering facility near the site to process the dredged materials, returning clean water to the river and sending the dried toxic sediment by train to a landfill in Texas.

DIOXIN (TCDD)

In the wet spring of 1983 public apprehension about the dangers of dioxin soared when the U.S. Environmental Protection Agency announced that inhabitants of the tiny riverside community of Times Beach, Missouri, should abandon their homes and evacuate the town. Soil analyses had revealed high levels of dioxin contamination due to oiling of roads for dust control in the early 1970s; the oil had been scavenged from a trichlorophenol factory by a waste hauler and was heavily laced with the toxic chemical.

Times Beach is but one of numerous places around the world where industrial accidents, deliberate dumping, or inadvertent use of dioxin-tainted pesticides have resulted in environmental contamination. Public con-

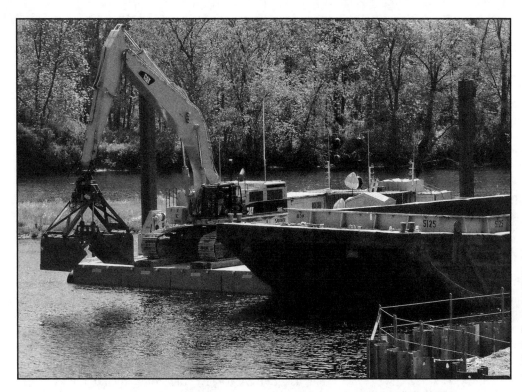

Dredging operations to remove PCB-laden sediment from the Upper Hudson River commenced in May 2009. The second phase of this Superfund remediation effort is scheduled to get underway in 2011. [*AP Photo / Hans Pennink*]

cerns have been heightened by debatable statements by some researchers that "dioxin is the most toxic substance ever created by humans," and by allegations of a wide range of health problems and genetic disorders among American servicemen who, during their tour of duty in the Vietnam War, were exposed to dioxin, a contaminant in the herbicide "Agent Orange," used in clearing jungle vegetation. Nearly four decades after the end of that conflict, lingering questions about such a cause-and-effect relationship prompted the U.S. Department of Veterans Affairs in 2009 to announce that it was adding Parkinson's disease, ischemic heart disease, and hairy-cell leukemia to a list of more than a dozen other ailments presumably linked to Agent Orange exposure. This action will facilitate claims by thousands of now-aging veterans suffering from any of these ailments that their condition is a direct result of military service in Vietnam, thus making it easier to secure medical benefits and disability payments from the government.

On the home front, widespread fears that serious human health damage can be caused by infinitesimally small amounts of the chemical have led to such controversial regulatory actions as the evacuation of Times Beach and the suspension of the selective herbicides 2, 4, 5–T and silvex, yet the results of numerous follow-up studies on exposed populations fail to show a single case where human death has resulted from dioxin exposure. What are the facts about this chemical whose very name provokes concern?

Chemically related to PCBs and other chlorinated hydrocarbons, dioxins form a large group of chemicals of widely varying levels of toxicity. The most dangerous dioxin is 2, 3, 7, 8–tetrachlorodibenzo-p-dioxin, generally referred to as TCDD or, simply, "dioxin." TCDD, unlike its chemical cousin PCB, has no industrial usefulness and has never been intentionally manufactured; it is formed as an unwanted by-product in the production of certain herbicides and the germ-killer hexachlorophene. Dioxin can escape into the atmosphere when it evaporates from TCDD-contaminated soil and water or when dioxin- or other chlorine-containing compounds are burned (EPA researchers say that municipal and medical waste incinerators currently constitute the leading source of dioxin emissions in the United States). Airborne dioxins can be carried long distances before they eventually are rained out or settle as dry deposits on soil, plant surfaces, or bodies of water. There they bind tightly to soil particles or sediment at the bottom of lakes and streams. Although TCDD undergoes rapid photolysis, if protected from light exposure dioxin breaks down very slowly—experimental evidence suggests that its half-life in soil may exceed 10 years. Thanks to regulatory controls on industrial emissions and the banning of 2,4,5–T, dioxin levels in the environment have fallen by about 50% since the late 1980s. Nevertheless, TCDD in minute quantities is still very widespread, present in soil, dust, chimneys of wood-burning stoves and furnaces, eggs, fish tissues, and animal fat. Most humans have accumulated small amounts of dioxin in their fatty tissues largely through consumption of meat, fish, and dairy products, with only 1% or less of the total body burden coming from exposure to contaminated air or water.

Statements asserting that dioxin is the "most toxic of all synthetic chemicals" are somewhat misleading because they are based on the observation that extremely low doses of TCDD are fatal to guinea pigs, by far the most sensitive species to the chemical's lethal effects. Hamsters, by contrast, can tolerate doses of dioxin up to 1,900 times the amount that would kill a guinea pig. For other test species, dioxin's lethality ranges somewhere between these extremes. However, dioxin is capable of producing many adverse effects other than death, and while any given species may exhibit a biological response at the far end of the range for a particular TCDD-induced problem, most species, humans included, respond similarly for most effects. For example, dioxin produces chloracne in rabbits, monkeys, mice, and humans at roughly equivalent levels of exposure. Interference with immune system function, fetal toxicity, and cancer are other adverse effects of dioxin exposure to which humans, rats, guinea pigs, and hamsters exhibit similar sensitivity. On the other hand, some of TCDD's effects are strikingly species-specific. Teratogenic effects of dioxin are apparent only in mice, which develop cleft palates at doses below the lethal level. Similarly, while dioxin acts as a liver toxin in a number of species, no signs of liver damage have yet been observed in highly exposed humans. By contrast, TCDD is carcinogenic in most species, producing malignant tumors at multiple sites—but only at high levels of exposure. Perhaps most significant among dioxin's long-term effects revealed by animal tests (presumed valid for humans as well) is the chemical's ability to disrupt the hormonal systems that control reproduction. Evidence from both wildlife and laboratory studies shows that exposure to dioxin (and to chlorinated organic chemicals in general) may result in reduced fertility, fetal loss, changes in sexual behavior, thyroid dysfunction, and suppression of the immune system. Indeed, some scientists conclude that these effects are far more significant than the carcinogenicity concerns that have been the focus of most toxicological research in relation to dioxin (Colborn, Dumanoski, and Myers, 1996; Birnbaum, 1994).

The implications of all this so far as human exposure is concerned remains somewhat problematic. Over the years thousands of people, particularly chemical industry workers, have had extensive exposure to the chemical at relatively high levels (e.g., a 1976 explosion at a trichlorophenol factory near Milan, Italy, released a toxic cloud that settled on the nearby suburb of Seveso, exposing 37,000 people of all ages to considerable amounts of dioxin). It is estimated that additional millions have been exposed to low concentrations (e.g., the farmers and ranchers using dioxin-contaminated herbicides, military personnel exposed to Agent Orange, residents of Times Beach and other communities where dioxin-laced waste oils were sprayed on dirt roads, consumers of TCDD-tainted fish, etc.). With the exception of a group of chemical industry workers whose dioxin exposure was 500 times greater than that experienced by the general public, the only confirmed human health problems associated with TCDD have been acute symptoms such as chloracne, muscle aches and pains, nervous system disorders, digestive upsets, and some psychiatric effects. TCDD's potential for causing such problems became international headline news in 2004, when Ukrainian presidential candidate Viktor Yushchenko was diagnosed with a severe case of dioxin-induced chloracne resulting from a bizarre assassination attempt.

Among the thousands of Seveso residents exposed to dioxin fallout from the 1976 industrial accident, the only health problems reported in the months following the explosion were about 200 cases of chloracne, almost all of them involving children, though over 200 animal deaths in the area were reported (Ottoboni, 1991). Nevertheless, a statistically significant increase in deaths due to soft tissue sarcoma (a type of cancer) and respiratory cancer has been confirmed among a group of men who were highly exposed while working for more than 20 years in chemical manufacturing plants. Among this group, workers who had been exposed to dioxin for the longest period of time had TCDD blood levels of 3600 ppt (parts per trillion). By comparison, for adults living in the industrialized world, the average blood level of dioxin is 6 ppt, while members of the U.S. military who handled dioxin-contaminated Agent Orange exhibited peak levels around 400 ppt (Fingerhut et al., 1991). In 1993, publication of a study carried out by a team of Italian researchers reviewing the medical records of thousands of Seveso residents documented an increase in soft tissue sarcomas, cancer of the gall bladder, and multiple myelomas among citizens exposed to the highest levels of dioxin ever recorded among civilian populations. However, the overall cancer rate for the region was lower than expected. Another study of U.S. chemical industry workers whose exposure to TCDD averaged less than one year revealed average blood concentrations of 640 ppt—a level 90 times higher than the national norm—yet the cancer death rate among these men 20 years after exposure was scarcely distinguishable from that of the general public (Dickson and Buzik, 1993).

In 1997 the International Agency for Research on Cancer officially classified TCDD as a group 1 human carcinogen, basing its designation on studies showing an excess of all cancers among several groups of highly exposed workers. Results from a follow-up study of one

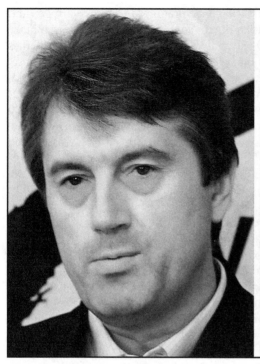
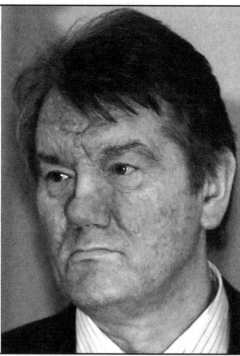

Former Ukrainian president Viktor Yushchenko is shown in photos from March 2002 (left) and December 2004 (right). When Yushchenko was a presidential candidate in 2004 he was scarred by deliberate dioxin poisoning. [*AP Photo/Viktor Pobedinsky/ Efrem Lukatsky*]

of these groups, involving over 5,000 U.S. chemical workers, confirmed an increased cancer incidence due to dioxin exposure, but only among those who experienced doses 100–1,000 times higher than those encountered by the general public (Steenland et al., 1999). Such findings have led most researchers to the conclusion that while dioxin *does* cause cancer in humans at very high levels of exposure, it poses a minimal threat of malignancies at the low concentrations commonly encountered.

For those charged with protecting the public health and setting regulatory requirements regarding TCDD exposure, the dioxin issue presents some difficult decisions. Without question the chemical is acutely toxic to laboratory animals and produces serious chronic health problems in many animal species as well. However, in spite of extensive human exposure to TCDD, only a handful of transitory acute effects have been confirmed in people. It must be noted that one of the problems in determining the health effects of dioxin is the fact that TCDD virtually never occurs alone; rather, it is one of many chemicals in a mixture that may include PCBs, dibenzofurans, chlorophenols, and other dioxins. Since the identity of these other chemicals is frequently not known or not reported, it could be risky to attribute a given observed health effect to TCDD alone. While some investigators argue that dioxin presents less of a health threat to humans than to other animal species, others are convinced that the subtle effects observed in laboratory animals are having an impact on people as well. Citing animal data regarding TCDD's adverse impact on repro-

duction and on immune system function as justification for continued regulatory controls, such authorities are convinced of the necessity to limit human exposure to dioxin as much as possible (Colborn et al., 1996).

ASBESTOS

Probably no other hazardous substance has resulted in so many deaths and cases of disabling disease as has asbestos, the collective term for a group of six fibrous silicate minerals (amosite, chrysotile, tremolite, actinolite, anthophyllite, and crocidolite) found almost worldwide. The major asbestos producers currently are Canada, Russia, China, Brazil, Zimbabwe, and Kazakhstan.

Utilized by humans ever since Stone Age potters employed the substance to reinforce their clay, asbestos was woven into cloth during Greek and Roman times and was regarded as having magical properties because of its invulnerability to fire. In modern times asbestos has acquired great economic value as an essential component in over 3,000 commercial products. By the period of peak production in the late 1970s, over 5 million tons of asbestos were being produced each year worldwide. Production of asbestos has declined significantly since then, with somewhat over 2 million tons being mined annually at present. Over 80% of the asbestos produced today is used in a relatively small number of countries in Asia, South America, and the former Soviet Union; China is currently the world's leading consumer of asbestos, closely followed by Russia (Virta, 2006). Although asbestos has been used in brake linings, insulation, textiles, roofing paper, ironing board covers, caulking compounds, floor tiles, and a host of other products, over 85% of all asbestos produced today is incorporated into asbestos-cement construction materials (LaDou, 2004).

Unfortunately, in addition to being very useful, asbestos is an occupational hazard of major proportions. Public health experts estimate that until asbestos exposure is eliminated, as many as 10 million people—the majority of them individuals occupationally exposed to asbestos fibers—may die of asbestos-related cancer. The number of workers exposed to asbestos far exceeds those involved in mining and processing the ore; an estimated 20–40% of adult men worldwide report some degree of occupational contact with asbestos, primarily through the replacement, repair, or maintenance of materials containing the fibers (Tossavainen, 2004). Exposure to asbestos is primarily through inhalation of tiny fibers suspended in the air. While airborne fibers may occur naturally in regions characterized by outcroppings of the mineral, they are more commonly associated with the deterioration of manufactured asbestos-containing materials or with the demolition or renovation of buildings containing asbestos. Fiber levels tend to be highest near asbestos mines or factories and are higher in cities than in rural areas, but virtually any air sample, regardless of where it is taken, will contain some asbestos fibers. Once inhaled, asbestos fibers are deposited in the air passages and cells within the lungs. Most of these are quickly carried away by the mucus that lines the respiratory tract, being transported up to the throat where they are swallowed, carried to the stomach, and eventually excreted with the feces. Some, however, remain trapped deep in the lungs and may never be removed.

Although inhalation represents the primary route by which asbestos enters the human body, people may also be exposed to the mineral in drinking water. Asbestos fibers can be released into water supplies when cement asbestos pipes corrode or when asbestos-containing wastes piled near mine sites are washed into lakes or rivers. Asbestos that is swallowed, fortunately, presents much less of a health hazard than that which is inhaled. Most fibers are simply carried through the stomach and intestines and are excreted within a few days. A small portion, however, may lodge in the cells lining the gastrointestinal tract, while a few may move through the intestinal lining and enter the bloodstream. These may either become trapped in other tissues or be excreted in the urine.

Asbestos-Related Diseases

Several different types of asbestos-related diseases are known, the most significant being the following.

Asbestosis

A chronic disease characterized by a scarring of the lung tissue, asbestosis most commonly occurs among workers who have been exposed to very high levels of asbestos dust. It is an irreversible, excruciatingly painful, progressively worsening disease, the first symptom of which is shortness of breath following exertion. Lung function is adversely affected, the maximum volume of air a victim can inhale being reduced. In most cases, it takes 10–40 years of exposure to asbestos before symptoms of the disease appear; unfortunately, by this time asbestosis has usually reached an advanced state. The severity of asbestosis is influenced not only by the duration of exposure, but also by the type of asbestos fibers inhaled and by the synergistic effects of cigarette smoking. Until the 1940s, when concerns about workers' health led to regulations regarding dust levels in asbestos factories, asbestosis was the leading cause of death among asbestos workers. Since then, rates of asbestosis have been reduced, but the U.S. Department of Labor reports that an estimated 1.3 million American workers continue to experience asbestos exposure on the job. Those particularly at risk of premature death due to asbestosis include insulation workers, plumbers, pipe fitters, and steamfitters. Although the majority of cases being diagnosed today were caused by exposure to large quantities of asbestos fibers years ago, health authorities warn that the fact that cases of asbestosis are still occurring in younger persons indicates an ongoing need for efforts to prevent and eliminate this occupational disease (CDC, 2008b).

Lung Cancer

With the gradual reduction in dust levels in asbestos factories, deaths due to asbestosis have been decreasing, allowing workers to live long enough to develop today's leading cause of asbestos-related mortality, lung cancer. Approximately 5–7% of all lung cancer cases today can be attributed to occupational exposure to asbestos, with roughly 20,000 new victims diagnosed each year in developed nations with a long history of asbestos production and use (Tossavainen, 2004). It is estimated that as many as 20–25% of asbestos workers now succumb to this disease. The risk is especially great when exposure to asbestos fibers is accompanied by exposure to cigarette smoke. Studies have shown that while asbestos exposure alone increases an individual's risk of lung cancer death by a factor of seven, exposure to both asbestos and cigarette smoke entails a 60 times greater risk of lung cancer.

Mesothelioma

This previously rare cancer of the lung or stomach lining today kills more than 5% of all asbestos workers. Like many other forms of cancer, mesothelioma is character-

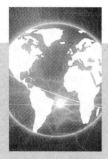

· · · · · · · 7-2 · · · · · · · ·

Deadly Dust

No community in the United States is suffering more grievously from the ravages of asbestos-related disease than the small town of Libby, Montana, located in the scenic northwest corner of the state. Today Libby is the site of an extensive EPA hazardous waste cleanup effort under the federal Superfund program, a belated response to seven decades of massive contamination with tremolite asbestos fibers from a nearby vermiculite mine, an economic mainstay of the community from the 1930s until its closure in 1990. By 2001, shortly before remediation efforts got underway, over 200 residents of the area had died of asbestosis or asbestos-caused cancer and nearly 1,400 were being treated for asbestos disease. According to a 2000 report from the federal Agency for Toxic Substances and Disease Registry (ATSDR), the number of asbestos-related deaths in Libby is 60 times higher than the U.S. average and, given the long latency period associated with the onset of asbestos disease symptoms, the toll is likely to increase further in the years immediately ahead.

The events culminating in this tragic situation began with the discovery in 1919 of one of the world's largest deposits of vermiculite a few miles outside the town. The economic potential of Libby's immense vermiculite deposits prompted an entrepreneurial mining engineer to stake a claim in the early 1920s to approximately 1,200 acres of mineral-rich land and to open a mine which, by the 1930s, was shipping out ever-increasing quantities of a vermiculite product the company dubbed "Zonolite." By the early 1970s the Libby mine was producing over 200,000 tons of vermiculite each year—80% of the world's total.

Throughout these years, mine workers, grateful for well-paying jobs, seldom complained that the workplace environment subjected them to enormous quantities of airborne particulates as the ore was crushed and processed. Miners would return home covered with a thick layer of white dust on their clothes, skin, and hair, exposing family members to the material. To the workers, such conditions were simply an unavoidable part of their job—nothing to worry about, since company officials assured them it was nothing more than "nuisance dust," certainly not a health threat. Vermiculite itself is, indeed, harmless; but what the workers and townspeople were never told was that the vermiculite deposit at Libby was highly contaminated with asbestos, formed by the same geologic processes responsible for the presence of vermiculite. Although the dangers weren't recognized when the mine first opened, by 1956 asbestos had been officially listed as an ingredient in the Libby mine dust, with concentrations noted as ranging from 8–21% of the total (a subsequent analysis in 1982 revealed concentrations in the 21–26% range). State regulatory officials as well as mine owners were aware of the fact, yet workers were never told of the problem nor given protective equipment other than paper masks, which none of them wore. By 1959 chest X-rays showed that over one-third of the mine workers exhibited lung abnormalities. A few years later, laboratory analysis identified the type of asbestos fibers in the mine dust as tremolite, one of the most dangerous forms of asbestos.

The cover-up continued after W. R. Grace purchased the mine in 1963 and expanded production. Occasional inspections of the facility by state regulators revealed that miners were being exposed to levels of asbestos far higher than the so-called "safety limit" (in fact, there is *no safe* level of asbestos exposure), yet no government enforcement action was taken against the company. Although W. R. Grace installed a new ventilation system intended to eliminate indoor dust, smokestacks at the mill were emitting an estimated 5,000 tons of dust and fiber daily. At the same time, Grace was allowing waste vermiculite to be spread throughout Libby—in homes and gardens, on schoolyards, children's ballparks, and the high school running track. Grateful Libby residents admired Grace as a good corporate citizen, helping to improve community life; they never realized until it was too late that, as a result of the company's largesse, everyone in town was now in direct daily contact with one of the world's most pervasive environmental hazards.

By the 1960s overt signs of asbestos disease began to appear among individuals who had started working at the mine several decades earlier. As the years went by, more and more people became ill—not only miners, but wives and children as well. At first many attributed their poor health to "bronchial problems," but eventually those who traveled to Seattle or Spokane to seek medical advice were informed they had asbestosis, a disease many of them had never before heard of.

Elsewhere in the country, growing awareness of the extent of asbestos-related disease and of the massive industry cover-up of the problem (in legal terms, the "failure to warn") had resulted in a steady escalation in legal action against asbestos companies. Since the late 1970s, approximately 600,000 lawsuits have been filed in the U.S. With irate juries awarding plaintiffs first hundreds of thousands and, later, millions of dollars in compensatory and punitive damages, even the wealthiest corporations began to buckle under the financial pressure. Eventually more than fifty U.S. corporations, including W. R. Grace in 2001, sought protection under Chapter 11 bankruptcy proceedings. Demand for products containing asbestos underwent a steady decline in most developed nations and in 1990 W. R. Grace ceased operations at its plant in Libby.

By the 1990s, several Libby asbestos victims had filed suits against Grace, but all settled with the company out of court, agreeing to accept a monetary award in return for a promise not to talk about their case. It was only in 1998 that a claimant who had lost both parents to asbestosis and was determined to bring Grace to justice insisted on her lawsuit going to trial. During the proceedings some of the most influential testimony came from an asbestos expert from Brown University, who told the court that among men who had worked at the mine for twenty years, 92% were diseased: "The highest reported rate of lung disease in any group of workers exposed to an asbestos form of mineral that I've seen." The woman won her case, becoming the first Libby resident to sue W. R. Grace successfully. To her disappointment, however, the world outside Libby continued to ignore what was happening there. Even among community leaders, concern about the town's image created pressure to downplay the severity of local health and environmental problems.

Although Grace had closed the mine and ceased its operations in Libby, the company had been ordered to remediate the site and had posted a cleanup bond, as required, to ensure that it would do so. In 1999 the local newspaper carried an article stating that Grace considered its work complete and was filing a request to recover the unused portion of its bond. The same resident who had successfully sued Grace the previous year spotted this story and decided to see for herself whether the cleanup had truly been finished. Driving to the site, she found few signs of reclamation; mine tailings were exposed to wind and rain, ensuring further dissemination of deadly asbestos fibers. Furious, she repeatedly contacted the appropriate Montana state regulatory agencies, insisting they come to Libby to view the mess for themselves. When they finally arrived several weeks later, they found conditions just as she had described them. At that point, the press was contacted and suddenly—finally—Libby's plight became national news.

Shortly thereafter an EPA Emergency Response Team arrived from the Denver regional office and launched what turned out to be a two-year investigation. Federal agents were amazed at the community-wide extent of the contamination, in numerous cases affecting whole families. Almost 20% of the people who submitted to testing exhibited abnormal lung X-rays, a sure sign of asbestos-related disease. None of the investigators had ever before encountered such widespread poisoning, particularly among residents who had never themselves worked with asbestos. By the end of 2001, intervention by Montana's governor resulted in Libby being placed on the National Priority List for Superfund remedial action (Bowker, 2003). Cleanup got underway in the summer of 2002; the major source areas of contamination have now been cleaned up and EPA has shifted its focus to remediation of smaller sources around homes and businesses. In 2008 W.R. Grace agreed to spend $250 million for environmental cleanup of the town and to pay $3 billion in compensation to asbestos victims. Libby residents finally have reason to believe that the end is in sight to their decades-long nightmare of pollution and disease.

ized by a long latency period, onset of disease symptoms occurring 25–40 years after initial exposure. For this reason, peak levels of mortality from mesothelioma may not occur until 2010–2020, when workers exposed during the asbestos production boom of the late 1970s begin to sicken and die. Some health officials predict that western Europe alone will experience 250,000 mesothelioma deaths during the first three decades of the 21st century as a result of past asbestos exposure (LaDou, 2004). About half of all victims will be construction workers and men employed in shipyards, where for almost half a century asbestos materials were used on virtually every ship (Tossavainen, 2004). Even very low levels of asbestos can result in mesothelioma, as evidenced by cases among young adults whose only contact with the mineral involved childhood exposure to their fathers' asbestos-contaminated work clothes.

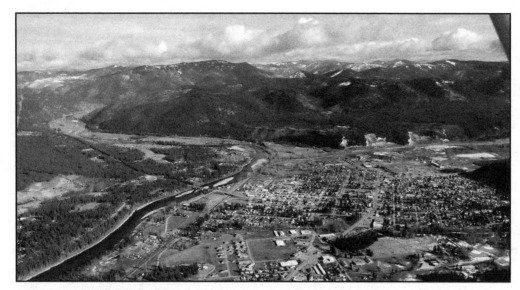

Libby, Montana, a town of 3,000 along the Kootenai River, has emerged as the deadliest Superfund site in U.S. history due to decades of contamination with asbestos fibers from a nearby vermiculite mine. [*AP Photo/ Rick Bowmer*]

Mesothelioma is of special interest to researchers because, unlike other forms of cancer, the only known causative agent for this disease is asbestos. Thus mesothelioma is considered a "marker disease" indicating asbestos exposure. Since no effective treatment exists, mesothelioma is an invariably fatal ailment, with death generally occurring within two years of diagnosis.

Although research has not yet been able to establish conclusively the degree of asbestos exposure necessary to initiate cancer, evidence suggests that some individuals who were exposed to high levels of asbestos for only one day developed cancer years later as a result. For this reason the current presumption is that there is *no safe level for asbestos exposure.* Some scientists have argued that the development of asbestos-related disease is dependent on the mineral type of asbestos to which an individual is exposed. However, most researchers believe that fiber size is a more important determinant of asbestos' cancer-causing potential than are its chemical or physical properties. Experimental data suggest that long fibers (those exceeding 1/5,000 of an inch in length) are more injurious than short fibers (less than 1/10,000 of an inch).

While *any* amount of asbestos exposure entails some degree of hazard, the extent of that risk is determined by a combination of several factors, among the most important of which are:

- level and duration of exposure
- time since exposure occurred
- age at which exposure occurred
- personal history of cigarette smoking
- type and size of asbestos fibers

While asbestos workers constitute by far the largest percentage of victims, others may be affected through indirect exposure. Mesothelioma has claimed casualties among people living in the vicinity of asbestos factories and among children of asbestos workers. When asbestos is brought into the home, it becomes a permanent part of the domestic environment, embedded in carpets and draperies and suspended in the air where it constitutes a 24-hour/day source of exposure not only to the less vulnerable healthy adults of the household but also to the very young, the sick, and the elderly who are the groups most susceptible to any type of environmental irritant. For this reason, asbestos workers today are cautioned to shower and change clothes at the workplace in order to avoid inadvertent contamination of their homes with asbestos fibers.

Asbestos Problems in Public Buildings

Until the mid-1970s most asbestos-related health concerns were focused on the millions of workers who had experienced significant levels of occupational exposure to the hazardous fibers. It thus came as an unwelcome surprise when the EPA warned that the general public has been receiving asbestos exposure for years simply by working or living in any of the estimated 700,000 commercial, governmental, or residential buildings that contain friable asbestos ("friable" refers to asbestos material which, when dry, can be crumbled to a powder by hand pressure).

Of greatest concern was the revelation that as many as 2–6 million schoolchildren and 300,000 teachers in 31,000 primary and secondary schools across the nation might be inhaling asbestos fibers on a daily basis. During the years 1946–1973, asbestos-containing fireproofing materials were extensively used in constructing or renovating schools throughout the country. By 1973 increasing documentation of the health threats posed by asbestos had caused the EPA to ban all spray applications of asbestos in insulating and fireproofing materials, and in 1977 new restrictions totally halted the spray application of asbestos. Such regulation had no effect, however, on existing asbestos-containing materials which, by this time, were beginning to deteriorate in many schools, releasing potentially dangerous fibers into the classroom environment. When asbestos-contaminated dust is swept up by janitors or disturbed by students' coming and going, it becomes resuspended and can remain in the air—at breathing level—for as long as 80 hours. The high levels of asbestos fibers measured in the indoor air of many schools prompted concerns for elevated rates of lung cancer and mesothelioma among schoolchildren 20–40 years hence.

The initial EPA response to this perceived threat was to issue an advisory to school districts throughout the country, informing them of the situation and requiring that they inspect their buildings for the presence of asbestos-containing materials (ACM). If friable asbestos was found, the districts were to notify parents or the PTA of that fact. The federal authorities apparently assumed that if an asbestos hazard were identified, parental concerns about their children's safety would be sufficient to ensure prompt remediation of the problem. Such did not prove to be the case, however, as financially strapped school districts, in the absence of a firm federal mandate, postponed expensive remediation projects. By 1983, 66% of the nation's school districts had not yet even inspected for asbestos or had failed to report doing so to the EPA.

Consequently, in the fall of 1986, President Reagan signed into law the far-reaching Asbestos Hazard Emergency Response Act (AHERA), requiring that all primary and secondary schools be inspected for the presence of asbestos; if such materials were found, the school district was required to file and carry out an asbestos abatement plan. EPA was charged with promulgating rules detailing correct inspection procedures, establishing asbestos abatement standards, certification programs for contractors, and standards for the transportation and disposal of asbestos.

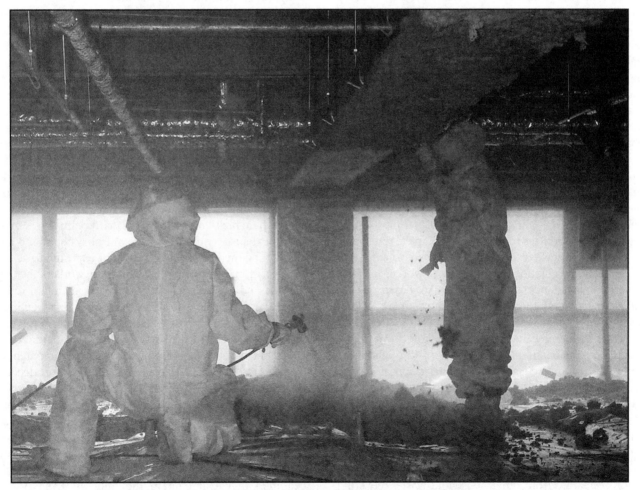

Workers in full-body protective gear dampen and remove asbestos-containing materials from a high school. [*AP Photo/Kyodo News*]

Asbestos Abatement

When an asbestos hazard is identified, those charged with remedying the situation have several options from which to choose:

1. *Encapsulation.* This is a technique in which exposed asbestos is heavily coated with a polymer sealant to prevent further release of fibers.

2. *Enclosure.* Feasible when the area affected is relatively small, this process involves building a nonpermeable barrier between the source of exposure and surrounding open areas.

3. *Removal.* A labor-intensive process whereby all asbestos containing materials are physically removed from the structure.

Of the various abatement alternatives, complete removal is the most expensive and time consuming. It also entails the risk of worker exposure to asbestos fibers and, if carelessly done, could endanger the public as well. However, since removal absolves a building's owner of future liability and because encapsulated asbestos requires periodic reinspection, removal may, in the long run, be cheaper than encapsulation. In addition, federal laws require that any buildings that are going to be demolished or renovated, other than private homes or apartments with four or less dwelling units, must be inspected for the presence of asbestos-containing material. If any friable asbestos is found it must be removed before work can commence. Essentially this means that if a school district chose encapsulation as its asbestos abatement option and subsequently decided to tear down or substantially renovate that building, it would first have to hire a contractor to remove all encapsulated asbestos materials, thereby paying twice to have the job done. For these reasons, even though encapsulation is an acceptable method of reducing asbestos exposure, most asbestos abatement projects today involve complete removal.

Asbestos removal projects must adhere to strict federal and state regulations to protect both workers and the general public. Under the Clean Air Act provisions for hazardous air pollutants, EPA has set a standard of "no visible emissions" for any asbestos removal activities. Asbestos-containing materials must be wet down before work commences and must be kept damp throughout the course of the project, right up to final disposal. Damp asbestos wastes must be containerized in thick plastic bags or plastic lined containers, tagged with an appropriate warning label, and transported in a covered vehicle to an approved sanitary landfill. Since asbestos is not classified as a hazardous waste, the EPA-approved method of asbestos disposal is to bury the material in an area of the landfill separate from other household wastes, covering the containers with at least six inches of soil or with some

other nonasbestos materials before compacting. Final cover of an additional 30 inches of nonasbestos material is required.

Legal Status of Asbestos

The mass of evidence documenting asbestos' adverse health impact prompted over 40 countries to institute full or partial bans on the use of asbestos and a vigorous "Ban Asbestos" movement has been working actively to persuade additional governments that the only solution to the worldwide epidemic of asbestos cancer is to discontinue all mining and use of the material (Harris and Kahwa, 2003). Among industrialized countries, the two major holdouts are Canada and the United States. As the largest exporter of asbestos, primarily to developing countries, Canada continues to promote asbestos use and to oppose international efforts to outlaw the material (LaDou, 2004). In the United States, an EPA-mandated phase-out of all asbestos-containing products was announced in 1989 but was subsequently overturned on a legal technicality in 1991; as a result, a number of asbestos products continue to be marketed in the U.S. with little government regulation (Bowker, 2003). Nevertheless, by 2003 general awareness of asbestos-associated health problems, as well as issues of legal liability, had resulted in a drastic decline in U.S. asbestos consumption to just 0.7% of the material's peak use in 1973.

In the absence of a total ban, action against asbestos in the U.S. is proceeding on several fronts. Occupational exposure, which in the 1970s was lowered first to 5 and subsequently to 2 fibers/cm^3 of air, has now been reduced to 0.1 fibers/cm^3 over an eight-hour time-weighted average. Employers are required to sample at factory sites every six months and daily at construction sites unless employees are wearing respirators. In situations where fiber levels exceed standards, employers must install exhaust ventilation, dust-control systems, and air-vacuuming methods to reduce worker exposure to asbestos dust. Employers also must monitor workers' health, provide and launder protective clothing, maintain respirators, and provide showering and changing facilities. For the protection of the general public, the federal government has banned the use of asbestos in a number of consumer products: certain pipe coverings and patching compounds, artificial fireplace logs, sprayed-on decorations, and hair dryers. Since 1997, production of asbestos-containing materials for home construction and use has been banned. In spite of these prohibitions, however, consumers cannot always assume that products they buy are asbestos-free. Items imported from countries without legal restrictions on asbestos (Canada being a notable example) may still contain the mineral. Even in the United States, asbestos-containing products are not legally required to be labeled as such and therefore buyers wishing to know product content are advised to contact the manufacturer or the U.S. Consumer Product Safety Commission.

LEAD

Lead poisoning is entirely preventable, yet it is the most common and societally devastating environmental disease of young children.

—Dr. Louis Sullivan,
former Secretary of Health and Human Services

Dr. Sullivan's remarks regarding the impact of lead on children's health were prompted by the recognition that 3–4 million American youngsters at that time had blood lead levels high enough to impair their brain function. This situation galvanized the public health community to redouble efforts to identify children affected by subclinical (i.e., lacking visible disease symptoms) lead toxicity and to remove sources of lead exposure. As a result of these initiatives, the number of children testing positive for elevated blood lead levels has been steadily falling. By 2003–2004, a national survey of children aged 1–5 reported that an estimated 250,000 children exhibited blood lead levels above the threshold at which medical intervention is recommended (i.e. $\geq 20\mu g/dL$); this represents an 89% decline since the late 1970s when the number so affected was estimated at 4.7 million (CDC, 2009b). Obviously the situation is improving, but with a quarter million children still lead-poisoned, the battle is far from over. Future med-

ical historians may regard it as ironic that in the early years of the 21st century, a substance whose toxicity has been well established for millennia is regarded as the single most important environmental health problem affecting American children.

Human contact with lead, a mineral element naturally occurring throughout the environment, dates back to at least 4000 BC when it was first smelted as a by-product of silver processing. Because it is malleable and easy to work; doesn't rust, corrode, or dissolve in water; and binds readily with other metals, lead has been widely used since ancient times as an alloy; as an ingredient in paints, glazes, and cosmetics; and for gutters and piping. Indeed, the word "plumbing" is derived from the Latin word for lead, *plumbum*—hence lead's chemical symbol, Pb.

Among those who worked with the metal, it early became apparent that in addition to being commercially valuable, lead is a potent human poison. Over the centuries, evidence of the multifaceted aspects of lead's toxicity has continued to mount. More than two thousand years ago, Roman doctors were describing patients suffering with symptoms of gout, an ailment associated with chronic lead poisoning; modern commentators theorize such problems may have been caused by the Roman practice of lining wine casks, cooking pots, and aqueducts with lead. Lead poisoning may also have contributed to the low birth rate and high incidence of mental retardation among the Roman aristocracy. A major source of exposure to the metal among wealthy Romans is thought to have been a grape juice syrup, *frumentum*,

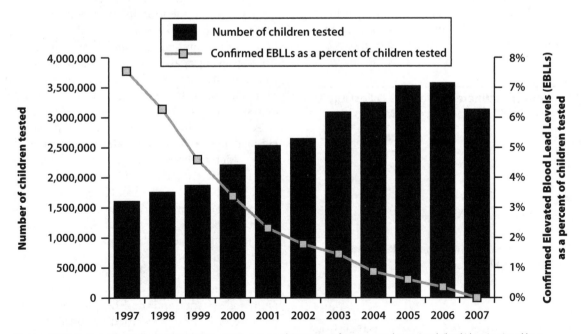

Source: CDC's National Surveillance Data (1997–2007). Accessed Sept. 2010 from www.cdc.gov/nceh/lead/data/national.htm

Figure 7-2   U.S. Blood Lead Surveillance Report, 1997–2007

which was brewed in lead pots and subsequently used to sweeten foods and wine; even one teaspoonful of this syrup would have been more than enough to cause chronic lead poisoning. Unfortunately, later generations learned little from the Roman experience; during medieval times, Europeans in large numbers fell victim to "Saturnine poisoning," a result of using soluble lead acetate to sweeten sour wine, and even in the 16th century widespread outbreaks of lead poisoning occurred in France as a result of storing wine in lead-lined vessels.

Sources of Lead

Today, as in centuries past, lead is used in a wide range of industrial products. The single largest use of lead, over 70% of total U.S. consumption of the metal, is for lead storage batteries (virtually every car on the road contains 20 pounds of lead in its battery); other lead-containing products include ammunition, brass, coverings for power and communication cables, glass TV tubes, solder, and pigments. With world production estimated at close to 4 million metric tons annually, lead is produced in larger amounts than any other nonferrous metal. Not surprisingly, lead is now found throughout the environment—in soils, water, air, and food. Until the mid-1980s, automobile emissions constituted the major source of environmental lead. With the phase-out of leaded gasoline in the United States and a number of other countries, amounts of lead entering the atmosphere have declined sharply.

Correspondingly, Americans' blood lead levels have fallen as well, down by more than 80% since the mid-1970s; by mid-2010, leaded gasoline for motor vehicles was still being sold in just 11 countries worldwide (The LEAD Group, 2010). While reduced exposure to lead

Table 7-1   Countries Where Leaded Gas Is Possibly Still Sold for Road Use as of May 2010

Africa	Middle East
1. Algeria	10. Iraq
2. Egypt	11. Yemen
Asia	
3. Afghanistan	
4. Korea, Dem. Peoples Rep of (N. Korea)	
5. Myanmar (Burma)	
Europe, C. I. S. (Commonwealth of Independent States)	
6. Bosnia and Herzegovina	
7. Montenegro	
8. Kosovo	
9. Serbia	

Source: Collated by The LEAD Group from matrices updated by the Partnership for Cleaner Fuels and Vehicles (PCFV), UN Environment Programme. Used with permission.

emissions from road traffic is good news for citizens in most nations, other sources of the toxic metal are sickening thousands of Chinese living near metal smelters. Mass poisonings affecting schoolchildren prompted angry demonstrations in at least three Chinese provinces during the summer and fall of 2009, with protesters demanding closure of smelters spewing toxic emissions into the air, in one case within 1,700 feet of a school (Wines, 2009). In two of the villages involved, 70% of the children tested positive for lead poisoning, with blood lead levels more than 10 times above those China considers safe. In the United States, airborne lead today originates primarily from the burning of lead-contaminated used oil, from the smelting of ores and other industrial processes, and from the incineration of municipal refuse. Currently more lead is released into soil than into the air, primarily as the result of lead-containing solid wastes being dumped in landfills (aware of this hazard, a number of states have passed laws banning landfill disposal of lead batteries). Weathering of lead-based paints, particularly around the foundations of older structures, and fallout of airborne lead further contribute to the buildup of lead in soils.

Route of Entry into Body

In years past, ingestion of lead-tainted food and water constituted the main source of lead intake for most Americans. Canned foods and beverages represented a significant hazard because over 90% of such cans had lead-soldered seams. Leaching of the toxic metal from the solder into the cans' contents was commonplace, especially when the food items were acidic (e.g., tomato products, citrus, or carbonated drinks). Airborne fallout of lead from automobile emissions onto vegetables or fruits growing near busy highways was responsible for lead concentrations as high as 3,000 ppm on such crops. Drinking water, too, has been identified as a source of exposure for as many as 40 million Americans whom EPA estimates live in homes where tap water contains elevated levels of lead due to the presence of lead pipes or lead solder in household plumbing. Other sources of drinking water contamination include brass faucets on kitchen or bathroom sinks and brass pump fittings in private wells, all of which can leach dissolved lead into tap water (see chapter 15). Fortunately, Americans' exposure to lead from all these sources has been declining sharply since the phase-out of leaded gasoline (a process completed in the U.S. by 1995), the substitution of plastic (PVC) for metal piping in new and replacement home plumbing systems, and the 1991 prohibition on the manufacture of lead-soldered food or soft drink cans. However, imported foods continue to pose a hazard since few other countries restrict the use of lead solder.

Ironically, house paint remains the most important source of lead poisoning problems, even though the use of lead in paints was halted years ago. Lead was used in residential paint in the U.S. from 1884–1978; until 1953 the use of paint containing as much as 50% lead by weight was common in the United States. In that year a consensus was reached within the industry to reduce paint lead levels, resulting in a steady decline in the manufacture and use of interior lead-base paint (most European countries had recognized the problem decades earlier, signing a treaty in 1921 to prohibit the use of *interior* paints containing lead). Exterior lead-base paint continued to be widely available until the mid-1970s, although its lead content by then was considerably less than that of paint produced prior to the 1950s. In 1977 the Consumer Product Safety Commission banned all house paints, interior or exterior, as well as paints on toys or furniture, which contained more than 0.06% lead by weight. Lead-base paint can still be used, even today, for painting bridges, ships, and other steel structures and for a variety of industrial and military applications and sometimes this paint ends up being applied in homes by workers who have access to the material and fail to realize its hazardous nature ("Preventing Lead Poisoning," 1991).

Although the use of leaded paint has been illegal for more than 30 years, the U.S. Department of Housing and Urban Development (HUD) estimates that approximately 24 million dwellings nationwide are still lead contaminated, 4.4 million of them home to one or more children under the age of 6 (CDC, 2001). In such structures, deterioration or renovation activities may expose older layers of paint, providing access to toddlers who may inadvertently consume the poison chips or paint dust. While at one time it was believed that chewing on windowsills or eating flakes of the sweet-tasting paint was the major lead-poisoning hazard to children, researchers are now convinced that the prime culprit is ordinary household dust, contaminated by tiny particles of lead from the gradually deteriorating paint. Simply by playing in their own homes and doing what children normally do—putting dirty fingers in their mouths—youngsters can swallow enough lead to cause serious health problems. Recognizing the extent of lead contamination in the nation's housing supply, the federal government now requires anyone selling or renting a home or apartment to sign a form disclosing any knowledge of lead-based paint in the structure and to agree, if requested by the buyer or renter, to have the building tested for the presence of lead.

Lead presents a hazard outside as well as inside homes. Soil or dust adjacent to housing once painted with lead-base paints may contain lead levels high enough to pose a risk to small children playing in such locations or to home gardeners consuming produce grown in lead-tainted soils (leafy greens, herbs, and root vegetables are more likely to accumulate lead than are tomatoes, squash, or beans). In both suburban and inner-city neighborhoods, the soil in gardens planted adjacent to structures built prior to 1978 when lead-based paint was taken off the market are likely to contain elevated lead levels; in such locations, residents hoping to plant vegetable gardens would be well-advised to contact their county extension office to inquire about having the soil tested. Orchard soils—or soils in areas where orchards formerly existed—are also frequently contaminated with high levels of both lead and arsenic, a legacy of widespread use of lead arsenate, the primary chemical used to kill insect pests prior to the introduction of DDT. Once deposited, such chemicals may remain in soils as long as 2,000 years (Mielke, 1999).

Interestingly, *ingested* lead poses a much greater hazard for young children than it does for adults. Whereas only 10% of lead swallowed by adults passes from the intestine into the bloodstream, 40% of the lead ingested by preschoolers remains within their bodies, making such youngsters the highest risk group for lead poisoning within our population. The fact that development of the blood-brain barrier isn't complete until a child reaches approximately three years of age means that lead can readily move into the central nervous system, further explaining why lead exposure is more hazardous for infants and toddlers than it is for other age groups. Par-

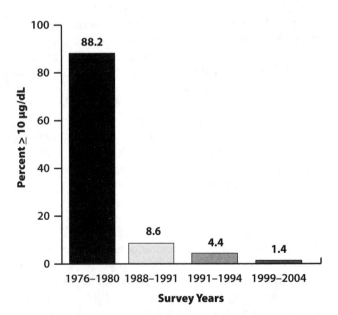

Source: CDC, *Fourth National Report on Human Exposure to Environmental Chemicals: Executive Summary.* Accessed Sept. 2010 from www.cdc.gov/exposure report/executive_summary.html

Figure 7-3   Percentage of U.S. Children 1–5 Years Old with Elevated Blood Lead Levels (≥ 10 µg/dL)

ticularly vulnerable are malnourished children; absorption of lead from the gastrointestinal tract occurs more readily among youngsters suffering from deficiencies of protein, calcium, zinc, or iron. Thus poor nutritional status is considered an additional risk factor for childhood lead poisoning (Chao and Kikano, 1993).

While young children constitute the primary victims of lead poisoning, people of any age are susceptible to the metal's toxic effects. The National Institute of Occupational Safety and Health (NIOSH) estimates that over 3 million Americans work in occupations involving potential lead exposure; of these, tens of thousands are estimated to suffer from lead poisoning each year, primarily through inhalation of airborne lead (30–40% of inhaled lead reaches the bloodstream and is deposited in the lower respiratory tract where it is almost completely absorbed). Occupational exposure to lead has been regulated since 1978 through specified **permissible exposure limits (PELs)** to airborne lead concentrations and by standards for allowable blood lead levels. Nevertheless, standards are not sufficiently enforced, with the result that significant worker exposure is an ongoing problem (Stauding and Roth, 1998). Those most at risk are construction workers who renovate or demolish bridges, approximately 90,000 of which in the United States are coated with lead-base paints. Such work is often performed without training or the use of personal protective equipment and may involve the use of acetylene torches or sandblasting, either of which can result in workers' inhalation of lead fumes or dust. After several weeks or months of such exposure, blood lead levels of workers can rise well above the point at which symptoms of acute lead poisoning are apparent.

In addition to bridge maintenance, other occupations that may involve excessive worker exposure to lead include battery manufacturing, shipbuilding, radiator repair, smelter and foundry operations, and certain crafts. Police or military personnel working at firing ranges have also reported symptoms of lead toxicity, a result of inhaling fumes released when lead-containing ammunition is fired (CDC, 1993a; Franklin, 1991). Occasionally, some rather bizarre instances of lead poisoning illustrate the challenges facing those in the environmental health profession: over a period of seven months during 1991, eight individuals in Alabama were diagnosed with various symptoms of lead poisoning (e.g., anemia, abdominal pains, weakness in the arms, seizures, and nervous system damage) which developed as a result of drinking illegal "moonshine" distilled in an old automobile radiator containing lead-soldered components! Such a practice, which results in the leaching of lead from the solder into the home-brewed liquor, is a frequent source of lead poisoning in some rural Alabama counties and accounts for the fact that moonshine may contain up to 74 µg/L of lead (CDC, 1992).

Although lead concerns understandably focus on human health problems, it shouldn't be overlooked that environmental lead constitutes a hazard to other species as well. Especially vulnerable are waterfowl, large numbers of which have died after eating lead fishing sinkers lost by anglers. In the mid-1990s, EPA banned the manufacture and distribution of lead sinkers in order to alleviate this problem.

Regardless of whether the route of exposure is ingestion or inhalation, upon entering the body, lead first moves into the bloodstream where its half-life is estimated at 36 days. For this reason, measurements of blood lead levels, calculated as micrograms of lead per deciliter of blood (µg/dL), are considered to give the most accurate indication of short-term lead exposure. Some lead makes its way into soft tissues such as the brain and kidneys; approximately 50–60% of the lead that enters the body is excreted relatively quickly, mainly through the feces but also in urine. Over a period of time the remaining lead is slowly deposited and stored in the bones, particularly in the long arm and leg bones where it can remain for years (the estimated half-life of lead in bones is 27 years). Lead also accumulates in children's baby teeth, which have been used in research to indicate a child's lead burden. Lead in bones can act as a cumulative poison, becoming increasingly concentrated over an extended time period. Although once thought to be inert, it is now known that lead in bones can be suddenly released back into the bloodstream by a number of conditions such as high fever, osteoporosis, or pregnancy, resulting in cases of acute lead poisoning.

Biological Effects

A potent toxin that can adversely affect people in any age group, lead can damage human health in a number of ways. It interferes with blood cell formation, often resulting in anemia; lead can cause kidney damage, sterility, miscarriage, and birth defects. Because lead has a strong affinity for nerve tissue, injury to the central nervous system is perhaps the most serious manifestation of lead poisoning. Depending on the degree of exposure, lead poisoning can be reflected by hyperirritability, poor memory, or sluggishness at lower levels all the way to mental retardation, epileptic convulsions, coma, and death at high levels.

Lead is a poison that exhibits what health experts refer to as a **continuum of toxicity;** any amount of exposure, however small, carries with it some degree of harm. Not surprisingly, as levels of exposure increase, risk of adverse health effects rise correspondingly (as is the case with exposure to any hazardous substance, identical levels of lead may provoke a varying range of responses in different people). Until about the 1960s, it was widely believed that a diagnosis of "lead poisoning" was appropriate only when blood lead levels were high enough to cause such overt symptoms as anemia, kidney disease, brain damage, or death. Such conditions can be manifested when blood lead levels exceed 70 μg/dL (typically, brain damage only occurs at blood lead levels above 100 μg/dL). At that time, levels of blood lead below 60 μg/dL weren't regarded as dangerous enough to warrant monitoring or treatment. By the early 1970s, however, new evidence regarding lead's harmful effects on biological systems prompted a reevaluation of the U.S. Public Health Service's level of "undue lead absorption"—the blood lead level at which medical intervention is recommended. In 1971 that level was lowered to 40 μg/dL, further lowered to 30 μg/dL in 1975, to 25 μg/dL in 1985, and, most recently, in 1991 was again reduced to 10 μg/dL (CDC, 2003c; Florini, 1990).

The justification for the steadily declining levels of blood lead that define a case of lead poisoning can be found in the results of numerous studies carried out over the last several decades, which have conclusively shown that even at levels previously considered safe, chronic low-level exposure to lead can inhibit the normal development of children's intellectual abilities. A landmark study launched in 1979 in the Boston suburbs of Somerville and Chelsea among second-grade students revealed that those whose baby teeth (which they had willingly withheld from the Tooth Fairy to contribute to science!) had a relatively higher lead level also exhibited a greater incidence of unruly classroom behavior, a lesser ability to follow instructions, and lower scores on I.Q. tests than did classmates with low lead levels in their teeth (Needleman et al., 1979). Yet none of the children would have been categorized as lead-poisoning victims based on the prevailing view at that time regarding "safe" levels of lead. Eleven years later, in 1990, a follow-up study was carried out to see whether the effects of low-level childhood lead poisoning persist into young adulthood. In light of the millions of children who have experienced some lead exposure, the results of this investigation were depressing: in comparison with classmates whose baby teeth had minimal levels of lead, the higher-lead students, by then 18-year-olds, exhibited a significantly greater school drop-out rate, higher incidence of reading disabilities, lower class rank, and higher absenteeism—all a legacy of childhood lead exposure (Needleman et al., 1990).

Lead Poisoning: Treatment and Prevention

Children with blood lead levels of 45 μg/dL or higher typically are treated through the use of chelation, a process that employs a drug that binds to lead, sequestering the metal and facilitating its excretion from the body. Most commonly, chelating agents are administered in a hospital setting where the patient must remain for a five-day period of treatment and testing (another type of chelating agent that can be given orally at home has been approved for use in less serious cases). Some forms of chelation therapy can be quite painful and the process, while essential in forestalling further impairment to the nervous system, cannot reverse damage that has already occurred. Nor is chelation a one-time solution to lead-poisoning problems. Since the chelating agent is generally unable to reach all of the lead stored in bones and teeth, blood lead levels frequently rebound following chelation therapy, the result of additional lead moving from bony tissues into the bloodstream. Many lead-poisoning victims are forced to suffer repeated bouts of hospitalization for years after the initial treatment. Children whose lead-poisoning symptoms are relieved by chelation therapy frequently require special education and therapy long after cessation of treatment and, in the all-too-common situation where they return to the same lead-contaminated environment responsible for the initial poisoning, their symptoms will promptly recur. For this reason, removal of the child from the source of exposure or, conversely, removal of lead from the child's environment, constitutes the prime strategy in restoring a lead-poisoned child to good health. Unfortunately, evidence suggests that mild brain damage persists in lead-poisoned children even after their blood lead levels were markedly reduced (Tong et al., 1998).

Preventing Childhood Lead Poisoning

Since the health impact of lead, even at very low levels, has been shown to be so devastating and because damage, once it occurs, may never be completely reversed, *prevention* of lead poisoning should be a high-priority societal goal. As mentioned previously, the near-total phase-out of the use of lead in gasoline, paint, food containers, and home plumbing has drastically reduced human exposure to this toxic metal in recent years. Nevertheless, 250,000 U.S. preschoolers continue to exhibit elevated lead levels due to lead-contaminated paint and dust still present in millions of homes. Other household items may present a threat as well. Vinyl mini blinds, introduced to the U.S. in the late 1980s, include several brands containing lead. A study of childhood lead poisoning cases in North Carolina revealed that for 9% of the children surveyed, mini blinds were the main source of exposure. While no-lead blinds are now available, a product recall on the lead-containing versions has never been issued and the latter remain in widespread use (Norman, 1998).

Food or juice served from improperly fired pottery or china coated with a lead-containing glaze has caused sporadic cases of lead poisoning, as has consumption of wine or other alcoholic beverages stored in lead-crystal decanters. Lead hazards continue to surface from unexpected sources; in 2003, health officials in both California and New Jersey issued health advisories targeted at "chapulines"—salty fried grasshopper snacks imported from Oaxaca that were popular among Mexican immigrants, unaware they were contaminated with high levels of lead. That same year public health workers in Rhode Island reported several cases of severe lead poisoning caused by a medicinal powder called "litargirio," widely used among immigrants from the Dominican Republic for purposes as varied as eliminating body odor and as a cure for sore feet (several of the Rhode Island victims were teenagers who had been using litargirio as a deodorant). One brand of litargirio tested by Rhode Island authorities contained 79% lead (Pérez-Peña, 2003; Urbina, 2003). Children may be inadvertently exposed when a family member engages in such hobbies as making pottery (lead glaze), stained glass, oil painting (some artists' paints contain lead), or furniture refinishing. Parents who work in occupational settings involving lead exposure may unintentionally carry lead dust home on work clothes, thereby exposing children to the toxic metal. A two-pronged national effort has been launched to combat childhood lead poisoning through environmental intervention to remove sources of lead exposure, and through screening programs to identify at-risk youngsters.

For the most part, environmental intervention entails removal of lead paint and lead dust from those structures where lead-poisoned children are living; prevention of future lead-poisoning cases would require removing lead paint from all homes, with special emphasis on residential units where such paint is deteriorating and presents an imminent and constant hazard (EPA, 1995b). Since soils around homes with exterior lead-base paints commonly exhibit elevated concentrations of lead (in some cases as high as 11,000 ppm), a number of health authorities also recommend soil abatement programs for neighborhoods where childhood lead poisoning is prevalent. Such efforts would involve removing the top 6–7 inches of soil, replacing this with clean dirt, and then revegetating the area. However, epidemiologic studies have shown that in urban areas where children were experiencing low-level lead exposure, blood lead levels declined only slightly when soil abatement activities were carried out. Thus, although lead in soils *does* contribute to children's body burden of the metal (studies have shown that blood lead levels rise by 3–7 µg/dL for every 1000 ppm increase in soil or dust concentrations), the considerable expense of contaminated soil removal may not be cost-effective; significantly greater health benefits can be achieved by targeting available funds to interior paint abatement.

In many situations where potential exposure to lead in soil is a concern, simply covering bare soil with sod, indoor-outdoor carpeting, or planting foundation shrubs along the base of the structure can eliminate or greatly reduce the opportunity for children to come into contact with contaminated soil—and at a much lower cost than removal activities would entail. However, in situations where soil lead levels are extremely high or where a child suffering from lead poisoning has a condition called pica—a tendency to eat nonfood items, including soil—then soil abatement could effect beneficial results (Mielke, 1999; Weitzman et al., 1993; Xintaras, 1992).

In the absence of a strong federal commitment to environmental lead remediation, the focus of prevention efforts on the part of government has shifted to blood lead screening to identify children at risk and to provide prompt treatment to those with elevated blood lead levels before damage becomes irreversible. Since many youngsters live in areas where the risk of lead poisoning is extremely low, screening efforts are being targeted at children living in older homes and children from low-income families. Although the prevalence of lead poisoning and its more severe manifestations have steadily declined since the 1970s, the fact that the disease still affects large numbers of young children means that society must persevere in efforts to eradicate humanity's most ancient toxic hazard.

MERCURY

This liquid metal, the "quicksilver" of ancient times, has been used for a wide variety of purposes for at least 2,500 years—and has been contributing to illness and death among those exposed to it for an equal period of time. Although at very low levels of exposure mercury does not appear to be damaging, the margin of safety is small. Mercury is a valuable constituent of many industrial products and processes. It has been used as a catalyst in the manufacture of plastics, as a slime retardant in paper making, in fluorescent lightbulbs, as a fungicide in paints, as an alloy in dental fillings, as an ingredient in many medicinal products (mercury's first medicinal use was for the treatment of syphilis when that disease reached epidemic proportions in 16th-century Europe), in the manufacture of scientific instruments, and for many other purposes.

Mercury has always been present in the environment in trace amounts, entering soil or water from vaporization and weathering of mercury compounds in the earth's crust or via volcanic activity. However, concentrations have increased three-fold in modern times due to coal combustion, mining and smelting of mercury-containing ores, and incineration of mercury wastes. Industrial processes such as electroplating, paper milling, mining and ore processing, chlorine and caustic soda production, textile manufacturing, and pharmaceutical production produce a mercury-laden effluent that is sometimes discharged into waterways. Evaporation of mercury from paints during the drying process can add significant quantities of this substance to the air; studies have shown that mercury concentrations in indoor air may be one thousand times higher immediately after a room is painted than they were before painting. Several well-publicized cases of children developing symptoms of mercury poisoning after mercury-containing latex paints were applied to their homes led to an agreement among U.S. paint manufacturers to stop adding mercury to their products. Nevertheless, although the production of interior paints containing mercury halted in 1990, followed by similar action regarding exterior paint in 1991, the fact that many people keep partly used containers of paint for future use means that paint will remain a potential source of mercury exposure for years to come.

Today, both in the United States and around the world, humans are most likely to encounter health-threatening levels of mercury exposure through consumption of mercury-tainted fish. Results of a U.S. Geological Survey study conducted from 1998–2005 revealed that all the fish sampled from 291 streams across the nation contained detectable levels of mercury (see table 7-2). At 27% of the sites sampled, concentrations of the toxic metal exceeded the EPA's human health criterion of 0.3 μg/gram wet weight, while over two-thirds of the fish sampled contained mercury at levels high enough to pose a threat to fish-eating mammals. The primary source of this ubiquitous contaminant is fallout of atmospheric mercury, most of which originates from the smokestacks of coal-fired power plants; some of the waters sampled in Western states were thought to have been impacted by gold and mercury mining operations as well (Scudder et al., 2009).

Some lake and ocean fish also pose a threat of mercury poisoning to those who eat them. The EPA and FDA have issued advisories to the public on fish species exhibiting the highest levels of mercury contamination and have recommended limits on their consumption. Warnings are targeted primarily at pregnant women, since children exposed *in utero* are at increased risk of subtle developmental delays and learning disorders. The EPA estimates that as many as 10% of U.S. women of childbearing age have blood mercury levels high enough to put a baby at risk; the government also estimates that as many as 630,000 children born in the U.S. each year are at risk of neurological problems related to mercury.

While most fish and shellfish contain at least some traces of mercury, authorities agree that for most people

Table 7-2   Summary Statistics for Mercury in U.S. Streams, 1998–2005: Total Mercury in Fish (EPA human-health criterion: ≤ 0.3 micrograms mercury per gram on a wet-weight basis)

| Parameter | Site grouping | Mercury concentration | | | | |
		Mean	Median	Minimum	Maximum	n
All fish	All sites	0.261	0.169	0.014	1.95	291
	Sites in unmined basins	0.238	0.165	0.014	1.80	232
	Sites in mined basins	0.351	0.235	0.020	1.95	59
All fish, by family						
Sunfish family	All sites	0.304	0.213	0.020	1.95	203 (33)
Trout family	All sites	0.109	0.089	0.014	0.588	53 (20)
Catfish family	All sites	0.200	0.097	0.036	1.58	19 (3)
Pike family	All sites	0.344	0.288	0.060	0.769	6 (0)
Perch family	All sites	0.517	0.635	0.250	0.666	3 (3)
Other	All sites	0.078	0.060	0.030	0.175	7 (0)
Species most commonly sampled						
Largemouth bass	All sites	0.460	0.333	0.081	1.80	62 (10)
Smallmouth bass	All sites	0.245	0.204	0.020	1.95	60 (9)
Rock bass	All sites	0.175	0.139	0.039	0.506	17 (0)
Spotted bass	All sites	0.485	0.420	0.148	0.943	14 (5)
Pumpkinseed	All sites	0.139	0.111	0.042	0.379	18 (2)
Rainbow-cutthroat trout	All sites	0.110	0.070	0.014	0.588	26 (7)
Brown trout	All sites	0.113	0.091	0.014	0.457	22 (9)
Channel catfish	All sites	0.084	0.080	0.036	0.131	12 (2)

Notes: Mercury concentrations are in micrograms per gram on a wet-weight basis; n = number of samples (with number of samples from mined basins in parentheses).
Source: Scudder et al., *Mercury in Fish, Bed Sediment, and Water from Streams Across the U.S., 1998–2005*, U.S. Geological Survey Report 2009–5109.

the nutritional benefits of eating fish far outweigh any health risk due to the toxin. Several of the most popular fish species, in fact, exhibit low mercury levels and up to 12 ounces of these can safely be eaten each week: catfish, salmon, pollock, shrimp, and light tuna (by contrast, albacore, or "white tuna," has higher levels and should be limited to one serving a week). The relatively short list of fish that shouldn't be eaten at all because of high mercury levels includes: shark, swordfish, king mackerel, and tilefish from the Gulf of Mexico. In some parts of the country, certain game fish may have high mercury concentrations, so those who enjoy recreational fishing should check local or state advisories regarding the safety of eating particular fish (all 50 states have mercury monitoring programs). If no information is available, the best advice is to eat no more than 6 ounces (one average-size meal) of locally caught fish per week and none from other sources.

Health Effects of Mercury Exposure

The action of mercury on the human system depends primarily on the form of mercury to which the victim is exposed, either inorganic metallic mercury or the far more toxic organic mercury.

Inorganic Metallic Mercury

This form of mercury frequently attacks the liver and kidneys; it also can diffuse through the alveolar membranes of the lungs and travel to the brain where it can cause such neurological problems as lack of coordination. Inorganic mercury can enter the system either by inhalation of mercury vapors or by absorption of mercury compounds through the skin after prolonged contact. Examples of human poisoning with inorganic mercury include a malady prevalent among hatmakers in 17th-century France called the "Mad Hatters' Disease" (immortalized by a character of the same name in Lewis Carroll's *Alice in Wonderland*). This neurological disorder, manifested as tremors and mental aberrations, resulted from the practice at that time of soaking animal hides in a solution of mercuric nitrate for purposes of softening the hairs. Since the hatmakers' bare arms and hands were in frequent contact with the solution as they manipulated the hides, skin absorption of mercury led to development of the disease symptoms.

Poisoning by inhalation is more common than skin absorption, however, and represents the most common form of occupational exposure to mercury. A survey conducted by NIOSH estimated that 70,000 American workers may be exposed to mercury vapors on the job. These include nurses, lab technicians, machine operators, miners, plumbers, dentists and dental hygienists, and many others. Even the families of potentially exposed workers may be at risk if mercury is carried home from the occu-

pational setting on contaminated work clothing. Exposure to mercury vapors from dental fillings (standard amalgams are approximately 50% mercury by weight) has provoked concern about the potential for chronic poisonings, but there is no convincing evidence to support such worries. In 2009, after reviewing more than 200 scientific studies, the Food and Drug Administration affirmed the safety of mercury-containing dental fillings, at least for adults and children ages 6 and above, concluding the amount of mercury in fillings is too small to pose any credible health risk. (The FDA said there is insufficient data regarding mercury's effects on children under age 6 to make any definite conclusions regarding infants and preschoolers.) Many people have become ill and some deaths have been reported among people exposed to mercury fumes when large quantities of mercury were accidentally spilled within confined, inadequately ventilated areas. If such an accident should occur, the mercury should be cleaned up as quickly as possible, regardless of how small an amount is involved, because vaporization of the metal over time could pose a serious health hazard to anyone in the vicinity, particularly small children and pregnant women (ATSDR, 1999).

In contrast to the serious dangers posed by *inhalation* of mercury, *swallowing* the metal—as could occur if a child bites down on an oral thermometer—poses no health threat. Metallic mercury is poorly absorbed by the gastrointestinal tract and is soon excreted in the feces.

Organic Mercury

Far more toxic than elemental mercury are the organic mercury compounds such as methyl mercury which, being extremely soluble, can readily penetrate living membranes. Organic mercury circulates in the bloodstream bound to red blood cells and gradually diffuses into the brain, destroying the cells that control coordination. Symptoms of organic mercury poisoning generally don't appear until a month or two after exposure, showing up initially as numbness in the lips, tongue, and fingertips. Gradually speech becomes slurred and difficulty in swallowing and walking becomes apparent. As mercury levels rise, deafness and vision problems may develop and the victim tends to lose contact with his or her surroundings. Before the nature of mercury poisoning was understood, such people were often thought to be neurotic or mentally ill and were occasionally placed in insane asylums.

Several tragic episodes involving methyl mercury poisoning have been documented in past decades. In 1972 more than 6,500 Iraqi villagers became seriously ill and 459 died after eating bread that had been made from seed wheat coated with an organic mercury fungicide. Contributing to this tragic accident was the fact that the brightly colored warning dye typically used to indicate

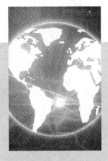

· · · · · · · *7-3* · · · · · · ·

Safety Tips for Mercury Cleanup

Compact fluorescent lightbulbs (CFLs) are highly recommended as long-lasting, energy-efficient replacements for traditional incandescent bulbs, and "green" consumers across the country are rapidly making the switch. The only drawback of CFLs, from an environmental health perspective, is the fact that they contain a small amount of elemental mercury—a problem if the bulb accidentally breaks. To avoid potential health damage caused by inhalation of mercury vapors, Energy Star, a program jointly sponsored by the U.S. EPA and the Department of Energy, recommends the following steps for safe cleanup of a broken CFL bulb:

1. *Before cleanup:*
   - Have everyone, pets included, leave the room without walking through the breakage area.
   - Open a window and leave the room for at least 15 minutes.
   - Turn off the central heating/air conditioning system.

2. *Cleanup of hard surfaces:*
   - Carefully scoop up glass fragments and mercury powder using stiff paper and place them in a sealed plastic bag or glass jar with metal lid.
   - Use duct tape to pick up any remaining small fragments.
   - Wipe area clean with damp paper towels and place them in the plastic bag or glass jar.
   - Do *NOT* use a vacuum or broom to clean up the broken bulb—this will only disperse the mercury.

3. *Cleanup of carpeted surfaces:*
   - Carefully pick up glass fragments and place in sealed container.
   - Use duct tape to pick up any remaining glass fragments and mercury powder.
   - After all visible materials are removed, if needed, vacuum the area where bulb was broken.
   - Remove the vacuum bag (or empty and wipe the canister) and put the bag or vacuum debris in a sealed plastic bag.

4. *Cleanup steps for clothing, bedding, etc.*
   - If clothing or bedding materials come in direct contact with broken glass or mercury powder that may stick to the fabric, those items should be discarded. *Do not wash* such items because mercury fragments in the fabric may contaminate the machine and/or pollute the wastewater.
   - Materials that have been exposed only to mercury *vapors* from a broken CFL (e.g., the clothing worn while cleaning up the broken bulb) can be washed, so long as it hasn't come into direct contact with materials from the broken bulb.

5. *Disposal of cleanup materials:*
   - If such disposal is not prohibited, immediately place all cleanup materials outdoors in a trash container or protected area for the next trash pickup.
   - Wash your hands after disposing of the containers of cleanup materials.
   - Check with your local or state government about disposal requirements, as some states require that mercury-containing bulbs, broken or unbroken, be disposed of at a local recycling center.

6. *Future cleaning of carpet:*
   - The next several times you clean the carpet, shut off the central heating/air-conditioning system and open a window prior to vacuuming.
   - Leave the window open and keep the central heating/air-conditioning system turned off for at least 15 minutes after vacuuming.

treated seed had been washed off and the instructions on the bags were printed only in English (Bakir et al., 1973). A similar situation, fortunately on a much smaller scale, occurred in the United States three years earlier when several members of a family in Alamagordo, New Mexico, suffered permanent neurological impairment after they butchered and ate a hog that had been fed fungicide-treated seed corn.

Undoubtedly the most infamous episode of mass poisoning with methyl mercury occurred during the years 1953–1961 in the coastal town of Minamata on the Japanese island of Kyushu. A plastics factory, Chisso Corporation, had for a number of years been discharging inorganic mercury wastes into the waters of Minamata Bay where many of the local residents earned their livelihood by fishing. In the anaerobic conditions among the sediments at the bottom of the bay, the inorganic mercury was converted into highly toxic methyl mercury by the bacterium *Methanobacterium amelanskis*. Readily soluble, the methyl mercury thus began moving through the aquatic food chain, being passively absorbed by microscopic algae which were subsequently eaten by zooplankton, which were eaten by small fish, etc. The methyl mercury became increasingly concentrated at each higher trophic level (mercury concentrations in predator fish at the top of aquatic food chains commonly reach levels 100,000 times higher than those present in the surrounding water).

Trouble first became apparent in Minamata when the town cats developed what residents first thought must be a strange viral disease, yowling continuously and sometimes leaping into the sea to drown. When the townspeople themselves started to complain of vague maladies such as extreme fatigue, headaches, numbness in their extremities, and difficulty in swallowing, it was first suspected that they were contracting some sort of illness from the sick cats. Eventually the true nature of their mutual problem was discovered—methyl mercury poisoning derived from a diet composed primarily of mercury-contaminated fish. By this time more than 100 people had been stricken with such symptoms as mental derangement, inability to walk or use chopsticks, visual disturbances, and convulsions. Forty-four of the Minamata victims died during this period and many others were permanently disabled. As this sad episode unfolded, the teratogenic properties of methyl mercury became apparent. Twenty-two brain-damaged babies were born during this period to mothers who themselves exhibited no outward signs of mercury poisoning, though several mentioned experiencing a slight numbness of the fingers during pregnancy and analysis showed a high level of mercury in their hair. Subsequent studies have revealed that methyl mercury has a special affinity for fetal tissue, easily crossing the placental barrier where it severely damages the developing child while leaving the mother unharmed.

The ultimate human toll of Chisso's poisoning of Minamata Bay included 700 deaths and 9,000 individuals left with varying degrees of paralysis and brain damage. Estimates are that as many as 50,000 people living within 35 miles of the bay who consumed its fish have suffered at least mild symptoms of mercury poisoning (Weisskopf, 1987). After years of legal wrangling over compensation, several thousand plaintiffs reached a settlement with Chisso in 1996, agreeing to drop lawsuits in return for a $24,200 lump sum payment to each Minamata Disease victim, plus additional payments to five national victims' groups. A year later, in 1997, the regional government (Kumamoto Prefecture) declared that Minamata Bay was again safe for fishing, with mercury in the waterway's marine life having fallen below the level the government considers dangerous (Pollack, 1997).

Ironically, as Japan's tragic episode of methyl mercury poisoning draws to a close, Minamata Disease is now claiming new victims along the Amazon. Brazil is in the throes of a modern-day gold rush, with an estimated half-million prospectors roaming the Amazon basin, searching along riverbeds for traces of the precious metal. Employing methods that would have looked entirely familiar to California's "Forty-niners" a century and a half ago, prospectors utilize mercury to separate gold from the muck dredged from the river. In doing so they are releasing an estimated 250 tons of mercury into the Amazon watershed each year. Following the same sequence of events that transpired decades ago in Minamata, mercury has reached high concentrations in Amazonian fish. Villagers who eat the tainted fish are now showing signs of neurological disorders and have detectable body burdens of methyl mercury.

Regulating Mercury

As evidence regarding mercury's adverse impact on neurological development of fetuses and young children has mounted over the years, pressure has increased on governments to impose regulatory controls on the major industrial sources of emissions. Attention first focused on municipal and medical waste incinerators, and between 1995 and 1997 those in the United States were required to reduce their mercury output by 90–94%. Regulatory attention then shifted to the nation's coal-burning power plants that currently contribute slightly over 40% of total U.S. mercury emissions—approximately 48 tons per year. Not affected by the restrictions imposed on waste incinerators and cement kilns in the mid-1990s, power plants were the target of regulations promulgated in 1995 under EPA's Clean Mercury Rule. Although the agency had originally proposed that new and existing coal-fired utilities be required to curb mercury emissions using the "maximum achievable control technology" standard which would have sharply lowered emissions by 2007, the Bush Administration opted instead for a more industry-friendly approach intended to reduce power plant emissions of the toxic metal by almost 70% from 1999 levels by 2018. In 2006 a federal court struck down this rule as both inadequate and invalid. Under the Obama Administration, the EPA in 2009 embarked upon a rule-making process that could require some power plants to reduce emissions by as much as 90%.

A year earlier, then-Senator Obama (D-IL) and Senator Lisa Murkowski (R-AK) cosponsored the Mercury Export Ban Act of 2008—legislation that was approved overwhelmingly in both houses of Congress and signed into law by President Bush in October 2008. Stressing the need to protect people around the world from mercury poisoning, the bill's supporters argued that while use of mercury is gradually being phased out by industry in the United States, inexpensive surplus supplies are being sold and shipped overseas to developing countries where mercury use by highly polluting industries goes largely unregulated and where the waste management infrastructure is underdeveloped. As a result, workers and ordinary citizens in those countries are suffering health damage due to excessive mercury exposure. In addition, the resultant airborne emissions contaminate fish harvests, endangering not only local people but also consumers elsewhere, Americans included, who eat imported seafood. The U.S. ban on export sales of elemental mercury takes effect in 2013; a similar regulation proposed by the European Commission would prohibit mercury exports from European Union countries by 2011.

To manage the surplus stocks of mercury that can no longer be sold abroad, the Mercury Export Ban Act requires the Department of Energy's Office of Environmental Management to have a long-term mercury storage site available by 2013. By mid-2009 the DOE had identified sites for consideration in seven different states, but failed to meet the Act's deadline of January 1, 2010, for deciding which one should be chosen as the nation's mercury storage site. Predictably, local concerns about hosting a facility that will be home to 7,500–10,000 metric tons of elemental mercury for more than 40 years have provoked a "not-in-my-backyard" response in all but one of the locations under consideration, the one exception being a private disposal facility owned by Waste Control Specialists (WCS) in Andrews County, Texas, whose CEO expressed interest in the project (Anderson, 2009a).

In addition to the toxic materials discussed in this chapter, there are many other substances capable of causing health damage in humans when present in more than trace amounts or when exposure to even very low levels persists over an extended time period. Cadmium, fluorides, selenium, copper, nickel, chromium, and arsenic are but a few of the naturally occurring toxins that are known, under certain conditions, to affect human health adversely. Unfortunately, because the symptoms of exposure to toxic substances are often so vague or so similar to those of other more common ailments, they are frequently either ignored or misdiagnosed. Thus it would not be surprising to find that health damage due to such toxins is more prevalent than commonly assumed at present.

8

Rats!
They fought the dogs and killed the cats,
And bit the babies in the cradles,
And ate the cheeses out of the vats
And licked the soup from the cooks' own ladles.
—Robert Browning, "The Pied Piper of Hamelin" (1845)

Pests and Pesticides

The tale of the mythical rat catcher of Hamelin, who rid that medieval town of its plague of rodents—and subsequently of its children as well—has been told and retold for centuries. Whether based on historical fact or not, the legend accurately conveys the sense of dismay and helplessness experienced by preindustrial societies when confronted with disastrous pest outbreaks. History records countless incidents of the devastating impact that certain insects, rodents, fungi, and so forth, can have on human health and well-being. Such organisms are typically referred to as "pests," a term derived from the Latin word pestis ("plague"), which was applied to a number of deadly epidemic diseases that periodically swept through the ancient world.

WHAT IS A PEST?

Biologically speaking, there is, of course, no such thing as a "pest"; no classification system divides living things into categories labeled "good species" and "bad species." The term "pest" is a purely human concept and refers broadly to any organism—animal, plant, or microbe—that adversely affects human interests. Pest species comprise only a small percentage of the total number of organisms on earth, the vast majority being either beneficial or, more commonly, neutral so far as their impact on humans is concerned. Pests are not restricted to any one taxonomic group; representative species can be found among such invertebrates as insects, mites, ticks, and nematodes. Several bird species such as starlings, pigeons, and English sparrows can be considered pests, as can some mammals—rats, mice, moles, rabbits, and, in some situations, deer, coyotes, or even elephants! Many types of microorganisms, such as disease-causing bacteria, viruses, rickettsia, and fungi, are pests, as are weeds—any "plant out of place," growing where it's not wanted.

PROBLEMS CAUSED BY PESTS

Conflict between people and pests has existed since time immemorial and is generated primarily when such organisms compete with humans for the same resources, cause us discomfort, or are vectors of disease. The need to protect human interests by limiting pest damage has created a demand for better methods of combating such problems and constitutes the chief justification for the development and use of chemical pesticides. Although

183

the use of such toxic compounds has, for a variety of reasons, come under increasing scrutiny and criticism, it is important to review the types of problems caused by pests in order to understand why suggestions to limit or abolish the use of chemical pesticides generates such controversy.

Resource Competition

According to some experts, insects, weeds, and plant pathogens (fungi, nematodes, bacteria and viruses) are responsible for the loss of an estimated 35–42% of the global harvest each year, despite more than 50 years of escalating chemical warfare against agricultural pests (Pimentel, 1997). Insect problems are particularly severe on cotton, tobacco, and potatoes, as well as on most fruit and vegetable crops. Fungal diseases cause significant losses primarily to fruits and some vegetables, while yield reductions due to weed infestations are most pronounced on acreage devoted to corn and soybean production. In addition to such losses in the field, about 6% of the annual harvest in the United States (and a substantially larger share in developing nations) is lost to pests while in storage or transit.

A reduction in current pesticide use would undoubtedly result in a further increase in crop loss due to pest depredation—a cause for concern both to farmers and to humanitarians worried about feeding a hungry world. The extent of such loss is hotly disputed, however. Some scientists estimate that without pesticides or alternative protective measures, U.S. agricultural production would drop by 24–57%, depending on the particular crop. Farm exports would be cut by half and American consumers would see their annual grocery bill rise by almost $230 (NRC, 2000). Others, however, calculate that preharvest losses of all crops resulting from a significant reduction in pesticide use would be minimal. A noted entomologist at Cornell University estimates that if American farmers were to adopt a variety of nonchemical control techniques they could cut current levels of agricultural pesticide use by 50% without experiencing any decline in yields. Under this scenario, substituting nonchemical for chemical controls would result in food price increases of less than 1% (Pimentel, 1991).

Although loss in farm production is the major example of resource competition between humans and pests, many other instances of conflict can be cited: **termites** cause incalculable damage to structures, especially in the tropics; in the United States alone, controlling termites and repairing the damage caused by these wood-destroying pests cost property owners an estimated $11 billion each year (Raloff, 2003). **Cockroaches**, the bread-and-butter of the structural pest control industry, are found worldwide and are universally despised for contaminating food and materials in homes, restaurants, supermar-

kets, cruise ships, warehouses—literally every place where careless humans provide them with a source of food and water. **Rats and mice** cause enormous economic losses, consuming as much as one-third of the world's harvest and rendering many stored food supplies unusable due to contamination with rodent hairs, droppings, and urine (Mallis, 1997).

Sources of Discomfort

Itching, buzzing, creeping, and crawling may not seem like serious concerns, but the creatures responsible have been driving people to distraction for millennia and have been the targets of a great deal of pesticide use in recent decades. Some of the major villains involved in producing acute human discomfort, if not illness, include the following.

Lice

Head lice, body lice, and crab lice are all human parasites that can cause severe itching, secondary infections, and scarred or hardened skin. Lice are typically associated with people living in crowded conditions where opportunities for bathing and laundering clothes are limited. With the introduction of DDT following World War II, the incidence of lice infestations dropped to low levels. As the use of this insecticide became restricted, however, cases of head lice among schoolchildren have increased.

Fleas

Aside from the flea species that transmit the deadly plague bacterium (see next section), fleas commonly found on domestic animals can cause severe irritation, loss of blood, and discomfort. Although most fleas prefer to feed on their animal host, they frequently bite humans if the normal host is absent. Such bites can be extremely painful and may cause swelling and a reddening of the skin.

Mites

These tiny insect relatives are responsible for the serious skin condition known as scabies, as well as a number of other forms of dermatitis such as "grocers' itch," acquired by handling mite-infested grain products, cheese, dried fruits, and so on. Mites that normally live as ectoparasites on birds may become very serious pests of humans when they migrate in large numbers into homes after starlings or sparrows leave their nests. For this reason, homeowners should discourage birds from nesting on eaves or windowsills or other locations in close proximity to homes. **Chiggers**, a type of mite inhabiting many parts of the southern or midwestern United States, can cause extreme skin irritation lasting for a week or more when they attach themselves to a human host, usually around the waist or armpits.

Bedbugs

During the day these small, lentil-shaped insects are seldom seen, hiding among bedsprings or the tufts of mattresses, in cracks in the bed frame or headboard, under loose wallpaper or area rugs—indeed, any place that is dark, secluded, and in close proximity to a blood meal. At night bedbugs emerge to feed on an unwary sleeper, leaving large, intensely itchy welts on sensitive victims and bloodstains on sheets when an engorged bug is inadvertently crushed as its human host rolls over in bed. Once a common pest almost everywhere, bedbugs largely disappeared in more affluent societies after World War II, due in part to the widespread use of DDT, but also thanks to fashion trends toward less elaborate bedroom furniture (i.e., fewer hiding places) and better vacuum cleaners (more efficient cleaning = fewer bedbugs).

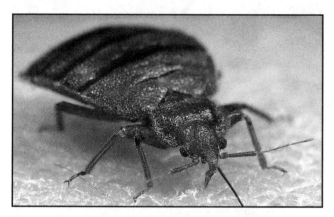

The small, lentil-shaped bedbug is making an unwelcome comeback due in large part to a surge in international trade and travel. [*CDC/Harvard University*]

In recent years, however, bedbugs—like head lice—are making a comeback, owing in large part to the surge in international trade and travel. New York and Chicago were among a number of U.S. cities where residents reported a record number of bedbug infestations in 2010, provoking panic among some citizens not accustomed to worrying about nighttime marauders. Since bedbugs can live for half a year or more without food, they can easily stow away in luggage or shipping crates, emerging hale and hungry in hotels, university dorms, hospitals, and homes half a world away. Bedbug infestations can be particularly bad in densely populated apartment buildings where landlords may spend tens of thousands of dollars for extermination services. The old bedtime admonition, "Sleep tight, don't let the bedbugs bite!" has new relevance in this age of globalization; fortunately, bedbugs are not known to transmit any diseases, though a few people develop severe allergic reactions, hives, or asthma after being bitten by bedbugs.

Spiders

Although many people harbor an irrational antipathy toward spiders, the vast majority of these eight-legged creatures are quite harmless to humans. Even the fearsome-looking tarantula—the loathsome villain in many a B-grade Hollywood thriller—is actually rather docile. Now widely sold as pets, tarantulas can be handled with ease and rarely bite; even when they do, their venom is of little harm to most people. Only three U.S. species present any real danger: the **black widow** (female only), the **brown recluse** (both sexes), and the **aggressive house spider** (males are more venomous and more likely to bite than females). The black widow, though more abundant in warmer regions of the country, can be found throughout the United States; primarily an outdoor spider, the black widow is typically found around piles of wood or other debris where the female spins a nondescript-looking web. Black widow venom acts as a nerve poison, but while bites may be quite painful they are very seldom fatal, even in the absence of medical attention. Contrary to popular myth, the diminutive male black widow is not devoured after mating by his much larger bride—unless she is unusually hungry!—but generally spends a parasitic post-nuptial existence in the vicinity of her web, waiting for any leftovers that may come his way.

The brown recluse spider, whose range covers much of the south-central and southeastern United States as far north as Missouri, Illinois, and Indiana, is most often encountered within dwellings where it hides in attics, closets, and other dark, seldom-disturbed places. It is a shy species that bites only when provoked—usually when rolled on at night or when clothes are taken out of storage. The poison injected by the bite of a brown recluse differs from that of a black widow in that it is cytotoxic, causing tissue death in the vicinity of the wound. Scarcely noticeable at first, the bite gradually becomes

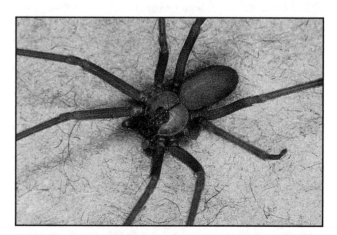

The brown recluse spider is found throughout much of south-central and southeastern United States. It often can be identified by the violin-shaped marking on its back. [*CDC*]

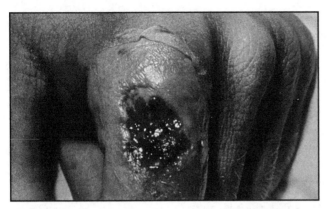

The poison injected by the bite of a brown recluse spider is a cytotoxin, causing tissue death in the area of the wound. [*CDC Archive, Bugwood.org*]

very painful and frequently develops into an open ulceration that persists for weeks and eventually leaves a large ugly scar.

The aggressive house spider (alternatively referred to as the "hobo spider"), a European immigrant whose range in North America is currently limited to British Columbia and five states in the northwestern U.S., has only recently been identified as the source of spider bites long attributed to the brown recluse (which doesn't live in that part of the country). Like brown recluse venom, that of the aggressive house spider is a cytotoxin. *Unlike* the brown recluse, however, aggressive house spiders are true to their name and tend to bite without provocation. Large (40 mm in length) and fast running, these spiders tend to live in or near houses, often in rock walls, along foundations, or in woodpiles (many bites occur when firewood is being carried inside). Large numbers of males enter basements and ground floor rooms of homes in the autumn and dogs and cats are frequently bitten on the face as they attempt to investigate, occasionally dying as a result. These are not nice spiders! (Akre and Myhre, 1994).

In addition to the above, the buzzing of flies, mosquitoes, gnats, cicadas, June bugs, or wasps—even when these insects are not carrying disease organisms—can provoke extreme annoyance. Certain plant species, particularly poison ivy and its relatives, also have been prime targets of chemical herbicides because of the intensely irritating rash which contact with these plants can produce.

Vectors of Disease

Public health practitioners, along with farmers, were among the first to greet the introduction of synthetic chemical pesticides with great enthusiasm. Compounds such as DDT were viewed as perhaps the ultimate weapon in freeing humanity from the threat of a number of insect- or rodent-borne diseases responsible for millions of deaths and illnesses each year. Quite appropri-

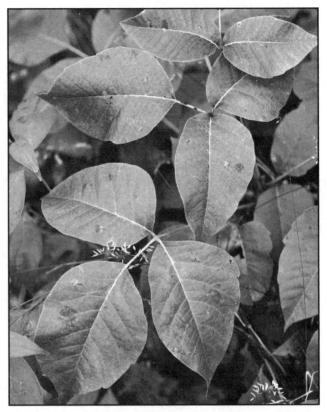

Poison ivy, which usually can be identified by its 3-leaf clusters, causes an uncomfortable, itchy rash.

ately, the first use to which DDT was put involved the wartime dusting of refugees in Italy to curb an outbreak of typhus fever. The success of this effort led to extensive spraying campaigns in many parts of the world against the vectors of such dreaded killers as malaria, yellow fever, river blindness, bubonic plague, and encephalitis. Although the medical community's high hopes for complete eradication of the carriers of these diseases have proven overly optimistic, pesticide use has played a significant role in lowering death rates and improving public health in many parts of the world. Some pests of particular public health importance include mosquitoes, flies, body lice, rat fleas, and ticks.

Mosquitoes

Mosquitoes have probably been responsible for more human deaths than any other insect, though their role as disease-carriers was not recognized until late in the 19th century. Worldwide, even today millions of people become ill each year due to such mosquito-borne ailments as malaria, yellow fever, dengue, filariasis, and encephalitis. In the past, there have been major outbreaks of all these diseases, particularly **malaria** and **yellow fever**, in parts of the United States. In recent years, infected immigrants or tourists returning from regions where malaria is still endemic have been responsible for approximately 1,500 cases each year of malaria acquired abroad but diagnosed and reported in the United States (CDC, 2009d). Since the mosquito vectors responsible for transmitting malaria in the U.S. are common species (*Anopheles quadrimaculatus* and *A. freeborni*), the opportunity still exists for future outbreaks.

Until recently, **dengue fever** and **dengue hemorrhagic fever**, carried by *Aedes aegypti*, also the vector of yellow fever, were considered relatively mild ailments. However, in recent years dengue has emerged as a major cause of death and disease throughout the world's tropics, particularly among children. Dengue is now considered the most important mosquito-borne *viral* disease of humans (malaria is caused by the Plasmodium parasite), sickening tens of millions of people annually. Reasons for the sudden emergence of dengue as a serious public health problem are complex, but according to the Centers for Disease Control and Prevention (CDC), widespread discontinuance of effective mosquito control efforts in the early 1970s due to concerns about the environmental impacts of chemical pesticides played a significant role in fostering the reestablishment of *A. aegypti* populations.

In the United States and Canada, **West Nile Virus** today presents the most serious mosquito-borne health threat. Mosquitoes pick up the virus when they feed on the blood of infected birds, subsequently transmitting the pathogen to a human victim. In its most serious form (less than 1% of cases), West Nile Virus causes a fatal inflammation of the brain (encephalitis). The vast majority of cases are far less severe, generally manifested as a mild, flu-like ailment that persists for only a few days. Although the first human cases were diagnosed only in 1999 in the U.S. and 2002 in Canada, by 2003 West Nile disease was being reported from coast to coast, with the number of people affected that year soaring to 9,000 confirmed cases and 240 fatalities. In subsequent years the number of cases has declined significantly, with 620 reported to the CDC by the end of 2010, including 23 deaths. Several other forms of viral encephalitis can be transmitted from infected birds to humans via mosquito bites, typically during the summer months and early fall. Of these, Eastern equine encephalitis exhibits the highest mortality rates (50–60%), but cases are quite rare, averaging just four per year. A few dozen cases of St. Louis encephalitis, LaCross encephalitis, and Western encephalitis occur sporadically each year, primarily in midwestern states; fatality rates for these diseases are low, but victims may experience long-term central nervous system damage.

U.S. Public Health Service officials striving to prevent outbreaks of vectorborne disease fear their task may be complicated by the arrival in 1985 of *Aedes albopictus*,

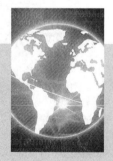

······· *8-1* ·······

Avoiding the Bite

In summers past, many a child took perverse pleasure in allowing a hungry mosquito to alight on his or her arm and begin feeding, slowly swelling up like a tiny red balloon until given a triumphant whack, splattering blood in all directions! Since the arrival of West Nile Virus (WNV) in the United States a few years ago, however, such "fun" now entails considerable health risk. Mosquito-borne West Nile disease has made the avoidance of mosquito bites an important aspect of summertime preventive health care. West Nile Virus was first reported in the United States in the summer of 1999, with most cases occurring in the New York metropolitan area. Since then, the virus has spread rapidly across the country, with California, Texas, Colorado, and Arizona reporting the largest number of cases in recent years.

While insecticidal spraying or fogging to reduce populations of adult mosquitoes may occasionally be justified in areas where disease outbreaks are severe, doing so is of limited usefulness and can itself raise health and environmental concerns. A much safer and more effective approach to reducing the risk of mosquito-borne disease is to focus on two complementary strategies:

1. reducing the size of the mosquito population and

2. using repellents to avoid being bitten.

The former primarily involves removing, to the greatest extent possible, any standing water around the house or yard where mosquitoes can lay their eggs. Some potential breeding places are fairly obvious:

- infrequently changed birdbaths or ornamental garden ponds (unless these contain larvae-devouring fish)
- neglected wading pools or swimming pool covers that have collected rainwater

Other egg-laying sites may not be so readily apparent:

- drainage saucers under well-watered planters
- pet water bowls
- leaf-clogged rain gutters that fail to drain adequately
- hollow stumps or tree holes
- rain-collecting tires or debris lying around the yard
- a child's wagon or wheelbarrow that hasn't been moved since the last downpour

While eradication of breeding sites can substantially reduce the number of mosquitoes in an area, it's unlikely to eliminate them altogether, making judicious repellent use another important approach for avoiding mosquito bites. Many products claim to be effective repellents, but CDC has long advised that only those containing the chemical compound popularly known as **DEET** keep mosquitoes at bay for any length of time; in 2005 CDC expanded its list of recommended mosquito repellents to include those containing the chemical picaridin or the oil of lemon eucalyptus. Plant-based mosquito repellents such as citronella have very limited effectiveness, deterring mosquitoes, on average, for only 3–20 minutes following application. One soybean-oil-based repellent is a bit better, providing protection up to about one hour. The much-touted moisturizer, *Skin-So-Soft Bath Oil®*, keeps mosquitoes away for less than 10 minutes. Wristbands impregnated with repellent, despite advertising claims, don't work at all, nor do "ultrasonic" devices or Vitamin B.

By contrast, DEET-containing products give complete protection against bites for several to many hours, depending on the concentration of the active ingredient. Rising concentrations of DEET are directly proportional to the duration of the bite-free period, with products containing 6–7% DEET protective for about 2 hours, 20% DEET for 4 hours, 24% DEET an average of 5 hours. Beyond 50%, increasing concentrations of the active ingredient do not further extend the length of protection.

Although in the past some pediatricians warned that the concentration of DEET in formulations used on young children should never exceed 10% (some advised against using DEET on small children at all), an extensive safety evaluation of DEET by the Environmental Protection Agency concluded that, when used in accordance with label directions, DEET can be safely used by people of all ages and at all concentrations. Certain safety precautions should, of course, be followed:

- When used directly on skin, apply only to exposed areas, avoiding the mouth, eyes, or any place where the skin is broken. DEET may also be sprayed on clothing, but should not be applied to skin underneath; clothing treated with DEET should be laundered before being worn again.
- When repellent is used on a child, it should be applied by an adult; avoid child's eyes, mouth, and hands (since children tend to put hands in their mouths) and use sparingly around the ears.
- Don't over-apply; a small amount, when evenly spread, is adequate for protection. Wash off repellent with soap and water after coming indoors.

Mosquito repellents can be used in conjunction with sunscreen but a single combination sunscreen/repellent lotion is not recommended because DEET shouldn't be applied as frequently as is necessary for sunscreen. The CDC advises that sunscreen be applied first, followed by a DEET-containing repellent. Sunscreen can subsequently be reapplied without reapplying repellent (Fradin and Day, 2002).

For optimum protection, insect repellent should be used whenever a person is going to be outdoors in a situation where mosquito bites are likely, especially at dusk or dawn when the largest numbers of hungry females are present. Mosquitoes have always been a summer presence; their new threat as vectors of West Nile Virus makes it more important than ever that we take active precautions to keep them as far away from us as possible!

the **Asian tiger mosquito**. A number of these alien invaders entered the port of Houston that year as stowaways in a shipment of used tires. They quickly spread from Texas throughout much of the eastern U.S., presumably hitchhiking on the truckloads of used tires that travel the interstate highway system (the female lays her eggs just above the waterline in tree holes or artificial containers—like tire casings). Because tiger mosquito eggs can overwinter, *A. albopictus* has had no difficulty in becoming established in northern states (there is now an established infestation in the region around Chicago), as well as in warmer regions of the country. By 2000 it was firmly established in 26 states and had also spread to parts of Mexico, Central America, and the Caribbean. *A. albopictus* was independently introduced to Brazil in 1986 and is now widespread in that country as well (CDC, 2005). Unlike many other mosquito species, it thrives in close proximity to people and can live inside houses year-round, breeding in pet water dishes and in the saucers under houseplants. The tiger mosquito is a vicious biter and, in its Asian homeland, is an important disease vector. Although as yet no disease outbreaks have been attributed to the newcomer, researchers have determined that the tiger mosquito has the ability to pick up and transmit the viral pathogens for dengue fever and encephalitis and fear that it has the potential to become the most important carrier of mosquito-borne diseases in the United States.

Flies

Many species of flies, particularly the common housefly, are important carriers of serious gastrointestinal diseases such as **typhoid fever**, **cholera**, **dysentery**, and **parasitic worm infections** due to their

Table 8-1   2010 West Nile Virus Human Infections in the United States

State	Human Cases Reported to CDC		Total cases	Deaths
	Neuroinvasive disease cases	Nonneuroinvasive disease cases		
Arizona	67	47	114	7
New York	72	31	103	3
California	37	23	60	1
Texas	39	6	45	3
Colorado	10	28	38	0
Nebraska	10	27	37	1
Michigan	17	4	21	2
New Jersey	12	8	20	2
South Dakota	4	16	20	0
Illinois	14	4	18	1
Louisiana	12	6	18	0
Pennsylvania	10	3	13	0
New Mexico	9	3	12	0
Georgia	4	7	11	0
Maryland	8	1	9	0
North Dakota	2	6	8	0
Florida	6	1	7	2
Connecticut	6	1	7	0
Kansas	1	5	6	0
Indiana	1	5	6	0
Arkansas	5	0	5	0
Minnesota	3	2	5	0
Mississippi	2	3	5	0
Wyoming	1	4	5	0
Missouri	4	0	4	0
Massachusetts	3	1	4	0
Iowa	1	2	3	0
Alabama	1	2	3	0
Virginia	2	0	2	1
Tennessee	1	1	2	0
Ohio	1	1	2	0
Kentucky	1	1	2	0
Wisconsin	0	2	2	0
Nevada	0	2	2	0
Idaho	0	1	1	0
Oklahoma	0	0	0	0
Totals	**366**	**254**	**620**	**23**

Notes:

Neuroinvasive disease cases refers to severe cases of disease that affect a person's nervous system. These include encephalitis, which is an inflammation of the brain; meningitis, which is an inflammation of the membrane around the brain and the spinal cord; and acute flaccid paralysis, which is an inflammation of the spinal cord that can cause a sudden onset of weakness in the limbs and/or breathing muscles. Nonneuroinvasive disease cases refers to typically less severe cases that show no evidence of neuroinvasion—primarily West Nile fever.

Total Human Cases Reported to CDC: These numbers reflect both mild and severe confirmed and probable human disease cases occurring between January 1, 2010 and December 31, 2010 as reported through November 9, 2010.

The high proportion of neuroinvasive disease cases among reported cases of West Nile virus disease reflects surveillance reporting bias. Serious cases are more likely to be reported than mild cases. Also, the surveillance system is not designed to detect asymptomatic infections. Data from population-based surveys indicate that among all people who become infected with West Nile virus (including people with asymptomatic infections) less than 1% will develop severe neuroinvasive disease.

Source: CDC, "West Nile Virus: Statistics, Surveillance, and Control." Accessed Oct. 2010 from www.cdc.gov/ncidod/dvbid/westnile/surv&controlCaseCount10_detailed.htm

habit of feeding on human and animal wastes. If such wastes contain pathogenic organisms, the fly can pick these up either on the sticky pads of its feet or on its body hairs or mouthparts and mechanically transmit them to humans when it alights on food materials. Fly vomitus and feces also frequently contain pathogenic bacteria that can inoculate human food, multiply rapidly in the food medium, and subsequently result in outbreaks of intestinal diseases when the food is consumed by people.

Cockroaches

Contrary to common belief, cockroaches have not been implicated as important vectors of infectious disease, even though laboratory studies have repeatedly shown these insects harbor a wide range of pathogenic microbes on their feet and can mechanically transmit these organisms to food. Some researchers have attributed cases of Salmonella food poisoning and other diarrheal illnesses to the presence of large numbers of cockroaches in or near food preparation areas, but the evidence for a cause-and-effect relationship is inconclusive. Undisputed, however, is the fact that heavy cockroach infestations can cause severe allergic reactions and precipitate asthma attacks. Secretions produced by roaches can induce symptoms ranging from skin irritations and runny nose to difficulty in breathing. Acute reaction to cockroach allergens has recently been recognized as the leading cause for the high incidence of **asthma** among inner-city children in the U.S. These findings suggest that vigorous cockroach control programs should be an integral part of public health efforts to combat asthma, the incidence rates of which have been dramatically rising worldwide (Rosenstreich et al., 1997).

Body Lice

As mentioned in the previous section, body lice can be a source of intense discomfort, but they are of special public health concern because they are vectors of several serious epidemic diseases. **Typhus fever**, characterized by elevated temperature, severe headache, and a rash, has been a major killer in past centuries, particularly during wartime when perhaps as many soldiers died from typhus as from swords or bullets. French researchers, analyzing remains from a mass grave in Lithuania where thousands of French troops were buried during Napoleon's disastrous 1812 retreat from Moscow, found that roughly one-third had died of louse-borne diseases (Raoult et al., 2006). The rickettsial pathogen responsible for the disease is passed from louse to human by the feces of the insect, not its bite. When a person infested with lice scratches the affected area, minor abrasions on the skin permit entry to the rickettsia. Other lice subsequently feeding on a person infected with typhus ingest the pathogen and spread it as they move from person to person. This method of transmission explains why typhus outbreaks are most prevalent when people are living together in crowded, unsanitary conditions. Insecticidal dusting of louse-infested persons has proven to be an effective method for controlling the spread of typhus fever. Two other louse-borne diseases, also most common during wartime but with much lower fatality rates than typhus, are trench fever and relapsing fever.

Rat Fleas

Aside from the enormous economic damage caused by rats, these pests are of great public health concern because they are vectors of a number of diseases, the most deadly of which is **plague** (the "Black Death" of medieval times). In September 1994 the first major plague outbreak in half a century terrorized residents of the Indian city of Surat, killing more than 50 people. Even before the Surat incident, plague rates had been steadily rising worldwide since the early 1980s. In addition to the 1994 plague outbreak in Surat, several other major outbreaks have occurred since then in Indonesia (1997), India (2002), and Algeria (2003). The vast majority of recent human plague cases and deaths, however, have been in Africa, most notably in the Democratic Republic of the Congo, Mozambique, Madagascar, Uganda, and Tanzania; a few Asian countries account for most of the remainder. Since 1989, the World Health Organization (WHO) has reported the average number of plague cases worldwide at slightly over 2,700 per year, with approximately 200 plague deaths annually. WHO admits these figures may underestimate plague's true human toll, however, in part because some countries are reluctant to acknowledge the extent of the problem, as well as due to the lack of facilities and medical personnel to provide diagnoses and clinical confirmation of suspected cases (WHO, 2004).

The plague bacterium actually is carried by fleas on rats, not by the rats themselves. When infected fleas feed on their rat hosts, the rats too sicken and die. If rats are living in close proximity to humans, a flea whose rat host has died may then hop onto a person for a blood meal and thus spread the plague organism to human populations. Because of the tendency of fleas to substitute hosts when necessary, rat-poisoning campaigns should always be preceded by insecticidal spraying of rat-infested areas to kill the fleas first. If this precautionary measure is not taken, one runs the risk of transferring rodent diseases to humans.

While most Americans tend to think of plague as a remnant of the Middle Ages, rat fleas infected with the plague bacterium were introduced into California early in the 20th century and quickly became endemic among wild rodent populations in the region. Since that time the focus of plague infection has expanded steadily eastward; today plague-infected rodent populations have been identified in 13 western states and in southwestern Canada. Each year an average of 10–15 human cases of plague are reported from this region, mostly in scattered rural areas. The incidence of plague outbreaks in the United States seems to be increasing, as rapid suburbanization results in growing numbers of people living in close proximity to wild rodent habitat. A worrisome trend noted in recent years is a rise in the number of human cases in which domestic cats were the source of infection. Because cats typically are allowed to roam freely, those living in areas where plague-infected rodents are common have ample opportunity to contract the disease and subsequently transmit the ailment to their human companions (CDC, 1994a). For this reason, CDC advises pet owners living in areas where plague is endemic to keep dogs and cats indoors and free of fleas through regular use of flea powders. People living, camping, hiking, or hunting in areas where plague is endemic should take precautions to avoid contact with wild rodents and rodent burrows (where infected fleas may be present) and should never approach or handle obviously sick or dying wild animals. Even recently dead rodents can present a disease hazard: one plague death in the Southwest involved a housewife who picked up a dead ground squirrel that her cat had proudly deposited on the doorstep. She presumably was bitten by a hungry flea who found her an acceptable alternative host and subsequently contracted a fatal case of bubonic plague; another case, fortunately with a happier outcome, involved a young woman living in an urban Los Angeles neighborhood who contracted bubonic plague after handling raw meat from a rabbit that had been killed and brought to her from a rural area where a die-off of jackrabbits and cottontails had been observed. The woman recovered after receiving antibiotic treatment (CDC, 2006b).

Ticks

Among our most common parasites, ticks are a source of profound annoyance to campers, hunters, dog owners, and livestock raisers who frequently discover themselves or their pets providing a blood meal to these tiny pests. Ticks are far more than a nuisance, however. They are vectors of several serious human diseases such as **Rocky Mountain spotted fever**, a condition that frequently results in death within two weeks and which, contrary to its name, is not restricted to mountainous areas but is found throughout the continental United States, with the largest number of cases being reported from North and South Carolina.

The most common tick-borne ailment in the United States today—indeed, the most common vectorborne ailment in this country—is **Lyme disease**, with cases reported from all 50 states, the District of Columbia, and several U.S. territories, as well as from various locations along the border in Canada. In spite of its wide geographic distribution (researchers hypothesize that birds are carrying the tick from one region of the country to another, since tick larvae frequently feed on avian hosts), Lyme disease poses a significant risk of infection in just 10 states in the Northeast and upper Midwest, where 93% of all cases between 1992–2006 were reported (CDC, 2008d).

Caused by the spirochete bacterium *Borrelia burgdorferi*, Lyme disease is transmitted to humans by the bite of an infected black-legged tick, *Ixodes scapularis;* on the West Coast a related species, *I. pacificus*, is the vector. The black-legged tick, once inaccurately referred to as the "deer tick," is a tiny arthropod that feeds on the blood of birds, small mammals like the white-footed mouse, deer, and—if they happen to be around—humans who venture into the ticks' woodland habitat. Because the tick is so small and inconspicuous, human victims may not even realize they've been bitten until disease symptoms appear, generally several days to a month later.

The first and most characteristic symptom of Lyme disease, observed in 60–80% of patients within 30 days after being bitten, is a circular, spreading red rash resembling a rosy "bull's eye" because of the pale area of skin in the center (in some cases the rash is uniformly red, without a central clear area). This rash, which usually develops on the torso of the body, though not necessarily at the location of the tick bite, is often accompanied by a splitting headache, fever, chills, muscle or joint pains, and extreme fatigue. At this stage the disease can be effectively treated with antibiotics, which generally produce a quick and complete cure. If not caught at this stage, Lyme disease can progress to a second stage characterized by nervous system dysfunction and muscle pains. The onset of arthritis, usually in the knees or other large joints, typifies the third stage of the disease and can be very painful. Unfortunately, antibiotics may not be particularly effective in combating these later stages of Lyme disease—perhaps as many as 50% of patients who develop chronic symptoms don't respond to antibiotic therapy. In 1998 the first vaccine for preventing Lyme disease, *LYMErix*, was approved by the FDA. Although this product was both safe and efficacious, the manufacturer withdrew it from the market in 2002 due to low consumer demand. The lack of a vaccine increases the importance of personal protective measures for hikers, campers, or those living in tick-infested areas.

The same tick species that carries the Lyme disease pathogen can also transmit a sometimes fatal bacterial ailment known as **anaplasmosis**, about 800–1000 cases of which are reported to the CDC each year. Symptoms generally occur within 5–21 days after being bitten by an infected tick and usually include fever, chills, severe headache, and muscle pains. Depending on the victim's age and general state of health, the condition can be life-threatening, so prompt treatment with antibiotics is highly recommended. **Ehrlichiosis**, another rickettsial tick-borne disease with symptoms similar to those of anaplasmosis though generally less severe, is carried by the Lone Star tick (*Amblyomma americanum*). Annual incidence of ehrlichiosis has quadrupled over the past decade, with approximately 800 cases reported in 2008, primarily in southern and south-central states (CDC, 2009a). Q-fever, relapsing fever, tularemia, and tick paralysis are just a few of many ailments that can be transmitted by ticks. Species that most commonly feed on humans generally are found in areas of wild vegetation such as woods, high grass, parks, and along paths frequented by wild animals. Here they cling to bushes or tall weeds, ready to latch onto an unwary passer-by (contrary to popular belief, they don't drop onto victims from trees). People planning outdoor activities in tick-infested areas should take such precautions as applying tick repellent to exposed areas of skin, wearing socks and long trousers, and avoiding sitting on the ground or on logs. They should also be diligent about checking their bodies for the presence of ticks at least twice a day and immediately removing them, since most tick-borne diseases are transmitted only after the creature has been feeding for several hours.

Although the previous discussion is by no means a complete listing of the human health problems caused by various pest species, it should convey some realization of the need for pest control and an understanding of why many public health officials feel that abandoning chemical pesticides would entail the risk of increased mortality and morbidity rates due to vectorborne disease.

PEST CONTROL

Early Attempts at Pest Control

Human efforts to control pest outbreaks date back to the development of agriculture approximately 10,000 years ago, when relatively large expanses of a single crop and sizeable numbers of people living close together in unsanitary conditions favored an increase in pest populations that wouldn't have been possible among small, scattered societies living a nomadic, hunter-gatherer lifestyle. Early attempts to reduce pest damage included purely physical efforts—stomping, flailing, and burning—as well as the offering of prayers, sacrifices, and ritual dances to the local gods. A few effective measures were discovered even at such early dates, however. The Sumerians, in what now is Iraq, successfully employed sulfur compounds against insects and mites more than 5,000 years ago; over 3,000 years ago the Chinese were treating

seeds with insecticides derived from plant extracts, using wood ashes and chalk to ward off insect pests in the home, and applying mercury and arsenic compounds to their bodies to control lice. Among the Chinese is found the earliest example of using a pest's natural enemies to control it: by AD 300 the Chinese were introducing colonies of predatory ants into their citrus groves to control caterpillars and certain beetles.

During the peak of Greek civilization, records indicate that some of the wealthier citizens used mosquito nets and built high sleeping towers to evade mosquitoes. They also used oil sprays and sulfur bitumen ointments to deter insects. The Romans designed rat-proof granaries, but relied largely on superstitious practices such as nailing up crayfish in different parts of the garden to keep away caterpillars. In medieval Europe people increasingly relied on religious faith to protect them from pest depredations; as late as 1476, during an outbreak of cutworms in Switzerland, several of the offending insects were hauled into court, proclaimed guilty, excommunicated by the archbishop, and banished from the land!

Not until the 18th and 19th centuries did efforts at pest control make any meaningful progress. This was a time when European farming practices were becoming more productive and scientific, and help in combating agricultural pests was eagerly sought. Botanical insecticides such as pyrethrum, derris (rotenone), and nicotine were introduced at this time. Heightened interest in improved pest control methods was propelled during the mid-19th century by several of the worst agricultural disasters ever recorded—the potato blight in Ireland, England, and Belgium in 1848, caused by a fungal disease; the fungus leaf spot disease of coffee in Ceylon (now Sri Lanka), which completely wiped out coffee cultivation on the island; and the outbreak of both powdery mildew and an insect pest, grape phylloxera, which nearly destroyed the wine industry in Europe. Such problems led to the development of new chemical pesticides and ushered in a whole new era of pest control. Two of the first such compounds, Bordeaux mixture (copper sulfate and lime) and Paris Green (copper acetoarsenite), were originally employed as fungicides but were subsequently found to be effective insecticides as well. Paris Green became one of the most widely used insecticides in the late 19th century and Bordeaux mixture even today is the most widely used fungicide in the world. Early in the 1900s arsenic-containing compounds such as lead arsenate, highly toxic to both insects and humans, became the most widely sold insecticides in the United States and retained their leading position until the advent of DDT after World War II (Flint and VandenBosch, 1981).

In 1939, Paul Müller, a Swiss chemist working for the Geigy Corporation, discovered that the synthetic compound dichlorodiphenyltrichloroethane (referred to as DDT for obvious reasons!) was extremely effective in killing insects on contact and retained its lethal character for a long time after application. Müller had simply been looking for a better product to use against clothes moths, but the outbreak of war in Europe gave far wider significance to the new chemical. Military authorities, recognizing that extensive campaigns would be carried out in the tropics where insect-borne disease threatened high troop losses, made the search for better insecticides a top priority. DDT, highly lethal to every kind of insect yet harmless to humans when applied as a powder, was just what the military needed. Initially, production of DDT was exclusively for use in the armed forces where it was employed first as a louse powder and later for mosquito control. At the end of the war DDT was released for civilian use, both in agriculture and for public health purposes. Its use quickly spread worldwide, amidst high expectations of complete eradication of many diseases and greatly reduced crop losses due to insects. Müller was awarded the 1948 Nobel Prize in Physiology and Medicine in recognition of his contribution. The enthusiastic reception given to DDT encouraged chemical companies in their search for new and even more effective synthetic pesticides. By the mid-1950s at least 25 new products that would revolutionize insect control practices were put on the market, among the more important of which were chlordane, heptachlor, toxaphene, aldrin, endrin, dieldrin, and parathion (Perkins, 1982). The age of chemical warfare against pests had begun.

Types of Pesticides

Pesticides, substances that kill pests, are subdivided into groups according to target organism. For example, insecticides kill insects, herbicides kill weeds, rodenticides kill rats and mice, nematicides kill nematodes, and so forth. Within each of these groups there may be further subdivisions based on such characteristics as route of intake of the poison or physiological effect on the target organism. A brief survey of some of the most common groups of pesticides currently in use would include the following.

Insecticides

The largest number of pesticides is employed against a wide variety of insects and includes **stomach poisons** (taken into the body through the mouth; effective against insects with biting or chewing mouthparts like caterpillars); **contact poisons** (penetrate through the body wall); and **fumigants** (enter insect through its respiratory system).

The earliest insecticides were inorganic compounds, most containing heavy metals or arsenic, and acted as *stomach* poisons. This meant that they were effective only against pests such as beetles or caterpillars that ingested the insecticide while feeding on treated crops, or against insects like cockroaches that might ingest pesticidal dusts while grooming themselves. Many of these products were quite toxic to humans as well, posing serious health hazards to the applicator and to farm workers; under certain environmental conditions they could also damage crop foliage, and they were relatively expensive. For all these reasons, when the new synthetic organic insecticides

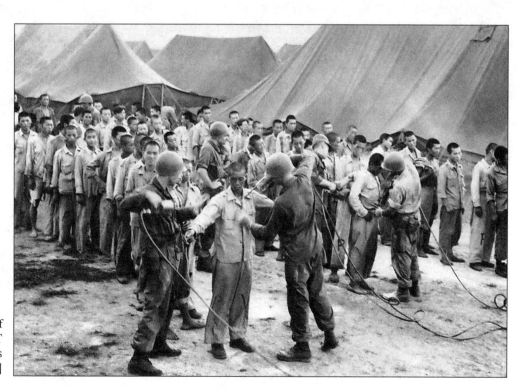

North Korean prisoners of war are sprayed with DDT powder by American soldiers circa 1950. [*AP Photo*]

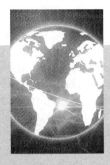

. . . . *8-2* . . . .

Battling Malaria

Although HIV/AIDS garners more media attention these days, malaria continues to take a more fearsome toll in terms of morbidity and mortality. Disease statistics are truly alarming. The CDC estimates that as many as 500 million new cases of malaria are contracted each year, with approximately one million people, mostly children, dying of the disease. While the number of countries affected by malaria is substantially less than it was prior to the mid-1900s (in the past large areas of southern and southeastern Europe were malarious, as was the Mississippi River Valley and all of the southeastern U.S.), 40% of the world's people today live in regions where the threat of malaria is ever-present. On the Indian subcontinent, in Southeast Asia, and in tropical South America the incidence of malaria has been rising rapidly since the 1980s, when government-sponsored mosquito abatement efforts were curtailed. It is in Africa, however, where the disease is taking its heaviest toll—today fully 90% of all malaria victims live in sub-Saharan Africa. Malaria is now the cause for 10% of hospital admissions and 20–30% of all doctors' visits in Africa. Public health workers there report that, thanks to climate change, malaria outbreaks are now occurring even in previously malaria-free regions, such as the highlands of Kenya, where the elevation and cooler climate once rendered the area inhospitable to disease-carrying mosquitoes.

That one of humanity's most ancient plagues should resurge in the early 21st century seems tragically ironic, considering the high hopes that greeted the Global Malaria Eradication Program launched by the newly created World Health Organization in 1955. With a powerful new weapon—DDT—and more than 60 nations providing financial support for establishing factories to produce the insecticide in poor countries, the worldwide assault against mosquitoes was initiated amid optimistic declarations that malaria would soon be banished forever. From the beginning, realists conceded that killing every last mosquito was impossible. However, it was believed that if insect populations could be reduced enough to limit the frequency of bites (and thereby transmission of the malarial parasite), within a few years the parasite would die out among the human population. After that, so it was reasoned, a resurgence in mosquito numbers would represent nothing more than an irritation, since the insects would no longer harbor the malaria pathogen. For several years the strategy seemed to be working brilliantly. By 1961 the incidence of malaria had plummeted in 37 countries; in some areas—notably Taiwan, Jamaica, and Sardinia—the disease was totally eliminated and they remain malaria-free to this day. However, by 1969 problems with insecticide resistance among some mosquito populations and growing concerns about health and environmental side effects of DDT use (*Silent Spring* had become a best-seller just a few years earlier!) led the WHO to abandon its campaign.

Over the next several decades, despite growing evidence that the disease was making a comeback, malaria control remained relatively low on the list of international public health priorities. Policy makers, distracted by new concerns like HIV/AIDS, lost interest in malaria and drastically cut funding for control efforts and basic research. By the late 1990s, however, the re-emergence of malaria as a major cause of death and disease in poor countries, and its corresponding deleterious impact on efforts to spur development and reduce poverty there, prompted a renewed commitment by international donors to battle the disease. Since 2000, groups such as the Global Fund for AIDS, Tuberculosis, and Malaria (referred to simply as The Global Fund), the President's Malaria Initiative (an effort launched by former President George W. Bush and managed through USAID), the World Bank Booster Program for Malaria, the Bill & Melinda Gates Foundation, and the U.K.-based Department for International Development are now cumulatively spending approximately $1 billion annually on malaria control efforts—up from just a few tens of millions a decade ago.

Among the various options for easing human suffering caused by malaria, the most obvious solution— and one long-sought by medical researchers—is a malaria vaccine. Unfortunately, for a variety of reasons, this appears to be a distant dream, though the decoding of the parasite's genome several years ago may offer valuable information to assist in this effort. In the meantime, efforts to combat the disease are focused on three main tools: insecticide-treated bednets, indoor residual spraying with insecticides, and anti-malarial drug therapies.

Numerous field trials and experience in countries like Uganda, Tanzania, and Zanzibar have repeatedly shown that bednets treated with pyrethroid insecticides, when used properly and consistently, can sharply reduce childhood deaths from malaria. Improvements in bednet technology have yielded models that incorporate insecticide into the net fiber itself, as opposed to older versions that had to be retreated every 3 months, making their use more convenient and less expensive over the long term. Because many families living in poor countries can't afford even the relatively modest cost of bednets, a number of charitable service organizations in developed countries, such as Rotary International, have made the provision of treated bednets to such families an integral part of their outreach program.

A second key component of current malaria eradication efforts is the resumption of DDT use on the interior walls of homes and the back side of furniture, leaving a residual that can kill adult mosquitoes alighting on such surfaces for a period of several months after application. Although renewed use of DDT has generated a fair degree of controversy due to its adverse environmental impact (proper use of DDT has resulted in few, if any, confirmed human health problems), the World Health Organization in 2006 forcefully endorsed wider use of the chlorinated hydrocarbon insecticide across Africa as a valuable weapon for fighting a disease that kills 800,000 African children each year, 2000 every day.

The third vital component of the war against malaria is effective drug therapy. Many experts attribute the post-1960s gradual comeback of malaria not only to termination of DDT use but also to the parasite's growing resistance to chloroquine, for decades the medicine of choice for malaria sufferers. Inexpensive, fast-acting, safe, and available over-the-counter, chloroquine has been so overused that it is now considered virtually useless in most parts of the world, including sub-Saharan Africa (though it is still widely used there, simply because it's the only drug many people can afford). By the 1990s, another drug, sulfadoxine/pyrimethamine, was introduced as a replacement for chloroquine, but within a few years the parasite developed resistance to it as well.

Malaria treatment is now focused exclusively on a combination drug containing artemisinin, a wormwood derivative from China, along with another drug, lumefantrine, that lingers longer in the blood, killing parasites that may have evaded artemisinin and thus helping to prevent drug resistance (Gelband, 2008). These new artemisinin-based combination therapies (ACTs) are now the basis for malaria treatment worldwide; one ACT, marketed by Novartis under the trade name Coartem, recently received FDA approval, making it available to military personnel and tourists traveling to areas where malaria is endemic (Coartem is intended for use only after a patient develops malaria, not as a preventive). Since ACTs have been hailed in recent years as humanity's greatest hope for eradicating malaria, reports from the Thai-Cambodian border area in 2008 of emerging parasite tolerance to the drug provoked dismay among health workers and researchers, one of whom termed the development "a global disaster." With no other malaria drugs to fall back on, and none in the pipeline, widespread resistance to ACTs could cause malaria cases to soar and dash all hopes of eradicating the disease. To date, the resistance problem is restricted to one limited geographic area; to prevent it from spreading further, malaria-control agencies in both Thailand and Cambodia are mounting a vigorous effort to wipe out malaria from the region where resistant parasites were found and to greatly reduce disease transmission in a large surrounding area. To achieve these objectives they are pursuing all the strategies described above, as well as mounting intensive public education efforts. The world can only hope they will be successful and that ACTs remain an effecting and enduring weapon in the ongoing battle against malaria (Enserink, 2008).

became commercially available soon after World War II, they were enthusiastically welcomed by pesticide users.

All of the new compounds—the **chlorinated hydrocarbons**, **organophosphates**, **carbamates**, and **pyrethroids**—acted as *contact* poisons, making them (unlike the inorganic insecticides) **broad-spectrum** poisons capable of killing virtually any insect they touched. These new weapons meant that a farmer no longer needed a shelf full of various chemicals to combat the pests in his fields—one insecticide would kill them all. The chlorinated hydrocarbons have an additional feature that initially seemed like a major plus—once applied, they are **persistent** in the environment, leaving a residue that breaks down very slowly, providing protection for a long period after the initial application. For the farmer, persistence meant that he didn't need to worry about re-treating his fields every time it rained—the DDT or aldrin or heptachlor would still be there. Chlordane, a member of this group that for many years was the structural pest control industry's termiticide of choice, was so persistent that, once applied around the perimeter of a home, it provided up to 40 years of protection from these wood-destroying insects.

Unfortunately, persistence was found to have a serious down-side as well; because the long-lasting residues are not water-soluble, they accumulate in fatty tissues when taken up by living organisms and may remain in the body indefinitely, becoming increasingly concentrated over time. For this reason, and because of human health concerns associated with this group of pesticides, most of the chlorinated hydrocarbons have been banned in the United States and many other countries. An international treaty ratified in 2004 (the Stockholm Convention on Persistent Organic Pollutants) obligates signatory nations to discontinue the production and use of nine chlorinated hydrocarbon insecticides included on the "Dirty Dozen" list of proscribed **Persistent Organic Pollutants ("POPs")**. A group of new chemicals to be added to the Convention was agreed upon at a conference in 2008 and took effect in August 2010.

Organophosphate and carbamate insecticides, unlike DDT and its kin, are not persistent in the environment, usually breaking down two weeks or less after application. However, some of these products are acutely toxic to humans and must be used with great care (those available to the general public, such as malathion and carbaryl have relatively low human toxicity and shouldn't cause problems when used according to label directions). These chemicals now dominate the insecticide market, along with the increasingly popular pyrethroids, synthetic chemical analogs of pyrethrum, a natural insecticide derived from chrysanthemum flowers. Providing quick knockdown of insects, the pyrethroids are probably the best choice for home or garden use because of their very low toxicity to humans and domestic animals. For this reason, they are among the few insecticides that can be safely used indoors, even in the kitchen. While these products are generally somewhat more expensive than other insecticides, they can be used effectively at much lower rates of application. If it is necessary to use an insecticidal dust, shampoo, or flea collar on young puppies or kittens, a product containing one of the pyrethroids is recommended.

Natural pyrethrum (*Pyrocide*) is still available, as is rotenone (*ChemFish*), a poison derived from a tropical legume. **Neem**, an extract of a South Asian tree of the same name, is another botanical insecticide registered for use on ornamental plants and vegetables. Valued in India since ancient times for both insecticidal and medicinal properties, neem seeds and leaves contain nine or more different liminoid compounds that exhibit potent repellent and pesticidal properties effective against at least 200 different species of insects. Like the other botanicals, neem is quite safe for humans—in fact, for centuries South Asians have used neem extensively for dental hygiene and a variety of other medical purposes (National Research Council, 1992).

Herbicides

Weeds in a field may not appear as threatening as hordes of insects, yet the economic losses caused by these unwanted species can be very high. Weeds compete with crop plants for vital mineral nutrients and water, thus reducing crop yields; they make harvesting more difficult and some species, when consumed, poison livestock.

Wide-scale application of chemicals for weed control is a relatively new phenomenon. Although a few inorganic compounds such as iron sulfate and sodium arsenite were used against broadleaf weeds as long ago as 1896, hand-weeding, mechanical cultivation, tillage, crop rotation, and the use of weed-free seeds were the most common methods of reducing crop losses due to weed infestations. After World War II, the first synthetic herbicide (2,4–D) was introduced and has been followed by a succession of more than a hundred different chemical weed killers. Today herbicide use has considerably surpassed insecticide use and is still increasing, while the use of insecticides has leveled off or declined.

Although herbicides are used most extensively for agricultural purposes, they also are used by public health workers to control weeds that harbor insects and rodents, and to eradicate nuisance plants such as ragweed or poison ivy.

Herbicides may be classified in various ways, including how and when they are applied or by their mode of action. The first of these categories include **preplanting** herbicides—products applied to the soil before a crop is planted; **pre-emergents**—herbicides applied to the soil shortly before weeds are expected to germinate; and **post-emergents**—those applied to the soil or directly onto the foliage of the weeds after the crop and/or the weeds have sprouted. A familiar example of a pre-emergent herbicide is Preen® (trifluralin), widely used by home gardeners to prevent weeds from germinating in their flowerbeds. Grouped by mode of action, herbicides can be categorized as **selective**—those that kill only certain types of plants (usually broad-leafed dicotyledonous species, a group to which many of the common weeds belong); **contact**—poisons that kill any actively growing plant part with which they come into contact; and **translocated**—herbicides that are absorbed from the soil via the roots or through the foliage into the plant's vascular system, through which they are carried to all parts of the plant. The numerous 2,4–D-containing products used for decades to kill dandelions and other turfgrass weeds while leaving the lawn undamaged are prime examples of selective herbicides (they also could be classified as post-emergents, since they are sprayed directly on the growing weeds). In recent years, sales of the contact herbicide glyphosate (Roundup®) have soared, due to its usefulness in "burning down" weeds prior to planting in no-till fields and for clearing vegetation from roadsides, fence-rows, cracks in the sidewalk, or any place where complete plant removal is desired. The recent proliferation of "Roundup Ready" crops has created a steadily expanding agricultural market for this contact herbicide.

Although most herbicides are thought to be only slightly toxic to humans, in recent years there have been several studies suggesting that herbicide exposure can cause genetic mutations, cancer, and birth defects. Farm workers occasionally blame health problems such as weight loss, nausea, vomiting, and loss of appetite to contact with herbicides. In 1986 researchers reported that Kansas farmers who used 2,4–D for more than 20 days per year had a six times greater risk of non-Hodgkin's lymphoma than did a control group with no exposure to herbicides (Blair et al., 1987). In 1991 the *Journal of the National Cancer Institute* reported that dogs, too, are at risk from 2,4–D. If their owners apply the weed killer four times or more each summer, canines are twice as likely to develop malignant lymphoma as are dogs whose owners abstain from herbicide use. More recently, several studies have reported an association between herbicide exposure and the development of persistent asthma among infants under one year of age (Salam et al., 2004) and between mixing and applying herbicides and infertility in women (Greenlee, Arbuckle, and Chou, 2003). Pregnant women who use herbicides during their first trimester triple their risk of bearing a child with a specific type of severe congenital heart defect (Loffredo et al., 2001). Countering these assertions, in June 2004 the EPA released a draft health and environmental risk assessment that concluded 2,4-D does not present a risk to human health nor is there evidence that would implicate the herbicide as a cause of cancer.

During the late 1970s and early 1980s a great deal of public controversy surrounded the use of 2,4,5–T and silvex, selective herbicides that contained traces of dioxin formed as an unavoidable contaminant during the manufacturing process. Notorious as a component of **Agent Orange**, the chemical defoliant used by U.S. military forces during the Vietnam War, 2,4,5–T (actually, the dioxin contaminating 2,4,5–T) was blamed for a wide range of physical and emotional problems among South Vietnamese living in the target areas, as well as among American servicemen who had come into contact with the herbicide during their tour of duty. Although independent studies of veterans' complaints have never been able to confirm an association between the alleged health effects and Agent Orange exposure, production of 2,4,5–T and silvex was terminated in the early 1980s, and in 1984 seven chemical companies agreed to an out-of-court settlement for $180 million with a veterans' group claiming health damage. Rapid growth in the commercial lawn-care industry has provoked a vociferous response in many communities by antipesticide activists who warn of the dangers posed to people, pets, and wildlife by toxic lawn chemicals ("Dandelions won't kill you—pesticides do!"). The increasingly common use by lawn-care firms of post-application warning signs, accompanied by recommended safety precautions, has been a positive, if limited, industry response to citizen concerns.

Rodenticides

Although good sanitation and rat-proofing of buildings and food storage facilities provide the only effective long-term control of domestic rodents, use of poisons is an important additional tool in keeping rat populations low. Because some rodenticides used in public health work are extremely toxic to humans as well as to rodents, their use in the United States is restricted to certified applicators. The hazard these chemicals pose to humans is evident in news accounts from China, where rat poison has become the murder weapon of choice in a land where private ownership of guns is illegal; readily available rodenticides also are blamed for a significant percentage of suicides in that country. According to the World Health Organization, intentional or accidental poisoning ranks among the top 10 causes of death among young Chinese (Yardley, 2003).

General-use rodenticides, chemicals that should not present a serious hazard either to the user or to the environment when used in accordance with instructions, can be purchased by the public. Even these may not be entirely safe, however; the same study that indicated a tripling of risk for congenital heart defects among children born to women using herbicides during their first trimester of pregnancy showed a quadrupling of risk for that same abnormality for women using rodenticides (Loffredo et al., 2001).

The rodenticides most commonly recommended for use by householders act as anticoagulants—compounds that, when consumed over a period of several days, cause internal hemorrhaging, causing the rodents to bleed to death painlessly. These poisons provide excellent control of both rats and mice, although up to two weeks may be required to get an effective kill.

ENVIRONMENTAL IMPACT OF PESTICIDE USE

In the early 1950s, bird-watchers in both the United States and Western Europe were confronted with a baffling mystery—a sudden, inexplicable decline in the populations of bald eagles, pelicans, and peregrine falcons appeared to threaten the very survival of these well-loved species. Investigations into the unanticipated population "crash" ultimately revealed that the villain was not a disease, nor overkilling, nor a scarcity of food, but rather was the presence of surprisingly high concentrations of the new insecticide DDT in the tissues of these birds. Although DDT did not appear to have a direct lethal effect on the adult birds, it interfered with their ability to metabolize calcium, thereby resulting in the production of eggs with shells so thin they broke when the nesting parents sat on them. Thus, pesticide-induced reproductive failure—the inability of the birds to produce viable offspring—was ultimately shown to be the factor responsible for the population decline.

This episode represented one of the first glimmerings of awareness on the part of the scientific community that the advent of the new wonder chemicals was not an unmitigated blessing. The public at large, however, remained largely unaware and unconcerned about such matters until the publication in 1962 of Rachel Carson's literary bombshell, *Silent Spring*. This best-seller represented a scathing indictment of pesticide misuse and for the first time made the average American aware of the havoc such chemicals could wreak on the environment and on human well-being. In retrospect, the publication of *Silent Spring* made "ecology" a household word and was probably the most important single event in launching the environmental movement of the 1970s. Carson and many subsequent researchers clearly demonstrated that extensive use and near-total reliance on chemicals for pest control have been accompanied by unanticipated and undesired side effects, many of which have raised problems serious enough to threaten the continued usefulness of these products.

Development of Resistance

Those who dreamed that the new pesticides might completely eradicate certain insect or other pest species were obviously ignorant of the principles that govern how the forces of natural selection act upon chance variations occurring within any population—particularly insect populations, whose long evolutionary history demonstrates the remarkable ability of these organisms to evolve and adapt rapidly to changing environmental conditions. The widespread, frequent, and intensive application of chemicals such as DDT in the post-war years was initially successful in drastically reducing pest populations, but eventually was responsible for providing the selective forces that would produce new strains of "super bugs," rendering the original poisons worthless.

The mechanism by which this occurs can be visualized by considering a hypothetical population of, say, boll

weevils ravaging a field of cotton. Aerial insecticide spraying may kill perhaps 99% of the weevils, but a few will survive, either by chance (perhaps an overhanging leaf shielded them from the spray) or because something in the genetic make-up of a particular individual somehow made it less vulnerable to the poison. Such a hereditary trait might be the production of a particular enzyme capable of detoxifying the pesticide, a less permeable type of epidermis which prevented penetration of the contact poison, a behavioral characteristic that allowed the individual to avoid fatal exposure, or some other factor of this nature. In a pesticide-free environment (the type of situation prevailing prior to the introduction of DDT) such a genetic trait would confer no special advantage to the individual carrying it, so the frequency of such a gene within that population would remain low. Once DDT came into widespread use, however, the boll weevils' environment was radically altered and those few individuals possessing the gene for immunity suddenly enjoyed a tremendous selective advantage. As the accompanying diagram (figure 8-1) indicates, successive sprayings largely eliminated boll weevils susceptible to the insecticide, but promoted the build-up of a population in which the vast majority carried the gene (or genes) conferring resistance. Those seeking to control pest outbreaks were thus forced to turn to newer and more powerful chemicals, only to witness the same cycle of events.

Since pesticide resistance had appeared as a localized problem even with the old-fashioned insecticides, it shouldn't have come as a total surprise when insects resistant to DDT began to appear in the late 1940s and early 1950s. Among the first species to display immunity were certain populations of houseflies and mosquitoes which, as early as 1946, could no longer be controlled with DDT. In 1951, during the Korean War, military officials were alarmed to discover that human body lice, vectors of typhus, had become resistant to DDT. Among agricultural pests, spider mites, cabbage loopers, codling moths, and tomato hornworms developed resistance to several of the common insecticides; by the mid-1950s when the boll weevil became resistant to many of the chlorinated hydrocarbons, the need for alternative control methods became obvious (Perkins, 1982).

At present, more than 500 species of insects and mites are resistant to common pesticides—more than double the number that were resistant just a few decades ago. Largely due to problems of pesticide resistance, crop losses due to insects are nearly twice as high now as they were when DDT was first brought onto the market, in spite of a quantum increase in pesticidal applications by farmers over the past half century. In the public health field, as in agriculture, growing pesticide resistance is causing serious concern. Worldwide, incidence of malaria is now on a sharp upswing as approximately 64 species of mosquitoes have become resistant to insecticides, according to WHO officials. Closer to home, bedbug populations are showing an alarming increase in resistance to pyrethroid insecticides, among the few bug-killers safe for use in the home ("Creatures of the Night," 2009).

Problems of pesticide resistance are not restricted to species of arthropods. Some rat populations, particularly those in cities with long-established rodent control programs, no longer respond to warfarin, the most extensively used rodenticide in the world. More than 150 species of plant pathogens (fungi and bacteria) are now resistant to at least one pesticide, as are 286 weed biotypes (GAO, 2001; WSSA, 2004). Although herbicide resistance is a relatively recent development and has received

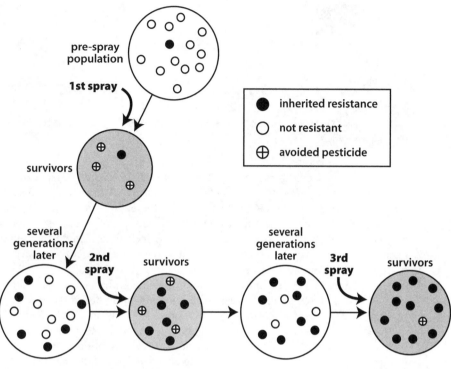

Figure 8-1   Pesticide Resistance Cycle

considerably less attention among agricultural experts than has insecticide resistance, weed scientists warn that the phenomenon is already widespread. In Australia, wheat growers by the early 1980s were reporting the emergence of new weed biotypes resistant to every selective herbicide that can be used on wheat. More ominous in recent years has been the emergence of weed resistance to glyphosate (*Roundup®*), the world's best-selling herbicide. Since the late 1990s, glyphosate-resistant weed populations have been reported from over a dozen U.S. states as well as several South American countries, Malaysia, Spain, and South Africa. This news is particularly worrisome to farmers because new commercial varieties of wheat, cotton, potatoes, sugar beets, canola, and soybeans have now been genetically engineered to survive direct field applications of glyphosate intended for weed control. Although glyphosate-resistant weed species are still quite limited in number and in their geographic distribution, many agricultural researchers are convinced that in areas where glyphosate is used intensively, it is inevitable that an increasing number of weeds will develop resistance to the herbicide. To reduce the rate at which this is happening, they advise against using glyphosate on the same acres every year, instead recommending an annual rotation of both crops and herbicides. At the same time, they point out that fears of the emergence of "superweeds" resulting from excessive glyphosate use are exaggerated, since effective alternative herbicides are available for most weed species (Hartzler and Owen, 2003).

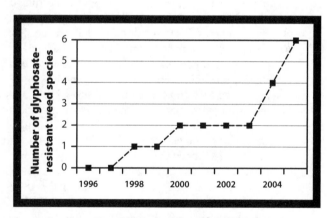

Source: Boerboom, C., and M. Owen, "Facts About Glyphosate Resistant Weeds." Accessed Sept. 2010 from www.ces.purdue.edu/extmedia/gwc/gwc-1.pdf

Figure 8-2   Increase in Glyphosate-Resistant Weed Species in the United States

Killing of Nontarget Species

Only a small percentage of insect species are considered pests, yet the most widely used synthetic insecticides are broad-spectrum poisons, killing both friend and foe alike. The destruction of many beneficial predator insect species as well as the target pest has led to two related types of problems. The first of these, referred to as **target**

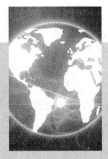

· · · · · · · *8-3* · · · · · · ·

Dengue Fever Spreads as the World Warms Up

"Climate change is the biggest global health threat of the 21st century"—so proclaims an alarming report published in May 2009 by a leading British medical journal, *The Lancet* (Costello et al., 2009). Citing numerous factors contributing to the devastating human health impacts of global warming, the authors of the study place the spread and increased transmission rate of several vectorborne diseases near the top of the list. Among the insect-transmitted ailments we're likely to hear more about in future decades as global temperatures rise is dengue (pronounced DEN-gay) fever, once a menace only in the tropics but now on the move into more temperate climes.

Sometimes called "breakbone fever" because of the excruciating joint pains experienced by some victims, dengue fever is a viral disease transmitted by mosquitoes. Its principle vector is *Aedes aegypti*, the same species that carries yellow fever, but it can also be transmitted by *Aedes albopictus*, the Asian tiger mosquito—a species accidentally introduced into the United States in 1985 and now well-established in many parts of the country. Disease symptoms generally develop within 3–14 days after being bitten by an infected mosquito and, in acute cases, typically include a high fever, chills, severe headache and eye pain, a rash, nausea, vomiting, and the characteristic joint and muscle pains mentioned above. Victims seldom die of dengue fever, but the disease can be extremely painful and disabling. In a small percentage of victims—about 1%—dengue fever may develop into dengue hemorrhagic fever (DHF), a potentially fatal illness that first manifests itself as fever lasting up to a week, with subsequent gastrointestinal bleeding. If not treated promptly, DHF may progress to sometimes lethal dengue shock syndrome (DSS). Interestingly, 50–80% of those infected with the dengue virus remain completely asymptomatic—not even aware they are carrying the disease—while others have relatively mild cases, experiencing little more than fever, fatigue, and general malaise (Larsen, 2009). For this reason, dengue is often difficult to diagnose and impossible to quarantine, and since symptoms don't develop until several days after the victim has become infectious, precautions to prevent further transmission of the disease may come too late.

The number of people infected with dengue fever has increased 30-fold over the past half century, due in part to the phase-out of DDT for mosquito control but also because the globalization of trade and travel has facilitated the spread of mosquito vectors and virus-infected humans from one part of the world to another, thereby increasing the risk of disease outbreaks. It's estimated that dengue now sickens 50–100 million people in more than 100 countries each year, resulting in 500,000 hospitalizations and 22,000 deaths. Large outbreaks of dengue were reported in 2007 in Thailand, Malaysia, India, Brazil, Mexico, Honduras, Costa Rica, and several other Latin American nations. Tropical countries account for the vast majority of victims at present, but that could change in the future as climate change accelerates. Researchers estimate that by 2080, 6 billion people around the world will be at risk of contracting dengue fever as a consequence of global warming, compared with 3.5 billion if the climate were to remain as it is today (Costello et al., 2009).

Epidemic outbreaks of dengue in the United States thus far have been limited to the U.S.-Mexico border and Hawaii, though isolated cases of dengue have been reported from nearly every state due to infected tourists returning home from abroad. From 1995–2005, close to 10,000 reports of "imported" and locally transmitted dengue cases, including those in the Texas/Mexico border region, were received by the CDC. Those numbers could rise sharply in the years ahead, however, since one or both of the mosquito species that carry the dengue virus are now well-established in at least 28 states and the District of Columbia. The entire southern United States, as well as a good portion of the central Midwest and mid-Atlantic region, now harbors *A. aegypti* and *A. albopictus* populations; it's estimated that close to 174 million Americans currently live in counties where dengue could become endemic—and the threat continues to spread northward as temperatures rise.

How could the warmer, wetter conditions resulting from climate change affect the range and incidence of dengue? Several interacting factors are involved:

- Warmer winters create conditions favorable to mosquito vectors, permitting them to expand their range; already the Asian tiger mosquito can be found as far north as Chicago and it continues to spread rapidly. The yellow fever mosquito, now well-entrenched in 16 southern states, is likely to find other regions equally congenial as temperatures rise.

- The mosquito goes through its life cycle more rapidly when the weather is warm; higher temperatures thus mean larger mosquito populations during the breeding season.

- The dengue virus replicates and becomes infective faster inside the mosquito when temperatures are high, thus increasing the number of days the mosquito can transmit pathogens during its 3–4 week lifespan.

- Female mosquitoes bite more often when conditions are hotter.

- Mosquito adults and eggs have better survival rates when humidity levels are high.

Given these realities, what can public health authorities—and health-conscious individuals—do to meet the future challenge posed by dengue fever? Since at present there is no vaccine, nor any medicine to cure dengue, the focus of control efforts is mosquito abatement. Accomplishing this through insecticidal spraying of adult mosquitoes is *not* recommended, however, in part because it's generally ineffective (and costly!) over the long-term due to the development of resistance among targeted mosquito populations, but also because the primary vector, *A. aegypti*, typically lives and breeds inside homes in warm, dark, enclosed spaces—inappropriate places for applying pesticides. The preferred approach is to implement community-wide programs to eradicate mosquito breeding sites, emptying or removing stagnant water containers, and disposing of waste tires (a favorite breeding place for *A. albopictus*).

Also needed are government initiatives to improve housing conditions and municipal services in poor neighborhoods: dengue is sometimes referred to as a "disease of poverty" since the majority of locally acquired dengue cases in the U.S. and elsewhere have thus far been in areas where homes lack intact window and door screens, trash is left uncollected and catching water, and where the lack of dependable piped water causes residents to collect and store water in uncovered containers. A survey taken in Brownsville, Texas, after a large dengue outbreak there in 2005 found that less than two-thirds of homes had window and door screens; numerous used tires and water buckets strewn about the area contained mosquito larvae; and less than a quarter of the citizens said they regularly used mosquito repellent.

These results indicate that another important component of dengue prevention efforts is public education, not only for the residents most at risk, but for municipal officials and medical personnel as well. Clinicians and health departments need information on how to recognize and treat a disease they may not have encountered in the past. The need for a nation-wide surveillance system to collect and test blood samples from suspected dengue cases is also widely acknowledged; in this context, the fact that CDC in 2009 added dengue to its list of nationally notifiable infectious diseases was welcome news. Tourists and business travelers setting out for tropical destinations should consult the CDC or WHO Web sites for information on whether the areas they plan to visit are experiencing dengue outbreaks. If so, they should be diligent about applying an insect repellent containing 20–30% DEET to exposed skin areas and to book rooms only in well-screened or air-conditioned hotels. And if they experience any of the tell-tale symptoms of dengue after returning home, they should immediately inform their local physician and health department of the situation—and make sure no hungry mosquito transmits their infected blood to an unwary neighbor!

The final element in an effort to restrict dengue fever's expanding range is to halt further climate change. Through myriad individual lifestyle choices and collective lobbying of elected representatives to enact mandatory reductions in greenhouse gas emissions, we all have a role to play in restricting the spread of vectorborne tropical diseases that are otherwise likely to characterize our warming world (Knowlton, Solomon, and Rotkin-Ellman, 2009; Larsen, 2009).

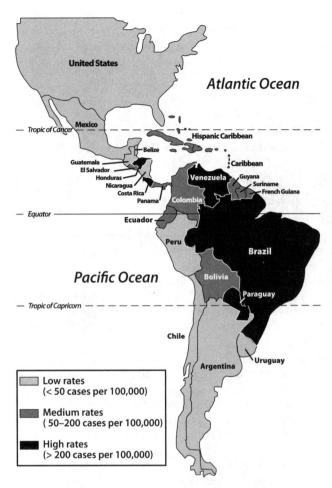

Source: Redrawn from Knowlton, K., G. Solomon, and M. Rotkin-Ellman, *Fever Pitch: Mosquito-borne Dengue Fever Threat Spreading in the Americas,* NRDC Issue Paper, July 2009. Used with permission of the Natural Resources Defense Council (NRDC).

Figure 8-3   Incidence of Dengue in the Americas, 2007

pest resurgence, occurs when an insecticide application that initially resulted in a drastic reduction in the pest population is quickly followed by a sudden increase in pest numbers to a level higher than that which existed prior to the spraying. This occurs because the natural enemies of the pest, which formerly kept its numbers under control, were also heavily decimated by the spraying. Since any predators that survived the pesticide would subsequently starve or migrate, the pests would then confront ideal conditions—no natural enemies and an abundance of their favorite food (i.e., the crop that had been sprayed). As a result, their populations can increase in size very rapidly, above and beyond the original level.

A second situation, known as **secondary pest outbreak**, involves the rise to prominence of certain plant-eating species which, prior to the spraying, were unimportant as pests because natural enemies kept their popu-

lations below the level at which they could cause significant economic damage. After pesticides eliminated most of their predators, such insects suddenly experience a population explosion and become major pests in their own right. In 1995 Texas cotton growers in the lower Rio Grande Valley experienced a devastating outbreak of several secondary pests after some 200,000 acres were targeted for aerial spraying with malathion to control boll weevils. Predictably, the spraying decimated beneficial insects along with the target pest, resulting in an unanticipated outbreak of cotton aphids that spread rapidly through the fields. Shortly afterwards, a beet armyworm infestation mushroomed as well, causing severe losses to the cotton crop. The armyworms were followed by whiteflies, which further reduced yields. In spite of as many as 25 insecticidal sprayings on some farms, many growers lost their entire crop and cotton yields in the area that year plunged 80% (Meister, 1996).

Beneficial insects are not the only nontarget species adversely affected by broad-spectrum poisons. Many kinds of birds, small mammals, fish, and other aquatic organisms are extremely sensitive to chemical pesticides and die immediately after coming into contact with such substances. Indeed, the numerous examples of mass die-offs of robins and other songbirds, squirrels, house cats, salmon, and many other well-loved species vividly documented by Rachel Carson provided the emotional images that explain *Silent Spring*'s profound impact on the national psyche. No one could read passages such as the following and remain unmoved:

> It was a spring without voices. On the mornings that had once throbbed with the dawn chorus of robins, catbirds, doves . . . there was now no sound; only silence lay over the fields and woods and marsh. (Carson, 1962)

Environmental Contamination

Liberal use of pesticides on a worldwide basis has resulted in a more thorough contamination of the biosphere than anyone in 1945 would have dreamed possible. Today pesticide residues, especially those of the chlorinated hydrocarbons, are found virtually everywhere in the tissues of creatures as diverse as Antarctic penguins, fish in deep ocean trenches, decomposer bacteria, and every human being. Since no one deliberately sprayed pesticides in Antarctica or in the middle of the Pacific, how could this have happened? Because the chlorinated hydrocarbons are persistent pesticides (meaning that they break down very slowly), they can circulate through the ecosystem for a long time, often traveling long distances from their point of origin. When such chemicals are aerially sprayed on forest, field, or pastureland, less than 10% of the pesticide actually hits the target; the remainder is carried off by air currents and is subsequently deposited miles away where it will eventually be washed into waterways or taken up by living organisms in the food they eat. Even when carefully applied according to label directions, pesticides can vaporize into the air, be washed off the land into lakes and streams during heavy rains, or percolate downward through the soil. The results of this unintended contamination include the following.

Indirect Killing via Depletion of Food or Habitat

When pesticides are targeted against insects, plants, or rodents that serve as a major food source for another group of organisms, the long-term effect can be just as devastating as direct poisoning would be. In New Jersey, populations of certain forest bird species declined by 45–55% after carbaryl spraying for gypsy moth control deprived the birds of their supper. Herbicide use similarly reduces both forage and habitat for many plant-eating insects and can have a "domino effect" when plummeting populations of arthropods adversely impact the food supply of insectivorous birds. On the high plains of Wyoming, a population of native sparrows crashed after herbicidal spraying of sagebrush to enlarge pasturelands for grazing. Unfortunately for the sparrows, the sagebrush supplied essential cover and nesting sites without which the birds couldn't survive (Parker, 1994).

Groundwater Contamination

The discovery in 1979 that 96 wells on Long Island were contaminated with a highly toxic carbamate insecticide, aldicarb, came as unwelcome news to a public that assumed that however polluted our rivers and lakes might be, groundwater supplies were safe from chemical contamination. Any hopes that the New York situation might be an isolated aberration were shattered by the revelation that 3,000 miles to the west, more than 2,000 wells in the fertile San Joaquin Valley were tainted with the nematicide DBCP, a chlorinated hydrocarbon that had earlier made headlines for causing sterility among male pesticide workers exposed to the chemical. In the late 1980s the EPA launched a nationwide survey to determine the extent of pesticide contamination of groundwater supplies. In 1990 the agency released a report showing that 14% of all public and private drinking water wells sampled had measurable levels of at least one pesticide. Two years later the agency reported new results indicating that nearly one-third of rural wells sampled showed unsafe levels of pesticide contamination, with aldicarb and the herbicides atrazine (*Aatrex®*) and alachlor (*Lasso®*), both suspected human carcinogens, posing the most widespread problems. Agency surveyors reported finding nearly 100 different pesticides in groundwater supplies and concluded that heavy agricul-

tural pesticide use was the main cause of the problem ("EPA Study," 1992; Curtis, Profeta, and Mott, 1993).

Additional studies carried out in the late 1990s found pesticide residues in over half the samples of well water taken at over 1,000 locations, both rural and urban. While numerous different chemicals were detected, their concentrations in most cases were quite low. Of those for which EPA has established drinking water standards, only one pesticide at one of the many locations sampled exceeded the allowable level. The fact that pesticides were detected almost as often in urban wells as in those from rural areas is an indication that pesticide contamination of groundwater is not a problem confined to agricultural areas. Although such studies show that the problem is widespread, the fact that concentrations are relatively low makes assessment of the potential human health threat problematic (NRC, 2000).

Due to concerns over groundwater contamination, several European countries have banned the use of atrazine—one of the world's most popular herbicides—and in 2003 the EU withdrew regulatory approval for this chemical. That same year, the Environmental Protection Agency made the opposite decision, re-approving registration of atrazine in the United States despite the opposition of environmentalists (but to the relief of farmers worried about losing an effective and relatively cheap herbicide). In the developing nations, where the rate of pesticide use is increasing even faster than in the industrialized world, virtually no groundwater monitoring is being carried out at present; it is quite likely that current agricultural activities may be seriously degrading underground water supplies over vast areas without anyone recognizing the potential threat to future generations (Nash, 1993).

Indirect Contamination via Food Chains

Since the chlorinated hydrocarbons are not water-soluble, they are not excreted from the body when ingested but instead are stored in fatty tissues such as liver, kidneys, and fat around the intestines. Toxic substances present in minute amounts in the general environment can thus become quite concentrated as they move along a food chain, sometimes reaching lethal doses in organisms at the highest trophic levels. This process, known as **biomagnification**, was the phenomenon responsible for the reproductive failure in the various birds of prey referred to earlier in this chapter. Eagles, pelicans, and falcons are all top carnivores, fish eaters, at the end of relatively long food chains. As such, they had accumulated amounts of DDT sufficiently high to interfere with important bodily processes.

A classic example of biomagnification occurred at Clear Lake, California—a favorite fishing spot about 90 miles north of San Francisco. Recreational anglers had long been annoyed by the swarms of nonbiting gnats that were frequently present at Clear Lake. The new synthetic pesticides seemingly offered an easy solution, so in 1949 officials decided to spray Clear Lake with a dilute solution of DDD (a chemical cousin of DDT which is less toxic to fish). After the first spraying, gnat populations dropped to barely detectable levels, but by 1951 the pesky insects were back in bothersome numbers, so the spraying was repeated. Several more sprayings followed in succeeding years as the gnat populations displayed increasing resistance to the poison. Then some strange side effects became apparent. By 1954 visitors to Clear Lake began reporting significant numbers of carcasses of the Western grebe, a type of waterfowl, around the lake. By the early 1960s, the grebe population at Clear Lake had plummeted from 1,000 nesting pairs to almost none. Suspecting that the repeated pesticide applications might somehow be related to the birds' demise, biologists began to measure DDD concentrations in various components of the lake ecosystem. Although the lake water itself contained traces of DDD in barely detectable amounts (0.02 ppm), concentrations of the pesticide increased dramatically when the tissues of living organisms were examined. The facts they uncovered are entirely consistent with the basic principles of a food chain:

Organism	DDD Concentration in Tissues (ppm)
Phytoplankton (producers)	5
Herbivorous fish (primary consumers)	40–300
Carnivorous fish (secondary consumers)	up to 2500
Western grebes (secondary consumers)	1600

The pesticide that had been sprayed on the lake, in what everybody at the time assumed was a safely dilute amount, was absorbed and concentrated by the plankton, which were the producer organisms of Clear Lake. When these were consumed by the herbivorous fish (primary consumers), the DDD became more concentrated. By the time these fish were eaten by grebes or by bullheads, the DDD had become sufficiently concentrated to cause the death of the birds.

By the late 1960s the futility of spraying to control the now-resistant gnats became obvious and a gnat-eating fish was introduced into the lake in what subsequently proved to be a very successful method of biological control. As pesticide levels gradually dropped, the grebes returned to Clear Lake and today are once again thriving at approximately their pre-1954 population levels. Numerous other examples of biomagnification involving other chlorinated hydrocarbons and heavy metals (methyl mercury at Minamata, for example) have since been described and illustrate the unanticipated effects that toxic substances can have as they move through ecosystems.

HAZARDS TO HUMAN HEALTH

Although pesticides are used specifically to kill pests, many of them are quite toxic to humans as well. Between 1998–2005 researchers identified over 3,000 cases of acute pesticide poisoning among U.S. agricultural workers—the group at highest risk of occupational pesticide exposure. The majority of these poisonings were of low severity, with only one fatality during this period. Nevertheless, the study highlighted the need for greater efforts to protect farm workers from pesticide exposure, given that 75% of pesticide use in the United States occurs in agriculture (Calvert et al., 2008). Poison control centers in the U.S. report over 100,000 pesticide poisonings each year, with 23,000 victims sick enough to visit hospital emergency rooms. Approximately 20 Americans, mostly children, die annually from accidental pesticide poisoning (Benbrook, 1996).

On a global basis, pesticides take a much higher toll. The WHO acknowledges that estimates of the incidence of acute pesticide poisoning in the developing world are unreliable, in part due to the lack of standardized case definition, but also because many cases are never reported, since affected field workers seldom seek medical treatment when they fall ill on the job. While increased emphasis on pesticide safety and improved application equipment has contributed to a marked decline in acute pesticide-related deaths and serious illness in the industrialized nations, such is not the case in most developing countries. Many of the farm chemicals used in these countries are highly toxic products now banned by industrial countries and farm workers seldom receive any training in their proper use. Adequate protective gear is seldom worn or even provided. Worse yet, workers often manually apply pesticides (sometimes by reaching bare-handed into a container of pesticidal dust and broadcasting it onto the target area) or spread them by tractor, affording ample opportunity for dusts, mists, or vapors to be inhaled or absorbed through the exposed skin of the applicator. Since field workers seldom have access to running water while working, quick removal of pesticides spilled on garments or on the skin is not possible and workers frequently wear contaminated clothing home, exposing their children, pregnant wives, or elderly parents (those most vulnerable to health damage from these poisons).

Additional exposure to family members may occur when workers, unaware of the danger, bring home empty

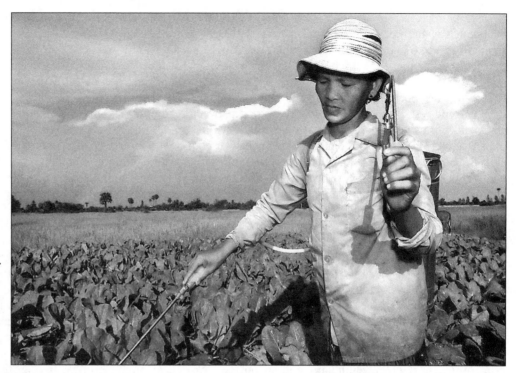

An unprotected Cambodian farmer sprays a cocktail of pesticides on her vegetable crop, unaware of their toxicity because she is unable to read the foreign language instructions on the containers. [*AP Photo/Andy Eames*]

pesticide containers to use for storing food or water. Although strict adherence to label directions could prevent some of the problems associated with improper handling, storage, and application practices, in fact farm workers in developing countries seldom read the label instructions, either because they are illiterate or because labels are printed in a language they don't understand (the latter situation poses a safety concern even in the United States where many agricultural laborers read only Spanish and are thus unable to heed warnings printed in English). Even worse, in many developing countries pesticides are often transferred from the original container to another unlabeled receptacle so that the user, even if literate and multilingual, has no way of knowing what hazards the material might present—or even its identity. Finally, a future threat that hasn't received the attention it deserves is the question of what to do with sizeable stocks of outdated or unusable pesticides—many of them persistent chlorinated hydrocarbons such as dieldrin and DDT—more than 15 million pounds (7 million kg) of which have accumulated in 35 developing countries. In many cases the containers in which these are stored are unlabeled, corroded, and leaking, posing serious pollution and health problems. Yet, the countries involved have no proper means for disposing of such toxins nor the resources for cleaning up contamination that has already occurred (World Resources Institute, 1994).

To cause harm, a pesticide must be taken internally through the mouth, skin, or respiratory system. Most oral exposure is due to carelessness; for example, leaving poisons within reach of young children, smoking or eating without washing hands after handling pesticides, using the mouth to start siphoning liquid pesticide concentrates, eating unwashed fruit that was recently sprayed, or accidentally drinking pesticides that were poured into an unlabeled container. Deliberate ingestion of highly toxic pesticides for the express purpose of committing suicide is responsible for a significant percentage of pesticide-related fatalities, most notably in China and Sri Lanka (NRC, 2000).

Exposure through the skin can occur when pesticides are spilled on the body or when wind-blown sprays or dusts come into contact with skin. Reentering a field too soon after pesticide application or careless handling of discarded containers can also result in absorption of pesticides through the skin. The larger the skin area contaminated and the longer the duration of contact, the more serious the results. Theoretically, dermal exposure could be reduced significantly through the use of protective clothing and equipment. In practice, however, such precautions are frequently ignored. Such gear is often expensive, cumbersome, and uncomfortable, especially during hot weather. All too often, applicators who know better fail to comply with safety recommendations and have been observed, in some instances, plying their trade wearing little more than bathing suits! Poisoning due to inhalation is most common in enclosed areas such as greenhouses but also can occur outside when pesticide mists or fumes are inhaled during application or if the applicator is smoking.

Symptoms of **acute** exposure (i.e., "one-time" cases) include headache, weakness, fatigue, or dizziness. If poisoning is due to one of the organophosphate insecticides, the victim may experience severe abdominal pain, vomiting, diarrhea, difficulty in breathing, excessive sweating, and sometimes convulsions, coma, and death. In contrast, **chronic** pesticide poisoning (low-level exposure over an extended time period) is characterized by vague symptoms that are difficult to pinpoint as having been caused by pesticide exposure. The greatest concern regarding chronic pesticide exposure, particularly to chlorinated hydrocarbons, is their potential for causing cancer or reproductive problems.

For many years **cancer** was the prime focus of concern regarding chronic effects of pesticide exposure. Extensive testing during the 1980s revealed that, on the basis of amounts applied, 60% of all herbicides, 90% of fungicides, and 30% of insecticides are either carcinogens or potentially carcinogenic (NRC, 1987). Beginning with its prohibition on the use of DDT in 1972, the EPA has gradually banned or restricted most of the chlorinated hydrocarbon pesticides, including endrin, aldrin, dieldrin, mirex, heptachlor, chlordane, and so on, largely because tests showed them to be carcinogenic to laboratory animals. The environmental consequences of this phaseout have been dramatic. In the United States, concentrations of these persistent pesticides in animal tissues have been steadily declining since the 1970s; certain bird populations that had nearly vanished by the late 1960s due to bioaccumulation of chlorinated pesticides have now largely rebounded. DDT levels in human breast milk also have plummeted by 90% since the EPA ban took effect (Schneider, 1994).

The impact of pesticide exposure on cancer incidence is still provoking debate among the experts (in California, the largest case-control study to date, published in April 1994, contradicted results of previous research by finding no association between breast cancer and DDT exposure). Meanwhile, a growing body of evidence supports the contention that **disruption of the endocrine and immune systems**, not cancer, constitutes the most serious long-term pesticide-related health concern. Since the endocrine hormones regulate a wide spectrum of bodily functions, including fertility and fetal development, compounds that interfere with such hormones have the potential for serious reproductive effects even at low levels of exposure. Scientists have now identified a number of pesticides, including many of the chlorinated hydrocarbons as well as some synthetic pyrethroids and triazine herbicides, as potent hormone disruptors. Studies of wildlife populations have shown that exposure to these compounds can lead to abnormal sexual behavior (especially feminization of males), birth defects, and impaired fertility among the offspring of pesticide-exposed parents (Curtis et al., 1993). Several of the more notorious pesticide-related tragedies have involved problems caused by the reproductive effects of chronic pesticide exposure. The nematicide DBCP (1,2–dibromo-3–chloropropane), for example, is known to have caused sterility among men in the California factory where it was manufactured, as well as among 1,500 male banana plantation workers in Costa Rica.

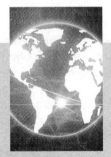

• • • • • • • *8-4* • • • • • • •

"EPA-Registered"—Synonymous with "Safe"?

The war against insects, rodents, and weeds is waged as vigorously on the home front as it is on the farm. An estimated 85% of American households harbor pesticidal products—three to five different chemicals, on average—that are used in prodigious amounts. Unfortunately, unlike farmers and structural pest control operators who are required to pass competency examinations, the average householder purchasing such pesticides has little or no idea of the health and environmental hazards such chemicals pose. After all, the reasoning goes, if the label says "EPA-Registered" it must be safe! This conviction reflects a dangerous ignorance of how pesticides are regulated and leads to a degree of complacency on the part of the general public that isn't warranted by the facts.

Early laws regulating pesticides focused almost exclusively on protecting farmers from untested, ineffective products, requiring truthful labeling but ignoring issues pertaining to human health or environmental impacts. By the late 1940s, as pesticide use began to grow rapidly, Congress enacted legislation requiring that chemical companies register their pesticide labels with the designated federal agency (originally with the U.S. Department of Agriculture; in 1970 that role was transferred to the newly created Environmental Protection Agency). Thus the fact that a particular product is government-registered simply means that it is legal to sell and use in the United States—nothing more.

By 1972, mounting evidence of human poisonings and environmental damage convinced policy makers that a shift in regulatory focus was needed. In that year, the old Federal Insecticide, Fungicide, and Rodenticide Act (FIFRA) was amended to incorporate health and environmental considerations into the regulatory process for the first time. These amendments mandated that henceforth chemical manufacturers must submit health and safety test results for new pesticides when they seek EPA registration for those products. Basic risk-benefit standards were developed for evaluating data submitted, the intention being to exclude high-risk pesticides from the market. Also in 1972, EPA canceled the registration of DDT, thus ending its legal use in the U.S., and shortly thereafter the agency took similar action with eight additional chlorinated hydrocarbon insecticides (Schneider, 1983).

With this seemingly protective regulatory framework in place for nearly 40 years and with most of the notorious cancer-causing insecticides banned from the U.S. marketplace, why shouldn't average citizens assume that pesticides currently in use pose negligible health risks? Several reasons:

1. The requirement for safety testing prior to registration was not retroactive; hundreds of acutely hazardous pesticides were already registered for use at the time the new law was enacted. The vast majority of these remain on the market. Only through a lengthy process of collecting scientific data and proving that these "grandfathered" chemicals pose "unreasonable adverse effects" can EPA end their legal use.

2. Safety testing data is required only for the active ingredients in a given pesticidal product, yet the largest part, by volume, of many pesticides is made up of so-called "inert" ingredients, for which no safety testing is required. Some of these inerts are themselves known to be toxic, yet label requirements don't even require that they be identified by name. Pesticide legislative reform efforts regularly target the issue of inert ingredients, so far to no avail.

3. Many pesticides introduced since 1972 obtained EPA approval on the basis of fraudulent testing data. A scandal that made headlines in the early 1980s revealed that the largest independent laboratory in the nation, Industrial Bio-Test (IBT), had contracts with a number of chemical companies to supply the toxicological test data required for EPA registration. Only after more than 200 pesticides had been registered on the basis of falsified test results did it become known that the company had perpetrated the most massive scientific fraud ever committed in the United States. The IBT executives involved in the deception eventually received prison sentences, convicted of conducting and distributing fake scientific research and then attempting to cover-up their crimes. Nevertheless, many of the products registered during this period remain on the market today. A 1988 amendment to FIFRA requires EPA to speed up the re-registration process for pre-1972 pesticides and for those originally tested by IBT, but that project is far behind schedule; EPA estimates the work will be completed in 2014.

4. Pesticides like DDT and chlordane, which were removed from commercial use due to concern for their *chronic* health effects, particularly cancer, were replaced largely by organophosphate or carbamate products that were often more acutely toxic than the chemicals they replaced, and are thus more dangerous to use. A number of these compounds are still commonly purchased for home or garden use, largely because they are cheaper than the less toxic pyrethrins.

In spite of many decades of pesticide regulation, overall use of chemical poisons continues to increase and the health and environmental risks they pose are as great as ever. Following common-sense safety precautions certainly can reduce the chance of injury or illness: follow label directions when using pesticides; keep pesticides in their original containers; keep them out of reach of children and pets; always wear protective clothing when applying chemicals; and avoid spraying when conditions are windy. Nevertheless, the decision to use chemical poisons always entails some degree of risk. Undeniably, pest problems need to be managed, but where nonchemical IPM approaches are equally effective, they represent the wiser, safer choice (Benbrook, 1996).

Immune system dysfunction can be provoked by either acute or subchronic exposure to many commonly used pesticides, including the herbicide 2,4–D and the insecticides malathion, parathion, aldicarb, carbofuran, and most of the chlorinated hydrocarbons (though most of these are no longer used in the United States, their residues persist in the environment). Young children, especially when malnourished, as well as elderly adults appear most vulnerable to pesticides' immuno-suppressive effects and tend to contract infectious diseases more frequently than individuals not exposed to pesticidal compounds. Pesticide-induced immunotoxicity may also be manifested as allergic contact dermatitis, a skin inflammation caused by immune system response to a foreign substance—in this case to pesticide exposure. Allergic reactions to contact with even minute amounts of pesticides can become chronic and in some cases have resulted in farm workers becoming permanently disabled due to chemical intolerance.

The adverse health and reproductive effects induced by endocrine-disrupting pesticides are further compounded when exposure to two or more such chemicals occurs simultaneously. The insecticides endosulfan and DDT, for example, interact synergistically to produce estrogenic effects 160–1,600 times greater than those of either pesticide alone. Inasmuch as humans are constantly exposed to numerous endocrine-disrupting chemicals (including PCBs and dioxins as well as pesticides) in air, food, and water, levels of exposure until now regarded as "safe" may need to be reassessed (Arnold et al., 1996).

Yet another health problem for which pesticide exposure has been implicated as a causative agent is **Parkinson's disease**, a neurogenerative condition usually manifested only in older people. An epidemiological study conducted in California's Central Valley focused on people living in residential areas exposed to "pesticide drift" from nearby agricultural fields over a 25-year time span. While not conclusive, results suggested that residents exposed to the herbicide paraquat or to the fungicide maneb when young incurred an increased risk of Parkinson's disease later in life; moreover, there was a fourfold to sixfold increase in risk for those exposed to both pesticides in combination, as compared with residents who hadn't been exposed to either (Costello et al., 2009).

The human health impact of **dietary exposure** to pesticides via residues on food has attracted intense public scrutiny since the 1987 publication of a study by the National Research Council (NRC), estimating that traces of carcinogenic fungicides, insecticides, and herbicides on the nation's fruits, vegetables, and meat could result in an additional 20,000 cancer deaths per year in the United States. These findings were hotly disputed by agrichemical interests but generated intense public concern over how pesticides are regulated. Demands for reform

received added impetus following publication in June 1993 of a long-awaited study by the NRC on pesticides in the diets of infants and small children. NRC scientists were critical of the EPA's outmoded approach for setting pesticide tolerance levels on agricultural produce (a system based on the estimated amount of any given pesticide the "average person"—i.e. an adult—is likely to consume as part of a typical American diet), and concluded that the youngest members of society are at enhanced risk because they consume more calories per unit of body weight and because their diet is less varied than that of adults.

Immediately after publication of the NRC report, a second study dealing with the same issue was released by the Environmental Working Group (EWG), a nonprofit research organization, stating that up to 35% of an individual's lifetime dose of dietary pesticides occurs before the age of 5, largely because young children consume proportionately far more residue-laden fruits and vegetables than do adults (EWG, 1998). Preschoolers, for example, eat six times the amount of fruit consumed by their parents and drink 31 times more apple juice in relation to their body weight than do adults. Thus pesticide residue safety levels based on presumed "average" diets may greatly underestimate the actual amount of exposure received by a young child. These reports also emphasized the fact that most foods contain residues of several different pesticides (a laboratory analysis performed on one pear identified 11 different pesticidal compounds), not just one, and that the sources of pesticide exposure are not restricted to food, but frequently include drinking water, lawn chemicals, and household insecticides as well.

All of these factors suggested that the existing regulatory framework for ensuring food safety was inadequate to protect infants and children (NRC, 1993; Curtis et al., 1993). In response to these concerns, the U.S. Congress in 1996 enacted comprehensive legislation to reform and modernize the nation's laws dealing with food safety and the setting of pesticide tolerance levels. The **Food Quality Protection Act of 1996** now requires that when the EPA sets tolerance levels for pesticide residues on food, it must take into account available information on consumption habits of infants and children, as well as the neurological differences between adults and children that make the latter uniquely sensitive to the harmful effects of pesticide exposure. The law also requires EPA to take into account the cumulative effect of multiple residues when establishing pesticide tolerance levels in food, incorporating an additional tenfold margin of safety to protect children, infants, and babies *in utero* (Benbrook, 1996). As required by the Food Quality Protection Act, EPA has reevaluated all food tolerances to ensure they meet the law's "reasonable certainty of no harm" standard, particularly in regard to children's health. The agency points out that although 19–29% of food samples tested between 1994 and 2001 contained detectable levels of organophosphate pesticide residues (the highest rates were detected in 1996 and 1997), during that same period the amounts of insecticides used on the foods most frequently eaten by children dropped by 44%. In 1999–2000, out of concern for children's pesticide exposure, EPA imposed new restrictions on the use of several organophosphate poisons on certain food crops, as well as in and around the home (EPA, 2003a).

ALTERNATIVES TO CHEMICAL PEST CONTROL

As increasing numbers of pest species become resistant to available chemicals and as concerns over the long-range effects of pesticide exposure on human health and the environment continue to grow, the advisability of continuing to rely exclusively on chemicals for pest control is increasingly being questioned. In recent years a different philosophy of pest control has gained support, a strategy known as **Integrated Pest Management (IPM)**. After ascertaining that a pest problem does indeed exist, IPM practitioners combine various compatible methods to prevent pest populations from reaching economically damaging levels while causing the least harm to human health and the environment. In 1977 the U.S. Department of Agriculture (USDA) adopted an official policy of encouraging IPM practices, sponsoring numerous research, development, and demonstration projects to promote IPM. In 1993 USDA set a goal, not yet achieved, of implementing IPM on fully 75% of total U.S. crop acreage by 2000 in order to reduce pesticide use and the environmental health risks posed by overreliance on chemicals for pest control (GAO, 2001).

While the emphasis in IPM is on utilizing natural controls such as predators, food deprivation, or weather to increase pest mortality, it also can include pesticide application, but only after careful monitoring of pest populations indicate a need. Unlike the total chemical control approach, IPM recognizes the extraordinary adaptability of insects and does not attempt to eradicate a particular pest entirely, but rather aims to keep pest populations below the threshold level at which they can cause significant economic loss. Among the methods that could be included in an IPM strategy are the following.

Natural Enemies

Many of our most serious insect and weed pests (such as Japanese beetle, gypsy moth, fire ant, kudzu, water hyacinth, and so on) are foreign imports that rapidly multiplied here in the absence of their natural enemies. Other native pests have caused serious problems only after their predators were eliminated by indiscriminate use of pesticides. Since the late 1800s, the government has imported more than 500 insect predators in an attempt to control alien species; more than 70 of these are now providing significant control of several important insect pests and weeds (Vail et al., 2001). Laboratory breeding of large populations of insect predators in hopes of overwhelming certain pests is also being conducted. Great success in controlling scale insects and mealybugs in citrus orchards was obtained by mass rearing and release of vedalia beetles and certain parasitic wasps. Home gardeners and organic farmers can assist natural predators in keeping pest insects at low levels by avoiding the use of broad-spectrum insecticides and by planting a diverse assemblage of species that provide alternative food sources and habitat for beneficial insects (see box 8-5). It is *not* recommended, however, that IPM enthusiasts purchase insect predators such as ladybird beetles or praying mantises for release in their home gardens. Doing so is basically a waste of money because commercially sold ladybirds, once released, typically disperse and fly elsewhere, providing minimal levels of control for the purchaser; praying mantises are general feeders and will eat other beneficials (even each other!) as well as pests. In addition, because of their low survival rates and territorial nature, mantids have a negligible impact in controlling pest outbreaks.

Microbial Pesticides

A further step in biological warfare against insects involves introducing various disease agents into a pest population. A number of microbial pathogens are now being marketed commercially and more are in the research and development stage. To date, the most successful and widely used is the bacterium, *Bacillus thuringiensis (Bt)*, an organism that produces a toxin fatal to over 100 species of caterpillars. Use of *Bt*-based biopesticides has been increasing rapidly in response to consumer concerns about pesticide residues on food, as reflected in mounting demand for organically grown produce. In addition to *Bt*'s use on food crops, variants of this pathogen are widely employed against a number of other insect pests. *Bt kurstaki (Btk)* is the most widely used insecticide against forest pests such as the gypsy moth, spruce budworm, and tent caterpillar; *Bt tenebrionis (Btt)* is being targeted against various beetles such as the Colorado potato beetle, an insect now resistant to virtually every chemical pesticide; and *Bt israelensis (Bti)* is quite effective as a mosquito larvicide.

Fungal pathogens also have been enlisted in the war against insect pests. These organisms produce spores capable of penetrating the insect's exoskeleton, growing

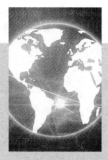

······· *8-5* ·······

IPM in Your Own Backyard

Although agriculture accounts for approximately three-fourths of all pesticide use in the United States, sales of herbicides and insecticides for home lawn and garden use have soared in recent decades. Millions of homeowners and backyard gardeners each year purchase and apply prodigious amounts of toxic chemicals to their property with little or no understanding of how to use, store, or dispose of such products in a safe manner. Increasing parental concerns about potential harm to children and pets from dangerous pesticide residues, confrontations among neighbors when "spray drift" from one property kills the flowers next door, and recognition that bird and butterfly populations plummet where insecticide use is profligate have prompted some to look for a better way to control weeds and insects in residential areas.

Integrated Pest Management (IPM) is a concept initially developed within the context of commercial agriculture, but its basic precepts are equally applicable and practical for the home gardener. Admittedly, it is much more demanding than conventional reliance on chemical pesticides, requiring an understanding of the life cycle and habits of the target pest. In the long run, however, IPM is a safer, more effective, and more sustainable approach to managing pest populations than conventional chemical treatment.

In a home lawn and garden environment, IPM is a process consisting of several steps:

1. **Determine whether a problem actually exists**. There's no point in automatically treating a lawn for grubs or spraying roses for aphids if none are present. Regular, systematic monitoring for the presence of pests prior to taking action is an essential component of any IPM program. This requires careful visual inspection of plants for signs of insect or disease problems or can involve the use of traps to determine whether certain pests are in the vicinity.

2. **Accurately identify the pest causing the problem**. Remember, not every insect present on a plant is a pest, nor is every discolored leaf evidence of a disease. Determination of the cause of damage can, in some cases, be tricky; injury due to herbicide spray drift, adverse weather conditions, or nutrient deficiency may produce symptoms similar to those of insect damage. Brown patches in the lawn, for example, may have many possible causes: drought, chemical burn, grubs, sod webworms, inadvertent spraying of dandelions with Roundup® (it happens!), or urination by a female dog. Determine the cause before taking appropriate action. If insects are spotted on a plant, note whether they appear to be causing any damage (chewing on leaves? sucking plant juices?); they may simply be harmless species "passing through" or a predator insect waiting to pounce on one of the "bad guys." Some knowledge of insect life cycles is important, since many pest species are damaging only during their larval stage or only as adults; attempting to control an insect at the wrong stage is generally a waste of effort. Similarly, spraying to control an insect that isn't a pest is environmentally bad and a waste of time and money—and may result in a worse problem if the victim happens to be a "good bug" who was helping to keep the pest population in check. Novices who don't feel capable of identifying presumed pests accurately can generally obtain help without charge at their county extension office or from a local Master Gardener group.

3. **Decide if the problem is serious enough to warrant action**. Once the problem is correctly identified, a decision must be made as to whether the pest is causing enough damage to warrant the effort and expense of controls. In an outdoor residential setting, this involves a subjective determination of the "aesthetic threshold"—how bad does a tree, lawn, or garden have to look to make rescuing it worthwhile in terms of time, money, and potential health risks due to pesticide exposure? It must be kept in mind that some types of infestations (e.g., spittlebugs or columbine leaf miners) may look threatening but really aren't significantly harming the plant. Decisions on whether or not to take action should also be influenced by the time of year when the infestation occurs; for example, insects defoliating trees in late spring represent a much more serious problem than would defo-

liation in late summer when the tree has already accumulated food reserves for winter and will soon lose its leaves anyhow. Application of pest control measures are probably appropriate in the former situation, but may not be recommended in the latter, even when the extent of leaf damage is the same. In some cases, weather conditions alone may take care of the problem—infestations of turf-destroying sod webworms may be completely eliminated during cool wet springs, thanks to a fungal pathogen of webworms that thrives under those climatic conditions. It should also be kept in mind that healthy, vigorous plants can sustain a considerable amount of insect feeding without much lasting damage. For all these reasons, doing nothing is one valid option.

4. **If the pest problem is deemed severe enough to warrant control, utilize a combination of methods best suited to the specific pest in question**. Such controls include many of the same strategies relied upon by farmers—planting cultivars that are resistant to pests or diseases known to be a problem in the area (e.g. scab-resistant crabapple trees, mildew-resistant Phlox 'David'); maintaining plants in good health by proper fertilization and watering practices; and, when all else fails, judicious chemical pesticide applications, using the "littlest gun" that will do the job, applied in a manner least likely to harm nontarget organisms.

A number of additional IPM strategies have been successfully practiced by home gardeners for generations:

Mechanical controls include hand-picking, stomping, and squashing (it's unlikely bugs will ever evolve resistance to being stepped on nor weeds to being ripped from the ground!). Floating row covers can protect young plants from flea beetles, cabbage moths, and a host of other flying insect pests, while stiff paper collars or bottomless coffee cans around tender transplants can effectively deter cutworms. Similarly, the use of nets or chicken wire to block access to plants may offer the only reliable approach to keeping birds and rabbits away. Pruning off infested plant parts (e.g., cutting off the ends of tree branches harboring fall webworm nests, removing infected iris rhizomes when dividing overgrown clumps, using scissors to cut bagworms off tree branches before the eggs hatch in the spring) can be far more effective than pesticide spraying in certain situations.

Cultural practices include adjusting the planting time of certain crops (e.g., potatoes) so that critical periods in plant development (in this case, blossom initiation) don't coincide with peak pest populations. Another highly recommended practice, especially in vegetable gardens, is the removal of all plant debris at the end of the season to reduce overwintering habitat of such common insect pests as squash bugs, flea beetles, and iris borers. A thorough fall cleanup also helps prevent fungal problems the following year. During the growing season, fungal diseases in general can be minimized by spacing plants far enough apart to maintain good air circulation; watering in the early morning rather than in the evening so that wet foliage will dry quickly also helps to avoid conditions favorable for fungal pathogens. To suppress weed growth, a 1–2″ layer of organic mulch (shredded bark, leaf mold, grass clippings straw, etc.) applied around the base of plants in early spring is quite effective in preventing weed seeds from germinating and smothering young weed seedlings; weeds that do manage to grow through the mulch are easily removed by hand. Black plastic can also be used to control weeds, especially in vegetable gardens where transplants can be inserted and grown through slits in the plastic cover.

Biological controls involve using natural enemies to keep pest populations at tolerable levels. The most important way to do this is to avoid, wherever possible, the use of chemical insecticides, since most of those on the market are broad-spectrum poisons that make no distinction between harmful and beneficial species. In addition, to encourage the "good guys" to take up residence in close proximity to where the pests are, gardeners need to provide harborage and alternative sources of nutrition for these species (have you ever considered what ladybugs eat in the early spring before the aphids arrive?—dandelion pollen, among other things!). This can be done quite easily by planting a variety of flowers nearby; some of the best species for this purpose include members of the mustard family (*Cruciferae*) like sweet alyssum and dame's rocket; members of the carrot family (*Umbelliferae*), including dill, coriander, and Queen Anne's lace; various legumes such as alfalfa and sweet clover, and many members of the aster family (*Asteraceae*)—marigolds, coneflowers, goldenrod, and, yes, even dandelions! "The more, the merrier" in terms of species in a garden seems to be the best approach to a chemical-free method of managing garden pests.

Inevitably there comes a time when gardeners must make a choice between allowing some plants to be destroyed by an out-of-control pest explosion or the judicious application of chemical pesticides (under an IPM regimen, unlike true organic gardening, chemical use is permitted as a last resort). However, adherence to an IPM program will minimize the need for such painful decisions and will result in a healthier backyard environment for plants and gardeners alike.

inside the host and digesting its tissues, resulting in death within a few days. One of these, *Metarhizium anisopliae*, is used extensively in Brazil for control of spittlebugs on sugar cane. Another, *Verticillium lecanii*, has been employed against greenhouse pests such as whiteflies, thrips, and aphids that are now resistant to almost all the chemical insecticides registered for use in greenhouses.

Pathogenic viruses also offer a promising method of pest control, since viral diseases in nature are frequently devastating to pest populations. A number of companies are currently conducting research on insect viruses that they hope to market against specific pests, but few are commercially available at present. The most widely used viral pesticide currently is a nuclear polyhedrosis virus, *Anticarsia gemmatalis*, used to combat the velvetbean caterpillar on nearly 15 million acres of Brazilian soybean fields (NRC, 2000). Researchers with the Canadian Forest Service are hopeful about developing an insect virus effective against the spruce budworm, pine sawfly, and other pests that periodically devastate Canadian forests.

A naturally occurring protozoan, *Nosema locustae*, has been successfully employed to control grasshoppers and Mormon crickets. When *Nosema* spores sprayed on a wheat-bran bait are consumed, they germinate inside the insect's stomach, multiply rapidly, and devour the pest from inside.

Sex Attractants

Certain chemical stimulants (pheromones) control many aspects of insect behavior, including mating. Sex pheromones may be excreted by the female to attract the male, or vice-versa. Some of these female pheromones have been synthesized in the lab and used to bait traps that can attract males from miles around. When the males enter the trap, expecting to encounter a receptive female, they are caught by a sticky substance on the bottom or sides of the trap. A variation on this method has yielded encouraging results in efforts to manage the codling moth, an insect whose larvae cause serious economic losses to pear and apple growers. To disrupt mating of adult moths, farmers place 10-inch-long twist-ties impregnated with female moth pheromone high in the branches of their orchard trees. When approximately 400 of these devices are used per acre, the "come hither" scent so pervades the area that male moths are thoroughly confused, not knowing in which direction to fly to find a mate. In this situation, most females remain unmated, lay infertile eggs, and over time the pest populations decline (Benbrook, 1996). The increasingly popular Japanese beetle trap marketed for home gardeners is baited with both a sex pheromone to attract males and a floral lure to entice female beetles. Although they are quite effective in doing just that, agricultural advisers rec-

ommend that homeowners not use them. Because they attract beetles from far and wide, many of which wouldn't have come otherwise, and because many of the arriving beetles evade the trap, gardeners who use these devices often experience more plant damage than they would have incurred without them.

Because the use of sex attractants as just described is effective only against adult insects, the technique is of limited effectiveness, since much crop damage is caused by insect larvae. In addition, because most pest species concentrate on a single crop, the market demand for any particular pheromone is relatively small. If the prospects for sales profits are not sufficiently attractive, manufacturers have no interest in producing them! Therefore, in recent years the prime strategy regarding sex attractants has shifted from using them to capture or confuse pest insects to employing pheromones to lure "good bugs" (i.e., predator species) into problem areas where they will then encounter—and eat—the "bad bugs." Since most predators eat a wide variety of pests, the same predator species could be a useful control agent in many different situations, a fact that significantly enhances the market demand for its pheromone. A patented product (The RESCUE®) being marketed through nurseries and hardware stores features a pheromone attractive to the spined soldier bug—a predator of approximately 100 different insect pests (ARS, 2004).

Insect Growth Regulators (IGRs)

Sometimes referred to as "biorational" insecticides, IGRs are chemicals that are identical to or closely mimic growth substances produced by the target pest. IGRs act either as **chitin inhibitors**, preventing proper development of the exoskeleton after molting, or, more commonly, as **juvenoids**. When the larvae of insects with a complete metamorphosis (fleas or mosquitoes, for example) contact or ingest juvenoids, these synthetic analogs of natural insect hormones prevent them from emerging as adults after pupating, thus effectively disrupting their life cycle. For insects characterized by a gradual metamorphosis (such as cockroaches) in which there is no pupal stage, nymphs may progress to adulthood but are abnormal in appearance and incapable of reproducing.

Several IGRs are now widely used in structural and public health pest control operations (usually in combination with standard insecticidal formulations to provide a "double whammy"), offering long-term control of such troublesome pests as cockroaches, fleas, ants, and floodwater mosquitoes. An obvious limitation to the use of insect growth regulators is that they are only useful against insects that cause damage as adults; many of the worst agricultural pests are larvae (such as caterpillars and grubs) against which IGRs are ineffective.

Sterile Insect Technique

This method relies on the mass rearing and release of huge numbers of male insects that have been sterilized by chemicals or radiation, usually gamma rays or X-rays. Subsequent mating of a normal female with a sterile male thus results in the production of infertile eggs. If the ratio of sterilized males to normal males is sufficiently large, most matings will be unsuccessful and over several generations pest populations will die out (the technique is most effective against target pest species in which the females mate only once). This technique was employed with great success on Zanzibar's Unguja Island to eradicate a tsetse fly population that for decades had caused devastating losses to livestock herds. Over a two-year period, from 1995–1997, an average of 50,000 male flies, mass-reared in laboratories and sterilized with a 28-second dose of gamma radiation, were released from airplanes across the island. With sterile males outnumbering the natural population of normal males by 50 to 1, induced sterility among females increased rapidly and the density of fly populations steadily dropped. The ultimate result was the total elimination of tsetse flies from the island (Kinley, 1998). Earlier SIT programs had been similarly successful in eradicating the screw-worm fly from Curacao, Florida, and parts of Central America, as well as the Mediterranean fruit fly from Chile, Mexico, and California. Not applicable in every setting, SIT is most effective when the pest population is geographically isolated, making reinvasion of the area with normal males unlikely.

Host Plant Resistance

Selective use of crop plant species that exhibit genetic resistance to pests is probably the most ecologically sound method for reducing losses due to plant diseases and nematodes. Practical applications of this IPM technique are numerous. For example, savvy home gardeners, as well as commercial growers, insist that the tomato seeds or plants they purchase be varieties bearing code letters that indicate resistance to several important tomato pathogens (e.g., the designation "**VFNT**" informs a prospective buyer that the plant in question is resistant to *Verticillium* wilt, *Fusarium* wilt, **N**ematodes, and **T**obacco mosaic virus, and thus is unlikely to require chemical pesticide applications to keep the plant disease-free). Host resistance also has been successfully employed against insect pests such as the Hessian fly, grape phylloxera, spotted alfalfa aphid, rice stem borer, and corn earworm.

More recently, genetic engineering has provided new and faster techniques for introducing desired characteristics from one species into another. In 1995, EPA approved the first **transgenic** corn variety engineered for resistance to the European corn borer (ECB), a moth whose larvae cause significant crop losses throughout the Corn Belt each year. Scientists spliced a gene for toxin production from the bacterium *Bt* into the DNA of corn, creating a hybrid plant that can poison an invading corn borer larva on the first bite. A crop that "fights back," killing its enemy before sustaining damage itself, offers big benefits to farmers in terms of increased yields, reduced exposure to chemical toxins, and reduced expenditures for insecticides. Environmental benefits are obvious as well, since pesticide contamination of streams and groundwater in agricultural areas should be significantly reduced on *Bt*-crop acreage.

However, most observers concede that there is a serious potential problem associated with the rapid proliferation of *Bt* crops; that is, the near-certainty that within a few years widespread resistance to the *Bt* toxin will develop among populations of target insects. To slow down what is generally regarded as an inevitable consequence of widespread exposure to *Bt*, farmers are being urged to reserve approximately 20% of their total acreage for non-*Bt* crop varieties. By doing so, it is hoped, pests within the reserve won't be under selective pressure to develop resistance; if resistant individuals from outside the reserve subsequently encounter and mate with one of these nonresistant pests, large-scale resistance within the population can at least be delayed. Unfortunately, anecdotal evidence from farm country suggests that the majority of growers are not setting aside enough of their cropland to make a significant difference. Hence it is likely that *Bt*'s unquestioned value for organic growers and large commercial farmers alike will be short-lived, undermined by increasing *Bt*-resistance within pest populations.

Sanitation

For control of insect and rodent pests in residential areas or business establishments, the most effective way to reduce pest numbers and keep them low is to apply the basic principles of sanitation. To survive and multiply, pests need a source of food, water, and harborage. If these are in short supply, large pest populations cannot be maintained. Strict observance of the rules of good housekeeping—promptly cleaning up spilled food, storing foods in tightly sealed containers, keeping garbage cans covered, avoiding use of mulch immediately adjacent to building foundations, mowing tall grass or weeds near structures, locating woodpiles at some distance from dwellings, regularly collecting and disposing of animal feces—will be far more effective in eliminating flies, rodents, and roaches over the long term than will pesticidal spraying. Similarly, structural alterations such as screens, metal or cement barriers, and caulk applied to cracks and crevices can assist in "building out" certain household pests. Habitat modification such as changing water in birdbaths frequently, keeping roof gutters free of twigs and leaves to permit complete drainage of rainwater, and maintaining premises free of discarded articles that could collect water can be very effective in reducing mosquito breeding. Pesticide use can provide a quick fix, but without adherence to good sanitary practices, control will be temporary at best.

None of the above methods alone is the total answer to effective pest management. However, in the proper combination after an accurate assessment of a specific pest situation, IPM techniques promise a safer, more ecologically sound, and ultimately more successful approach to limiting pest damage than does total reliance on chemicals.

9

It was no uncommon occurrence for a man to find the surface
of his pot of coffee swarming with weevils after breaking up
hardtack in it.... If a soldier cared to do so, he could
expel the weevils by heating the bread at the fire.
The maggots did not budge in that way.
—John Billings ("Hardtack and Coffee," 1887)

Food Quality

A Civil War veteran's reflections on the insect-infested fare common to both Yankee and Confederate armies during that historic conflict gives evidence that concerns about food contamination and food quality in general are nothing new. From time immemorial, humans have grappled with the problem of protecting stored food supplies from insects, molds, and rodent infestations; they learned through sad experience about natural toxins in certain foods and found they could minimize risk of food poisoning through proper processing and cooking practices. Until the mid-1800s however, problems related to food quality were relatively limited and localized because most people raised their food at home or purchased it from local producers. Consumers carefully inspected purchased items for signs of insect infestation, sniffed meat and fish to detect spoilage, and in general served as their own food inspectors. Government regulation of food quality prior to the 20th century was extremely limited, focusing primarily on commercially baked bread. Early bread laws were designed to standardize the weight of loaves in relation to the price of wheat; i.e., they were essentially price-fixing laws. Other regulations prohibited adding foreign substances such as ground chalk or powdered beans to flour. Subsequent laws provided for inspection of weights and flour quality (Janssen, 1975).

In the United States, prior to the 1900s the federal government had no role in regulating food safety, that issue being regarded as solely a prerogative of state or local authorities (NRC, 1998). However, in the decades following the Civil War, the close-to-home food production, distribution, and marketing systems that had prevailed virtually everywhere in the world up to that time began experiencing revolutionary change. The explosive growth of cities and the expansion of transportation networks—especially the railroad—during these years gave birth to an organized food industry that became national, and eventually global, in scope. The subsequent introduction of refrigerated railcars (and later refrigerated trucks and air freight) made possible the shipment of hitherto unavailable fresh meat and produce to markets thousands of miles distant from their place of origin. This rapid development, in the absence of regulation, was marred by deplorably unhygienic conditions and frequently unethical practices.

The biggest scandal of 19th-century food establishments involved the widespread practice of **adulteration**—the deliberate addition of inferior or cheaper material to a supposedly pure food product in order to stretch out supplies and increase profits. Adulteration has undoubtedly been practiced on a small scale for millennia by unscrupulous merchants, but the anonymity of large, unregulated corporations selling foodstuffs to faceless consumers hundreds of miles away gave great impetus to the proliferation of this age-old practice. Substances used as adulterants in some cases were harmless ingredients, cheating consumers only in a financial sense; in other instances, the adulterants consisted of toxic substances that posed a serious health threat. Some foods commonly adulterated during the 18th and 19th centuries included: (1) black pepper, commonly mixed with such materials as mustard seed husks, pea flour, juniper berries, or floor sweepings; (2) tea, adulterated on a large scale with leaves of the ash tree which were dried, curled, and sold to tea merchants for a few cents per pound. Green China tea was often adulterated with dried thorn leaves, tinted green with a toxic dye; black Indian tea was more easily adulterated by collecting used tea leaves from restaurants, drying and stiffening them with gum and then tinting them with black lead, also toxic, to make them look fresh; (3) cocoa powder "enriched" with brick dust; (4) milk supplies extended with water; (5) coffee blended with ground acorns or chicory.

Perhaps even more alarming were revelations in the late 19th century that many of the food colors and flavorings in widespread use were poisonous; e.g., pickles colored bright green with copper, candies and sweets brightly tinted with lead and copper salts, commercially baked bread whitened with alum, beer froth produced by iron sulfate. By the early 20th century, more than 80 synthetic agents were being used to color foods as diverse as mustard, jellies, and wine. Many had never been tested for adverse health effects and all were being used without any monitoring or regulatory controls; amazingly, some of these chemical additives had been developed as textile dyes and were never intended to be used in food products! Not surprisingly, contemporary accounts document a number of human illnesses and a few deaths attributable to consumption of toxic food colorants in those years (Tannahill, 1973; Henkel, 1993).

A growing awareness of such problems led to congressional passage in 1906 of the **Pure Food and Drugs Act**, one of the first federal laws intended to protect consumers against adulteration, mislabeling of foods, and harmful ingredients in food. As a result of this act and of subsequent food quality legislation, instances of adulteration in the United States are now much rarer, though regulations have had to be instituted from time to time to prevent the gradual degradation of foods, such as the increase in fat or ground bone content of hot dogs or the decrease in fruit content of jams or fruit pies. However, occasionally flagrant abuses still occur. In the fall of 1993 the Flavor Fresh Foods Corporation of Chicago, as well

as 11 of its corporate officials, pled guilty to charges of defrauding consumers of more than $40 million through sales of adulterated orange juice. For 12 years Flavor Fresh had been marketing a product labeled as "100% pure orange juice from concentrate," which in reality contained 55–75% beet sugar, along with other adulterants added to conceal the substitution (Ropp, 1994).

In 2007 an adulteration scandal originating in China outraged American pet owners and prompted one of the largest pet food recalls in U.S. history. After more than 14,000 dogs and cats were sickened and some died of kidney failure, American regulators found that two Chinese companies supplying wheat gluten to U.S. feed manufacturers had laced their product with melamine, a cheap nitrogen-containing plasticizer that makes the gluten's protein content appear higher than it actually is—and thereby increased their profits. Subsequent investigations revealed that a second adulterant, cyanuric acid, had also been used to boost apparent protein levels, contributing to pet deaths and illnesses by impairing kidney function. Unfortunately, this wasn't the first international incident involving tainted Chinese products; in 2006, Chinese cold medicines adulterated with the toxic sweetener diethylene glycol, added as a substitute for more expensive glycerin, killed several hundred people, mostly children, in Panama (Hoffman, 2007; Barboza, 2007a).

Within recent years the focus of public attention regarding food quality has shifted from adulteration to a concern over contaminants and additives in our food supply. The fact that few people today produce their own foods at home means that almost all of us, to a greater or lesser degree, have no choice but to rely on foodstuffs produced by a massive food industry—foods that contain many kinds of additives and, in some cases, contaminants over which we have very little control. The widespread interest in "health foods" is due, in no small measure, to the feeling of many people that industrially produced food is somehow less safe and less nutritious than the "natural" foods of yesteryear. Representatives of the food industry and, indeed, many scientists, counter that chemical additives are both safe and essential to ensure an abundant supply of food at affordable prices to a still-growing population. In an attempt to understand the nature of the debate and the rationale behind existing or proposed regulations, it is helpful to distinguish between those substances accidentally introduced into foods and those deliberately added to prevent deterioration or to enhance taste or attractiveness.

FOOD CONTAMINANTS

Substances accidentally incorporated into foods are called **contaminants**. Such contaminants include dirt, hairs, animal feces, fungal growths, insect fragments, pesticide residues, traces of growth hormones or antibiotics, and so on, that are introduced into food during the harvesting, processing, or packaging stage. They serve no useful purpose in the finished product and are presumed to be harmful unless proven otherwise. (In many cases, however, common food contaminants constitute an aesthetic affront to consumers rather than an actual health threat; for example, the thought of eating a fly wing hidden among the oregano leaves on a frozen pizza may be repugnant, but it won't make you sick—at least not if you don't see it!) Certainly every effort should be made to keep our foods as free from contamination as possible; however, it has never been, and probably never will be, possible to grow, harvest, and process crops that are totally free of natural defects. In order to ensure that foods are never contaminated by even a few insects, rodent hairs, or droppings, etc., we would have to use much larger amounts of chemical pesticides and would thus risk exposing consumers to the potentially greater hazard of increased levels of toxic residues.

Current philosophy holds that it is wiser to permit aesthetically unpleasant but harmless natural defects rather than pouring on more synthetic chemicals. For this reason, the Food and Drug Administration (FDA) has established what it terms **defect action levels**, specifying the maximum limit of contamination at or above which the agency will take legal action to remove the product from the market. It is important to understand that such defect action levels are not *average* levels of contamination—the averages are considerably lower—but represent the *upper limit* of allowable contamination. Defect action levels are set at that point where it is assumed there is no danger to human health. Some examples of existing defect action levels are shown in table 9-1.

Food contaminants that are less visible but more worrisome are the traces of antibiotics (see box 9-1) and growth hormones in meat products and toxic pesticide residues on fruits and vegetables. The issue of hormone-treated meat has been rankling relations between Europeans and major meat-exporting countries (primarily the U.S., Canada, Australia, and New Zealand) since 1989, when the European Community banned imports of meat from animals treated with growth hormones. Such hormones, illegal in Europe, are widely used by American beef producers, administered in the form of slow-release pelleted implants inserted under the skin on the backside of the earflap when cattle enter the feedlot and again

Table 9-1 Examples of Food Defect Action Levels

Product	Defect	Action Level
Apricots, canned	Insect filth	Average of 2% or more by count insect-infested or insect-damaged
Beets, canned	Rot	Average of 5% or more by weight of pieces with dry rot
Broccoli, frozen	Insects and mites	Average of 60 or more aphids, thrips, and/or mites per 100 grams
Cherries, maraschino	Insect filth	Average of over 5% rejects due to maggots
Corn, canned	Insect larvae (corn ear worms, corn borers)	Two or more 3 mm or longer larvae, cast skins or cast skin fragments of corn ear worm or corn borer, the aggregate length exceeding 12 mm in 24 pounds
Cornmeal	Rodent filth	Average of 1 or more rodent hairs per 25 grams or average of 1 or more rodent excreta fragment per 50 grams
Curry powder	Insect filth	Average of more than 100 insect fragments per 25 grams
	Rodent filth	Average of more than 4 rodent hairs per 25 grams
Macaroni and noodle products	Insect filth	Average of 225 insect fragments or more per 225 grams in 6 or more subsamples
	Rodent filth	Average of 4.5 rodent hairs or more per 225 grams in 6 or more subsamples
Olives, pitted	Pits	Average of more than 1.3% by count of olives with whole pits and/or pit fragments 2 mm or longer measured in the longest dimension
Peanuts, shelled	Multiple defects	Average of more than 5% of kernels by count are rejects (insect-infested, moldy, rancid, otherwise decomposed, and dirty)
Peanut butter	Insect filth	Average of 30 or more insect fragments per 100 grams
	Rodent filth	Average of 1 or more rodent hairs per 100 grams
	Grit	Gritty taste and water insoluble inorganic residue is more than 25 mg per 100 grams
Tomatoes, canned	Drosophila fly	Average of 10 fly eggs per 500 grams; or 5 fly eggs and 1 maggot per 500 grams; or 2 maggots per 500 grams

halfway through the 100-day fattening period prior to slaughter. Approximately 90% of feedlot cattle in the U.S. are implanted, as are a smaller percentage of sheep (neither hogs nor chickens receive hormone implants). Beef producers have used hormones for decades to hasten weight gain of their animals while using less feed, thereby adding over $80 in extra profit per animal, and to produce meat with a lower fat content. Europeans justify their prohibition of hormone-treated meat as a consumer safety measure, insisting that lingering traces of hormones in meat at the time of slaughter could pose human health risks. Although some U.S. scientists agree that hormone-tainted beef presents an increased cancer risk to consumers, the FDA has approved the use of hormones in livestock, arguing that numerous studies indicate negligible health risks. Regulators in the U.S. and Europe continue to hold opposite views on the safety of hormone-treated meat, but a compromise of sorts on the trade dispute was reached in 2009. Negotiations that year concluded with a 4-year deal in which the U.S. agreed to allow the European Union to retain its ban on hormone-containing beef in return for the EU consenting to accept duty-free imports of organic beef free of hormones.

Early in 1994 a genetically engineered growth hormone intended to boost milk production was introduced onto the market by Monsanto under the trade name Posilac, a move that provoked an outpouring of concern from some consumer groups (as well as from some dairy farmers worried about milk surpluses and falling prices). The hormone, alternatively known as **rBGH** (recombinant Bovine Growth Hormone) or **rBST** (recombinant Bovine Somatotropin), is injected into dairy cows every 14 days, resulting in a 10–20% increase in milk production. After extensive studies evaluating its safety and efficacy, the FDA approved sale of the hormone, making rBGH the first commercially important product of agricultural biotechnology to be incorporated into the nation's food supply.

In spite of FDA assurances that there is no human health risk associated with rBGH, many consumer groups remain wary. Critics charge that, by raising milk output per cow, the hormone puts additional stress on the animals, increasing the likelihood of udder infections, foot problems, and injection site reactions. For these reasons, in 1999 the Canadian regulatory agency for food safety, Health Canada, prohibited the sale of rBST; by

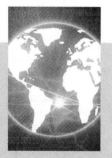

· · · · · · · *9–1* · · · · · · ·

Abusing a Valuable Resource

Antibiotics represent one of the great medical advances of the 20th century, relegating once-dreaded bacterial killers to the status of easily curable diseases. Unfortunately, overuse and misuse of these valuable pharmaceutical resources have contributed to the build-up of antibiotic resistance in an ever-increasing number of bacterial populations. Blame for this is widely shared by physicians and patients alike. For years microbiologists have criticized the overuse of antibiotics to treat conditions that would soon be resolved without medication, as well as the misuse of these drugs against viral infections or other health problems that don't respond to antibiotic treatment. The need for more judicious medical use of antibiotics in the face of increasing bacterial resistance is now generally accepted by doctors and by the general public, but few people are aware that another source of microbial exposure to these drugs is posing a major human health threat.

For decades the widespread use of antibiotics in the livestock and poultry industries has sparked bitter controversy between agro-pharmaceutical interests and food safety experts. According to the Union of Concerned Scientists, 70% of the antibiotics used in the United States are targeted to poultry, pork, and beef production. Of this amount, about one-fifth is administered for veterinary purposes, to treat animal diseases, while the remainder is incorporated in subtherapeutic amounts into animal feed and trough water to enhance growth and weight gain, as well as to maintain the health of animals living in overcrowded, unsanitary conditions. Both of these uses have the potential for fostering development of antibiotic resistance among bacterial populations, yet livestock producers have vigorously—and successfully—lobbied against regulatory controls. Claiming that antibiotic use is necessary to produce affordable meat and poultry, industry spokespersons long argued that no scientific evidence exists to show the practice has adversely affected human health. That argument can no longer be made; since the late 1990s, irrefutable proof of humans infected with antibiotic-resistant foodborne microbes has been traced to drug-resistant bacterial strains in animals.

In 1998, CDC researchers reported that one strain of *Salmonella* (DT104) had acquired resistance to five of the antibiotics commonly used against it: ampicillin, chloramphenicol, streptomycin, tetracycline, and the sulfonamides. In just seven years—from 1989 to 1996—the percentage of DT104 samples testing positive for multidrug resistance climbed from 0.6 to 34%, even though the number of human *Salmonella* infections remained relatively constant during the same time period. Although the majority of *Salmonella* infections run their course without need for medication, a small percentage (3–10%) result in bacteremia (i.e., bacteria invading the bloodstream), requiring antibiotic treatment. If the causative pathogens fail to respond to such treatment, the situation could become life-threatening (Glynn et al., 1998).

Further evidence of a cause-and-effect relationship between human disease and antibiotic use in meat production made news in 1999 when resistant bacterial isolates from people stricken with *Campylobacter* food poisoning were shown to have the same "DNA fingerprint" as *Campylobacter* strains found on chicken products. Currently among the most common forms of bacterial food poisoning in the U.S., *Campylobacter* infections are generally treated, when necessary, with fluoroquinolone antibiotics such as ciprofloxacin. In the early 1990s, fluoroquinolone-resistant *Campylobacter* was quite rare—slightly over 1% of all reported cases—and virtually all of these were acquired during foreign travel. In 1995, the use of fluoroquinolones to treat respiratory infections in poultry flocks was approved by the FDA over the vigorous objections of CDC scientists concerned about the wide-scale exposure of chickens to a relatively new human drug that the medical community hoped would remain effective for many years. As the CDC had feared, within a year after licensure of fluoroquinolone for use on poultry farms, cases of domestically acquired ciprofloxacin-resistant human *Campylobacter* infections began to climb in the U.S., reaching 14% by 1998 (Smith et al., 1999). By 2001, researchers sampling meats from local supermarkets reported finding antibiotic-resistant bacteria in packages of chicken, beef, and pork. These pathogens could still be found 1–2 weeks later in the intestines of consumers who ate them. If they had been present in sufficient numbers to induce illness, treatment with antibiotics would have been useless. Since pharmaceutical companies have no new wonder drugs currently in the pipeline, health authorities are increasingly worried that the livestock industry's profligate use of the same antibiotics needed to treat human disease is a reckless squandering of a vital resource (of the 17 classes of antibiotics used as growth promoters in food animals, 6 are also used to treat human diseases).

In response to increasingly vocal concerns being expressed by medical authorities, environmental organizations, and concerned consumers, some segments of the food industry have begun to take action on this issue. In 2001 McDonald's Corporation told its poultry suppliers to phase out use of fluoroquinolones in the chickens it purchased from them; the following year, without any fanfare, two large poultry producers began reducing the use of growth-promoting antibiotics. Most significant, however, was McDonald's declaration in June 2003 that it was calling on its direct suppliers worldwide to phase out use of all animal growth-promoting antibiotics that are also used in human medicine; indirect suppliers are similarly encouraged to eliminate these drugs and to reduce other antibiotic usage as well (McDonald's Corporation, 2003). Certification of compliance with the new standards must be provided each year and suppliers must maintain records of antibiotic use and make them available for company audit and review. The importance of McDonald's policy shift reflects the company's marketplace dominance; as the world's largest fast-food chain, McDonald's uses over 2.5 billion pounds of meat and chicken annually. When McDonald's speaks, meat producers listen. The impact has been greatest in the poultry industry, where suppliers such as Tyson Foods directly control the stages of production where decisions about antibiotic use are made. Tyson supported McDonald's decision, as did Cargill, another major supplier, and both promised vigorous efforts to comply with the new standards. Whether other fast-food chains decide to follow McDonald's lead remains to be seen; several have said such action is being considered.

At the governmental level, FDA's stance is that the use of antibiotics in farm animals is both safe and effective; nevertheless, agency officials concur that "less is better." The situation is quite different in Europe, where increasing numbers of human illnesses blamed on use of antibiotics for meat production led to a ban on this practice by the European Union; the World Health Organization also has recommended a phaseout. Although a number of consumer groups and some members of Congress have repeatedly called for a prohibition on all nontherapeutic antibiotic use in U.S. farm animals, political pressures and seeming public indifference have stymied passage of legislation requiring such action.

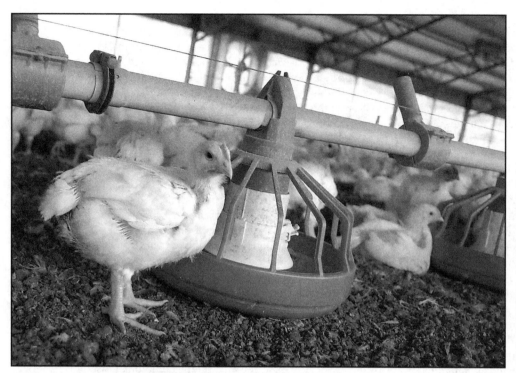

Mounting evidence indicates that routine use of antibiotics in the poultry and livestock industries is creating antibiotic-resistant bacteria that also cause disease in humans. Concern over the health implications prompted McDonald's Corp. to ask its meat suppliers to phase out use of growth-promoting antibiotics that also are used in human medicine. [*AP Photo/April L. Brown*]

2000 most of the European countries, as well as Japan, Australia, and New Zealand had done likewise. In 1998, after examining new evidence, the Joint Expert Committee on Food Additives, comprised of representatives of the United Nations' Food and Agriculture Organization (FAO) and World Health Organization (WHO), reconfirmed its position that use of rBGH is safe. Nevertheless, the United States remains the only major country to permit use of the hormone, with the FDA still insisting that there's no discernible difference in milk from rBST-treated cows and those that have not received the hormone. Many American consumers remain unconvinced, and demand in the U.S. for organically produced, rBST-free milk has increased markedly since the introduction of Posilac (Nestle, 2003; FAO, 1998). Because of the continuing widespread negative public attitude toward rBST, several major U.S. food retailers, including Walmart, Kroger, Costco, and Safeway, have chosen not to carry milk produced with rBST.

Pesticide residues in food occur when crops are sprayed directly or when livestock consume pesticide-contaminated fodder, traces of which can then be translocated into meat, eggs, or milk. EPA has established **tolerance levels** for all pesticides used on food crops representing the maximum quantity of a pesticide residue allowable on a raw agricultural commodity. Such tolerances constitute the federal government's principle means of regulating pesticide residues in food. These levels are based on results of field trials performed by pesticide manufacturers and reflect the maximum residue

concentrations likely when farm chemicals are applied properly. In essence, tolerance levels are set on the basis of good agricultural practices and not on considerations of human health.

In 1987 the National Research Council (NRC) of the National Academy of Sciences published an alarming report estimating a significant increase in cancer mortality among American consumers due to ingestion of certain pesticide residues on food, even when the amounts of such chemicals are within the established tolerance levels. A subsequent NRC report issued in 1993 questioned whether existing tolerance levels, established on the basis of estimated adult food consumption patterns, were sufficiently protective of children's health. The report pointed out that youngsters consume more chemically tainted fruit in relation to their body size than do adults and, because of their rapid rate of growth and development, they are more vulnerable than older people to toxic chemicals in food (NRC, 1993; 1987). These concerns led Congress to include a provision in the 1996 **Food Quality Protection Act** that EPA consider the consumption habits and unique vulnerability of children when setting tolerance levels and must be able to guarantee that any tolerance level approved by the agency is safe for children (Merrill, 1997).

While the findings contained in the 1987 and 1993 NRC reports demonstrate the need for strict controls, the National Academy of Sciences contends that under the current U.S. regulatory system, pesticide residues on food pose a negligible health threat to the general population. In a 1996 report, the NRC pointed out that although traces of pesticide residues are detectable in food and water virtually everywhere, the amounts present on U.S.-grown crops are typically very low and do not present a significant risk of cancer or other health problems. In recent years both the concentration of pesticide residues in food and the frequency with which they are found has steadily declined, due in part to the pesticide industry's shift to chemicals that break down quickly and hence are no longer present at harvest time. Since many of the newer chemicals are effective against pests at much lower concentrations than those applied in years past, the absolute quantity of residues present on pesticide-treated crops today is one-tenth or less that found on crops sprayed with the chemicals formerly used in U.S. agriculture (NRC, 2000; 1996).

Nevertheless, public perception of risk has given added impetus to a burgeoning consumer demand for organically grown food. Although the health benefits of organic foods have yet to be scientifically proven, organic foods represent the most rapidly growing segment of the food market. While they still represent a small portion of total U.S. food production, organic foods are increasing their market share by 20% annually (in contrast to a 1% per year growth rate for conventionally grown foods). In response to a request by organic farmers that Congress establish standards for designating food as organic, the federal government several years ago promulgated a list of practices that would be regarded as incompatible with the "organically grown" label. In addition to requiring chemical-free production methods, the new standards also prohibit application of the term "organic" to animals fed antibiotics, to any genetically modified foods, foods that have been irradiated, or those grown in soils amended with sewage sludge ("biosolids"). Incorporating the latter three criteria provoked a great deal of controversy; they were not included in the rules as originally proposed but were subsequently added in response to an unprecedented deluge of negative public comments following publication of the proposed, less restrictive criteria (Nestle, 2003).

Globalization of the marketplace poses additional challenges to food safety regulators. In recent years numerous food imports have been halted at the border due to unacceptable levels of contamination. Among the problems identified have been *Salmonella* bacteria in black pepper and other spices from India; unacceptable levels of filth on Mexican candies, cheese, fruit juice, and chili peppers; pesticide residues on fresh produce from the Dominican Republic; and illegal veterinary drug residues in Chinese farm-raised fish. As free-trade agreements open up borders to a worldwide food marketplace, food imports continue to soar; however, without a corresponding increase in funding for FDA inspectors at bor-

der crossings it will be increasingly difficult to ensure that the food Americans eat is relatively free from contaminants (Martin and Palmer, 2007; Barboza, 2007b).

FOOD ADDITIVES

More controversial than the accidental, often unavoidable, food contaminants are the approximately 2,800 food **additives**, substances intentionally added to food to modify its taste, color, texture, nutritive value, appearance, resistance to deterioration, and so forth. The years since the end of World War II witnessed explosive growth of the food chemical industry, as food processors responded to public demand (or occasionally created public demand) by promoting a host of new products—convenience foods, frozen foods, dehydrated foods, ethnic foods, low-calorie foods. Many of these products could not exist in a world free of additives. Nevertheless, a great many people are automatically suspicious of additives with long, often unpronounceable names. However, there's nothing inherently evil about using additives, provided that the chemical in question has no adverse effect on human health and performs a useful function.

Many substances that can technically be termed "additives" have been in use for thousands of years—sugar, salt, and spices are just a few examples. Some additives come from natural sources; lecithin, derived from soybeans or corn, is used as an emulsifier to achieve the desired consistency in products such as cake mixes, non-dairy creamers, salad dressings, ice cream, and chocolate milk. Other food additives are factory made but are chemically the same as their natural analogs. The synthetic vitamins and minerals added to foods to improve nutritive value are examples of these; identical in chemical composition to natural vitamins and minerals found in food, they are preferentially used because they are less expensive and more readily available. Such synthetic additives frequently are more concentrated, more pure, and of a more consistent quality than some of their counterparts in the natural world. The use of synthetic vitamins and minerals in food over the past half century has had a profound impact on public health in the United States, virtually eliminating certain deficiency diseases that formerly afflicted large numbers of Americans. The addition of vitamin D to milk, iodine to table salt, and niacin to bread has relegated rickets, goiter, and pellagra, respectively, to nearly nonexistent status in this country. Other additives perform such useful functions as retarding spoilage, preventing fats from turning rancid, retaining moisture in some foods and keeping it out of others.

Most people don't quarrel about additives used for these purposes. What does concern many scientists and consumers is that a significant number of chemicals are

Table 9-2   Common Types of Food Additives

Group	Purpose	Examples
Antioxidants	• prevent fats from turning rancid and fresh fruits from darkening during processing • minimize damage to some amino acids and loss of some vitamins	BHA, BHT, propylgallate
Bleaching Agents	• whiten and age flour	benzoyl peroxide, chlorine, nitrosyl chloride
Emulsifiers	• to disperse one liquid in another • to improve quality and uniformity of texture	lecithin, mono-and diglycerides, sorbitan monostea-rate, polysorbates
Acidulants	• maintain acid-alkali balance in jams, soft drinks, vegetables, etc., to keep them from being too sour	sodium bicarbonate, citric acid, lactic acid, phosphoric acid
Humectants	• maintain moisture in foods such as shredded coconut, marshmallows, and candies	sorbitol, glycerol, propylene glycol
Anti-caking compounds	• keep salts and powdered foods free-flowing	calcium or magnesium silicate, magnesium carbonate, tricalcium phosphate, sodium aluminosilicate
Preservatives	• control growth of spoilage organisms	sodium propionate, sodium benzoate, propionic acid
Stabilizers	• provide proper texture and consistency to ice cream, cheese spreads, salad dressings, syrups	gum arabic, guar gum, carrageenan, methyl cellulose, agar-agar

used as food additives for purely cosmetic purposes—and many of these have been shown to be toxic, carcinogenic, or both.

Until 1958, food processors wishing to use a new additive were free to do so unless the FDA could prove that it was harmful to human health. With the passage of the Food Additives Amendment to the Food, Drug, and Cosmetic Act in that year, the situation was reversed: the manufacturer of any proposed food additive or new food-contact chemical (e.g., packaging materials, equipment liners) now has to satisfy the FDA that the product is safe before it can be approved for use. Proof of safety must include such considerations as: (1) the amount of the additive that is likely to be consumed along with the food product, (2) the cumulative effect of ingesting small amounts of the additive over a long period of time, and (3) the potential for the additive to act as a toxin or a carcinogen when consumed by humans or animals (Foulke, 1993). Approval can be rescinded by the FDA at any time if new information indicates that the additive is unsafe.

While protection of public health is the main intent of the Food Additives Amendment, the law is also designed to prevent consumer fraud by prohibiting the use of preservatives that make foods look fresher than they really are. A case in point is the regulation forbidding the use of sulfites on meats, since these restore the red color, deceptively lending a just-slaughtered appearance to a variety of meat products. On the other hand, sodium nitrite, another additive recognized for its ability to "fix" the red color of fresh meats, can legally be added to meat, fish, and poultry because its primary purpose is to act as a preservative, deterring both spoilage and botulism, a

deadly disease caused by the presence of a bacterial toxin. Because it is now known that nitrites can react with other compounds in food to produce **nitrosamines**, substances known to be carcinogenic, food processors wishing to use the additive must take precautionary measures to severely limit nitrosamine formation (Foulke, 1993).

Undoubtedly the section of the Food Additives Amendment that has generated the most heated controversy is the **Delaney Clause**, which flatly prohibits the use in food of any ingredient shown to cause cancer in animals or humans. (People who question why the FDA bans certain moderately carcinogenic food dyes yet takes no action against cigarettes have to be reminded that the Delaney Clause pertains solely to carcinogenic food additives, not to carcinogens in general; if a food processor should propose to add cigarette smoke as a flavoring to, say, cured meats, this would undoubtedly be prohibited under the Delaney Clause.) While many environmental groups feel that the Delaney Clause constitutes the public's sole line of defense against the deliberate addition of carcinogens to the nation's food supply, critics charge that the "zero tolerance" standard is unrealistic and an example of regulatory overkill which fails to recognize enormous advances in analytical techniques. Whereas the best efforts at chemical analysis during the 1950s yielded results in the parts per million range, today's monitoring devices routinely detect the presence of chemical residues in the parts per trillion. New evidence for the existence of threshold levels of exposure for at least some carcinogens has added fuel to the debate as well (when the Delaney Clause was enacted in 1958 it was presumed that any amount of exposure to a carcinogen, no matter how small, could result in cancer). The Food Quality Protection Act attempted to address these concerns to a limited extent when it amended the Delaney Clause in 1996 by excluding pesticide residues in processed food from regulation as food additives. The revised mandate now permits EPA to approve a tolerance level for residues of a carcinogenic pesticide so long as the agency determines that doing so presents a "negligible risk" (defined as no more than one cancer death per one million population) to consumers. For all other food additives, the zero-tolerance standard explicit in the Delaney Clause remains intact (Merrill, 1997).

Since many hundreds of food additives were already in widespread use at the time the 1958 amendment was passed, a portion of this legislation exempted such substances from the rigorous safety testing demanded for new additives. Instead, additives already in common usage were designated "generally regarded as safe" and placed on what is referred to as the **GRAS list**. In order to remove a food additive from the GRAS list, the FDA must demonstrate that the substance is harmful. Screening of existing food additives to determine whether they should be placed on the GRAS list was done rather haphazardly, and by the 1970s it was recognized that longtime use is no firm guarantee of safety. More thorough studies of certain substances included on the GRAS list have resulted in removal of such once-common food additives as cyclamates (artificial sweeteners suspected of being carcinogenic); safrole (mutagenic and carcinogenic extract of sassafras root, formerly used to give root beer its characteristic flavor); and a number of coal-tar dyes (long used as food colorings but delisted because they were shown to be carcinogenic or to cause organ damage).

Numerous other additives still on the GRAS list are considered of dubious safety by many researchers, yet remain in use due to lack of conclusive evidence or because of industry pressure on FDA regulators. Critics of current policy insist that food additives require a higher standard of care than other environmental chemicals and shouldn't be used if they present a health risk. They base this judgment on the fact that everyone is exposed to chemicals in food, not only those who voluntarily assume the risk. Varying levels of susceptibility among individuals and the effects of simultaneous exposure to other chemicals, including synergistic effects, have to be taken into consideration. Both MSG (monosodium glutamate), a flavor enhancer that can cause the headache, dizziness, nausea, and facial flushing sometimes referred to as "Chinese Restaurant Syndrome," and a group of sulfur-containing compounds known collectively as "sulfites" or "sulfiting agents," added to certain foods, drugs, and wine to prevent discoloration and spoilage, are examples of food additives that serve a useful purpose and pose no danger to the majority of consumers but which can provoke severe allergic reactions among a sizeable minority of sensitive individuals. Because of the vast processed food market, any miscalculation of risk can have far-reaching implications. Nevertheless, although some health authorities recommend avoiding foods containing nonessential additives (such as artificial colors and flavorings) wherever possible, and the European Union requires that a warning label appear on most foods that contain dyes, little evidence exists at present to indicate that the health of Americans is suffering due to the chemical food additives currently in use.

FOODBORNE DISEASE

Ironically, while questions dealing with the safety of chemical additives or pesticide residues generate most of the public's concern regarding food quality these days, most cases of illness or death due to food involve a number of old-fashioned foodborne diseases commonly referred to as "food poisoning." Food poisoning can result from a variety of causes.

Natural Toxins in Food

The widely prevalent notion that all natural foods are safe and nutritious is a dangerous misconception. There are many common plants, both wild and cultivated, that are poisonous, capable of causing ailments ranging from mild stomach disorders to a quick and painful death. In addition, certain marine fish and shellfish species may contain toxins that induce severe illness or death. Some examples of plants or animals capable of causing a toxic reaction if eaten include the following.

Mushrooms

Mushrooms are a gourmet's delight, provided, of course, that the item in question is a nonpoisonous variety. Unfortunately, there is no simple rule of thumb for distinguishing between wild mushrooms that are safe and those that are not. Although only a relatively few of the thousands of species found in North America are poisonous, they may look very much like nonpoisonous species and frequently even grow together. One of the most poisonous types, the amanitas (one species of which is called the "Death Angel"), grows commonly in "fairy rings" in woods and on lawns. Just one or two bites of these alkaloid-containing amanitas can be fatal to an adult and, in fact, the vast majority of deaths due to mushroom poisoning are caused by these.

Water Hemlock (Cicuta maculata)

Sweet-tasting but deadly, this relative of carrots, parsley, celery, and parsnips (to which it bears a strong resemblance) is the most toxic of all native North American plants. Because it is found throughout the continent, is quite similar in appearance to edible plants for which it is commonly mistaken, and is lethal even in small amounts, water hemlock is responsible for more deaths due to misidentification than is any other plant species. **Cicutoxin**, the poisonous substance in water hemlock, is a neurotoxin present in all parts of the plant and at every stage of development. Concentrations of the toxin are at peak levels in springtime and are highest in the root. In the fall of 1992, a 23-year-old Maine resident died three hours after taking just three bites from the root of a water hemlock plant he had collected in the woods (CDC, 1994b). Children have occasionally suffered fatal poisonings after playing with toy whistles made from the hollow stems of water hemlock. Since there is no antidote for cicutoxin, about 30% of reported poisonings have resulted in the death of the victim.

Castor Bean (Ricinus communis)

This attractive shrub-like plant is commonly grown as an ornamental foundation planting as well as commercially for its oil. The leaves of the plant are only slightly toxic, but the colorful mottled seeds can be deadly, containing a toxin called **ricin**. Children who chew on the seeds experience intense irritation of the mouth and throat, gastroenteritis, extreme thirst, dullness of vision, convulsions, uremia, and death. Only one to three seeds can kill a child; four to eight are generally required to cause fatality in adults.

Jimsonweed (Datura stramonium)

This common weed contains toxic alkaloids in all parts of the plant. The seeds and leaves are especially dangerous; children have been poisoned by sucking nectar from the flowers, eating the seeds, or drinking liquid in which the leaves have been soaked. A very small amount can be fatal to a child.

Ergot (Claviceps purpurea)

This fungus, which frequently infects cereal grains, especially rye, produces a toxic alkaloid, ergotamine, responsible for the serious type of food poisoning known as ergotism or "St. Anthony's Fire." When the fungal sclerotia growing on the rye grain are ground up with flour and subsequently consumed in bread, violent muscle contractions, excruciating pain, vomiting, deafness, blindness, and hallucinations can follow. One type of ergotism is characterized by severe constriction of the blood vessels, development of gangrene, and a painful death. Outbreaks of ergotism resulting in thousands of deaths were common until the 20th century, when the decrease in home milling and institution of quality control in commercial mills reduced the level of flour contamination. Even so, small outbreaks of ergotism are still reported from time to

time. Interestingly, federal controls do not apply to rye grown for the organic foods market (Klein, 1979).

Aflatoxin

Another mycotoxin (fungal poison) already discussed in chapter 6, aflatoxins are produced by the mold *Aspergillus flavus*, which grows on a wide variety of nuts, grains, and peanuts. When consumed, they can cause serious liver damage and are some of the most potent carcinogens known.

Certain Fish and Shellfish

Several different types of food poisoning are associated with eating various marine organisms. **Ciguatera fish poisoning**, responsible for numerous food poisoning outbreaks in Florida and Hawaii, is caused by eating certain large reef-dwelling fish such as barracuda, amberjack, and red snapper containing a potent algal toxin and is one of

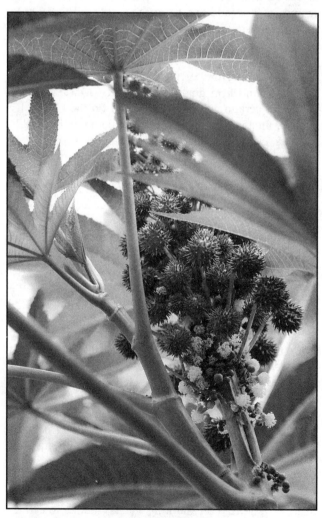

The leaves of the castor bean plant are only slightly toxic, but the colorful seeds contain a toxin called ricin that can be fatal if ingested.

the most common seafood-related illnesses in the United States; worldwide, up to 50,000 cases are reported each year, mainly in countries bordering the Indian Ocean, the Caribbean, and tropical and subtropical regions of the Pacific basin. Ciguatoxin is not destroyed by cooking, nor is its development related to spoilage, so the usual precautions for avoiding foodborne disease don't apply in the case of ciguatera fish poisoning. Symptoms of the disease become evident within 4–48 hours after eating contaminated fish and typically include a reversal of hot and cold sensations, fatigue, itching, and muscle pain, in addition to the usual gastrointestinal problems. In some victims, symptoms may persist for many months after the initial attack.

Scombroid poisoning, generally associated with deep-sea fish such as tuna and mackerel, is caused by ingestion of a toxin produced by certain bacteria acting on the flesh of fish that aren't refrigerated and handled properly after catching. Onset of symptoms—a flushing of the skin, headache, dizziness, a burning sensation in the mouth, hives, and the usual gastrointestinal discomfort—generally occurs very quickly, averaging 1/2 hour after eating. Unfortunately, scombrotoxin cannot be broken down by cooking, freezing, smoking, or canning.

Paralytic Shellfish Poisoning (PSP) results from eating shellfish such as oysters, clams, or scallops contaminated with saxitoxin, a nerve poison produced by microscopic dinoflagellates (algae). PSP is characterized by numbness in the mouth and extremities, gastroenteritis, and in severe cases, difficulty in speaking and walking; such symptoms occur within 30 minutes to 3 hours after eating. In a small percentage of cases death may result. Protection of the public against PSP depends on effective shellfish sanitation and inspection programs in the states where harvesting occurs.

Microbial Contamination

Microbial pathogens are responsible for the vast majority of food poisoning incidents; in the United States alone, the CDC (2010c) estimates that 48 million people each year contract a foodborne illness, 128,000 are hospitalized as a result, and 3,000 die; economic costs to society from microbial foodborne disease are difficult to quantify but have been estimated in the billions of dollars. Since the CDC's estimates are based on a voluntary reporting system, many health experts are convinced that the actual number of cases is considerably higher (Nestle, 2003). Whatever the case, authorities agree the problem is a serious one, as evidenced by numerous well-publicized food-poisoning outbreaks and food recalls in recent years.

Although the toll in human suffering is immense, food-poisoning cases are often misdiagnosed by victims ("I just had a touch of 24-hour flu") or stoically endured (". . . it'll pass in a day or two"). As a result, this entirely preventable malady fails to arouse the public attention it deserves and is perpetuated by widespread carelessness and ignorance of safe food-handling principles. Although food poisoning can, and frequently does, occur with foods prepared and consumed at home, public health officials are most concerned with the potential for large-scale poisoning inherent in the current trend toward more frequent eating outside the home and with the rapid growth and sheer size of the food service industry in the United States today (in 2009 the National Restaurant Association reported that on a typical day in the United States, 945,000 food service establishments serve over 130 million patrons). Institutions such as day care centers and nursing homes, as well as congregate feeding centers for the indigent or homeless, also serve meals to large numbers of people on a daily basis. Diners at these facilities comprise many of those most vulnerable to foodborne disease: the very young, the very old, the ill, and the immunocompromised. As the number of meals eaten away from home increases, the task of preventing foodborne disease grows more challenging.

It should be noted that food *spoilage* is not the same thing as food poisoning. Spoilage involves the decompo-

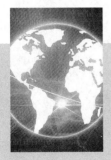

· · · · · · · *9-2* · · · · · · ·

Petting Zoo Perils

Tainted produce and undercooked poultry top the list of "what's to blame?" for symptoms endured by those stricken with *E. coli* poisoning, salmonellosis, and *Campylobacter* infections. However, for a number of victims—the majority of them young children—the cause of gastrointestinal distress has nothing to do with what they *ate*, but rather with what they touched or fondled. Specifically, it has to do with children's love of creatures cute and cuddly and with the proliferation of opportunities for bringing young animals and young people together at petting zoos, carnivals, county fairs, educational exhibits at schools, and a host of other such venues. According to the CDC, public settings like these have been responsible for approximately 100 infectious disease outbreaks reported from 1996 to 2008. In the home environment as well, ill-advised though well-intentioned gifts of newly hatched chicks or baby turtles given to small children present serious risk of acute salmonellosis.

Unfortunately, such problems persist due to widespread lack of understanding among the general public regarding the potential for disease transmission inherent in human-animal interaction—with gastrointestinal illness ranking first and foremost among possible problems. As with more conventional forms of human food poisoning, the fecal-oral route of transmission is responsible for disease outbreaks traced to contact with animals in public settings. While scarcely anyone would deliberately handle animal manure, let alone put it in their mouth, simply petting or holding a calf, lamb, chick, or duckling and subsequently engaging in inadvertent hand-to-mouth contact can have the same ultimate effect. Fecal pathogens are commonly present on animals' hair, fur, skin, and in their saliva; thus, stroking, holding, feeding, or being licked by an animal means a person likely will come in contact with fecal organisms. Nor is the potential for such contact limited directly to the animals themselves—animal bedding, the flooring and sides of animal pens, shoes that have walked through animal confinement areas, water troughs—all are likely to contain microbes shed by infected animals. Pathogens can survive for months or even years in such environments; an *E. coli 0157:H7* outbreak in Ohio sickened 23 people who came into contact with contaminated sawdust while attending a dance held in a barn where animals had been exhibited a week earlier.

The threat of contagion is always present, since animals that appear completely healthy can harbor intestinal pathogens. Animal exhibits present a greater-than-normal risk, however, for several reasons. Among these is the fact that the prevalence of pathogenic microbes is higher in young animals than in older ones—and young animals are the ones most likely to be encountered at petting zoos and other such venues. In addition, the increased stress levels experienced by animals due to confinement, crowding, and unaccustomed handling cause them to shed larger numbers of bacteria than would be the case under less stressful conditions. Finally, even in normal situations, shedding of *E. coli* and *Salmonella* is more prevalent in the late summer and early fall than it is at other times during the year—yet this is the time when traveling exhibits and petting zoos are most common. Added to all these risk factors is the innate behavior of pre-school children whose interactions with baby animals are often accompanied by thumb-sucking, pacifier use, or eating snacks (which they often share with their four-legged friends and which increases the likelihood of subsequent illness). All too frequently the adults supervising such events lack awareness of the inherent disease threat and fail to pay close attention to children's risky behavior, while inadequate or nonexistent handwashing facilities increase the potential for infection.

Certainly the education, enjoyment, and entertainment derived every year by millions of people of all ages through contact with animals in public settings precludes any attempt to limit such opportunities due to fear of possible illness. Nevertheless, awareness of the risk should prompt both parents and those managing such events to take some common-sense precautions. While it will never be possible to eliminate all risk from animal contact, lessons learned from past outbreaks show that infections could be minimized by providing hand sanitizers or well-maintained facilities for visitors to wash their hands with soap and water immediately after leaving animal confinement areas—and to install such facilities at a height accessible to children. Visitors should be prohibited from bringing food into animal areas and toddlers should be closely watched to make sure they don't put anything into their mouths while there. Transition zones between animal/nonanimal areas should be maintained; in several instances outbreaks have occurred when animal displays were located next to farm stands, Christmas tree lots, or a pumpkin patch visited by preschoolers.

Beyond the public venue, parents need to ensure that young children not be allowed to handle baby chicks or other live poultry, nor should turtles and other reptiles be given to children as pets. Even home aquariums may present an infection hazard, as several multidrug-resistant cases of salmonellosis have been linked to contact with contaminated water from home aquariums containing tropical fish. Awareness of potential risk, plus a few basic sanitary precautions, will help to ensure that human-animal contact remains a pleasurable experience and not the prelude for a trip to the doctor's office (Blackmore, 2009; CDC, 2009e).

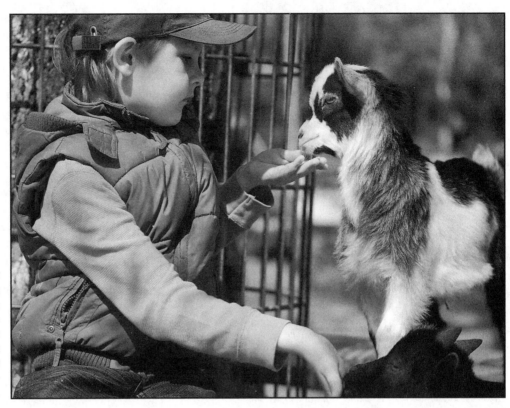

Petting zoos bring together young animals and young children, the result of which may be an unpleasant episode of microbial illness unless parents ensure that children promptly wash their hands after handling the cuddly creatures.

sition of foods due to the action of natural enzymes within food, to chemical reactions between food and containers, or to the activities of certain types of bacteria, fungi, or insects, resulting in unpleasant odors, taste, or appearance of the food. However, spoilage organisms do not produce toxins that would cause human illness if they were consumed, nor does eating food containing such live organisms induce sickness. The same cannot be said of food-poisoning bacteria, whose presence is not betrayed by the appearance, smell, or taste of the food. The old term "ptomaine poisoning" often used in reference to food poisoning is a misnomer—there is no such thing. Ptomaines are foul-smelling chemical compounds produced by bacterial decomposition of proteins. Eating food containing ptomaines will not produce any illness.

The microbial culprits responsible for food poisoning can be grouped into three general categories: bacteria, viruses, and parasites.

Bacteria

Of the various foodborne diseases, the greatest number of outbreaks can be traced to ingestion of food containing certain pathogenic bacteria or bacterial toxins preformed in the food before it was eaten. Bacterial foodborne diseases are classified either as **infections** or **intoxications**, depending on whether illness is caused by consuming large numbers of live organisms or by ingesting preformed bacterial toxins, respectively. The more

common types of bacterial food poisoning have rather similar symptoms: diarrhea, abdominal pain, vomiting, dehydration, prostration, and often fever and chills in the case of bacterial infections (not, however, with intoxications). Onset of such symptoms usually occurs within 1–24 hours after eating the contaminated food, depending on the type of bacteria involved and the amount of food ingested. Examples of foodborne bacterial infections include the following.

Salmonellosis. Often referred to by more descriptive appellations such as "Delhi Belly" or "The Tropical Trots," salmonellosis is one of the most common bacterial foodborne infections in the United States. Although incidence of the disease has been gradually declining since 1996, presumably as a result of a new food safety system imposed on slaughterhouses and meat processing plants in 1997 (see box 9-5), the CDC reports that approximately 40,000 cases of salmonellosis are laboratory-confirmed each year—a figure that the CDC estimates at just 3% of the actual number of illnesses, since most cases are never reported to the National *Salmonella* Surveillance System.

Caused by a number of species of the genus *Salmonella*, the disease is typically associated with eating poultry, meat, or eggs harboring large numbers of the rod-shaped bacterium. Nevertheless, numerous outbreaks have been traced to foods not generally associated with the disease:

Table 9-3 Recent Salmonella Outbreaks

2010

Shell Eggs	*Salmonella* Enteritidis
Frozen Mamey Fruit Pulp	*Salmonella* Typhi (Typhoid Fever)
Alfalfa Sprouts	*Salmonella* Newport
Cheesy Chicken Rice Frozen Entrée	*Salmonella* Chester
Frozen Rodents	*Salmonella* I 4,[5],12i:
Red and Black Pepper/ Italian-Style Meats	*Salmonella* Montevideo
Restaurant Chain A	*Salmonella* Hartford and *Salmonella* Baildon

2009

Alfalfa Sprouts	*Salmonella* Saintpaul
Pistachios	*Salmonella* (multiple types)
Water Frogs	*Salmonella* Typhimurium

2008

Cantaloupes	*Salmonella* Litchfield
Malt-O-Meal Rice/Wheat Cereals	*Salmonella* Agona
Peanut Butter	*Salmonella* Typhimurium
Raw Produce	*Salmonella* Saintpaul

2007

Banquet Pot Pies	*Salmonella* I 4,[5],12:i:
Dry Pet Food	*Salmonella* Schwarzengrund
Peanut Butter	*Salmonella* Tennessee
Veggie Booty	*Salmonella* Wandsworth

2006

Tomatoes	*Salmonella* Typhimurium

Source: CDC, "Salmonella Outbreaks." Accessed Sept. 2010 from www.cdc.gov/salmonella/outbreaks.html

the largest salmonellosis outbreak in U.S. history, affecting an estimated 200,000 people (16,000 laboratory-confirmed cases, many more unreported) in Illinois and several other Midwest states in the spring of 1985, was traced to milk. Although potentially an excellent medium for the growth of *Salmonella* and other foodborne pathogens, milk today is considered one of our safest foods due to pasteurization and high standards of sanitation in the dairy industry; less than 3% of all foodborne disease outbreaks in recent years have been traced to contaminated milk. Alfalfa sprouts tainted with *Salmonella* have caused widespread food-poisoning outbreaks in recent years. Though many people regard raw sprouts as a healthy and nutritious food item, sprouts seeds can be contaminated on the farm with *Salmonella*-tainted water, animal feces, improperly composted manure used as fertilizer, or dirty harvesting or processing machines. The same conditions that promote seed germination are also ideal for the multiplication of *Salmonella* organisms. As a result, government food safety agencies recommend that sprouts always be cooked before eating to reduce the risk of illness (CDC, 2002a).

Another unpleasant surprise has been the emergence since the early 1980s of *Salmonella enteritidis* (SE) infections associated with whole, uncracked eggs. Most recently, during the summer of 2010, thousands of victims across the U.S. were sickened and half a billion eggs recalled due to SE-contaminated eggs traced to five farms in Iowa, all owned by one of the largest egg producers in the country—and the same individual whose eggs were the source of the nation's first SE outbreaks in the 1980s! Contamination occurs when the bacteria are transmitted from infected hens via their ovaries into the developing egg; short of laboratory testing, neither egg producers nor home cooks have any way of identifying which eggs are tainted. It is estimated that one out of every 10,000 eggs (approximately 4.5 million/year) is contaminated. Although the problem was originally confined to the northeastern U.S., it is now nationwide. As a result, today eggs are near the top of the list as prime contributors to food-poisoning outbreaks in the United States. According to federal researchers, each year over 130,000 people in the U.S. are sickened and 30 die from eating *Salmonella*-contaminated eggs. For this reason, much to the dismay of Caesar salad and homemade eggnog lovers, health agencies now strongly advise against the consumption of raw or undercooked eggs—hard-boiled is the only guarantee of safety!

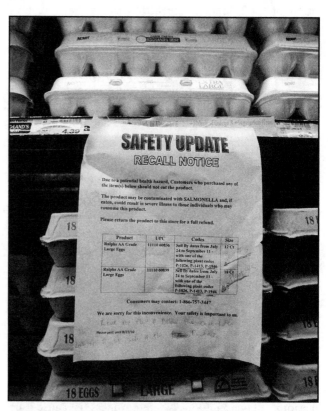

An outbreak of *Salmonella enteritidis* during the summer of 2010 sickened thousands and prompted the recall of about a half billion eggs. [*AP Photo/Reed Saxon*]

In 2007 and again in 2008, *Salmonella* outbreaks traced to tainted peanut butter were reported from 44 states across the United States. Peanut butter is another food seldom associated with food-poisoning problems, since the peanuts are typically roasted at temperatures high enough to kill any bacteria within a few minutes. Subsequent investigations revealed that the problem in both outbreaks involved lack of proper sanitation in the processing plants, with contamination of the product occurring after the final heat treatment but prior to sealing the peanut butter in jars. In each of these situations, mammoth product recalls reminded American consumers that the safety of even our most iconic "comfort foods" can't always be taken for granted (Hoffman, 2007).

Inside the small intestine, colonies of *Salmonella* continue to grow and invade the host tissue, irritating the mucosal lining. Sudden onset of disease symptoms most commonly occurs within 12–24 hours after eating the contaminated food, with 18 hours being the most common time interval; discomfort may persist for several days and some victims may remain carriers for months after all outward symptoms have disappeared, shedding bacteria in their feces and remaining capable of infecting others. Severity of the disease ranges from very mild to very severe, with young children, the elderly, and travelers often the most adversely affected. Among otherwise healthy adults, fatalities due to salmonellosis are rare (victims only wish they were dead!). However, salmonellosis can be life-threatening to the elderly, to patients in hospitals and nursing homes, and to people whose immune systems are compromised. Hundreds of Americans, most of them from one of these highly vulnerable groups, die of salmonellosis each year.

In addition to the obvious short-term effects of the ailment, salmonellosis sufferers may also develop serious chronic disorders as a result of their infection. About 2–3% of victims later contract chronic arthritis, while a much smaller percentage develop painful septic arthritis when the *Salmonella* bacteria invade the joints.

Campylobacter jejuni.   One of several ailments often referred to as "Traveler's Diarrhea" because cases used to be most common among vacationers returning home from abroad, infections caused by *Campylobacter jejuni* are now among the most common forms of bacterial food poisoning in the United States. Like salmonellosis, however, *Campylobacter* incidence is lower than it was a decade ago and for the same reason—improved food safety practices in the facilities that kill and process poultry. *C. jejuni* infections are characterized by high fever and bloody diarrhea, along with the nausea and abdominal pain typical of most foodborne ailments; symptoms generally persist for about a week but may last much longer. Most worrisome is the fact that as many as 10% of sufferers develop serious, long-term complications such as Guillain-Barré syndrome, arthritis, or meningitis. Undercooked chicken or turkey is by far the leading source of *C. jejuni* infections, since the organism is almost always present on poultry carcasses. The marked shift from beef to chicken consumption in the U.S. over the past 30 years has been accompanied by a rapid increase in *Campylobacter* foodborne disease. Other sources of infection include raw clams and other shellfish, inadequately cooked pork, and unpasteurized milk products.

E. coli 0157:H7.   Among the most dangerous foodborne pathogens, this nasty relative of the harmless *E. coli* strains that are normal inhabitants of the human gut was first recognized as a newly emerging public health problem in 1982. Several sporadic outbreaks occurred during the 1980s, but it was only in 1993 that the disease hit the headlines when four children died and hundreds of people became ill after eating hamburgers at several Jack-in-the-Box restaurants in the Pacific Northwest. In late summer 2006, U.S. consumers were warned not to eat bagged fresh spinach after a multistate outbreak of *E. coli 0157:H7* that ultimately resulted in 199 victims sickened, 31 cases of kidney failure, and 3 deaths associated with ready-to-eat spinach. Eventually the contaminated product was traced to one 50-acre California organic farm, packaged in one processing plant during just one production shift, but the entire spinach crop was discarded and sales of spinach continued to suffer for months afterwards. A second *E. coli* outbreak, this time linked to prepackaged lettuce, sickened 80 people in December of the same year. Estimates for the number of *E. coli 0157:H7* infections occurring annually range from 10,000–20,000, resulting in approximately 50–100 deaths.

In recent years a new food safety threat has been emerging in the form of six other rare strains of *E. coli* for which, unlike *E. coli 0157:H7*, the government currently does not require testing by the meat industry. In April 2010 at least 26 people in five U.S. states were sickened when they ate romaine lettuce contaminated with the pathogen *E. coli 0145*; three of the victims suffered kidney failure as a result. Food safety experts are unsure as to how the bacteria were transferred from cattle to fresh produce, but suggest that wild animals could have tracked manure through the fields or that irrigation water may have been tainted with cattle feces. During the summer of 2010, 8,500 pounds of ground beef produced at a Cargill packing plant in Pennsylvania were recalled after three people were infected with *E. coli 026* traced to the contaminated hamburger. Due to the difficulty of testing for and identifying these rare *E. coli* strains, the USDA has been reluctant to ban their presence in beef until it can develop tests for rapid detection, a goal it expects to achieve by the end of 2011 (Neuman, 2010a, 2010b).

E. coli 0157:H7, as well as the other pathogenic *E. coli* strains, normally inhabits the intestinal tract of healthy cattle and is excreted with fecal material. It frequently is found on the udders of cows and thus can be readily transferred to raw milk or to milking equipment. When people come into direct contact with fecal material harboring the pathogen or with fecal-contaminated food or water, infection can result. Unlike most foodborne pathogens that must be present in very large numbers to cause illness, the infective dose for *E. coli 0157:H7* is extraordinarily low—as few as 50 organisms have been shown capable of inducing disease symptoms.

Once ingested, *E. coli 0157:H7* multiplies within the human digestive tract, producing a potent toxin that damages cells of the intestinal lining. These lesions permit blood to leak into the intestines, giving rise to the bloody diarrhea that generally develops within several days of eating contaminated food and is one of the characteristic symptoms of *E. coli* infection. Sufferers may also experience abdominal pains, vomiting, and nausea; only rarely will fever be present, however. In most cases the disease runs its course in 5–10 days and the victim recovers completely without treatment. Administration of antibiotics does nothing to improve a patient's condition and may cause kidney problems. Similarly, the use of antidiarrheal medicine is not advisable. For 2–7% of victims the consequences of infection are much more dangerous. If bacterial toxins pass through the damaged intestinal wall and enter the bloodstream, they travel to the kidneys where they can cause **hemolytic uremic syndrome (HUS)**, a serious ailment in which red blood cells are destroyed, leading to kidney failure and possible death. Such patients often require blood transfusions and kidney dialysis. Even with intensive care, 3–5% of patients who develop HUS die.

In the U.S., undercooked hamburgers were initially identified as the food most often implicated in *E. coli 0157:H7* outbreaks. Accordingly, public health agencies renewed their warnings to commercial food establishments and home cooks to cook beef to 160°F until no traces of pink remain in the center and juices run clear. Since the late 1990s, however, an even larger number of *E. coli* food poisonings have been traced to such seemingly harmless foods as alfalfa sprouts, spinach, lettuce, and unpasteurized fruit juices. In all these cases, poor sanitation at some stage of production or processing allowed food to become contaminated with *E. coli*-contaminated cow manure. Since the foods mentioned above are seldom cooked prior to consumption, live pathogens were present on the food when it was eaten. As a result of these incidents, people at high risk of serious consequences if they contract food poisoning (e.g., young children, the ill or elderly, AIDS patients) are being advised simply to avoid eating sprouts and unpasteurized juice.

Listeriosis. Caused by *Listeria monocytogenes*, a pathogen associated with an extremely wide range of hosts (mammals, birds, fish, ticks, crustaceans) and commonly found in food-processing environments, this disease, once considered rare in human populations, has become a subject of increasing concern in recent years. Listeriosis outbreaks have most frequently been associated with contaminated cold cuts, hot dogs, milk, soft cheeses, and other refrigerated products generally eaten without further cooking. Listeriosis is particularly dangerous in pregnant women, where infection often results in septicemia, miscarriage, or stillbirth. Apparently healthy babies born to infected mothers may develop meningitis within a few days or weeks after birth. Newborns infected with *Listeria* have high fatality rates, as do older victims suffering from diabetes or compromised immune systems (AIDS victims or people receiving corticosteroids, chemotherapy, radiation therapy, etc.).

Listeriosis, fortunately, is much less common than salmonellosis or *C. jejuni* diarrhea; 2,500 people in the U.S. fall victim to listeriosis each year, according to CDC, and of those stricken, approximately 500 die. Recognition that *Listeria*, unlike other microbial pathogens, grows vigorously at low temperatures makes this organism a subject of serious concern to regulatory agencies and to the food industry in general, since refrigeration provides no assurance against bacterial multiplication. The FDA has set a "zero tolerance" requirement for presence of *Listeria* in foods. A major problem in diagnosing listeriosis and in identifying its source is the fact that symptoms

---

Table 9-4 Expert Judgment-Based Estimates of the Incidence of Foodborne Illness and Death by Foods

Food Category	Percent of total cases*	Percent of total deaths**
Produce	29.4	11.9
Seafood	24.8	7.1
Poultry	15.8	16.9
Luncheon and other meats	7.1	17.2
Breads and bakery	4.2	0.6
Dairy	4.1	10.3
Eggs	3.5	7.2
Beverages	3.4	1.1
Beef	3.4	11.3
Pork	3.1	11.4
Game	1.1	5.2
Total	100	100

* Total cases: 12,908,605
** Total deaths: 1,765

Source: Sandra Hoffmann, "Attributing U.S. Foodborne Illness to Food Consumption," *Resources* 172 (Summer 2009). Used with permission of Resources for the Future, www.rff.org.

of the disease may not occur for as long as 90 days after consumption of the contaminated food; even the *average* time from exposure to illness is 30 days and few people can accurately recall what they ate that long ago.

Vibrio vulnificus. First described as a cause of human illness only in 1979, this free-living marine bacterium lives in unpolluted warm ocean waters. It is commonly found along the Gulf Coast in the southeastern U.S. where it may contaminate oysters and other shellfish. Most human illnesses result from consuming raw oysters, since the bacteria are readily killed by cooking. *V. vulnificus* infections are especially dangerous for individuals with preexisting liver disease resulting from alcoholism, viral hepatitis, or other causes, and for those with compromised immune systems (CDC, 1993b). One of the most deadly foodborne diseases, *V. vulnificus* kills approximately half of those infected, with the number of deaths averaging 15–20 annually since 2001. Survivors often suffer excruciating pain, skin loss, kidney failure, and lesions all over their bodies, sometimes necessitating the amputation of arms or legs. Eating raw Gulf Coast oysters is *not* a good idea!

Exhibiting characteristics of both an infection and an intoxication is:

Clostridium perfringens. Because outbreaks of this foodborne ailment are usually associated with quantity food preparation in institutions where meals are often prepared several hours before serving, *C. perfringens* is frequently referred to as "the cafeteria germ." This illness is sometimes categorized as a foodborne infection because live bacteria multiply within the host; alternatively, it may be classified as an intoxication because the disease symptoms are caused by a toxin which is either produced by live bacteria inside the body or is already present in the food at the time of consumption. In either case, very large numbers of bacteria or large amounts of toxin must be ingested to induce illness. Cooked poultry or meat left unrefrigerated for several hours have often been traced as the source of an outbreak (*C. perfringens* is the most common bacterial pathogen associated with poultry-related illness), as have meat pies, casseroles, stews, and gravies. The CDC estimates the incidence of *C. perfringens* food poisoning in the U.S. at about 250,000 cases each year. Disease symptoms generally become evident 8–22 hours after eating; fortunately, *C. perfringens* poisonings are relatively mild and of brief duration, discomfort generally lasting only a day or two.

Among bacterial foodborne intoxications the most important are:

Staphylococcus aureus. Sometimes known as "Roto-Rooter Disease" because of its violent onset, *Staphylococcus* intoxication is caused by a common bacterium pres-

Table 9-5   Microbial Foodborne Ailments

Because many people assume that food poisoning always occurs within a few hours after eating contaminated food, they frequently misdiagnose the cause of their illness or lay the blame on some innocent menu item in the last meal consumed before disease symptoms appear. In fact, most microbial foodborne ailments manifest themselves 24 hours or more after tainted foods are eaten. The elapsed time before a food-poisoning victim feels sick varies depending on the pathogen involved and the amount of contaminated food consumed. Listed below are the time periods typically required for signs of illness to appear for a representative group of foodborne ailments:

Pathogen	Time Frame for Onset of Symptoms
Campylobacter	1 to 10 days (usually 3 to 5 days)
Clostridium botulinum	12 to 36 hours
Clostridium perfringens	8 to 22 hours
E. coli 0157:H7	1 to 10 days (usually 3 to 5 days)
Hepatitis A	1 to 7 weeks (usually 25 days)
Listeria monocytogenes	4 days to 3 months (average 30 days)
Salmonella	6 hours to 3 days (average 18 hours)
Staphylococcus aureus	2 to 7 hours
Vibrio vulnificus	1 to 3 days

ent in pimples, boils, hangnails, wound infections, sputum, and sneeze droplets. People thus constitute the prime source of these organisms, which flourish in such proteinaceous foods as cooked ham, sauces and gravies, chicken salad, egg salad, cream pies and pastries, and so on. Growth of the bacteria within the food medium results in production of an enterotoxin (poison of the intestinal tract) that is not destroyed when the food is cooked. When consumed, the toxin causes irritation and inflammation of the stomach and intestine, resulting in vomiting and diarrhea. Since illness is produced by a poison already in the food at the time of eating rather than by bacterial growth within the victim's intestine, the effects of bacterial intoxication appear more rapidly than do those of an infection. People consuming *Staphylococcus* toxin may experience the sudden onset of vomiting and diarrhea within as little as 30 minutes after eating, although a period of 2–4 hours is more common. As is the case with most foodborne illness, individual differences in susceptibility will result in some people becoming quite ill after eating the tainted food, while others may be unaffected (Koren, 1980). Due to the nature of the symptoms and the fact that the illness is relatively brief, seldom persisting for more than a day or two, sufferers of staph intoxication frequently blame their miseries on "the 24-hour flu" rather than on the true culprit—contaminated food. Deaths from this foodborne disease are extremely rare and most victims recover quickly without any complications.

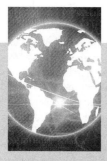

· · · · · · · *9-3* · · · · · · ·

Food Safety Reform

"Don't eat pistachios!" was FDA's unprecedented warning to U.S. consumers in April 2009—unprecedented because never before had the nation's food safety agency taken precautionary action *prior* to a foodborne disease outbreak. Prompted by repeated problems of *Salmonella* contamination in the country's second-largest pistachio processing plant, as well as by complaints from Kraft Foods that nuts shipped to them by the California-based processor often had to be rejected or destroyed due to the presence of *Salmonella*, the FDA, under new leadership, resolved to act preemptively. Shortly after the agency's announcement, the processing company agreed to recall its entire 2008 pistachio crop.

The strong government response to a potential public health threat signaled an abrupt departure from the anti-regulatory stance and lack of attention to food safety issues during the previous eight years and indicated that the FDA's formerly mild warnings to the food industry regarding sanitary lapses were being replaced by a more proactive approach. Such a change in direction is long overdue. While federal regulatory efforts during the latter half of the 20th century resulted in steady progress toward ensuring the safety of Americans' food supply, those gains have leveled off since 2004 and the number of large foodborne disease outbreaks has increased sharply during the past few years (Harris, 2009).

Underlying the current problem is the fact that U.S. food laws are antiquated, totally inadequate in an era of worldwide rapid distribution chains and an increasingly global food industry. The USDA still regulates meat and poultry under laws basically unchanged since 1906, when live inspection of animal carcasses was the main focus of quality control. All other foods—fruits and vegetables, seafood, shell eggs, packaged foods, dairy products—accounting for about 80% of the total U.S. food supply, are under FDA jurisdiction, regulated by a statute enacted in 1938. Adoption of Hazard Analysis and Critical Control Point (HACCP) standards by both USDA and FDA in the 1990s helped improve food product quality (see box 9-5), but broader reform is urgently needed, especially in terms of improved, regular collection and analysis of public data. More accurate and timely information is needed on the incidence of foodborne disease as well—current CDC estimates haven't been revised since 1999 (Hoffman, 2007).

As safety concerns about the American food supply grow with each new product recall, federal efforts to detect problems—or prevent them in the first place—have been severely compromised by tight budgets, an inadequate number of inspectors to handle the overwhelming workload, and by the archaic food safety regulatory system itself. An explosive increase in the volume of imported food products, spurred by consumer demand for year-round availability of fresh fruits and vegetables, has only added to the challenge. Numerous food-poisoning incidents over the past decade have been linked to fresh produce imported from countries where standards of health and hygiene are less rigorous than those in the U.S. Although both the USDA and the FDA maintain the position that imported food should meet the same standards of safety, composition, and labeling as U.S.-produced foods, their ability to ensure that such standards are met are sharply limited. While FDA inspectors can impound suspect imports, they cannot automatically block importation of food shipments from countries whose food safety system is known to be sub-standard (USDA can do so). FDA officials are not permitted to inspect foreign processing facilities and are not allowed to travel abroad to investigate an ongoing food poisoning outbreak unless invited to do so by the host government (NRC, 1998).

For years, the obvious need to overhaul the U.S. food safety system has been widely acknowledged by lawmakers and consumer groups. The food industry itself agrees that fundamental changes are needed, especially in light of the enormous financial burden food recalls are imposing on both growers and food processors. "The devil is in the details," however, and federal officials have been arguing since the 1980s about how to solve the problem. By late 2009, however, broad bipartisan support for meaningful reform raised hopes for passage of historic food safety reform. That year, the House of Representatives, by a wide margin, passed legislation incorporating many of the changes long-sought by consumer and health groups; several months later a similar bill emerged from a key Senate committee. In late November 2010, the Senate passed the bill, known as the Food Safety Modernization Act, by a 73 to 25 vote. In December 2010 the full Congress passed this legislation and it was signed into law in January 2011, though many of its most important provisions will only go into effect gradually over the next few years.

Among the most important provisions included in the legislation (focused exclusively on the FDA, since the USDA has long enjoyed stronger regulations) is a requirement for more frequent inspections of food-processing plants. Rather than visiting facilities just once per decade or more as has often been the case in recent years, the bill requires that processing plants deemed "high-risk" (i.e., facilities with a history of past problems or those that handle items that are inherently vulnerable to contamination) be inspected every 6–12 months; those of lower-risk (i.e., those handling dry packaged products with no history of problems), every 18–24 months. Another major change gives the FDA authority to order the recall of tainted food, rather than having to persuade producers to act voluntarily. The legislation increases inspection requirements for food imports, requires that processing plant records be made available to inspectors, and mandates that food manufacturers develop and implement proactive safety plans to prevent problems before they occur. The FDA also will be required to devise a system for tracing foods throughout the entire chain of production and distribution, so that the source of any foodborne disease outbreak can be quickly identified.

The new legislation does not solve all food safety problems; some advocates of reform argue that the FDA should be split into two agencies, with one working exclusively for consumers and food producers. Fragmentation of oversight among a number of different federal and state agencies will continue to impair the efficiency of food safety programs, while the need for significantly increased funding to implement the mandated reforms will be a perennial issue. Nevertheless, hopes are brighter now than they have been for decades that the drastic reforms essential for assuring Americans that the food on their table is safe to eat will soon become reality.

Botulism. The most serious of all bacterial food-borne diseases, botulism is caused by the spore-forming soil bacterium *Clostridium botulinum*, which, growing under anaerobic conditions, produces a deadly neurotoxin, the most poisonous substance known. Outbreaks of botulism have been most frequently associated with home-canned, low-acid foods such as beans, corn, beets, spinach, and mushrooms. This is because many home canners fail to realize that a long processing time (or a shorter time at high pressure in a pressure cooker) is necessary in order to kill the heat-resistant bacterial spores. If the spores survive, they can germinate and, in the absence of oxygen, multiply within the food medium, producing the deadly poison. If food contaminated with the botulism toxin is boiled for 15–20 minutes, the poison will be destroyed, but all too frequently such food is eaten uncooked or only briefly warmed, with disastrous results.

Commercially processed foods, mostly smoked fish or vacuum-packed items, occasionally have been identified as the cause of botulism outbreaks, as have some highly atypical sources such as commercially bottled carrot juice (CDC, 2006a). In the fall of 1983, one of the worst botulism outbreaks in U.S. history resulted in the hospitalization of 28 victims (one of whom subsequently died) who had eaten "patty melt" sandwiches at a restaurant in Peoria, Illinois. Surprised investigators ultimately identified sautéed onions as the cause of the problem.

Contaminated with *C. botulinum* spores from the soil in which they grew, the onions were fried in margarine, which provided a protective air-free shield for germinating bacteria. The bacteria proceeded to multiply in the incubating temperatures provided by the warming tray in the restaurant kitchen. By the time the onions were consumed many hours later, enough of the deadly *botulinum* toxin had been formed to cause the disease outbreak. In an unrelated incident in Baton Rouge, Louisiana, the following year, a restaurant patron was stricken with botulism after eating a foil-wrapped baked potato, warmed up from the previous day. The foil wrapping had provided the anaerobic conditions that permitted growth of bacterial spores on the potato skin, while remaining at room temperature overnight allowed the organism to multiply and produce the toxin (Miller, 1984).

Botulism is first evidenced by the usual gastrointestinal distress, which generally appears within 12–36 hours, followed by the onset of such neurological symptoms as double vision, stammering, and difficulty in breathing. If untreated, botulism can result in death due to respiratory paralysis. Another manifestation of the disease that has now become the most common form of human botulism in the United States affects only children under one year of age and is referred to as "infant botulism." This condition can occur when babies are fed honey (or when infant pacifiers are dipped in honey) containing *C. botulinum* spores. When these spores germinate inside the baby's intestinal tract, they release a nerve poison that may cause a weakening of the infant's muscles, resulting in a condition called "floppy baby." Other symptoms of infant botulism include excessive drooling, difficulty in swallowing, droopy eyelids, lack of facial expression, weak cry, constipation, and sometimes respiratory arrest. The condition often requires a lengthy period of hospitalization. Because infant botulism can be provoked by as few as 10–100 *C. botulinum* spores, parents are advised never to feed babies honey (Tarr and Doyle, 1996).

Viruses

Since viruses are unable to multiply outside a living host cell, these pathogens do not increase in number when they are introduced into food materials. Virus-contaminated foods simply serve as a route of transmission—a means by which virus particles can be transported from one host to another. Nevertheless, because the infectious dose needed to cause a viral disease is thought to be quite small, perhaps as low as 10–100 particles, viruses should never be allowed to contaminate food in the first place. Because the viruses associated with foodborne illness are of fecal origin, poor hygienic practices on the part of food handlers or food contact with sewage-polluted water are the most frequent causes of outbreaks. Since viruses are not utilizing the food as a growth medium, *any* type of food is a potential reservoir (i.e., pathogenic foodborne viruses, unlike bacteria, do not have any particular nutritional requirements for survival and hence are not restricted to certain "potentially hazardous foods"). Two of the more prevalent foodborne illnesses of viral origin are:

Noroviruses. Formerly called "Norwalk-like viruses," noroviruses cause more cases of acute gastroenteritis—about 23 million annually—than any other foodborne pathogen. As with *Staphylococcus* intoxication, victims often attribute the sudden and violent onset of nausea, profuse vomiting, cramps, and diarrhea to "stomach flu." Low-grade fever, chills, headache, muscle pains, and a general malaise also can occur. Fortunately, the illness generally lasts only a day or two and has no long-term health consequences. Fecal contamination of food or water is the primary means of transmission, with salads and shellfish the foods most often implicated in outbreaks, particularly when consumed raw or undercooked (Pierson and Corlett, 1992). Highly contagious, noroviruses can spread easily from person-to-person through direct contact (e.g., via airborne particles of vomitus) or by hand-to-mouth contact with virus-contaminated objects such as doorknobs. In recent years the cruise ship industry has been plagued by repeated norovirus outbreaks, demonstrating the environmental persistence of

the organism and the difficulty of controlling it through routine sanitary measures (CDC, 2002b).

Hepatitis A (HAV).   Most commonly associated with the consumption of raw clams or oysters harvested from sewage-tainted coastal waters, hepatitis A outbreaks also have been traced to foods as diverse as glazed doughnuts, strawberry sauce, sandwiches, orange juice, and salads. Uncooked green onions were identified as the cause of the United States' largest-ever outbreak of HAV in the fall of 2003, when over 550 patrons of a Chi-Chi's restaurant in western Pennsylvania were sickened and three died. Symptoms of the disease, which include jaundice (an indication of liver infection) as well as the usual gastrointestinal distress, generally don't appear until 10–50 days after eating the contaminated food. An infection typically persists for weeks or even months, and can, in some cases, lead to permanent liver damage.

An individual suffering from HAV can easily transmit the virus to others if he or she isn't conscientious about good hygienic practices, since the virus is shed in urine and feces. A victim is most contagious 10–14 days before the onset of disease symptoms and remains infectious until about a week after jaundice appears; thus rigorous adherence to routine hand-washing practices is of critical importance in preventing the transmission of HAV. A number of hepatitis A outbreaks have been attributed to direct person-food-person transmission, when an infected food handler failed to wash his/her hands after using the toilet, subsequently touched food that received no further cooking, and then served it to a customer (Applied Foodservice Sanitation, 1985). Although this was initially suspected as the cause of Pennsylvania's HAV outbreak, traceback investigations revealed that contamination of the onions likely occurred due to contact with HAV-infected fieldworkers or HAV-polluted water on the farm in Mexico where the onions were grown and processed prior to shipment (CDC, 2003a).

Parasites

Certain parasitic protozoan diseases such as amoebic dysentery or giardiasis are typically associated with ingestion of sewage-contaminated drinking water but have been known to occur when infected food service workers transmitted the microbes to food as a result of faulty hand-washing practices. Certain parasitic roundworm infections can occur when untreated sewage ("nightsoil") containing worm eggs is used to fertilize certain vegetable crops. If such produce is consumed raw, the eggs subsequently hatch inside the human host and perpetuate the cycle of infection. Other sources of helminthic (i.e., worm) foodborne ailments include the consumption of raw or undercooked fish. In recent years the United States has witnessed a small but increasing number of foodborne helminthic ailments traced to the growing popularity of ethnic specialties such as *sushi* or *ceviche*. Tapeworm infections are the most commonly reported problems, occurring predominantly along the West Coast where most victims admit to having eaten raw fish, mainly salmon. Symptoms of tapeworm infections, as well as time of onset, vary greatly from one person to another: some victims report experiencing severe cramps, nausea, and diarrhea almost immediately after eating; others may not develop symptoms for weeks or months. However, most victims experience no symptoms at all and only realize they have an infection when they pass the tapeworm, or segments of it, in their stool. Tapeworm infections can be eradicated with drugs, but roundworm infections (anisakiasis) are much more serious since there is no effective medication available. Such infections are very painful and may require surgery to remove the parasite. Consumers can easily avoid such problems simply by thoroughly cooking fish until it is flaky (internal temperature should be at 145°F for five minutes) or by freezing it at –4°F for 3–5 days before eating in order to kill the worms.

Trichinellosis, another foodborne illness caused by a parasitic roundworm, *Trichinella spiralis*, results primarily from the consumption of raw or undercooked meat containing encysted larvae of the pathogen. Inside the human host, larvae mature into adult worms and burrow into the intestinal wall, producing new larvae that travel via the circulatory system to muscle tissue. There they embed themselves and produce the typical symptoms of foodborne disease. Until recently, most cases of trichinellosis were associated with consumption of undercooked pork, a result of foraging pigs' propensity to eat rodents or other wildlife infected with *Trichinella*. Today the presence of the parasite in pork is much less common than it was years ago, thanks in part to prohibitions on feeding uncooked garbage to hogs—until the late 1940s a common practice that perpetuated the cycle of reinfection.

More recent changes in commercial swine production practices have also had an impact in reducing the incidence of pork-associated trichinellosis. Researchers have found that hogs raised in confinement almost always test parasite-free, while free-range hogs that spend time out-of-doors where they can interact with moist soil, rats, and other wildlife occasionally harbor disease-causing bacteria and parasites, including *Trichinella* (McWilliams, 2009).

Within the past decade, the epidemiology of trichinellosis has been changing, with more cases now being linked to meats other than pork, particularly bear meat and other wild game. Because *Trichinella* larvae are killed by high temperatures, the surest way to prevent trichinosis is always to cook pork, bear, venison, and other game meat until it is well done (160°F). Hunters and consumers of game meat also need to know that while *Trichinella* in pork is killed by exposure to 30 days or more of below-freezing temperatures, freezing does *not* kill all the species of *Trichinella* larvae found in wild game—thorough cooking is the only assurance of safety (Montgomery et al., 2009)

PREVENTING FOODBORNE DISEASE

> You won't be surprised that diseases are innumerable—count the cooks.
> —Seneca (1st century AD)

Microbial contamination of foods can occur at any time from the production of food in field or feedlot right up to preparation and serving of the meal. Thus strict adherence to principles of food sanitation are essential at every step from production to processing, transportation, storage, preparation, and service if food-poisoning outbreaks are to be avoided.

In theory, any food can be a route of transmission for foodborne disease. However, some foods are implicated in food-poisoning outbreaks much more frequently than others and are therefore designated by the U.S. Public Health Service as **potentially hazardous foods**—those that are capable of supporting rapid and progressive growth of infectious or toxigenic microbes. Most potentially hazardous foods are high-protein animal products such as poultry, meat, fish, dairy products, and eggs. However, in recent years fresh produce such as lettuce and spinach have, collectively, accounted for more foodborne disease outbreaks than any other high-risk food. Contamination of leafy greens commonly occurs in the field, due to contact with manure, wild animals, or fecally tainted water. Poor handling practices during or following harvest can also spread pathogens, and since these products are generally eaten raw, microbes that would otherwise be killed by cooking remain viable. Foodborne pathogens also grow well in cooked rice or beans, baked or boiled potatoes, and tofu. Because bacteria must obtain their nutrients in dissolved form, they can only multiply on moist food media, explaining why *cooked* rice, for example, is considered "potentially hazardous" while raw rice is not. The inability of bacteria to grow in foods with very low water content is the basis for preservation of such food products as beef jerky or dried apricots. Drying foods does not *kill* microbes, however—it merely prevents their multiplication. If these foods become wet, bacterial growth will resume and their consumption could result in foodborne illness. Food-poisoning bacteria also have specific pH requirements. Most species grow best at pH levels ranging from 4.6 to 9; highly acidic foods such as citrus fruits, tomatoes, most fresh fruits (low-acid berries and cantaloupe are excep-

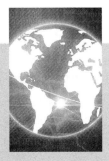

······· *9-4* ·······
Irradiating Foodborne Microbes

Reason and scientific facts triumphed over fear-mongering and misinformation in February 2000 when the federal government added raw beef and lamb to the list of foods that can be irradiated to control foodborne pathogens. This action followed FDA's determination in 1997 that irradiation does not make meat unsafe to eat, change its taste or smell, or significantly alter its nutritional value. Subsequently, in 1999, USDA's Food Safety Inspection Service gave its approval, allowing irradiated hamburger to make its debut the following year. USDA had already approved regulations governing irradiation of pork (1986) and of poultry (1992), but the action on raw beef marked a major milestone in gaining official acceptance of this technology. It should be noted that USDA's action does not require that meat be irradiated, but merely permits it for producers or marketers who desire to utilize the technology as an effective weapon against foodborne disease. The Centers for Disease Control and Prevention (CDC), most public health officials, private groups such as the American Council on Science and Health and the Food Safety Consortium, and food industry representatives, all hailed the government's action as an important step toward reducing the incidence of foodborne illness in the U.S. Some authorities liken the approval of food irradiation to the advent of pasteurized milk in terms of its potential benefit to public health.

Approval of meat irradiation came after many years of controversy over the advisability of using ionizing radiation to kill microbial pathogens or insect pests in food products and to delay spoilage of fresh foods. Irradiation was approved in 1963 to control mold in wheat flour and in 1964 to inhibit sprouting of potatoes. By the 1980s FDA had given the go-ahead to use irradiation to kill trichina worms in fresh pork, to control insects and to slow ripening in fruits and vegetables, and to kill pests in dry herbs, spices, and tea. As the range of food products approved for irradiation expanded, vociferous objections arose from some consumer and environmental groups fearful of possible health implications. Their concerns, expressed in a torrent of negative comments to the FDA in the late 1990s, were reflected in that agency's subsequent exclusion of irradiated products from its official definition of what foods can be marketed as "organic."

Public opinion elsewhere in the world appears to be more accepting of food irradiation. The process has now been approved in over 50 countries and is being used successfully on several types of food in more than 30. Many of these nations, including Canada, Japan, and most European countries, have a long history of high standards on food safety issues. Moreover, food irradiation has been endorsed by the World Health Organization, the American Medical Association, and a number of public health organizations. Nevertheless, until the early 1990s, efforts to expand the range of U.S. products approved for irradiation were stymied by perceived public opposition. Marketing research confirmed the impression of consumer reluctance to embrace the technology, and concluded that, in the absence of extensive public education on the food safety benefits of irradiated food, demand is likely to remain weak (Frenzen et al., 2000).

The event that galvanized supporters of food irradiation and sparked new interest in the issue was the 1993 *E. coli 0157:H7* outbreak. Food scientists are convinced that, other than thorough cooking, irradiation is the only method known that can completely eliminate pathogenic *E. coli* in raw meat. Numerous food-poisoning outbreaks and meat recalls due to contamination with *E. coli* and *Listeria* in the late 1990s reinforced the conviction among food safety experts that food irradiation's time had come (federal food safety agencies are now considering whether to approve irradiation of ready-to-eat processed meats such as cold cuts and hot dogs for *Listeria* control). Widespread outbreaks of *E. coli 0157:H7* food poisoning associated with uncooked leafy vegetables in 2006 prompted FDA to publish a new rule in 2008, allowing the irradiation of fresh iceberg lettuce and fresh spinach.

Government approval doesn't guarantee that irradiated foods will be widely accepted in the U.S. marketplace. Widespread public ignorance and misinformation about the technology has resulted in little demand for irradiated foods; although the number of U.S. supermarkets selling irradiated meat and produce is slightly higher now than it was a decade ago, those doing so nevertheless represent a very small minority.

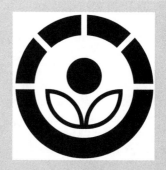

Irradiated chicken is purchased mainly by some hospitals and nursing homes where sick or elderly patients are more vulnerable than the general population to foodborne illnesses. Some consumers avoid irradiated food products due to erroneous ideas about what the process entails. The most common irradiation methods employ gamma rays (generally from a cobalt-60 source), X-rays, or electron beams which, unlike pesticides, accomplish the task for which they were intended without leaving any residue and without rendering the food itself radioactive (just as people receiving dental X-rays or luggage passing through an airport metal detector don't become radioactive as a result). The alleged "unidentified radiolytic products" raised as a concern by anti-irradiation activists have never been found by independent researchers. Ideally, the product is irradiated after it is packaged and sealed, thus preventing any opportunity for recontamination. Consumers handling or eating irradiated food are exposed to no radiation whatsoever. To ensure safe operations, food irradiation facilities must adhere to strict regulations promulgated by the Nuclear Regulatory Commission and the Occupational Safety and Health Administration. Some 50 years of experience using irradiation to sterilize medical devices, a process very similar to food irradiation, have demonstrated that the technology has performed extremely well in terms of safeguarding employee health and transporting radioactive material.

One consumer advocacy group, the Center for Science in the Public Interest, worries that widespread adoption of irradiation to control foodborne pathogens might tempt meat producers to become lax in maintaining high sanitary standards in processing facilities. Proponents, however, insist that irradiation will never be a substitute for hygienic processing and handling of food; indeed, they stress that irradiation's microbiocidal efficiency depends on the cleanliness of the food being treated. Similarly, they emphasize the importance of safe food-handling practices after the irradiated food package is opened, since recontamination then becomes a possibility. Contrary to much of the negative publicity surrounding the issue, irradiation is simply one additional tool—along with production of healthy animals, sanitary processing plants, and proper cooking—to ensure wholesome, pathogen-free food (ACSH, 2003).

tions to the rule), and pickles are seldom implicated in bacterial foodborne disease outbreaks.

The bacterial pathogens that cause foodborne disease are common inhabitants of the intestinal tracts of humans and domestic animals, present in healthy and sick individuals alike; some are naturally present in boils as well. When discharged in fecal material, these organisms can survive for long periods in litter, feces, trough water, and soil. Livestock feed is often contaminated with *Salmonella* organisms introduced when infected animal by-products are rendered and added to the feed mixture. Animals can become infected from any of these sources and thus bring such pathogens into slaughterhouses and poultry-processing plants. Just one infected organ or carcass or animal feces can contaminate cutting equipment or workers' hands and thereby can transfer the bacteria to other carcasses or foods, a process referred to as **cross-contamination**. Once in a processing plant or food establishment, pathogenic organisms can survive on the surface of equipment for long periods and thus constitute sources of food contamination over an extended time period. For this reason, cleaning and sanitizing of grinders, choppers, slicers, and other equipment after each use and frequent hand washing are important measures in preventing cross-contamination.

Foods, particularly those of animal origin, often contain pathogens such as *Salmonella* and *Campylobacter jejuni* when they enter the kitchen. Once in the kitchen, additional opportunity for contamination is presented by the food handlers themselves. The primary reservoir of the *Staphylococcus* organism is the human nose; if kitchen workers cough or sneeze near foods, the bacteria are readily transferred to an appropriate growth medium. If food handlers have infected cuts on their hands, boils, bad cases of acne, or other skin eruptions, *Staphylococcus* bacteria likewise can be transferred to food. Similarly, since approximately 40% of all healthy people carry *Salmonella* organisms in their gastrointestinal tract and regularly shed the live bacteria when they defecate, kitchen workers who do not wash their hands thoroughly after using the bathroom can contaminate foods with this pathogen. The low pay, lack of health benefits, limited education, and minimal employment opportunities that characterize the average food service worker complicate efforts to instill a strong commitment to safe food-handling practices.

Since so many foods contain at least some disease-causing bacteria, it is fortunate that the number of bacterial cells or concentration of bacterial toxins within the ingested food must be relatively high to induce the symptoms of most bacterial foodborne diseases (listeriosis and *E. coli 0157:H7* food poisoning are exceptions to this general rule). Thus the approach to preventing foodborne disease outbreaks must be two-pronged: (1) to the greatest extent possible, avoid microbial contamination of food in the first place through rigorous adherence to rules of good sanitation and hygiene; and (2) maintain environmental conditions that inhibit the multiplication of bacteria that may be present in small numbers within the food medium.

Sanitation

High standards of cleanliness and personal hygiene among those who handle or prepare food are of the utmost importance in preventing outbreaks of foodborne disease. Regulations that local and state public health agencies impose on more than a million retail food establishments in the United States highlight the responsibility of food service personnel for observing good sanitary practices—practices equally relevant to food preparation at home. In its model *Food Code*, a compilation of recommendations that state and local health departments can adopt when developing or updating their own regulatory requirements, the FDA recommends that food service workers be held accountable for lapses in personal hygiene. The *Code* places a special obligation on employees to notify supervisors if they are experiencing any symptoms of gastrointestinal illness or if they are suffering from boils, dermatitis, or other infections on the hands, wrists, exposed portions of the arms, or other parts of the body, unless covered by a proper bandage (such pus-filled infections are prime sources of *Staphylococcus* bacteria). Thus informed, a supervisor is required to restrict sick employees from direct contact with food or to exclude them from the establishment altogether until health problems have been resolved.

Perhaps the most important of all sanitary practices in protecting food quality is frequent and proper hand washing. The FDA cites germ-laden hands as a major

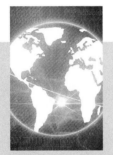

· · · · · · · *9-5* · · · · · · ·

HACCP—Preventive Approach to Food Safety

In confronting the challenge of how best to ensure the safety of food supplies from biological, chemical, or physical hazards, government regulators and food industry personnel alike traditionally relied on an approach that involved periodic inspections of food-processing facilities (e.g., mills, slaughterhouses, canneries, bakeries, supermarkets, restaurants, etc.) and random end-product analyses. The mandated inspection system for meat and poultry still relies heavily on visual examination, the inspector touching and sniffing carcasses to detect signs of disease or spoilage. Most food safety experts decry this approach as outdated and completely useless for identifying the presence of the foodborne pathogens that constitute today's most urgent food quality concerns. In recent years a paradigm shift has been occurring in the way regulatory agencies approach foodborne disease prevention. Moving away from a century-old reactive food safety strategy, regulators are turning instead to a science-based concept called the **Hazard Analysis and Critical Control Point system**, or **HACCP** (pronounced "hassip").

So what *is* this new approach? Essentially HACCP is a preventive system of quality control which, when properly applied, can be used to control any point in the food system that might contribute to a hazardous situation. The concept originated with the space program in the late 1950s, when NASA asked the Pillsbury Company to produce a food that could be eaten by astronauts in orbit. Such an undertaking presented a number of challenges, none more daunting than the imperative of ensuring that any food developed be 100% free of microbial, chemical, or physical contamination. The potentially disastrous consequences of a food-poisoning outbreak inside a space capsule had to be avoided at any cost. Pillsbury scientists realized that only a proactive preventive system could provide the high degree of safety assurance required. Pillsbury spent the following decade developing and refining its concept and in 1971 adopted the HACCP approach in its own facilities. That same year the FDA awarded Pillsbury a contract to conduct classes for its employees on the HACCP system, and in 1973 the company published the first comprehensive document on HACCP principles as a training manual for FDA personnel. In 1980, several federal agencies requested that the National Academy of Sciences examine the potential applications for microbiological criteria in food. The result was a 1985 NAS publication that strongly recommended the application of HACCP in regulatory programs, stating that HACCP "provides a more specific and critical approach to the control of microbiological hazards in foods than that provided by traditional inspection and quality control approaches."

Following this endorsement by NAS, an increasing number of federal, state, and local agencies have redesigned their regulatory approach in conformance with HACCP principles. In 1994 the FDA embraced HACCP as the best method for ensuring food safety, promulgating voluntary HACCP rules for seafood and shellfish (1997), raw sprouts and eggs (1999), and fresh juices (2001). USDA has instituted a mandatory HACCP requirement for meat and poultry, with rules specifically targeted toward reducing microbial levels in these products. The HACCP rules developed by these two federal agencies for the various segments of the food industry each regulates (meat, poultry, and processed eggs by USDA, all other foods by FDA) differ in several respects, most notably in USDA's requirement that the firms under its jurisdiction test for the presence of bacteria, while FDA has no such mandate. In addition, while USDA's HACCP requirements pertain to all meat and poultry operations, FDA has promulgated HACCP rules on a food-by-food basis, leaving many foods it regulates without any proposed controls. It should be mentioned that, even without government prodding, several large food companies have developed and implemented pilot HACCP systems for products as diverse as breakfast cereal, cheese, bread, and salad dressing. Results have been what food safety experts would have predicted: HACCP controls are quite effective in helping companies detect—and then correct—food safety problems.

While food producers must develop individualized HACCP systems tailored to their own processing and distribution conditions, each HACCP program consists of seven basic steps:

1. **Analyze hazard**, identifying potential hazards associated with the food in question, based on close observation of how the food is grown, processed, and distributed—right up to the point of consumption; an assessment is then made of the likelihood of those hazards occurring and preventive measures for controlling such hazards are identified.

2. **Determine critical control points (CCPs)** to minimize or eliminate the hazards identified; CCPs comprise operational steps or procedures such as cooking, chilling, sanitizing, employee hygiene, etc.

3. **Establish critical limits or tolerances** that must be met to ensure that the CCP is under control; some of the criteria most often used include temperature, time, pH, humidity, salt concentration, etc.

4. **Establish a monitoring system** through scheduled testing or observation to ensure that CCP is being controlled.

5. **Establish the corrective action** to be taken when monitoring indicates a deviation from appropriate controls; because of the wide range of possible critical control points, a specific corrective action plan must be developed for each one.

6. **Establish effective record-keeping systems** that document the HACCP plan.

7. **Establish verification procedures** that demonstrate that HACCP is working correctly; such procedures require minimal end-product sampling (due to safeguards built into the system), relying instead on frequent reviews of plan procedure and affirmation that the plan is being followed correctly. Both the food producer and the appropriate regulatory agencies have a role to play in verifying HACCP plan performance.

Implementing a HACCP program in any given setting is neither quick nor easy. HACCP is a technically sophisticated system requiring extensive site-specific research, discussion, and preparation prior to application. Intensive training of both in-plant personnel and regulatory agency inspectors, a high degree of industry/government cooperation, and rigorous enforcement efforts by the regulatory agency inspectors are essential prerequisites to the success of any HACCP plan. Nevertheless, ultimate results are well worth the effort. According to the NAS analysis, effective use of HACCP in food production systems is the one approach by which meaningful reductions in the incidence of foodborne disease can be achieved (National Research Council, 1998; Nestle, 2003).

vehicle of disease transmission, a situation resulting largely from negligence on the part of food handlers. Emphasizing that *rigorous hand-washing practices represent the single most effective means for breaking the chain of infection*, public health authorities recommend that immediately before handling food, food service workers and home cooks alike should engage in a vigorous 20-second scrub using soap and running water, followed by thorough rinsing under clean water. This procedure should be repeated as often as necessary during food preparation to remove soil and to prevent cross-contamination when changing tasks or after handling soiled equipment. Good hand-washing procedures, including using a fingernail brush to clean the fingertips and under the nails, are especially important after food handlers use the toilet, cough, sneeze, smoke, eat, or drink.

WARNING

EMPLOYEES MUST WASH HANDS BEFORE RETURNING TO WORK

Perhaps the most important practice in preventing foodborne illness is rigorous hand washing by food handlers.

Good sanitation of course involves attention to more than employee health and hygiene. General cleanliness of the facility, routine sanitization of cutting tools and food preparation equipment, safe food storage practices, effective dish-washing procedures, proper waste disposal and trash storage—all are important for ensuring that dangerous microbes and food never have a chance to meet.

Time-Temperature Control

When certain environmental preconditions such as optimum pH, moisture, essential nutrients, and temperature are met, populations of pathogenic bacteria in food multiply in accordance with the sigmoidal growth pattern described in chapter 2: after an initial lag phase of about one hour, during which there is negligible increase in numbers while the organisms adjust to new conditions, a period of extremely rapid increase in population

size continues until the supply of essential nutrients diminishes and toxic by-products accumulate. At this stage, growth levels off and the number of organisms remains relatively constant until eventually a progressive die-off of cells occurs. Perhaps the most crucial element in determining the rate of bacterial multiplication during this sequence of events is *temperature*. The bacteria responsible for the majority of foodborne disease outbreaks multiply most rapidly within a temperature range referred to as the **Danger Zone**, defined under the FDA's Food Code as 41–140°F (5–60°C). Temperatures above 140°F will kill most actively growing bacteria, though bacterial spores and a few thermophilic species may survive. At temperatures below 41°F, growth of the bacterial populations associated with common foodborne illnesses either ceases entirely or is extremely slow; however, the organisms are not killed by cold temperatures and can remain viable for long periods of time, resuming multiplication when temperatures rise. Therefore, the most effective way to prevent buildup of bacterial numbers is to keep foods refrigerated, especially those proteinaceous foods that most frequently harbor pathogenic bacteria. Heating such foods thoroughly will kill bacteria that may be present in the food; the higher the temperature above 140°F, the shorter the time the bacterial population will be able to survive (normal cooking times and temperatures are not sufficient, however, to break down *Staphylococcus* toxin).

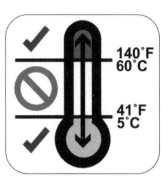

Copyright © International Association for Food Protection

To ensure complete heat penetration throughout the item being cooked, it is advised that internal temperatures reach the following USDA-recommended minimum levels to guarantee that any pathogens present within the food are killed:

Ground Poultry	165°F (74°C)
Ground beef, veal, lamb, pork	160°F (71°C)
Roast beef or lamb	145°F (63°C)
Roast pork	145°F (63°C)
Ham, fresh	160°F (71°C)
Ham, pre-cooked	140°F (60°C)
Roast chicken, turkey	180°F (82°C)
Chicken or turkey breast	170°F (77°C)
Stuffing	165°F (74°C)

It should be noted that the internal temperature of the item being cooked, rather than the temperature of the oven or burner, is the crucial factor. In many instances, large roasts of beef, ham, or turkey still harbor viable pathogens after cooking because they weren't in the oven long enough for temperatures at the center of the roast to reach the recommended level. In the same way, large pieces of cooked meat held in the refrigerator for cooling frequently have internal temperatures well within the growth range, even though the refrigerator thermostat registers at or below 41°F as advised. To promote rapid cooling, cooked meat should be sliced into thin layers and placed in shallow pans before being refrigerated.

The most effective methods that food handlers can follow to prevent foodborne disease, be it in the home, in restaurants, or at large public gatherings, is to complete the processing of food within an hour or two while the bacteria remain in the lag phase of growth and to cool foods rapidly if they are not to be consumed immediately.

Unfortunately, although good sanitation and proper time-temperature controls are relatively simple preventive concepts, they are all-too-frequently neglected by home-makers and commercial food establishments alike. Thus bacterial food poisoning, which fundamentally is a result of improper food-handling practices and should not even exist in affluent modern societies, will undoubtedly remain our most prevalent food-related health problem.

·······10·······

There is no evil in the atom; only in men's souls.
—Adlai Stevenson (1952)

Radiation

Late in the autumn of 1895, a German physics professor, Wilhelm Roentgen, was busily pursuing a line of research that would soon revolutionize medical science and transform our understanding of the nature of matter and energy. Roentgen was experimenting with a cathode-ray tube, a device perfected by the English scientist Crookes two decades earlier that consisted of a glass vacuum tube through which flowed a high voltage electric current. By chance, Roentgen noticed that emissions from the tube caused a nearby sheet of paper coated with a fluorescent chemical to glow, and he observed that these emanations could be blocked to varying degrees by materials of different densities. Calling his wife to place her hand on a photographic plate, Roentgen turned on the cathode-ray tube; when the plate was subsequently developed, Roentgen amazed the world with a picture of his wife's bones inside her hand. Realizing that he had stumbled upon a form of radiation whose existence was hitherto completely unsuspected, Roentgen appropriated the mathematical symbol for the unknown and called his discovery "X-rays." Within a few days after publication of his findings, the medical profession put the fluoroscope and "roentgenogram" to use—the shortest time gap between announcement of a major medical discovery and its practical application yet recorded.

The implications of Roentgen's announcement far transcended the field of medicine, however. Upon hearing of Roentgen's findings, the noted French scientist Henri Becquerel became intrigued by the relationship between X-rays and fluorescence and thereupon directed his attention to naturally phosphorescent minerals. In February of 1896, just two months after publication of Roentgen's report, Becquerel placed some crystals of a uranium compound on a photographic plate wrapped in black paper and demonstrated that the emanations from the uranium exhibited the same characteristics as Roentgen's X-rays. Becquerel's work was quickly picked up by Marie and Pierre Curie who termed the mysterious phenomenon "radioactivity" and who soon succeeded in isolating two new radioactive substances, polonium and radium, from uranium ore (Kevles, 1997). Thus the independent discovery of both artificial and natural radioactivity within a three-month time span quickly led to the birth of a whole new field of scientific inquiry with far-reaching implications in physics, biology, medicine, and, unfortunately, warfare.

IONIZING RADIATION

Early investigations of radioactivity quickly revealed that the observed emissions were of several different kinds. Some consisted of subatomic particles—protons, neutrons, or electrons—released when atoms spontaneously decay; these came to be known as **particulate radiation,** a group that includes **alpha** and **beta particles.** Other emissions, such as Roentgen's X-rays and naturally occurring **gamma rays,** were shown to consist of highly energetic short wavelengths of electromagnetic radiation, a form of energy that also includes ultraviolet light, visible light, infrared waves, and microwaves. Alpha and beta particles, as well as X-rays and gamma rays, are today referred to as **ionizing radiation** because the particles or rays involved are sufficiently energetic to dislodge electrons from the atoms or molecules they encounter, leaving behind ions, i.e., electrically charged particles. While certain forms of non-ionizing radiation such as ultraviolet light and microwaves can have an adverse effect on living organisms and will be discussed later in this chapter, ionizing radiation's ability to destroy chemical bonds gives it special significance in relation to both human health and environmental pollution. It is recognized today that when certain particularly vulnerable cells (e.g., fetal cells, sex cells) are exposed to ionizing radiation, birth defects or mutations can result; in any cell, radiation-induced alteration of DNA can lead to cancer. Although discovery of ionizing radiation was immediately hailed as a momentous medical and scientific event, subsequent investigations regarding what is frequently called our "most studied and best understood pollutant" have revealed the importance of extreme caution in dealing with radioactive materials.

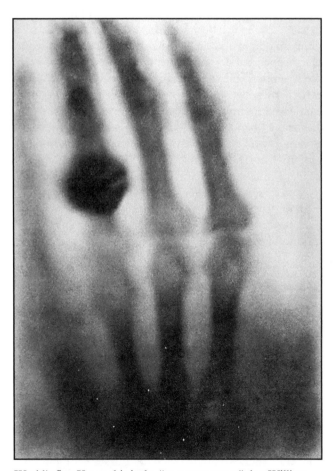

World's first X-ray; this is the "roentgenogram" that William Roentgen took of his wife's hand, thereby demonstrating the existence of the mysterious emanations that he named "X-rays." [*National Library of Medicine*]

Radiation Exposure

Exposure to ionizing radiation is an inescapable circumstance of life on this planet. Every individual, to a greater or lesser extent, comes into contact with ionizing radiation from three general types of sources: naturally occurring, naturally occurring but enhanced by human actions, and human generated.

Natural Sources

Although the fact was not realized until Becquerel's discovery in 1896, earth, air, water, and food all contain traces of radioactive materials that constitute a ubiquitous source of naturally occurring, or "background," radiation. Some of the more significant sources of background radiation include the following:

Cosmic radiation. High-energy particles composed primarily of protons and electrons continually stream toward the earth both from outer space and from the sun following episodes of solar flares. An appreciable amount of such cosmic radiation is blocked by the layer of atmosphere surrounding the globe, so that exposure to cosmic radiation is considerably less at sea level than at high altitudes (annual exposure to cosmic radiation approximately doubles with each 2,000-meter increase in altitude above sea level). For this reason, residents of Denver receive about twice as much cosmic radiation as do inhabitants of Los Angeles or Miami; citizens of La Paz, Bolivia, receive annual radiation exposures fully 7.5 times higher than do people living at sea level (Bennett, 1997). Flying long distances in an airliner also results in higher-than-average exposure to cosmic rays for those aboard. In fact, flight crews on airliners flying more northerly routes receive annual radiation doses in excess of those experienced by most hospital radiologists; as a result, they are classified as radiation workers by a number of European countries (Hall, 2000). While the natural tendency is to assume that something which has always been with us must be harmless, some biologists assert that perhaps 25% of all spontaneous mutations are caused by cosmic radiation.

Radioactive minerals in the earth's crust. Radioactive compounds of uranium, thorium, potassium, and radium are found in soils and rocks in many parts of the world. For example, people living along the Kerala coast in southwestern India, the Morro de Ferro and Meaipe regions of Brazil's Atlantic coast, and in Yangjiang, Guangdong Province in China are all exposed to significantly higher-than-average levels of background radiation due to emissions from thorium-rich monazite sands. Similarly, Floridians living near radioactive phosphate deposits, and residents of New Hampshire, the Rocky Mountain region of the United States, and parts of Sweden—all granite-rich areas—are constantly exposed to external radiation from the soils and rocks around them. In some localities, notably Badgastein in Austria and Mahallat and Ramsar in Iran, high levels of background radiation exposure are received internally due to the ingestion of naturally occurring radioactive minerals in drinking water and to the inhalation of radon gas when bathing in the hot springs for which these regions are famous (Sohrabi, 1998).

Coal deposits frequently contain a number of radioactive elements that are released into the atmosphere when the coal is burned. Ironically, the growing appeal of low-sulfur western coal as an economical approach to reducing sulfur emissions ignores the fact that western coal contains about 10 times more radionuclides than do eastern or midwestern coal deposits (Carter, 1977).

Radionuclides in the body.   A number of radioactive substances enter the body by ingestion of food, milk, water, or by inhalation and are incorporated into body tissues where their concentration may be maintained at a steady state or gradually increase with age. Plants growing in soil containing radioactive minerals readily take up potassium-40, a radioactive isotope believed to make a not-insignificant contribution to human radiation exposure. Some authorities hypothesize that potassium-40 ingested with food may be one source of human mutations (Hall, 2000). In regions where groundwater is in contact with radioac-

tive rock strata, well water used for domestic drinking supplies may constitute a significant source of indoor exposure to radioactive radon gas. Another unavoidable source of radiation exposure is carbon-14, a naturally occurring isotope of carbon, which is inhaled with the air we breathe and is incorporated into the tissues of all living organisms (a fact that has useful implications for scientists who employ C-14 dating techniques to ascertain the age of ancient plant and animal remains).

Enhanced Natural Sources

This category of sources, while not fundamentally different from the group just discussed, is considered separately because of the impact human activities have on levels of exposure that would, under other conditions, be much lower. Examples of enhanced natural sources include uranium mill tailings, phosphate mining, and jet airline travel (due to increased exposure to cosmic radiation at high altitudes). Experts consider radon gas, our single most significant source of radiation exposure, to be an enhanced natural source because, although naturally occurring, it reaches potentially dangerous concentrations only in enclosed environments such as houses and mine shafts ("Ionizing Radiation," 1987). For more information on radon, see the section on "Indoor Air Pollutants" in chapter 12.

Human-Generated Sources

Human beings have evolved and multiplied in an environment where constant exposure to low levels of ionizing radiation is a universal experience. With the exception of indoor radon concerns that are currently the subject of a great deal of attention and remedial action, most naturally occurring radiation is relatively constant and cannot be controlled or reduced in any feasible way. However, human-created sources of ionizing radiation have multiplied at exponential rates during the years since Roentgen first exhibited the X-ray of his wife's hand to an astonished world. It is these artificial sources, which can be controlled, that constitute the focus of a growing concern today about the impact of ionizing radiation on human health.

Medical applications.   By far the greatest source of exposure to artificial ionizing radiation for the average American comes from the use of medical X-rays and radio-pharmaceuticals for both diagnostic and therapeutic purposes. Today approximately 75% of all Americans receive one or more medical or dental X-rays annually. Radioactive isotopes of phosphorus, technicium, iodine, iron, chromium, cobalt, and selenium are widely employed in hospitals for therapy and diagnosis, with as many as one-fourth of all patients in some hospitals receiving applications of some form of nuclear medicine. In addition to X-ray machines and radionuclides, the

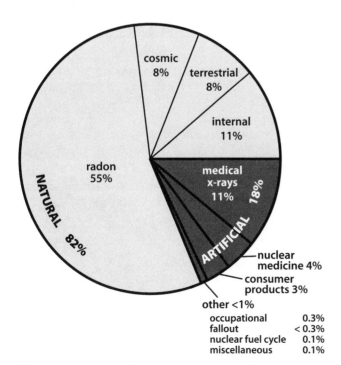

Figure 10-1   Contribution of Various Radiation Sources to the Total Average Effective Dose Equivalent in the U.S. Population

health professions utilize other such radiation-producing devices as Computerized Axial Tomography machines (CAT scans), teleradioisotope units, and accelerators (e.g., cyclotrons, linear accelerators) to generate subatomic particles for radiotherapy. While radiation has provided medical science with an extremely valuable tool, its occasional misuse has been accompanied by some serious health problems; thus a thoughtful weighing of risks versus benefits should precede any decision regarding the application of ionizing radiation for medical purposes.

Nuclear weapons fallout. Since the explosion of the first atomic bomb in 1945 until the signing of the Limited Test-Ban Treaty in 1963, atmospheric testing of nuclear weapons by several of the major powers, primarily the United States and the former Soviet Union, resulted in significant amounts of radioactive fallout worldwide. Such fallout consists of a number of atomic fission products, including strontium-90, iodine-131, cesium-137, and radioactive krypton. Weapons fallout is not always evenly distributed, however. Local fallout close to the test site can be quite intense for about a day following the explosion, a fact that became obvious after the March 1, 1954, detonation of a multimegaton U.S. bomb over Bikini Atoll in the Pacific. Heavy fallout of large radioactive particles and dust contaminated several inhabited islands nearby, as well as a Japanese fishing boat sailing in the vicinity. Many of the Marshall Islanders and the fishermen developed burns, skin lesions, and loss of hair as a result of radiation exposure, and one of the islands,

Rongelap, had to be evacuated and remained unoccupied for a number of years following the incident. In some cases air currents or rainstorms can cause radioactive particles and gases to precipitate unevenly.

The greatest concern about weapons fallout is focused on those isotopes that enter the human system in food and are incorporated into body tissues. Of these, the most significant health threat is the increased risk of thyroid cancer posed by exposure to iodine-131 in milk from cows or goats that grazed on pasturelands exposed to fallout (Institute of Medicine and National Research Council, 1999). During the peak period of weapons testing, an average individual's radiation exposure due to bomb fallout was 13 millirems annually, a figure that has been steadily falling since 1963 (Eisenbud, 1973). According to the National Council on Radiation Protection and Measurements (NCRP), annual fallout exposure currently averages less than 0.01 mSv (1 mrem) and, barring a resumption of atmospheric testing of nuclear weapons, will continue to decline. Having reached such negligible levels, nuclear weapons fallout need no longer be taken into account in calculating total human radiation exposure.

Nuclear power plant emissions. Public opposition to construction of nuclear power plants often centers around fears concerning radioactive emissions both to the air and in wastewater released from such plants. Radioisotopes such as tritium (H3), iodine-131, cesium-137, strontium-90, krypton, and others are indeed released into the environment during routine operation

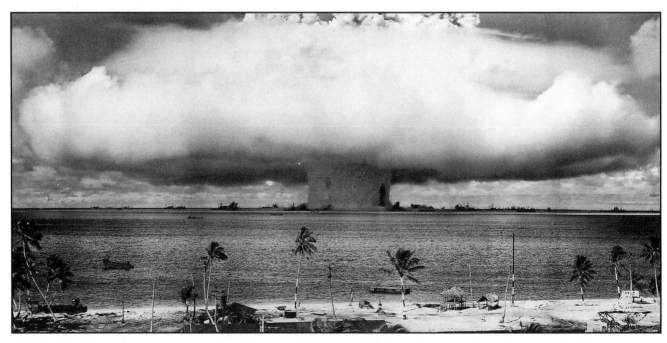

The U.S. military conducted its first underwater test of an atom bomb at Bikini Atoll in the Pacific in July 1946. [*AP Photo*]

of a nuclear power generator, but the quantities involved are extremely minute—the average annual dose to individuals living within a 50-mile radius of the plant being less than one millirem, an amount considerably lower than that received from background radiation ("Ionizing Radiation," 1987).

Consumer products.   In addition to the sources mentioned above, very small amounts of exposure are received from luminous instrument dials (radium, tritium), home smoke detectors (americium), static eliminators (polonium), airport security checks (X-rays), and tobacco products (polonium). Of these sources, the most significant is tobacco; the radioactive polonium particles in cigarette smoke lodge primarily in the bronchial epithelium of the upper airways—the site of most lung cancers—thereby further contributing to the health risk posed by other carcinogenic and toxic substances in tobacco smoke (NCRP, 1987).

Since radon exposure alone constitutes approximately 55% of the average American's annual radiation burden, natural (including enhanced) sources, contributing 82% of total radiation exposure, are far more significant than the 18% from artificial sources (NCRP, 1987). For any one individual, of course, the ratio can vary widely. A person living in an area of unusually high natural radioactivity (e.g., Salt Lake City, Denver) or sleeping in a basement bedroom where radon levels are exceptionally high might receive an even larger portion of his or her total exposure from background sources, while a person undergoing radiation therapy or working inside a nuclear power plant would receive a disproportionate share from artificial sources.

Health Impacts of Ionizing Radiation

The advent of X-ray technology for diagnosing and treating human illness, so eagerly and immediately seized upon by the medical profession, was soon shown to be a double-edged sword so far as its impact on human health was concerned. The first reported case of X-ray induced illness involved an American physician, Grubbe, who began self-experimenting with a homemade cathode-ray tube. Within a few weeks he reported acute irritation of the skin on his hand; later, cancer developed and eventually his hand had to be amputated. Grubbe's case was not an isolated one. By 1897, scarcely a year after the new technology came into use, 69 cases of X-ray induced injuries had been documented from various clinics and laboratories in different parts of the world (Eisenbud, 1973). One of the most famous early radiation victims was Clarence Dally, Thomas Edison's chief assistant, who "died by inches" after just a few years of working with X-rays. In 1896 Dally had begun experimenting with Roentgen's new device in Edison's West Orange,

New Jersey, laboratory, frequently holding his hand in front of the tube to make sure X-rays were being produced. Dally soon noticed slight burns and hair loss, but continued his work. By 1902 he was suffering from oozing ulcers on his hands and eventually had his left hand amputated; cancerous sores then appeared on his right hand and four fingers were amputated, followed by both arms. In such acute pain he couldn't even lie down, Dally died in agony in 1904 (Kevles, 1997). Reports of health damage due to radiation from natural sources were not long in following. Becquerel himself reported a reddening of the skin on his chest as a result of carrying a vial of radium in his vest pocket. He and the Curies subsequently used a radium extract to produce a skin burn on the forearm of a male volunteer, thereby demonstrating that X-rays and natural radioactivity have essentially identical biological effects (Cooper, 1973).

In spite of an increasing awareness of the hazards, as well as the usefulness, of ionizing radiation, the first few decades of the 20th century witnessed numerous cases of radiation-induced illness or death resulting from carelessness, faulty equipment, or simple ignorance. As early as 1903 a dangerous misconception of radiation's curative powers catapulted both X-rays and radium into prominence as the latest medical fads, regarded as modern panaceas for a wide range of ailments. Over a period of approximately 20 years, first in Europe and later in the U.S., radiation treatments were prescribed to hopeful patients both for destroying unwanted external tissue (e.g., warts, birthmarks, excess facial hair) and as an internal medicine. Many researchers during this period were convinced that radiation selectively destroyed diseased cells while actually promoting the growth of healthy ones. Some claimed that the radioactive element radium had germicidal properties, leading one scientist to propose the inhalation of radioactive gas as a treatment for tuberculosis! The discovery during this period that the mineral waters at many health spas were radioactive reinforced the notion that radioactivity must confer health benefits and encouraged promoters of such popular resorts as Saratoga Springs, New York, and Hot Springs, Arkansas, to claim their waters had the power to cure ailments ranging from rheumatism to malaria, alcoholism, chronic skin disease, anemia, and female sterility.

More surprising in retrospect was the medical practice, widespread during the 1910s and 1920s, of administering intravenous injections of radium salts as a treatment for such maladies as high blood pressure, arthritis, leukemia, sexual dysfunction, and senility; rather than curing such ills, the treatment all too often provoked the development of anemia or cancer (Clark, 1997). Outside physicians' offices, a wide variety of radium-based consumer products—candies, liniments, creams, and so on—were being marketed to a gullible public with assurances that

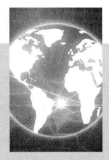

········ 10–1 ········

Tragedy of the Radium Dial-Painters

The most infamous example on record of fatal carelessness in the handling of radioactive materials involved scores of young female workers in the radium dial-painting industry in the 1920s and 1930s. The tragedy that befell these first victims of occupational radiation poisoning had its origin in the development, in 1915, of radium-containing luminous paint—a product that promptly found use in the watch-making industry for producing "glow-in-the dark" wristwatches. To supply the demand for this consumer fad, between 1917 and 1925 dial-painting factories were established in New Jersey, Connecticut, and Illinois, cumulatively employing 3,000–4,000 workers over the years they were in operation.

Offering what they touted as "ideal working conditions," firms such as U.S. Radium in New Jersey and Radium Dial Company (later replaced by Luminous Processes) in Illinois selectively recruited a workforce composed of women in their late teens and early twenties, regarding such employees as particularly well-suited for jobs requiring little physical strength but considerable manual dexterity. From moderately prosperous working-class families, these women felt fortunate to find employment in firms offering above-average wages in pleasant surroundings. They also found it exciting to be in daily contact with a substance as magical as radium. In more playful moments they applied the luminous paint to their fingernails, eyelids, and buttons; one particularly vivacious girl in New Jersey laughingly painted her teeth with radium to surprise her boyfriend with a glow-in-the-dark smile! Dial-painters often returned home from work with their hair and clothes liberally speckled with luminous powder and would sometimes amuse friends and family by standing in a dark closet where they cast off a ghostly glow.

The dial-painters' most ill-advised practice, however, was lip-pointing. As instructed by supervisors, each worker used her lips to maintain a fine point on the brush as she painted the tiny numbers on the watch dial; in doing so, she inadvertently swallowed small amounts of radium each time the brush touched her mouth. Although most of the ingested radium was subsequently excreted, some was absorbed into the bloodstream and eventually accumulated in the bones where it constituted a chronic source of internal radiation exposure. Knowing little about the properties of radium themselves, the women were reassured by management that the substance with which they were working was quite harmless. In the Illinois plant one worker interviewed years later recalled a supervisor telling her that radium would "put a glow in our cheeks"! Since radium in those years also was being marketed for medicinal use, such statements were readily believed. Unfortunately, they were untrue.

In 1922, a young New Jersey woman who had worked at U.S. Radium for only three years became the first dial-painter to die of radium poisoning; by then several of her coworkers were gravely ill and within a few years they were dead also. Each of these early deaths involved necrosis of the jawbone, followed by rampant infections that proved uncontrollable in that pre-antibiotic era. Several died of anemia, while other women experienced debilitating weakening of their bones, often resulting in arms or legs breaking from even modest pressure. The largest number of dial-painter fatalities, however, was due to bone cancer or multiple myelomas, which began to appear in the late 1920s. Word of the mysterious ailments plaguing their coworkers began to spread among dial-painters who were increasingly convinced they were confronting a new occupational disease. By 1925, after the death of a 21-year-old employee at the Connecticut plant, managers instituted a ban on lip-pointing, even though the company never officially acknowledged radium as the cause of this tragedy. With definitive scientific proof still lacking, neither industry, government regulators, nor medical researchers were ready to concede that radium was the culprit causing the health problems that were now appearing with increasing frequency.

By 1927, however, the mounting evidence could no longer be ignored; in that year a physiologist hired by industry to refute evidence of radium's harmful effects came to the conclusion that "radium is partially if not the primary cause of the pathological condition described." While the radium industry, much like modern-day tobacco company spokespersons, continued to deny any adverse health effects associated with its product, the medical and scientific community at last recognized radium as a major occupational hazard. With this acknowledgment, the focus of attention shifted to that of winning financial compensation for dying workers and their families. By contemporary standards, such compensation was surprisingly meager. In general, the dial-painters who were affected the worst and the earliest received most of the money awarded; many victims were given nothing at all. While records indicate that altogether 84 dial-painters died of radium-induced cancer and an undetermined but smaller number perished from jaw necrosis or anemia, compensation was awarded to just 13 women in Illinois, 16 in Connecticut, and 10 or 11 in New Jersey. The highest amount received was $5,700; most awards were for considerably lower sums.

During the 1920s, as the women desperately sought recognition for their plight, they received little support from male-dominated labor organizations; the State Health and Labor Department officials who might logically have been expected to take up their cause instead supported the politically influential radium industry. Scientists and medical researchers likewise tailored their reports to please the corporate sponsors who funded their research or paid their salaries. Nevertheless, publicity surrounding the mounting toll of dying and disabled workers raised general awareness of the problem and eventually resulted in improved worker safety precautions in the dial-painting facilities. The scientific investigations launched in response to an obvious problem gave birth to a new field of study—health physics—and in time yielded the information that formed the basis of health standards for a new generation of industrial workers, scientists, medical personnel, and patients (Clark, 1997).

the effects of radiation in trace amounts were beneficial to health, perhaps even necessary! One such bogus cure-all, "Radithor," was advertised as a panacea for impotence, high blood pressure, indigestion, and more than 150 other ills. Sold in the United States for over six years, Radithor was taken off the market only after it had induced fatal cancer in a well-known socialite, a Radithor devotee who was reported to have consumed 1,000 to 1,500 bottlefuls of the radium solution between 1927 and 1931. The legal restrictions on sales of radiopharmaceuticals currently prevailing in the United States were a direct result of the outrage provoked by the Radithor scandal (Macklis, 1993).

Another example of a practice that in retrospect seems inconceivably misguided started in about 1925, when some doctors began irradiating children's scalps to treat ringworm, their heads and throats for enlarged tonsils and adenoids, and their faces to banish acne. Even as late as the 1960s some physicians used low-voltage X-rays to shrink the thymus gland (located in the neck) of infants in the erroneous belief that such treatments would cure colds. Unfortunately, such X-rays could not be precisely focused. As they spread out they irradiated not only the target tissue but the thyroid gland as well. The thyroid is one of the most radiation-sensitive organs in the body, and about 10 or more years following exposure (19 years seemed to be the peak period) significant numbers of these now-teenagers or young adults developed thyroid cancer (Norwood, 1980).

One segment of the population at special risk during the early years of work with radiation was the medical community itself, particularly radiologists. A questionnaire sent to all American radiologists in 1928 revealed that a shockingly high percentage of respondents had been unable to father children and the rate of defective births among those who did have offspring was double that considered normal. Radiologists' mortality rates due to cancer, particularly leukemia, were several times higher than those of their colleagues in other areas of medicine, and the gloved or amputated hand became a macabre symbol of the radiologists' profession. Organizers of a 1920 banquet at a radiologists' convention blundered badly by including chicken on the menu because most of the guests present had lost at least one hand and were unable to cut their meat (Kevles, 1997).

Observations of radiation-induced health problems such as those just described led to extensive research into safer methods of utilizing this valuable but dangerous tool. Since the early 1940s, improvements in equipment design and increasingly stringent standards relating to allowable exposure have significantly reduced the incidence of overt cases of radiation damage. Nevertheless, concerns regarding unnecessary use of X-rays for diagnostic purposes and new understanding regarding long-term effects of low-level exposure require that individuals must be alert to the dangers implicit in any degree of radiation exposure and take an active role in deciding whether such exposure is justified.

Types of Ionizing Radiation

Although any exposure to ionizing radiation is potentially dangerous, the degree and nature of harm varies depending on the type of radiation involved. Early studies of radioactivity revealed that ionizing radiation comprises several different types of emissions, the most biologically significant of which include the following.

Alpha Particles

Basically helium nuclei consisting of two protons and two neutrons, alpha particles are relatively massive particles that are the most energetic type of radiation, yet are the least penetrating. Such flimsy barriers as a sheet of paper, clothing, or even human skin can stop them. The greatest threat to health involving alpha radiation occurs when alpha-emitting particles (e.g., plutonium, radium, radon) are inhaled, ingested with food or water, or taken into the body through a cut or wound. Once in contact with delicate internal tissues, alpha radiation can cause intense damage within a localized area. Theoretical projections of large numbers of lung cancer deaths following a nuclear power plant meltdown are based on assumptions of pulmonary damage caused by inhalation of alpha-emitting plutonium dust.

Beta Particles

Consisting of single electrons, beta particles are more penetrating than alphas, capable of passing through the skin to a depth of about a half-inch. Like alphas, however, they are most dangerous when ingested. Since several beta emitters (e.g., strontium-90, iodine-131) are chemically similar to naturally occurring bodily constituents, they may substitute for those elements and concentrate in living tissues (e.g., bones, thyroid), where they continue to emit radiation for an extended period of time, increasing the risk of cancer or mutations. Most fis-

sion products in spent fuel rods or in reprocessed nuclear wastes are beta emitters.

Gamma Rays

These are the most penetrating form of ionizing radiation and generally accompany beta radiation. Shielding with a dense material such as lead is necessary to prevent gamma radiation from penetrating the body and harming vital organs. Short-lived beta emitters such as krypton-85 generally exhibit the highest levels of gamma radiation.

X-Rays

Though slightly less penetrating, X-rays have basically the same characteristics as gamma rays.

Dosage

Since ionizing radiation can be neither seen nor felt, human exposure is measured in terms of the amount of tissue damage it causes. Under the International System of Units, the term gray (Gy) is the unit of absorbed dose, used to quantify the amount of energy from ionizing radiation absorbed per unit mass of material (the gray has replaced an older term, "rad"; a gray is equivalent to 100 rads, while what was formerly termed "one rad" is now called a centigray). The most common unit for measuring effective radiation dose in humans, however, is the **sievert (Sv)**, a figure obtained by multiplying the absorbed dose in grays by a factor called the **relative biological effectiveness (RBE)**. This measurement reflects the fact that the health impact of radiation depends not only on the amount of energy absorbed, but also on the

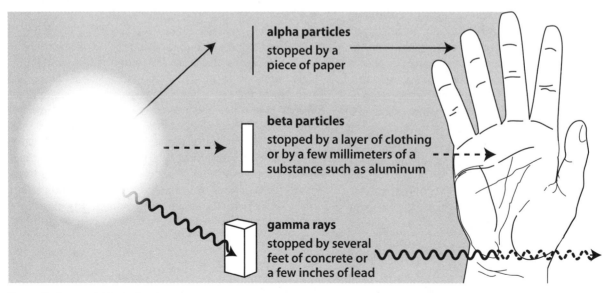

Source: Environmental Protection Agency.

Figure 10-2   Penetrating Power of Alpha and Beta Particles and Gamma Rays

form of that energy. For example, X-rays and gamma rays that pass through tissue striking only occasional molecules along their path have an RBE of 1; beta particles have RBEs ranging from 1 to 5, depending on their energy level, while the relatively massive alpha particles have an RBE of 10, indicating their greater potential to damage living tissue. For practical purposes, human radiation exposure standards are set in terms of **millisieverts (mSv)**, an amount one-thousandth of a sievert, since these represent levels of exposure most commonly encountered by the average individual. Just as the gray has replaced the rad, sieverts and millisieverts are replacing units, still used in many references, called "rems" and "millirems" (mrem). Under the new system a sievert is equivalent to 100 rems. The average amount of whole-body radiation exposure for a person in the U.S. from all sources is estimated to be 3.6 mSv (360 mrem) a year or 0.01 mSv (1 mrem) per day.

There is little evidence that present average levels of exposure to ionizing radiation are having any adverse effect on the health of the general public. It is well known, however, that higher doses can be extremely injurious to living tissues. Types of radiation-induced biological damage include mutations, birth defects, impairment of fertility, leukemia and other forms of cancer, infections, hemorrhage, cataracts, and reduced lifespan. Humans, and mammals in general, are far more sensitive to ionizing radiation than are lower forms of life. The same degree of damage that a dose of 0.5 Sv (50 rems) can cause in a mammalian cell requires 1,000 Sv (100,000 rems) exposure in an amoeba or 3,000 Sv (300,000 rems) in a paramecium. The frequent reference in old horror films to cockroaches inheriting the earth in the aftermath of all-out nuclear war is reflective of the fact that insects also have a very high level of tolerance to ionizing radiation.

Dose **rate**, the quantity of radiation received within a given unit of time, is thought to be very significant in determining the extent of tissue damage incurred, perhaps even more important than total dose. The prevailing view holds that radiation absorbed over an extended period is less harmful than the same amount delivered during a brief time span, due to the existence of bodily repair mechanisms. Furthermore, not only does the risk of damage (e.g., cancer) fall as the dose rate is decreased, but also the latency period becomes longer (Goldman, 1996). In relation to carcinogenesis, however, two noted British epidemiologists argue that numerous small doses of radiation exposure are more likely to induce cancer than is a single large dose. Basing their conclusions on a study of health records of 35,000 nuclear bomb production workers at the federal government's Hanford Reservation in Richland, Washington, these researchers hypothesize that large doses of radiation kill cells, while smaller doses simply damage the genetic material, giving rise to mutations that increase the likelihood of cancer (Kneale and Stewart, 1993).

High-Level vs. Low-Level Radiation Exposure

Health effects of ionizing radiation can be subdivided into those types of damage caused by high-level and low-level exposure, respectively. **High-level radiation exposure** is defined as a whole-body dose of 1 Sv (100 rems) or more, delivered within a relatively short period of time—minutes or hours. As soon as a few hours after exposure or as long as several weeks later, people receiving a dose of high-level radiation begin to exhibit obvious symptoms of radiation sickness, ranging in severity from nausea, vomiting, or hair loss to bloody diarrhea, convulsive seizures, and death. These effects are referred to as "deterministic," a term used to describe effects observed only after a threshold level of exposure has been exceeded and whose severity is directly proportional to the dosage received (Hall, 2000). Levels of ionizing radiation capable of inducing the above-mentioned effects would most likely occur only in such extreme situations as a nuclear bomb explosion, a nuclear power plant meltdown, or in severe industrial accidents involving mishandling of radioactive materials. Such effects are largely reflective of cell death which, if extensive, can be fatal to the organism. Human effects of high-level exposure have been determined from studies of victims of the Hiroshima-Nagasaki atomic bomb explosions, from experience with radiation therapy, and from observations of the results of nuclear accident victims. The 135,000 unfortunate Ukrainians and Byelorussians exposed to large amounts of radioactive debris resulting from the 1986 disaster at Chernobyl constitute a particularly valuable study group for radiation biologists because the radiation doses they received were measured at the time of the accident, unlike the wartime situation in Japan where exposures were estimated after the event (Hawkes et al., 1987).

Low-level radiation exposure, encompassing dosage levels below 1 Sv (100 rems), seldom results in immediately apparent health damage. It can, however, produce "stochastic" effects—problems whose ultimate severity (e.g., death due to cancer) is not related to dosage received but whose likelihood of occurring at all increases with increasing dose. It is assumed for purposes of regulation that there is no threshold for stochastic effects, although, as will be explained shortly, that assumption is no longer universally held. Because of its potential to damage the cell rather than to kill it outright, low-level radiation has the potential to induce mutations, congenital abnormalities, and cancer. Since almost everyone experiences low-level exposure at one time or another, the human health effects of low doses of radiation have been a prime focus of radiation research for many years.

Radiation-Induced Mutations

Exposure even to very low levels of ionizing radiation can result in gene mutations; indeed, experiments to date indicate that there is no threshold level below which no mutations would be expected (however, at very low levels of exposure the mutation rate will correspondingly be quite low). There is, rather, a direct linear relationship between increasing radiation dosage and an increased number of mutations, either at the gene or chromosomal level. Both diagnostic X-rays and radioactive isotopes used for treating various ailments have been shown to damage chromosomes. Nuclear power plant workers and medical personnel, particularly radiotherapy nurses, who receive small doses of radiation on a daily basis, have been shown to exhibit a marked increase in the frequency

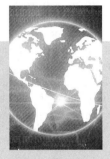

· · · · · · · 10-2 · · · · · · ·

Half-Life

Not all radioisotopes are dangerous for the same length of time. Each radioactive element is characterized by its own unique half-life (T½)—a period of time during which half of the amount originally present, undergoing radioactive decay, is transformed into something else. The concept of half-life, in essence, is the reverse of exponential growth. Assume, for example, that one has a gram of cesium-137 whose half-life is 30 years. After 30 years there would remain ½ gram of cesium-137 and ½ gram of cesium's nonradioactive daughter product, barium-137; the radiation now being emitted is only half the original value. After 60 years the radioactivity would be only ¼ the original amount; in 90 years ⅛ the original value, and so on.

Obviously the term half-life is not synonymous with safety—½ gram of cesium-137 still presents a hazard. Indeed, highly radioactive substances may have to go through 10 or more half-lives (i.e., 300 years in the case of cesium) before their level of radioactivity is low enough to pose no significant health threat. However, the half-life concept has considerable relevance in assessing relative hazards and in devising waste management strategies.

Isotopes with very short half-lives are intensely radioactive initially; that is, they are experiencing a very high number of disintegrations at any one point in time. However, within a few days or weeks they go through so many half-lives that they no longer present a significant risk. The best management strategy for such wastes is simply to isolate them from human contact during the brief period when they are dangerous. Isotopes with extremely long half-lives will be radioactive virtually forever, but the level of emissions at any one point in time is relatively low; one can briefly handle a piece of long-lived uranium or thorium ore with little concern for radiation injury. The most difficult management problems involve those isotopes with intermediate-length half-lives, elements such as plutonium which, with a half-life of 24,000 years, remains hazardous for hundreds of thousands of years. Human contact with such radioisotopes must be accompanied by stringent safety precautions and ultimate disposal of such material must be carried out in such a way that it remains isolated from the general environment for extremely long periods of time.

Some representative half-lives

Element	Half-life	Element	Half-life
Radon-222	3.8 days	Cesium-137	30 years
Iodine-131	8.1 days	Radium-226	1,600 years
Phosphorus-32	14 days	Carbon-14	5,800 years
Krypton-85	11 years	Plutonium-239	24,000 years
Tritium	12 years	Uranium-235	710,000,000 years
Strontium-90	29 years	Thorium-232	14,000,000,000 years

of mutations in their chromosomes (these can be observed as breaks or changes in chromosome number when chromosome smears are made from a sampling of white blood cells). The number of such abnormalities is generally highest among individuals who have been occupationally exposed to radiation for a number of years, indicating that the damaging effects of radiation exposure are cumulative.

Of greatest concern from a genetic standpoint, of course, are the mutations that accumulate in the gonadal cells, which are the precursors of eggs and sperm. The number of new mutations that an individual passes on to his or her children depends on the amount of radiation the sex organs have absorbed from the time of conception up to the moment each of his or her children are conceived. Most radiation-induced mutations are recessive; hence even though most are of a harmful nature, they are likely to persist in the human gene pool, increasing in frequency over several generations before carriers of the recessive gene mate, producing offspring who exhibit the mutant characteristic. Studies recently conducted on populations living downwind from the former Soviet Union's nuclear bomb test site at Semipalatinsk in Kazakhstan found that more than half the children of parents exposed to radioactive fallout during the early 1950s exhibit germline mutations—clear evidence that genetic damage caused by radiation can be passed on from one generation to the next (Dubrova et al., 2002).

In addition to inducing mutations in sex cells, X-ray exposure also has been shown to be capable of causing chromosomal damage in developing fetuses. Because the majority of such instances involved diagnostic X-rays of women in the very early stages of pregnancy who were not yet aware of their condition, it is now recommended that irradiation of reproductive-age women be limited to the first ten days after the onset of their last menstrual cycle to prevent exposure of an unsuspected embryo. Males and females alike should insist on being provided with a gonadal shield (e.g., lead apron) to reduce the risk of sex-cell mutations whenever X-rays are administered.

Radiation and Birth Defects

Laboratory experiments with animals, as well as direct observations of unintended consequences of humans exposed to ionizing radiation during fetal or embryonic development, provide ample evidence of radiation's teratogenic effects. The most tragic and widely studied cases of radiation-induced birth defects involve the Japanese children irradiated in utero at the time of the atomic bomb explosions over Hiroshima and Nagasaki and of children who received X-ray exposure while still in the womb. While these sources of fetal/embryonic exposure are now, hopefully, relics of the past, other less

acute sources of radiation exposure still pose safety concerns. Among these are natural radionuclides (potassium-40, carbon-14, radon and its daughter products) that can be inhaled or ingested by a pregnant woman with food or water. Radioactive fallout products, such as those released after the nuclear power plant explosion at Chernobyl, constitute another potential source of exposure. Occupational activities of the mother could result in exposure of the unborn child if her work involves production, distribution, or use of radiopharmaceuticals or the treatment and handling of patients undergoing nuclear medicine procedures. Similarly, administration of radiopharmaceuticals to pregnant patients for diagnosing or treating health problems may pose a radiation risk to the embryo/fetus (NCRP, 1998).

Sensitivity to radiation is many times greater during fetal development than at any subsequent period of a person's life, since rapid development and differentiation of tissues is occurring during this time (the more actively cells are dividing, the more vulnerable they are to radiation). In terms of lethal, as opposed to teratogenic effects, the radiosensitivity of the embryo/fetus steadily decreases during the period before birth. However, the nature and extent of fetal injury (i.e., congenital abnormalities as opposed to death) caused by radiation vary widely, depending not only on the dose absorbed but also on the precise stage of development. Because the fetal tissues are constantly growing and differentiating, the developmental response to radiation exposure on any given day may be quite different from what it would have been the day before or the day after. In addition, there are individual genetic differences in sensitivity to radiation that make it unlikely that any two fetuses would respond in precisely the same manner, even when the doses are identical.

In general, radiation exposure during the first 10 days after conception will either kill the fetus or, conversely, have no discernible teratogenic effect at all. Exposure during the following period of organ formation (organogenesis), extending through the eighth week of pregnancy, can result in severe malformations. Both the skeletal system and the central nervous system are especially radiosensitive, thus exposure to X-rays or other sources of ionizing radiation can result in babies being born with abnormally small heads (microcephaly), spinal deformities, eye problems, and permanent growth retardation (the latter effect can be produced by exposure at any time during prenatal development but is most pronounced when exposure occurs during organogenesis). After the second month of pregnancy, radiation does not cause major structural defects but can provoke severe intellectual disability, since the third and fourth months of pregnancy mark a period of rapid brain development. Studies of Japanese children irradiated at Hiroshima revealed that the period of highest risk for intellectual disability from *in utero* exposure is between the 8th and 15th weeks of pregnancy, with another slightly less sensitive period occurring between the 16th and 25th weeks. Late-term radiation exposure has not been linked to structural problems or functional disturbances, but has been shown to increase the risk of developing childhood cancer.

The severity of the effects described increase with increasing radiation dosage; however, the existence of a threshold dose (i.e., a "safe level" of exposure below which no teratogenic effects have been observed) in the range of 0.2 to 0.4 Gy is now generally accepted (Streffer, 1997).

Radiation-Induced Cancer

The potential for health damage as a result of radiation exposure was first recognized in connection with the development of skin cancers among early radiologists, of whom nearly 100 fell victim to this disease within 15 years following the discovery of X-rays. Since then other forms of cancer, most notably leukemia, bone cancer, lung cancer, and thyroid cancer, also have been linked to radiation exposure.

Leukemia is perhaps the classic example of X-ray-induced malignancy. As early as 1911 a report of 11 cases of leukemia among radiation workers suggested a connection between the disease and their occupational exposure. Subsequently, epidemiological studies among radiologists, Japanese survivors of Hiroshima and Nagasaki, patients treated with X-ray therapy, and children who were irradiated in the womb when their mothers received diagnostic X-rays, all confirm the association between exposure to ionizing radiation and the induction of leukemia. Leukemia, like other forms of cancer, is characterized by a latency period following the initial exposure, with development of disease symptoms in this case occurring, on the average, after 5–7 years (some as early as just 2 years after irradiation).

Evidence on the amount of radiation required to induce a malignancy is scarce, particularly at doses less than 0.5 Sv (50 rems). Radiation protection policies since the early 1950s have been based on the assumption that all radiation exposure, no matter how low, is harmful; low doses are regarded as having the same effects as high doses, though at a lower rate of incidence (a concept known as the **linear no-threshold theory**). The validity of this belief has been challenged in recent years by a growing body of evidence indicating that an exposure threshold for radiation-induced cancer does, in fact, exist and that, more surprisingly, exposure to very low levels of ionizing radiation may actually reduce the risk of cancer and enhance longevity, a phenomenon known as "hormesis." The scientific rationale for this point of view is that the ability of cells to repair minor genetic damage is stimulated by low-dose radiation, thus increasing the effectiveness of the DNA damage-control biosystem. Proponents of this argument point to the millions of people living in regions of higher-than-normal background radiation (e.g., those areas in India, Brazil, China, Austria, and U.S. described in an earlier section of this chapter) whom several epidemiologic studies have shown to have lower rates of cancer than people living outside those areas. A study conducted in 1993 on Japanese atomic bomb survivors revealed significantly greater longevity among those exposed to radiation than among unexposed Japanese; a 1991 report on U.S. nuclear shipyard workers showed a statistically significant decrease in mortality rates for deaths from all causes among men occupationally exposed to gamma radiation when compared with unexposed workers. These studies suggest to

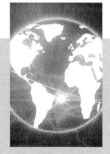

······· 10-3 ·······
"Loose Nukes" and "Dirty Bombs"

Of all the security threats confronting the United States, none is more nightmarish than the prospect of a terrorist group exploding a nuclear device in the middle of a large American city. In what later proved to be a false alarm, warnings in October 2001 that al Qaeda operatives inside the U.S. possessed a 10-kiloton weapon prompted alarming calculations of the damage a bomb that size could wreak. Easily transportable in an ordinary passenger vehicle, a 10-kiloton nuclear bomb, upon detonation, would vaporize everything within a radius of one-third mile; beyond that point to three-quarters of a mile away, buildings would be reduced to rubble; raging fires and massive levels of ionizing radiation would extend in a third circle out to

1½ miles from ground zero. Hundreds of thousands of people would be killed within minutes by collapsing buildings and fires. Within days many more would perish of radiation sickness. The blast-generated electromagnetic pulse would wipe out all forms of electronic communication and the ability of rescue personnel and medical facilities to deal with such a crisis would be overwhelmed. Over the long term, survivors would have to be evacuated and resettled, since the resulting radioactive contamination of the area would render it uninhabitable for years to come. And evacuation of the survivors wouldn't end their suffering—tens of thousands would inevitably die prematurely due to radiation-induced cancer.

Though most of us find it hard to imagine such a catastrophe actually occurring, a number of nuclear antiterrorism experts reluctantly conclude that "it's not a matter of *if*, it's a matter of *when*." Their pessimism stems from a realization of how many unsecured sources of weapons-grade material exist around the world (Russia, Pakistan, and North Korea constitute particularly worrisome potential sources) and how readily available, both on the Internet and in libraries, is the information necessary for any reasonably intelligent person to build a nuclear bomb.

Once obtained, there are numerous ways in which a bomb or nuclear material could be smuggled into the country and transported to its intended target. Many terrorism experts suggest that the most likely method would be to pack it inside one of the approximately 20,000 shipping containers that arrive at U.S. ports every day—fewer than one in 20 of which is inspected upon arrival. Another option might be airfreight, courtesy of FedEx or UPS. With less than 10% of air cargo on passenger and all-cargo flights subject to screening, the chances of a concealed bomb being detected are not great. Nuclear weapons inside shipping containers also could enter the U.S. by truck at one of approximately 300 crossing points along the 4,000-mile land border with Canada or the 2,000-mile Mexican border. Here again, chances of detection are slight; by land, sea, or air, incoming shipments on commercial carriers have about a 5% chance of being inspected—rather good odds for a terrorist. Of course other options exist in addition to commercial carriers. As criminal smugglers of drugs and illegal immigrants well know, there are many places to sneak across U.S. borders on land; backpacks can easily carry enough plutonium for making a bomb. Similarly, thousands of miles of unguarded coastline offer ample opportunity for small boats to bring deadly cargo ashore, even in full public view, since Customs officials routinely inspect fewer than 10% of noncommercial private vessels.

Although acquisition and detonation of a small nuclear bomb represents the ultimate horror, obtaining enough fissile material to make one could present some difficulties. For this reason, terrorists seeking to use radiation as a weapon might opt instead for a **radiological dispersion device (RDD)**, popularly referred to as a "dirty bomb." Designed to scatter radioactive materials throughout a localized area without a nuclear explosion, dirty bombs could take one of several forms. The simplest, and perhaps the most likely, might consist merely of several sticks of dynamite packaged with a small amount of radioactive material such as cesium-137; it could also take the form of a large truck packed with a fertilizer-based explosive wrapped in cobalt-60. In both cases, detonation of the explosive would pulverize the radioactive material, dispersing it into the surrounding environment. With this type of dirty bomb, the explosion itself would announce the terrorist attack, prompting a rapid evacuation of the area and thus limiting human exposure to the radioactive materials released. A more stealthy approach—and one likely to result in higher casualties—would be the nonexplosive release of certain radioactive isotopes via burning, vaporization, or by dissolving them in a solvent and spraying the liquid around an area. The threat represented by the latter tactic would be less immediately obvious, so widespread radiation exposure could occur before the danger was recognized.

The ingredients for a dirty bomb are much easier to obtain than are the plutonium or highly enriched uranium needed to build a nuclear device; approximately 2 million sealed radiation sources exist in the United States alone. The radioactive isotopes whose physical properties render them capable of causing immense harm (e.g., cesium-137, cobalt-60, strontium-90, radium-226, iridium-192) are used for a wide range of medical, industrial, and commercial purposes and are readily and legally available. They also can be stolen or simply scavenged when equipment containing radioactive sources is carelessly discarded. Many experts fear that lax monitoring and inadequate regulatory controls of these materials poses a serious threat, both to public health and national security, since there is little to prevent a determined terrorist from accessing such widespread, carelessly guarded sources. The General Accounting Office (GAO) reported more than 1,300 incidents between 1998–2002 in which sealed radioactive sources in the U.S. were abandoned, lost, or stolen; it's doubtful whether the record in more than 100 other countries utilizing such materials is any better. The International Atomic Energy Agency reported 27 sources of cesium-137 disappearing in Croatia during the war in the Balkans in the mid-1990s; in 2003 after the U.S. invasion of Iraq, cobalt and cesium sources were stolen from a nuclear research center south of Baghdad. Numerous "orphaned" materials in regions of the world plagued by war, civil unrest, or organized crime constitute additional potential sources of supply for terrorists wanting to fashion a dirty bomb.

The closest the world has come yet to a RDD attack occurred in 1995 when Chechen separatists called a Russian television station to say they had placed a radiological weapon containing dynamite and cesium-137 in a Moscow park. Although they didn't detonate their crude bomb, the act vividly demonstrated the capability of a dedicated terrorist organization to wreak havoc in the heart of their enemy's largest city. It was once assumed that such groups would be deterred from making a large RDD because, in doing so, those involved would themselves receive a lethal dose of radiation. Such assumptions no longer appear valid, given the willingness of many terrorists to sacrifice their own lives for their cause.

While a dirty bomb attack would cause far fewer human deaths and radiation-induced cancers than a nuclear explosion, it would have a devastating economic and psychological impact on the affected area. Several variables, including the size of the bomb, the type of radioactive material used, and whether the release occurs within a confined space or in the open air, can affect the number of casualties and the subsequent extent of radioactive contamination. The largest number of deaths, if any, is likely to be caused by the blast itself, not by the ensuing radiation exposure. Those who survive the initial explosion presumably would flee the affected area quickly enough to escape damaging doses of external radiation exposure. If they subsequently wash their bodies, hair, and clothing thoroughly, their chances of developing health problems related to radiation exposure are minimal.

A far greater threat than external exposure is the possibility of internal contamination if radioactive particles are inhaled (as could occur if large amounts of dust are generated) or ingested. Individuals who experience internal exposure themselves become radioactive, their body wastes and everything they contact becoming contaminated. People ministering to their needs must take special precautions and use shielding to protect themselves from the patient. Long-term elevated cancer risk in the affected region is difficult to predict, but since virtually everyone would be evacuated from contaminated areas and hence would not be subject to prolonged exposure, most health authorities doubt that the few additional radiation-induced cancers that might occur 20 or 30 years later could be identified among the 2,000 out of every 10,000 Americans who die annually of cancer from nonradiation related causes.

Experts estimate that, under the worst circumstances, fatalities due to a radiological dispersion device would number in the tens to hundreds; although such deaths would be tragic to the families involved, the most damaging societal impact of a dirty bomb attack would be economic. Due to the EPA's extremely stringent cleanup standards following a radioactive release (set with small-scale laboratory accidents in mind), after-the-fact decontamination efforts would be enormously expensive, probably requiring the removal of contaminated buildings and soil. Simply finding a location to dispose of enormous volumes of low-level radioactive wastes would pose an immense challenge. Economic activities would necessarily be suspended for many months following a dirty bomb attack and large numbers of people would have to be evacuated and resettled, perhaps permanently. Since virtually all insurance policies explicitly exclude radiation damage, losses suffered by businesses or homeowners would not be compensated, imposing great financial hardship on those involved. The fear created by radiological contamination would, in all likelihood, far exceed the actual danger and could severely hamper efforts to revive commerce, tourism, or agriculture in the affected area even after successful cleanup efforts.

Unarguably, the consequences of either a "loose nuke" or "dirty bomb" would be catastrophic. Far more could be done to ensure that nuclear weapons and radioactive materials in the former Soviet Union and elsewhere are secured, out of reach to terrorists and criminal gangs. Tighter U.S. border controls, including more stringent inspections of incoming shipping containers, are urgently needed, as are tougher licensing requirements for those legally buying and selling radioactive materials. Serious consideration should be given to increasing the allowable level of residual radiation following cleanup of a dirty bomb attack; doing so would reduce the otherwise astronomical costs of remediation with minimal impact on human health. Finally, civil defense authorities should be much more proactive in providing the public with accurate information about what to do in the event of an attack. In particular, they should educate citizens as to the difference between a nuclear weapon and a dirty bomb, assuring them of the high likelihood of surviving the latter without serious injury and with little additional cancer risk if they avoid panic and evacuate in a timely fashion. If we're lucky, the ultimate nightmare can be avoided, but more vigorous governmental efforts to reduce the odds are overdue (Allison, 2004; Zimmerman and Loeb, 2004).

their authors that while there is no question that at doses of 1 Gy or above cancer risk increases with increasing dosage, doses of radiation under 0.2 Gy are not carcinogenic. Indeed, they argue that very low levels of radiation not only present no health threat, but may actually be beneficial (Jaworowski, 1999; Pollycove, 1997).

However, in 2005 the Nuclear and Radiation Studies Board of the National Research Council took issue with such reasoning and, citing data generated over the last 15 years, reaffirmed the linear relationship between radiation exposure and human cancer incidence. According to Board Chairman Richard Monson, "The scientific research base shows that there is no threshold of exposure below which low levels of ionizing radiation can be demonstrated to be harmless or beneficial." Currently, federal standards set 1 mSv/year (100 mR/year), excluding medical exposure, as the upper limit for annual effective dose equivalent for continuous or repeated exposure for members of the general population as a whole, no more than 0.25 mSv (25mR) of which should come from a nuclear power facility. Individuals may receive up to 5 mSv/year (500 mR/year) as the maximum permissible annual effective dose equivalent when exposure is infrequent. Workers in radiation-related occupations are allowed average yearly exposures of 50 mSv (5 rems). People under the age of 18 are permitted no occupational exposure whatsoever (Hall, 2000).

Such standards have been set for the intended purpose of protecting human health against the long-term radiation effects of cancer and genetic defects. These standards do not reflect levels of absolute safety but rather attempt to strike a balance between possible adverse effects of low-level exposure and the known benefits of nuclear power and other uses of radioactive materials. In the late 1980s the safety of current exposure limits was called into question by new interpretation of data on exposure received by Japanese survivors at Hiroshima and Nagasaki. Post-war estimates of likely radiation levels at varying distances from ground zero, correlated with observed health effects, have formed the basis for radiation standards since the end of World War II. Results from studies conducted during the 1980s suggested that the original data overestimated the radiation dosage received by people in the affected area. Some researchers now believe that the observable health damage experienced by survivors was caused by approximately one-half the amount of radiation exposure calculated previously. These findings, if correct, imply that current radiation protection standards should be at least twice as stringent as they are now in order to protect public health.

It should be noted that the above-mentioned consequences of low-level radiation exposure may also be manifested at higher rates among survivors of high-level radiation doses. Mutations, birth defects among off-spring, a significantly heightened risk of leukemia and other cancers, as well as cataracts and a general shortening of life span due to premature aging, are realistic possibilities confronting individuals who have recovered from overt symptoms of radiation sickness.

Radiation and Nuclear Power Generation

While medical uses of X-rays and radioisotopes constitute by far the largest amount of non-background radiation exposure, it is not these sources but rather the perceived health and safety threat from nuclear power plants that has received the lion's share of public attention in recent years. Since 1957 when the first commercial nuclear power plant in the United States came on line in Shippingsport, Pennsylvania (the world's first civilian nuclear plant opened in 1954 in the former USSR), the percentage of electricity generated by nuclear energy in the United States grew rapidly until the mid-1970s, much more slowly since then. No new commercial nuclear reactors have been ordered by U.S. utility companies since 1977 and construction on the last was completed in 1996. At present, approximately 20% of the electrical energy in the United States is generated by 104 nuclear power plants at 66 locations in 31 states, operated by 30 different power companies (work resumed in 2008 on one additional nuclear plant whose construction had been suspended since 1985; this unit is expected to go on line in 2013). Outside the United States, there were an additional 331 nuclear reactors operating in 2009; worldwide, nuclear energy accounts for 15% of total electrical power generation. Canada currently has 18 operating nuclear reactors. Although the 40-year licenses of power plants currently in operation began to expire in 2009, by October of that year the Nuclear Regulatory Commission (NRC) had granted 20-year license extensions to 55 plants, with more applications expected by 2013. Overall, about 90 U.S. reactors are likely to receive authorization to operate over a 60-year life span.

In addition to these license extensions, by 2009 the NRC had received 17 license applications for 26 new nuclear power plants—the first such applications submitted in several decades. Indeed, after years of stagnation, the nuclear power industry may be on the verge of what some utility spokespeople refer to as a "nuclear renaissance," characterized by a revival of interest in expanding domestic reliance on nuclear energy for electricity generation that has spurred new license applications and a new generation in reactor and plant design. As a result, construction of new nuclear plants in the U.S.—at a standstill for many years—is expected to get underway early in the coming decade.

Given the past history of nuclear power in the United States, such a turnabout, if indeed it does occur, will

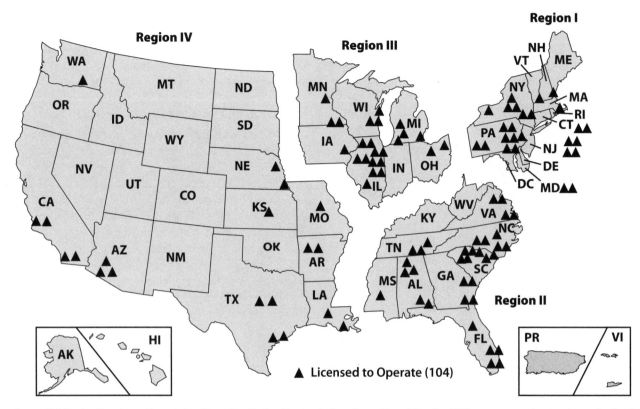

Source: U.S. Nuclear Regulatory Commission. "Operating Nuclear Reactors by Location or Name," October 2010, www.nrc.gov/reactors/operating.html

Figure 10-3   Map of the U.S. Showing Locations of Operating Nuclear Power Reactors

mark a radical departure from earlier trends, influenced both by environmental and security concerns. Even before the serious accident in 1979 at the Three Mile Island power plant near Harrisburg, Pennsylvania, and the catastrophe at Chernobyl in the former Soviet Union in 1986, concerns about the safety of nuclear power had given rise to an active and vocal anti-nuclear movement. TV footage of protest marches with demonstrators shouting "Hell, no, we won't glow!" became indelibly associated with the tumultuous period of the late 1960s/early 1970s. However, far more influential in pulling the plug on new nuclear plant orders by the mid-1970s was the realization by utility company executives and Wall Street financiers that the business risks and costs associated with nuclear power were excessive and not economically competitive. Many independent observers argue that assessment still holds and contend that a significant expansion of U.S. nuclear-generating capacity is unlikely because of the enormous costs involved—an estimated $9–12 billion per plant, depending on reactor size—making new nuclear technologies more expensive than virtually any other power generation option (Severance, 2009).

So why are some utility companies and government officials insisting that new nuclear power plants are essential for U.S. energy security? To a large extent, the sense of urgency grows out of concerns about pending climate change regulations and the realization that future coal-fired plants, notorious as major CO_2-emitters, may not be an option. Since coal today provides approximately half of all U.S. electrical power, utilities feel a need to diversify their sources of supply and are scrambling for alternatives. Recent large natural gas discoveries at several locations in the United States, as well as the efficiency of natural gas combined cycle gas turbines, provides a comfortable cushion for the necessary energy supply transition now underway in this country. However, some utility companies, particularly those in the southeastern U.S. where wind, solar, and geothermal potential is low, are looking to nuclear power as a clean, reliable replacement for coal—and one for which the cost is independent of oil prices. Ironically, unlike coal or other alternatives such as wind or solar power, nuclear energy cannot claim to rely exclusively on domestic sources of supply, since the bulk of the uranium oxide used for making nuclear fuel—over 92% in 2007—comes from foreign sources (Severance, 2009). It would undoubtedly come as a surprise to most Americans to learn that, according to the Nuclear Energy Institute, recycled uranium from old Soviet bomb cores currently accounts for 45% of the fuel in American nuclear reactors (Kramer, 2009).

The recent upsurge in enthusiasm for a "nuclear renaissance" is far from universal. Aside from the exorbitant costs which many observers believe will be the primary deterrent, detractors point to long-standing and still-unresolved radioactive waste management problems and to the worldwide shortage of skilled nuclear engineers and manufacturing facilities. Overshadowing these important issues, however, is widespread concern that a significant expansion of nuclear power production will inevitably increase the risk of nuclear proliferation. Fears that the enriched uranium fueling most modern nuclear reactors could be diverted for bomb production are not simply hypothetical worries. Israel, India, and Pakistan all secured the materials for their first nuclear weapons from "atoms for peace" programs involving civilian nuclear reactors; many suspect that Iran is now on the verge of following the example of those countries while continuing to insist that its only goal is nuclear electricity production (Crooks and Blitz, 2009).

Arguments supporting increased reliance on nuclear energy are aptly summed up by Hans-Holger Rogner at the International Atomic Energy Agency, who contends that "if we want to curb greenhouse gas emissions by 50–80% by 2050, and we don't use nuclear power for base load electricity, what can we use instead? It is not a quick fix: it depends on public acceptance and government support. It is not the whole solution to the problem. But it can make a contribution." Doubters concede that nuclear energy will, indeed, continue to be part of the world's energy mix but, due to the exorbitant costs involved, are skeptical that nuclear power will ever increase its share of global electricity-generating capacity. New plants coming online will simply be replacing old ones at the end of their useful lifespan, thus basically maintaining the status quo; emerging renewable energy technologies, they argue, will be cheaper, safer, and climate-friendly and are becoming major players in the world's energy economy much more rapidly than anyone believed possible just a few years ago.

It remains to be seen which of these lines of reasoning ultimately proves to be correct. The ongoing debate in the United States is echoed in many other countries, where pro- and anti-nuclear groups are making their voices heard as policy makers wrestle with the issue. Until quite recently, sentiment in Western Europe was overwhelmingly anti-nuclear; in fact, in 2002 the German parliament passed legislation mandating closure of all 17 of that country's nuclear power plants by 2022, in spite of the fact that nuclear power currently provides 23% of Germany's electricity. However, growing realization among the German electorate that the loss of

nuclear power would inevitably result in heavier reliance on carbon-intensive coal combustion or increased dependence on Russia for natural gas supplies led voters in Germany's September 2009 election to support candidates favoring extended use of nuclear power. Though anti-nuclear activists vow to fight any policy change, it appears likely that the existing reactors will be allowed to continue operating until renewable energy alternatives can fill the gap (Fuhrmans, 2009).

Elsewhere in Western Europe, widespread anti-nuclear sentiment persists; only in France, where nuclear power provides 80% of that country's electricity, and in Finland is there any new plant construction underway, with one new plant each. (Both facilities feature a new-generation reactor design, once touted as the "showpiece of the nuclear renaissance"; both projects are also months behind schedule and significantly over budget). In Eastern Europe and in Asia the situation is quite different; nine new plants are being built in Russia, two in Slovakia, six in India, five in South Korea, two in Japan, one each in Iran and Pakistan, and 16 in China—with 125 more proposed in that country (Crooks and Blitz, 2009). While these numbers appear impressive, a closer look reveals that not all is going according to plan. Nearly half the reactors currently being built around the world, like those in France and Finland, have encountered construction delays; nine don't even have designated start-up dates. In the United States, Congress has balked at giving utilities billions of dollars worth of requested loan guarantees, while resistance by some state governments to levy pre-construction utility rate hikes on customers in order to finance new plant construction has led to at least one suspension of a planned project.

Economists predict that advanced new reactors will be much slower coming on line than nuclear proponents had promised. The impact that increased reliance on nuclear power would have in combating climate change—the main rationale cited by nuclear proponents—is also being questioned. The Organization for Economic Cooperation and Development's (OECD) Nuclear Energy Agency asserts that, worldwide, an average of 12 new reactors would have to be brought on line every year from now until 2030 in order to have a significant impact on greenhouse gas reduction. Currently the number of new reactors being built isn't even sufficient to replace those units being retired; so, barring a major and unanticipated acceleration in the pace of new plant construction, the prospect of nuclear power saving the world from global warming is not very bright (Kanter, 2009).

While the public attitude toward nuclear energy has become somewhat more positive in recent years, in many countries, including the U.S., opposition to nuclear power by an influential segment of the population continues to stymie or delay efforts to build new facilities.

Arguments by proponents that nuclear power is urgently needed to curb greenhouse gas emissions are discounted by a public concerned about the absence of safe methods for permanent radwaste disposal, aware that "accidents can happen," and harboring a visceral fear of anything labeled "radioactive." Given the emotionalism involved, it is important that citizens clearly understand the extent to which nuclear power generation contributes to the overall radiation burden experienced by the general public. Although most attention is focused on the power plants themselves, nuclear power production is dependent upon a number of activities, collectively referred to as the **nuclear fuel cycle**. The three main components of this cycle, along with their environmental health impacts, are described in the following sections.

Front-End

Prior to the generation of power inside a nuclear reactor, the nuclear fuel itself must be mined, processed, and fabricated into fuel rods. Uranium-235 constitutes the fissionable fuel in most nuclear reactors and is mined in a number of locations around the world, including Australia, Canada, parts of eastern Europe, and several western states in the U.S. In the past, when uranium ore was obtained primarily from underground mines, the most significant radiation hazard was the increased risk of lung cancer among uranium miners, caused by the inhalation of alpha-emitting radon gas and radon daughters (radioactive isotopes of polonium and lead) attached to tiny particles of mine dust. Between 1950–1990, more than 500 miners, the majority of whom were Navajos recruited by the government to work for the nuclear weapons industry but never warned about the known health risks, died of lung cancer resulting from their occupational exposure—a death rate 4 to 5 times higher than that prevailing among the general population. Similarly, at least 20,000 East German miners, mobilized in the late 1940s and early 1950s to supply uranium for the former Soviet Union's nuclear arsenal, have died or are dying of lung diseases caused by their exposure to radioactive gases and dust (Kahn, 1993). Open-pit uranium mining avoids the occupational health risks entailed by underground mining; however, like strip-mining for coal, it is environmentally disruptive and often results in soil erosion and contaminated runoff.

The uranium ore extracted from underground or open-pit mines must subsequently be crushed and processed to produce the form of uranium dioxide known as "yellowcake." These milling operations and the enormous piles of sand-like tailings they create (for every ounce of uranium extracted from ore, 99 ounces of waste tailings are generated) are by far the most significant source of public exposure to ionizing radiation related to nuclear power production. In the United States, more than 140 million tons of radioactive tailings were left at abandoned mill sites scattered across seven western states, releasing radon into the air and leaching radium into the subsoil. In 1979, the rupture of an earthen dam at a uranium mine and mill site near Churchrock, New Mexico, released 1,100 tons of tailings sludge and 90 million gallons of radioactively contaminated water into a stream running through the Navajo reservation. Considered the worst radwaste spill ever to occur in the United States, this accident resulted in traces of radioactive materials being carried at least 75 miles downstream across the Arizona border.

In Grand Junction, Colorado, mine tailings were incorporated into concrete that was used for foundations of homes, churches, and schools. For nearly 20 years until the problem was recognized, approximately 30,000 people living in those dwellings were exposed to levels of radon up to seven times the maximum allowable level for uranium miners; subsequent cleanup efforts at the Grand Junction mill site and over 4,000 nearby properties cost the government close to $700 million. A number of other western communities, including Denver and Salt Lake City, also have used radioactive tailings in constructing roads and the foundations of buildings. Because of the radiation hazards posed by mill tailings (radiation levels 40–400 times above normal background levels), Congress in 1978 passed legislation authorizing the U.S. Department of Energy to remediate 50 uranium-processing sites, as well as nearby contaminated properties. While a number of mills were still active in 1978 when the law was passed, all are now closed and cleanup of surface contamination has been completed. In most cases site remediation involved enclosing the tailings in a containment cell, covering the cell with compacted clay to prevent the release of radon, and, finally, topping the area with vegetation or rocks. Cleanup of contaminated groundwater at these sites is ongoing and isn't expected to be finished until at least 2014 (Steinhardt, 1996).

Similar environmental problems associated with uranium milling operations continue to plague a number of European countries. In eastern Germany, Hungary, and the Czech Republic, large areas are today littered with abandoned piles of uranium tailings and other radioactive wastes, confronting the leaders of those countries with massive cleanup challenges.

Today almost all production of uranium in the United States, and in many places elsewhere in the world, utilizes an extraction process called **in-situ leaching (ISL)**. ISL is a closed-loop mining system whereby uranium is dissolved in place by a leaching agent—usually sulfuric acid—that is injected into the ore deposit, with the liquid subsequently being pumped to the surface where the uranium is recovered out of the solution. After processing, the fluid is returned to the well field to continue the leaching cycle. Unlike underground or open-pit mining, ISL methods eliminate worker exposure to radioactive gases, minimize surface disruption, and produce no tailings whatsoever; the only surface wastes associated with the process are small evaporation ponds. Nevertheless, while in-situ leaching is often described by advocates as an "environmentally benign" method of mining uranium, it isn't problem-free. The injection of massive amounts of acid into rock deposits can result in extensive groundwater contamination if proper precautions aren't followed. At an in-situ leaching site that has been operating for more than 25 years in the Czech Republic, highly contaminated liquids have migrated from the leaching zone, seeping along faulty wells to an upper-level aquifer. As a result of this, some 76 million cubic meters of drinking water in northern Bohemia's largest aquifer are now polluted (Perera, 1997).

Transforming the milled yellowcake into nuclear fuel requires several additional steps. First, the uranium is converted into gaseous uranium hexafluoride, then enriched to increase the concentration of the fissionable U-235 isotope from its original 0.7% (the bulk of uranium ore is U-238, a nonfissionable isotope) to 2–4%, the level necessary to sustain a fission reaction. Finally, at a fuel fabrication facility, the enriched uranium hexafluoride gas is converted into solid uranium dioxide pellets that are then loaded into fuel rods. Cumulatively, these processes have very minimal environmental health impacts, entailing the venting of small, regulated quantities of radioactive emissions into the air and very limited discharges of diluted liquid wastes; occupational exposure among workers in the plants where these activities are carried out likewise is very low.

In summary, the front-end of the nuclear fuel cycle is characterized by relatively low levels of radioactive emissions and minimal public exposure to radiation, the major exception to this being those people living in the vicinity of improperly managed uranium mill tailings and the unfortunate uranium miners whose untimely deaths due to lung cancer can be attributed largely to their workplace exposure to radioactive gases in underground mines.

Power Production

Under normal operating conditions, radiation exposure to the general public emanating from nuclear power plants comes primarily from the deliberate release of controlled amounts of radioactive gases to the atmosphere. Gaseous fission products such as tritium and krypton build up in the fuel rods, leak through the cladding into the reactor building, and must be periodically vented. In addition, small amounts of radioactive materials may be discharged with wastewaters. Overall, the radiation hazard to people living in the vicinity of a normally operating nuclear reactor is minimal, considerably less than that from natural background sources.

The main fear among those opposed to expansion of nuclear power, of course, is the potential, however remote, of catastrophic release of radioactive materials should a major accident occur. Most people today realize that it is physically impossible for a nuclear power plant to explode like a bomb—for this to occur the U-235 fuel would have to be enriched to a concentration far above the level necessary to sustain a fission reaction for power production purposes. However, a **core meltdown**, which represents a worst-type accident scenario, would be nearly as devastating. Overheating of the reactor core, such as might occur if water should cease to circulate among the fuel rods (a "loss-of-coolant" accident), could result in melting of the fuel rods and breaching of the containment vessel. The massive release of highly radioactive isotopes into the atmosphere, such as occurred at Chernobyl, or into groundwater supplies could cause widespread human exposure to lethal doses of radiation. Moreover, contamination of the general environment with radioactive fallout would initiate numerous leukemias and other cancers that would be manifested years later. Although physical destruction of buildings and property would not occur, the biological impact of a core meltdown would be nearly as serious as a bomb blast in terms of human health and environmental degradation. The "defense in depth" concept employed in the construction of nuclear plants, characterized by repeated layers of thick shielding materials and multiple safeguards designed to ensure safety even in the event of partial failure, are intended to prevent this situation from ever becoming a reality.

In spite of such precautions, thousands of mishaps have occurred both here and abroad since the advent of commercial nuclear power. Prior to the Three Mile Island incident, there were two serious U.S. accidents: (1) at the Enrico Fermi experimental fast breeder reactor near Detroit, part of the fuel in the core melted in early October 1966, and (2) at Browns Ferry, Alabama in March 1975, a fire ignited by an electrician's candle raged for seven hours, destroying all the emergency cooling systems in one of the reactors at the complex. In both cases, a core meltdown was only narrowly averted. Each major accident has led to a tightening of safety regulations; no accidents resulting in damage to the reactor core have occurred since the partial meltdown at Three Mile Island in 1979, nor have any off-site releases of large amounts of radioactivity taken place. In recent years the number of "safety-significant events" reported to the Nuclear Regulatory Commission has declined significantly; in 1990 they averaged around two per plant each year, but by 2000 had declined to less than one-tenth that number. The next generation of nuclear reactors should

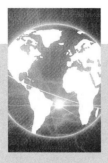

· · · · · · · 10-4 · · · · · · ·

Aftermath of Chernobyl

A quarter-century after the name "Chernobyl" became an internationally recognized synonym for an event the International Atomic Energy Agency calls the "foremost nuclear catastrophe in human history," the full impact of that disaster remains a subject of research and controversy. What is clear, however, is that the death tally of 31 persons killed in the explosion, as initially reported by Soviet authorities, significantly understates the accident's actual human health and environmental toll. On the other hand, more than two decades of intensive studies have revealed that apocalyptic forecasts of an enormous surge of radiation-induced cancer deaths and widespread environmental contamination were overblown—in fact, a 2005 report authored by a panel of UN experts concluded that the largest public health problem associated with the accident may be its mental health impact.

When reactor #4 of the nuclear power complex near the Ukrainian town of Chernobyl experienced a steam explosion and core meltdown on April 26, 1986, the resulting massive release of radioactive materials contaminated the environment with fallout equivalent to that of a hundred Hiroshima-type bombs. The graphite core of the reactor burned uncontrollably for ten days in spite of heroic efforts by firefighters to quench the blaze and prevent its spread to three nearby reactors. Of the 31 fatalities attributed to the accident by Soviet officials, 28 were among these men who knowingly braved lethal doses of radiation, standing their ground even as their boots stuck to the melting tar of the reactor roof.

By this time the radioactive plume rising from the stricken reactor had spread over much of Europe. Due to the wind direction at the time of the accident, approximately 70% of the radioactive fallout from Chernobyl was deposited in the neighboring republic of Belarus, where 21% of the national territory remains contaminated 25 years later. Significant fallout also affected northern Ukraine in the area surrounding Chernobyl, as well as in nearby regions of Russia.

Evacuation of the population living in the vicinity of Chernobyl was delayed for about 36 hours following the explosion due to administrative confusion and indecision, but eventually resulted in the permanent relocation of about 116,000 people from within a 19-mile (30 km) radius of the plant during the next few months, followed by another 230,000 in subsequent years. The evacuated region, officially designated as the "Scientific Exclusion Zone" (but commonly called the "Dead Zone"), now constitutes a living laboratory where scientists can study the long-term ecological effects of radioactive contamination on biotic communities.

Ukrainians and Belarussians also are subjects of interest to researchers, who will study the incidence rates of cancer and other radiation-related illnesses for years to come. Shortly following the explosion, government agencies in Russia, Ukraine, and Belarus reported between 25,000–100,000 post-accident deaths among the 600,000 "liquidators" who participated in the cleanup operations. A more recent exhaustive UN report says the true number will probably be closer to 4,000, including both those who have already died as well as those likely to die in future years due to radiation-induced cancer. Nevertheless, an estimated 100,000–200,000 people continue to experience after-effects of the disaster. It is known that many of the liquidators, as well as surviving workers at the power plant, received high radiation doses. Workers who suffered symptoms of radiation sickness such as hair loss or skin lesions have since recovered. Early assumptions about much higher Chernobyl-related fatalities are now attributed to the tendency among people in the region to blame all health-related problems on radiation exposure, even when other factors were actually responsible.

The main physical health impact of the Chernobyl accident has been the upswing in thyroid malignancies, especially among children. As cattle grazed on pasturelands contaminated by radioactive fallout during the weeks immediately following the accident, iodine-131 traveled via milk to children's thyroid glands where it concentrated to levels 100 times higher than in other tissues. Youthful thyroid glands are 25 times more sensitive to radioactive iodine than are those of adults and within four years of the disaster, cases of childhood thyroid cancer began to be reported with increasing frequency. Fortunately, because this disease is usually treatable, by 2005 only nine of the approximately 4,000 children stricken with thyroid cancer had died of the malignancy. Other than thyroid cancer, researchers have found only minimal physical health impacts among the millions of people exposed to low levels of radiation from the fallout of wind-blown particles. Contrary to expectations, except for a few cases among workers in the contaminated reactor building, there have been no reports of a rise in the incidence of leukemia—a form of blood cancer often associated with radiation exposure. Similarly, there has been no increase in the rate of birth defects, nor a decrease in human fertility.

In addition to its human health impact, the radiation released by the Chernobyl explosion inflicted a severe environmental and economic toll. Extensive areas of agricultural and forest lands have been heavily contaminated by radioactive fallout from the fire that raged for 10 days; relatively immobile and with a 30-year half-life, cesium-137 is especially problematic because it will persist near the soil surface in the root zone of plants for many decades to come. Radioactive contamination of forest plants utilized by villagers for food has raised serious public health concerns. In Belarus, wild mushrooms have long been a national dish, and even though fallout contaminated the mushrooms in half the country, villagers continue to collect and eat them. Cattle and goats bioaccumulate radioactive isotopes present on pasture grasses and incorporate these materials into milk and meat, while fish from contaminated lake waters present yet another source of dietary radiation exposure. Some 25 years since the accident, 5–7% of Ukraine's entire annual budget is spent on problems relating to Chernobyl—significantly more than it spends on health, education, or culture. The financial impact on Belarus has been equally severe—one expert estimates that in the years since the accident, Belarus' economic losses have been ten times greater than the country's annual budget.

Unfortunately, there's no end in sight to Ukraine's Chernobyl-related problems. A group of experts assembled by the World Health Organization to evaluate the health effects and medical care programs in the region concluded that the *mental* health impact of Chernobyl represents the biggest public health problem associated with the accident. Among people living in the affected areas, a sense of fatalism and widespread assumption that their lives are going to be cut short has led to a loss of initiative in solving their own problems and to dependency on the state for support. At the same time, it has led them to attribute all their health issues to presumed radiation exposure, discounting personal lifestyle choices such as heavy drinking, smoking, and—despite government warnings—consumption of contaminated forest products such as mushrooms and berries. The conviction that they are "victims" rather than "survivors" has produced a culture of dependency that has become a major barrier to the region's economic recovery (The Chernobyl Forum, 2005).

Perhaps the most urgent issue awaiting final resolution is the damaged reactor. The concrete "sarcophagus" built immediately after the accident to contain further radioactive releases from the molten core was hastily constructed without a structural margin of safety. Experts fear that the already cracked structure could collapse if overburdened with heavy snow—a troubling prospect since engineers have confirmed the presence of some 34 tons of radioactive dust within the sarcophagus. Moreover, the basement of the sarcophagus is flooded with about 3,000 cubic meters of radioactively contaminated water, due to infiltration of precipitation and routine spraying for dust suppression. There are fears that this water has the potential to contaminate groundwater, the level of which has been rising under the reactor since 1993. Pollution of groundwater in the vicinity is made even more problematic by the existence of large amounts of intensely radioactive wastes buried in shallow trenches on plant grounds and at various locations within the exclusion zone. These hastily constructed burial trenches are situated just 4 meters above the water table and lack waterproof barriers. Inside the sarcophagus, high humidity and standing water are dissolving fission products in the radioactive debris, causing it to crumble and leading to fears that a burst of neutrons (a "criticality incident") could result due to the increasing concentration of fission products.

Acknowledging that the damaged reactor was in desperate need of repair and that outside help was needed, in 1997 the Group of Seven (G7) industrialized countries, plus Russia, the European Union, and Ukraine launched the Shelter Implementation Plan—a project to build a new 20,000 ton structure to enclose the existing sarcophagus. Intended to provide safe confinement of the radioactive materials still inside the damaged reactor for at least 100 years, the new shelter is scheduled for completion by 2012. In the meantime, officials in Russia and Ukraine continue to argue publicly about the condition of the deteriorating sarcophagus, with Russia's top atomic energy official warning that the sarcophagus is in serious danger of collapse while Ukrainian officials insist the problem is under control. Regrettably, Chernobyl's lethal legacy of health and environmental threats will continue to bedevil policy makers, scientists, and the medical community for decades to come (Bradley, 1997).

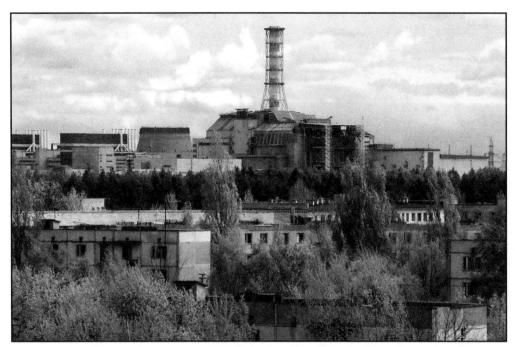

The long-shuttered Chernobyl nuclear power plant looms behind abandoned apartment buildings in this 2007 photo. The evacuated region, commonly called the "dead zone," nonetheless has seen some regrowth of vegetation. [*AP Photo/ Efrem Lukatsky*]

have an even better safety record, since new plant designs incorporate features intended to prevent accidents and to minimize the severity of those that occur (Lake, Bennett, and Kotek, 2002).

The operating record of nuclear power plants in Japan and the countries of western Europe roughly parallels that of the United States. Since the breakup of the former Soviet Union, however, numerous concerns have been raised about the deplorable conditions prevailing at a number of nuclear power plants operating in Russia and several of the former Soviet republics. Russian safety experts, nuclear plant workers, and Western scientists have all concluded that the nuclear power industry throughout the former USSR is on the verge of disaster. The tragic accident at Chernobyl in 1986, initially blamed on violations of operating procedures by plant personnel, is now attributed primarily to fundamental design faults in the reactor itself. This conclusion is troubling because 11 other reactors of similar design are operating in Russia, two more in Lithuania. These plants, in the view of many experts, are "accidents waiting to happen."

Neither the Chernobyl-style reactors nor the older Soviet-version pressurized water reactors are enclosed by the concrete and metal radiation containment structures that are a standard feature of reactor design in other industrial countries. (Russian reactors built after 1981 do have full containment structures, however.) An inventory of nuclear facilities conducted by Russia's State Committee for Nuclear and Radiation Safety Oversight (Gosatomnadzor) in 1993 revealed that many of the nation's older reactors were in dire need of radical reconstruction due to repeated failures of obsolete or worn-out equipment and system components. Some of these older facilities are characterized by such serious design flaws that Committee members concluded they could never be retrofitted to international standards and urged that they be closed. In the Moscow area alone, 50 nuclear reactors were judged to be unsafe, with the Committee concluding that "Russia's nuclear power plants are incapable of maintaining their equipment in a safe state" (Feshbach, 1995).

Back-End

After a fuel assembly has been in operation for about a year, waste fission products accumulate in the rods to such an extent that the fission reaction can no longer be sustained, necessitating replacement of these "spent" rods with fresh ones. Spent fuel rods, highly radioactive, are initially placed in swimming pool-like cooling tanks where the isotopes with very short half-lives decay within a relatively brief time. The rods are still highly radioactive (and physically hot as well) due to longer-lived fission products still present and also contain appreciable amounts of unused fuel in the form of U-235 and plutonium that formed during the fission process within the fuel rods. To separate these two useful products from the other isotopes that constitute high-level radioactive wastes, **reprocessing** of the material in the spent rods was once envisioned as a vital part of the nuclear fuel cycle. In this process the fuel is removed from the rods and dissolved in nitric acid, the solution then being treated chemically to separate it into uranium (95.6%), plutonium (1%), and waste components (3.4%). This operation represents a potential public hazard, since volatile radioisotopes, particularly krypton, are released into the atmosphere and other radioisotopes are discharged with liquid wastes. Workers inside the reprocessing plant also are exposed to higher levels of radioactivity than are nuclear power plant workers, though conceivably safeguards could be taken to reduce this risk.

Although reprocessing was considered an important means to reduce radioactive waste and extend the fuel supply, a moratorium on commercial reprocessing was imposed by President Ford in 1976 and continued by President Carter due to the concern that reprocessing plants would be tempting targets for attack by terrorists intent on obtaining weapons-grade plutonium. Although President Reagan subsequently lifted the ban, financial considerations deterred private interests from reentering the reprocessing business. Over the next two decades, little attention was paid to reprocessing, largely due to arguments by scientists and others that fuel reprocessing made no economic sense since permanent disposal of radioactive waste is far more cost-effective.

In 2006, President George W. Bush announced a major new initiative—the Global Nuclear Energy Partnership (GNEP)—as a way to promote nuclear power while avoiding nuclear proliferation by helping participating countries to obtain nuclear fuel so they don't produce it themselves. GNEP as initially proposed involved seven different elements aimed at jump-starting a worldwide nuclear renaissance, one of which was to resurrect commercial spent-fuel reprocessing at a facility in the United States. During the remainder of the Bush presidency, the Department of Energy aggressively lobbied lawmakers for funds to pursue its ambitious goals. Congress, however, was not to be persuaded, its aversion to committing billions of taxpayer dollars over many decades to such a project buttressed by testimony from scientists, environmental groups, the Nuclear Energy Institute (a private group representing the nuclear industry), and the General Accounting Office. All of these groups criticized GNEP's exorbitant price tag, unproven or nonexistent technology, and lack of industry participation in the decision-making process. Opponents argued that proceeding with GNEP could undermine nonproliferation efforts by legitimizing the commercial production and stockpiling of plutonium, while generating even more radioactive waste and diverting funds from existing radwaste management programs. Agreeing with these concerns and not persuaded by DOE's arguments to the contrary, Congress in 2008 cut all funding for GNEP and in 2009 the administration of President Obama let the GNEP initiative die a quiet death. Once again the U.S. has relegated commercial spent-fuel reprocessing to the back burner—at least for the moment.

Elsewhere in the world, France continues to reprocess spent fuel from nuclear reactors at its reprocessing plant in La Hague, serving its own 58 reactors plus a number of foreign customers as well. The United Kingdom has three reprocessing plants at Sellafield, one of which is due to close around 2015; there is no fixed closure date for the other two plants. Japan persists in its commitment to reprocessing, with a small facility at Tokai-Mura about 70 miles northeast of Tokyo, in operation since 1981, and another larger plant under construction at Rokkasho in northern Honshu. Plagued by numerous problems and many years behind schedule, the Rokkasho Reprocessing Plant was officially slated to open in October 2012—a time frame most outsiders considered questionable, given that the completion date for the plant had been extended 18 times over a 13-year period (Sawai, 2009). Not surprisingly, in September 2010 that date was postponed yet again, with no new completion date announced.

Russia has three formerly secret reprocessing plants, built primarily to obtain plutonium for weapons production during the Cold War years. In 1957 a high-level waste tank at the Mayak facility near the town of Kyshtym exploded, releasing about two million curies of radiation over the region. Although the outside world was not told of this event until three decades later, during the year following the accident 11,000 people were evacuated from the area and for many years farming was prohibited on 440 square miles of heavily contaminated land surrounding the site. Today Russia's Mayak reprocessing plant generates badly needed foreign exchange by reprocessing, for a fee, spent nuclear fuel from other countries. In 1993, another of the plants, Tomsk-7 in Siberia, experienced an explosion that contaminated 1,500 square meters of land in the vicinity of the plant; radioactive fallout from the accident was detected over a 120-square-kilometer area, with the most heavily contaminated areas registering gamma radiation readings 20 times above background levels (Perera, 1998).

Japan's nuclear complex at Tokai-Mura has experienced several serious accidents in recent years. A fire and explosion at the reprocessing plant in March 1997 exposed 37 workers to low levels of radiation and released some plutonium into the environment ("Reprocessing Facility," 1997). In the autumn of 1999, improper handling of enriched uranium at a nearby fuel processing plant resulted in a critical reaction that exposed three workers to life-threatening levels of radiation (one of these men subsequently died). Neutrons escaping from the facility irradiated a number of people outside the plant as well; the government's official count of people experiencing radiation exposure was 69, although some environmental groups insisted the actual number was much higher. Regarded as the worst accident to date in

Japan's nuclear program, the incident prompted a temporary evacuation order for residents living nearest the plant, while an additional 310,000 people within a six-mile radius were advised to remain indoors until radiation levels subsided (Landers, 1999). It should be noted that although reprocessing has been touted as a way to solve nuclear waste disposal problems, the nuclear by-products remaining after enriched uranium and plutonium have been removed from the spent fuel are themselves highly radioactive, requiring safe storage and disposal. In addition, when spent, the mixed oxide (MOX) uranium-plutonium fuel produced through reprocessing is even hotter and more radioactive than conventional spent fuel.

While reprocessing facilities may present radiation hazards both to their workers and to the environment, the most significant source of dangerous radioactive emissions from the back-end of the nuclear fuel cycle is the waste material produced by nuclear reactors. Nuclear power production generates large quantities of high-level and low-level wastes, the former primarily in the form of spent fuel from reactors, the latter consisting of contaminated clothing, clean-up solutions, wiping rags, hand tools, etc. **High-level wastes** are extremely radioactive, highly penetrating, and generate a great deal of heat, hence must be handled without direct human contact. Currently, most high-level commercial wastes in the U.S. are being stored in cooling ponds or aboveground containment casks at the power plants where they were produced; a relatively small percentage is in storage at facilities in Morris, Illinois, and West Valley, New York, once intended as reprocessing plants.

Responding to criticism that the lack of any clear-cut policy for permanent disposal of high-level radioactive waste could prove the Achilles' heel of the nuclear power industry, Congress in 1982 enacted the **Nuclear Waste Policy Act**. This legislation delegated responsibility for high-level radwaste management to the federal government and designated the U.S. Department of Energy as the lead agency to coordinate the effort to site, construct, and operate the nation's first permanent repository for such wastes. Convinced that deep geologic burial was the ultimate solution to safe high-level radwaste disposal, the government launched a politically sensitive search for an appropriate location for such a facility. Although a number of sites were initially being evaluated by DOE as potential candidates for the repository, politics intervened to influence the selection. With the choices narrowed down to sites in the states of Texas, Washington, and Nevada (at a time when both the Speaker of the House and the vice president were Texans and the House majority leader was from Washington) Congress voted in 1987 to designate Yucca Mountain, Nevada—land already owned by the federal government and adjacent to

a nuclear weapons test site—as the only location to be evaluated for the nation's first commercial high-level radwaste disposal facility (Wald, 2009a).

Cynics at the time referred to this legislation as the "Screw Nevada Bill" and over the years since then Nevada lawmakers from both political parties have done their utmost to delay progress on a project they feared would turn their state into a "national sacrifice zone." Nevertheless, over the next two decades extensive characterization studies to determine the geologic suitability of the site for deep burial of solidified radwastes were conducted by the DOE. Since the fission products in spent fuel rods will be dangerously radioactive for tens of thousands of years, it was understood that the suitability of any site chosen for an underground repository would depend on the ability of surrounding geological formations to absorb heat and to prevent radioactive emissions from escaping into the environment. Yet from a geologic standpoint, Yucca Mountain was always a problematic location because of its long-term potential for earthquakes or volcanic eruptions in an area of known seismic activity; other issues of concern were the possibility of groundwater intrusion into storage caverns in the eventuality of future climatic change.

In December 1998, DOE released its viability assessment for Yucca Mountain, concluding that while some uncertainties remained, there were no major problems that would disqualify the site from consideration. In 2002, President Bush approved Yucca Mountain as the nation's high-level waste disposal site, stating that the location was "scientifically and technically suitable for the development of a repository." Several months later, in spite of vehement objections from Nevada lawmakers, Congress voted to approve the site. The DOE announced its intent to submit a license application to the Nuclear Regulatory Commission by December 2004 and hoped to have Yucca Mountain operational by 2010. Those plans were thwarted in July 2004 when a federal appeals court, acting on a case brought by the State of Nevada and several environmental groups, declared that the government's radiation protection standards for the Yucca Mountain facility were insufficiently protective. The court ruled that DOE needed to demonstrate the wastes could be safely stored for one million years, not merely the 10,000-year period addressed in DOE's license application. This development derailed filing of DOE's license application, while perennial government underfunding of work at the site repeatedly delayed repository operations and further postponed a final decision on Yucca Mountain's ultimate fate.

By the time of the 2008 U.S. presidential election, the official opening date for Yucca Mountain had been pushed back to 2017—but once again politics intervened. With Nevada Senator Harry Reid by that time the Senate majority leader and Nevada in contention as a "swing state" in the election, the fate of Yucca Mountain became an issue in the presidential race. Victorious candidate Barack Obama followed through on his campaign pledge and, in his 2010 budget, drastically cut funding for Yucca Mountain, in effect terminating a 22-year, $10.5 billion effort to develop a deep geologic repository there. As U.S. Secretary of Energy Steven Chu remarked, Yucca is now "off the table." Unfortunately, there is no "Plan B" for permanent disposal of U.S. high-level radwaste. The 1987 law designating the Nevada location as the focus of characterization studies explicitly forbids consideration of any other site; for political reasons Congress, in essence, put all the nation's "eggs in one basket."

Following Obama's Yucca budget cuts, Energy Secretary Chu, in January 2010, recruited 15 leading scientists, former elected officials, and nuclear industry representatives to serve on the newly created "Blue Ribbon Commission on America's Nuclear Future." Charged with providing suggestions for storing, processing, and disposing of spent nuclear fuel from both civilian and military reactors—though under explicit instructions to disregard Yucca Mountain as an option—the panel is scheduled to submit an interim report to Secretary Chu in mid-2011 and a final report by 2012 ("Chu Presents 'Blue-Ribbon' Panel," 2010).

The future of high-level radwaste disposal became even murkier in June 2010 when the U.S. Nuclear Regulatory Commission's Atomic Safety and Licensing Board ruled that the Department of Energy lacks the authority to terminate the Yucca Mountain project because Congress authorized the repository-building process in 1982—hence only Congress can cancel it. As this book goes to press, the future of Yucca Mountain and of HLW management in general remains in limbo, since the president's proposed budget for 2011 contains zero funding for the repository and politicians are bitterly divided on what should be done to resolve the issue ("Licensing Board," 2010).

In the meantime, spent fuel rods continue to accumulate at power plants across the country; by 2010 approximately 60,000 metric tons of spent fuel had piled up at power plants and government facilities in 39 states, posing a major problem for the federal government as well as for the nuclear power industry. Under terms of the Nuclear Waste Policy Act, Washington has been collecting a one-tenth of a cent fee on every kilowatt-hour of electricity generated by nuclear power since 1983, with these revenues being deposited in a special fund earmarked for development of the permanent repository. In return, Washington made a contractual commitment to the utility companies that it would begin to move spent fuel from reactor sites in 1998. By the time the deadline date arrived, utilities had paid $14 billion into the Nuclear Waste Fund and were furious that the federal government had failed to meet its obligation under the law. By the time the Obama administration effectively cancelled the Yucca Mountain project, the Nuclear Waste Fund had grown to $22 billion. With no repository in sight, some utilities have told the government they should no longer have to pay into the fund, while some nuclear companies are urging that the money already collected be diverted to research on new waste processing technologies (Wald, 2009b).

For the foreseeable future, it now appears likely that as cooling ponds at reactor sites reach capacity, power plant operators will utilize on-site dry cask storage, sealing the radioactive spent fuel rods inside huge steel-lined concrete silos with 9-inch thick walls, placed outdoors on a barbed-wire enclosed concrete pad and constantly monitored by security personnel. Acknowledging the reality of this situation, the Nuclear Regulatory Commission now affirms that spent fuel can be safely stored in casks at reactor sites for many decades with no adverse environmental effects until a burial site someday becomes available (Wald, 2009a).

In contrast to the failed effort to bury commercial high-level radwastes at Yucca Mountain, a radioactive waste success story has unfolded in New Mexico. In March 1999, the **Waste Isolation Pilot Plant (WIPP)** opened its gates and in so doing became the world's first certified deep radwaste facility. Designed as a permanent repository for lower-level **transuranic wastes**—plutonium-contaminated rags, tools, and protective clothing from nuclear weapons production facilities—WIPP is a subterranean complex of shafts, tunnels, and rooms excavated more than 2,000 feet (655 meters) underground in a salt formation 25 miles east of Carlsbad, New Mexico. Site selection was driven by a search for the most secure salt bed in the country, salt considered most desirable because of its solid, impermeable nature and because of its tendency under pressure to flow, sealing up any excavated cavities. Although its development was repeatedly delayed by legal challenges related to technical and safety issues, WIPP has won the approval of scientists, regulators, and citizens of Carlsbad as a safe repository. WIPP's opening was welcome news for the ten national weapons laboratories where nearly 60,000 cubic meters of transuranic wastes had been in interim storage for years. While no radwastes from *commercial* nuclear power plants can be sent to WIPP (by law, the facility is reserved exclusively for *defense* radwastes), the opening of a final resting place for transuranic wastes was an important milestone in the federal government's efforts to implement a responsible radioactive waste management program (Kerr, 1999). During its first decade of operation, WIPP received 8,000 shipments of transuranic waste; the two million cubic feet of waste deposited in

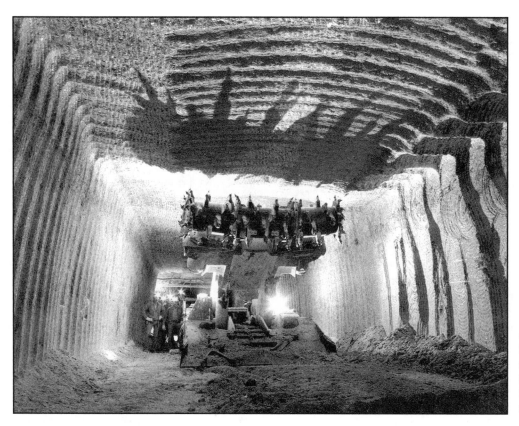

A portion of an underground tunnel at the WIPP facility is shown here, along with a machine used for excavation. [*Courtesy of U.S. Department of Energy*]

the facility during that period occupies one-third of the repository's capacity.

Elsewhere in the world, the 29 additional countries currently utilizing nuclear power face a similar radioactive waste disposal challenge. Although none have yet developed a permanent disposal facility, there is unanimous agreement that deep burial of such materials is the best option. As a result, in more than 20 countries efforts are now underway to identify appropriate locations for such facilities. In Japan the government is now searching—thus far unsuccessfully—for communities willing to host a high-level waste repository deep underground. As in the U.S., the Japanese government requires that radwaste generators pay into a fund to cover future disposal costs and estimates that a site will be ready to open around 2035. Sweden plans to store radwastes in 5-centimeter-thick copper pipes that will be embedded in clay in large underground caverns. In Finland, construction is underway on a 3-mile long, 1,600-foot deep tunnel into bedrock where spent fuel rods from that country's nuclear reactors will be sealed off for at least 100,000 years; completion of the project is expected by 2020. Czech officials have been searching since 1992 for a geologically suitable location for that country's radwaste, but in 2009 suspended research on the eight sites under consideration because of local opposition.

In Germany, plans for a nuclear waste repository since 1977 have focused on an abandoned salt mine near the small village of Gorleben. Over the past 30-plus years, the German government has spent nearly $2 billion to research an underground facility it had hoped to open by 2030, in the meantime utilizing the location as a temporary disposal site. Anti-nuclear protesters have long argued that the site is unsafe because the clay layers covering the salt dome are too thin to prevent water infiltration and have demanded that the site be closed. In 2009 Germany's environment minister—an ardent foe of nuclear energy—declared Gorleben "is dead," though German Chancellor Angela Merkel continued to insist it was an appropriate site (Vogel, 2009). Both in the United States and abroad, efforts to launch the awaited "nuclear renaissance" are unlikely to succeed unless and until high-level radwaste management challenges are satisfactorily resolved.

Low-level wastes, produced not only by nuclear power plants but also by hospitals, research labs, universities, and industries, exhibit low but sometimes potentially hazardous concentrations of radioisotopes. They differ from high-level wastes in having significantly lower levels of radioactive emissions; they are not physically hot, generally require no shielding, and, unlike high-level wastes that remain dangerous for millennia, most decay to harmless levels within 100–300 years. In the United States during the 1950s, many low-level commercial radwastes were buried on military reservations along with defense wastes or were simply dumped into the ocean—a practice that didn't cease entirely until 1970 (as recently as the fall of 1993, Russia defied world public opinion and infuriated the Japanese by brazenly dumping more than 900 tons of low-level radwastes into a prime squid fishing area in the Sea of Japan). From 1947–1970 at least 47,500 barrels of radwastes, primarily low-level wastes but also including plutonium wastes from atomic research labs, were dumped at three different sites near the Gulf of Farallones National Marine Sanctuary, an ocean wildlife preserve about 25 miles offshore from San Francisco. While the 55-gallon drums containing the wastes had a 10-year life expectancy in seawater and the concrete encasing the wastes was calculated to remain intact for 30 years, the radionuclides themselves have half-lives ranging from 30–24,000 years. By now virtually all of the barrels have reached their functional life span, but it isn't known for certain whether the radionuclides they contained remain deposited in or on nearby sediments or whether they have already been widely dispersed by ocean currents (Suchanek et al., 1996).

By the 1960s, the commercial nuclear industry was relying on shallow land burial for disposal of low-level wastes, utilizing six privately owned facilities specifically licensed for this purpose. By the late 1970s, three of these sites had closed due to migration of radioactive materials from the trenches, though no radioactive contamination was detected outside site boundaries. Because the states in which the three remaining sites were located (South Carolina, Nevada, and Washington) vigorously objected to being the "nuclear dumping ground" of the nation, Congress was persuaded to enact the **1980 Low-Level Radioactive Waste Policy Act**. This legislation placed responsibility for low-level radwaste management on state governments (as opposed to *federal* jurisdiction over high-level wastes), which were required to provide a means of safe disposal for all low-level wastes generated within their borders. Any states failing to do so could find their radwastes barred from disposal at existing sites in other states. However, recognizing that construction of 50 separate disposal facilities was neither necessary nor economically feasible, Congress permitted states to negotiate regional **"compact"** agreements among themselves to provide for the establishment, operation, and regulation of low-level radioactive waste facilities within each compact area. Currently 42 states are members of ten regional compacts approved by Congress; eight additional states, the District of Columbia, and Puerto Rico remain unaffiliated. Each regional compact is required to designate one of its members as the **"host state"**—i.e., the state in which the disposal facility is to be located—and to make numerous decisions regarding operational procedures, disposal fees, and type of facility to be constructed. The original 1986 deadline date for completion

of regional facilities was extended to January 1, 1993, but in every compact area, intense public opposition stymied efforts to carry out the requirements of the law.

Meanwhile, of the three ongoing sites, the small facility at Beatty, Nevada, closed its gates in December 1992, and the Hanford, Washington, landfill restricted access to all but 11 northwestern and Rocky Mountain states. This left only the facility at Barnwell, South Carolina—the largest of the three—to meet the radwaste disposal needs of generators from the remaining 39 states. A new radioactive waste landfill owned and operated by Envirocare of Utah, Inc., opened in 1988 at a site 80 miles west of Salt Lake City within a 100-square mile hazardous waste zone (neighbors include an Army nerve gas storage site and Dugway Proving Grounds), but facility operations are restricted solely to the management of naturally occurring radioactive materials such as slightly contaminated soil and certain types of low-activity, high-volume wastes.

In 2001 South Carolina passed legislation requiring that by mid-2008 access to Barnwell be restricted to the three members of the Atlantic Compact (South Carolina, New Jersey, and Connecticut), leaving the remaining 36 states with nowhere to send any but their lowest activity wastes (because of lower disposal costs, most of these are already being shipped to Envirocare). Indeed, in July 2008 Barnwell closed its gates to Atlantic Compact outsiders, sparking serious concerns among radwaste generators and regulatory officials alike. Closure was particularly troublesome for small generators such as universities and medical facilities with limited on-site storage space. A number of these institutions were forced to delay or even halt research projects due to the high cost of treating, storing, and disposing of low-level wastes.

Fortunately, such difficulties may be resolved by the anticipated opening of a new low-level radioactive waste repository in Andrews County, Texas, in early 2011. Fully licensed to manage the full range of low-level wastes (Classes A, B, & C) and operated by Waste Control Specialists, the facility, as of December 2010, was awaiting approval by the Texas Compact Commission to accept out-of-compact wastes, thereby resolving the dilemma created by closure of Barnwell (Anderson, 2009b). The recent disposal capacity crisis has prompted a number of observers to urge that Congress authorize development of a national low-level waste disposal facility. Others have suggested repealing the 1980 law that established the compact system, thereby motivating development of private sector radwaste management operations or, alternatively, requiring DOE to accept some commercial low-level wastes at its facilities ("Planned Barnwell Closure," 2005).

In the meantime, those engaged in the struggle to provide radwaste disposal options must continue public education efforts, aware that the contentious issue of where to

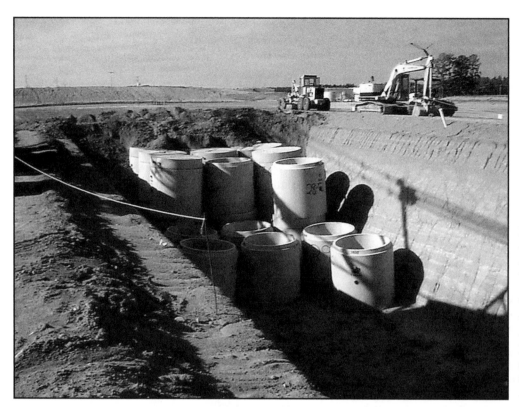

Low-level radioactive wastes are stored in concrete vaults and then placed in earthen trenches at the Barnwell, South Carolina, facility. When the trenches are full they are covered with an engineered cap of multiple layers of sand, clay, high-density polyethylene, and top soil. [*Courtesy of Chem-Nuclear Systems, LLC*]

locate needed facilities will continue to undermine efforts to manage low-level radioactive wastes in a responsible manner. While most radiation experts contend that low-level wastes, properly managed, pose minimal health or environmental hazards, the public's inability to distinguish between the vastly different risks presented by high-level vs. low-level radwastes contributes to the emotionalism surrounding the facility-siting issue, making resolution of the nation's radioactive waste disposal conundrum one of our most difficult public policy issues.

ULTRAVIOLET RADIATION

Wavelengths of the electromagnetic spectrum ranging between 40–400 nanometers in length are categorized as ultraviolet (UV) light. Although UV waves longer than 124 nanometers are not of sufficiently high energy to ionize atoms and molecules, certain portions within this range are strongly absorbed by living tissues, particularly by DNA that constitutes the major target of UV damage. Injury to the hereditary material of cells is the reason for the lethal or mutational effects which excess UV exposure can provoke in living organisms. Research has shown that the most detrimental effects to biological systems occur when UV radiation is in the 230–320 nanometer range (referred to as UVB, as opposed to longer-wavelength UVA), peak absorption by DNA occurring at 260 nanometers. Much of the ultraviolet light naturally

present in incoming solar radiation is filtered out by the layer of atmospheric ozone located about 20 miles above the earth's surface (see chapter 11). Living organisms have developed various defense mechanisms to protect themselves against the amounts that do penetrate—shielding devices such as fur, feathers, shells, or darkly pigmented skin, as well as light-avoidance behavior patterns among a variety of species.

Of equal importance to these defenses has been the evolution of enzymatic mechanisms for repairing UV-induced damage to DNA when levels of injury are not excessive. Without this cellular repair ability it is doubtful whether many organisms could survive existing levels of UV exposure. The importance of such mechanisms can be seen in the example of individuals suffering from the genetic disease xeroderma pigmentosum. Lacking the enzyme needed for repair of radiation-damaged DNA, victims of this ailment have to remain indoors throughout daylight hours or risk the development of multiple fatal skin cancers. There appears to be a tenuous balance between continual UV assault on the hereditary material and its biochemical repair. If the cell's capacity to deal with such damage is overwhelmed, the cell will die.

Since ultraviolet light cannot penetrate very deeply into living tissues, the major concern in reference to UV injury to humans involves the induction of skin cancers, particularly in lighter-skinned individuals who lack protective melanin granules in their epidermal skin layers.

Since the late 1940s, when the tyranny of fashion decreed that pale skin was "out" and the bronzed look "in," the apparently irresistible urge among fair-complexioned citizens to spend hours broiling themselves under the sun or at rapidly proliferating tanning parlors has resulted in an alarming increase in the incidence of skin cancer in Western countries due to increased exposure to UV radiation, a known carcinogen and mutagen. According to the American Cancer Society, three major types of skin cancer account for approximately half of all cancer cases diagnosed in the United States each year. The situation is even worse in Australia, where skin cancer rates are the highest in the world; an estimated two out of every three white Australians will be diagnosed with some form of skin cancer by the time they reach age 75. Skin cancer risk is highest among people with fair complexions and blonde or red hair; malignancies are lowest among African-Americans, who are 20 times less likely than whites to develop skin cancer.

Basal cell carcinoma and **squamous cell carcinoma** comprise the vast majority of all skin cancers—over 3.5 million new cases in the U.S. each year—and are increasing at a 5% annual rate. Chronic exposure to sunlight is recognized as the cause of over 90% of these two cancers. They appear, predictably, on portions of the body receiving the greatest sun exposure—face, neck, ears, back of the hands. Until recently such cancers were unusual in people under the age of 50; now, however, numerous cases have been diagnosed among people in their 20s and 30s and occasionally even in teenagers. Not surprisingly, they are also being found on the legs, chest, and back of victims as the sunbathing mania takes its toll. Fortunately, the majority of such cancers can be treated if detected early, but each year approximately 2,500 cases prove fatal when their neglect leads to invasion of underlying tissues.

Malignant melanoma is much less common than basal cell or squamous cell carcinomas, but far more deadly. According to the Skin Cancer Foundation, an estimated 68,720 new victims were diagnosed with malignant melanoma in 2009 and nearly 8,650 died of the disease. The incidence of melanoma continues to rise rapidly, with one out of every 55 Americans likely to be diagnosed with the disease during his or her lifetime. Melanoma is now the most common form of cancer for those aged 25–29 and the second-most common for teenagers and young adults.

Unlike the nonmelanoma skin cancers, in which risk is greatest among people receiving repeated UV exposure over a period of many years, malignant melanoma may be triggered by a single severe sunburn during childhood or adolescence. According to the U.S. National Library of Medicine and the National Institutes of Health, one blistering sunburn before the age of 20 doubles an individual's risk of developing malignant melanoma as an adult. At any age, the risk of melanoma doubles after five or more sunburns. More surprisingly, while basal cell and squamous cell carcinomas develop only on sun-exposed portions of the body, malignant melanomas frequently occur on areas normally covered. They also tend to occur at a younger age than do the other two forms of skin cancer; although the risk of melanoma increases with age, half of all cases occur among those under 50, with incidence rates rising most rapidly among people below 40 years of age. Because of the suspected link between childhood sunburn and melanoma, groups such as The Skin Cancer Foundation are urging parents to be particularly careful in protecting youngsters from excessive sun exposure.

Ill effects of UV-light exposure are not limited to cancer and sunburn. Premature wrinkling, drying, and mottling of the skin are among the less desirable consequences of UV exposure. In fact, the Skin Cancer

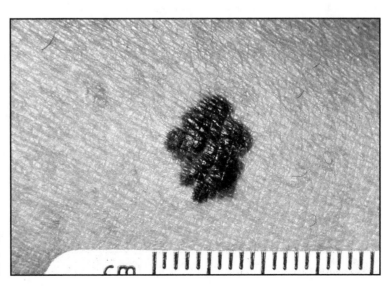

Melanoma has a characteristic blue-black color and borders that are uneven, ragged, or notched. [*Skin Cancer Foundation*]

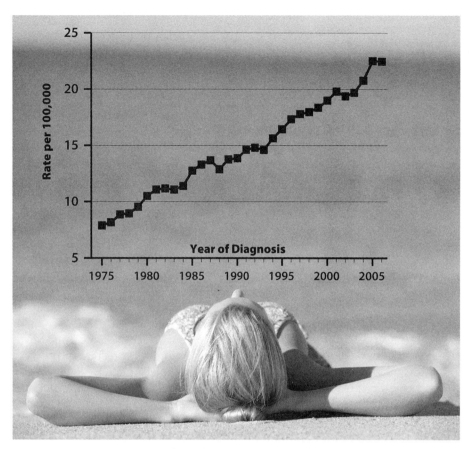

Source: Cancer Trends Progress Report—2009–2010 Update, National Cancer Institute. (http://seer.cancer.gov/registries/terms.html)

Figure 10-4   Rates of Increase of Melanoma of the Skin, 1975–2006

pills, even certain cosmetics. Such a toxic reaction is generally manifested as an unusually severe sunburn immediately following exposure to UV light.

Exposure to even moderate amounts of ultraviolet radiation can be dangerous for individuals suffering from *lupus erythematosus*, an autoimmune ailment. Between 40–60% of lupus patients experience aggravation of skin disease or systemic symptoms when exposed to either UVA or UVB light. Many researchers contend that the threat of UV damage to the body's immune system should be regarded just as seriously as its ability to induce skin cancer. Studies have shown that ultraviolet radiation from both natural and artificial sources can alter the proportions of various types of white blood cells and depress the activity of natural killer-T cells in the bloodstream. Immune system dysfunction caused by UV exposure is not related to the amount of pigmentation in a person's skin, as is the case

Foundation reports that up to 90% of visible skin changes widely assumed to be an inevitable consequence of growing old are actually caused by too much time spent in the sun. In recent years the growing popularity of tanning parlors has been accompanied by claims from their owners that they provide a safe alternative to sunbathing because they utilize UVA radiation rather than UVB and hence cannot result in burning. Nevertheless, tanning beds expose users to several other serious risks. Not only can UVA, like UVB, induce skin cancer, it also causes premature aging of the skin and development of cataracts. In addition, UVA enhances the effect of sunlight: individuals who sunbathe outdoors shortly after a stint in a tanning parlor often suffer extremely severe sunburns. People who frequent tanning parlors using new high-pressure sunlamps may be exposing themselves to as much as 12 times the yearly UVA dose they would receive from sun exposure. Photosensitive reactions to either tanning parlors or outdoor sunbathing can occur when sun-worshippers expose themselves to UV light while taking antibiotics (especially tetracycline), antihistamines, birth control

with skin cancer. Individuals with black or brown skin are just as likely to suffer immune system damage if they spend too much time in the sun as are fair-skinned people. Unfortunately, most sunscreens do not appear to be effective in preventing the type of immune system damage provoked by UVB exposure (Sontheimer, 1992; "Sunscreens," 1992). Weighing serious long-term health risks against short-term fashion benefits, dermatologists are unanimous in their recommendation that all UV exposure, whether on the beach or at a tanning salon, be avoided to the greatest extent possible.

Ultraviolet light has some beneficial as well as harmful effects. A certain amount of skin exposure is necessary to promote the bodily synthesis of vitamin D, a deficiency of which can result in the development of rickets, a bone deformity. The germicidal properties of UV light have recommended its use in operating rooms to reduce the danger of bacterial or viral infections. Ultraviolet light applications have also been successfully employed to treat such bacterial skin diseases as acne and boils.

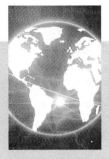

······ 10~5 ·······

Can Sunscreens Prevent Skin Cancer?

Health educators' efforts to promote sunscreen use among a sun-loving public have met with considerable success in recent years. It is now well recognized that sunscreens with an SPF (sun protection factor) of 15 or higher, when used properly, are very effective in preventing sunburn as well as protecting the skin against premature aging and wrinkling. However, their role in preventing skin cancer—the primary concern among most users—has been questioned by some researchers who point to the simultaneous rise in sunscreen sales and skin cancer rates. Some physicians go so far as to suggest that the use of chemical sunscreens is, in large part, responsible for the current skin cancer epidemic, pointing out that the highest rates of melanoma are being reported from countries where the use of chemical sunscreens has been strongly promoted (Garland et al., 1992).

Although the vast majority of dermatologists remain strong advocates of sunscreen use, some worry that users of these products may assume they can safely remain in the sun for long periods of time. Many of the sunscreens now in use are so-called "broad spectrum" products, providing varying levels of protection—depending on their rating—against both the short-wave UVB radiation that causes sunburn and the more deeply penetrating long-wave UVA rays linked to skin cancer and immune system damage. However, most experts agree that while sunscreen use is both desirable and recommended, it is not enough. Even more important are common-sense strategies such as staying indoors or in the shade during mid-day hours (10 am to 3 pm) when the sun is most intense and wearing a tightly woven long-sleeved shirt and trousers with a broad-brimmed hat when exposure is unavoidable.

Such precautions are particularly important for youngsters, who generally spend much more time outdoors than do adults. Parents should be especially careful not to allow infants or children to become badly sunburned, since childhood sunburns are widely considered to be a triggering factor for subsequent development of malignant melanoma. Extreme care should be taken to minimize sun exposure of infants; babies under 6 months of age have very sensitive skin and should be kept in the shade when outdoors. Conscientious parents will ensure that strollers are fitted with hoods and babies protected with wide-brimmed hats. Baby oil should never be applied to an infant's skin before going outdoors, since it makes the skin more translucent to harmful solar radiation. Toddlers and older children are somewhat less vulnerable than infants, but dermatologists advise that they, too, should wear protective clothing and hats while playing outdoors. Unfortunately, the inconvenience of these precautions makes it unlikely that such advice will be heeded; accordingly, parents need to do the next best thing and insist that their children regularly use sunscreen.

Dermatologists surmise that an additional explanation for the rise in skin cancer incidence among sunscreen users could be due to improper application of these products. For greatest effectiveness, sunscreen should be applied 30 minutes prior to sun exposure so that protective ingredients have time to be absorbed; it should then be reapplied every two hours or whenever perspiration or contact with water removes the original protective layer. Sunscreens should be liberally applied to parts of the body especially prone to sunburn—lips, nose, ears—and should be used on cloudy or hazy days as conscientiously as when the sun is shining brightly. Similarly, sunscreen should be worn when one is out in the snow, particularly at high altitudes. Use of products with an SPF value lower than 15 provides insufficient protection, regardless of skin type. Sunscreens with an SPF of 15 filter out 93% of UVB rays, a figure that rises to 97% for SPF 30, and 98% for SPF 50; the additional UVB protection afforded by sunscreens with an SPF greater than 50 is negligible, according to the Skin Cancer Foundation. To provide consumers with information on a sunscreen's ability to block UVA rays, the FDA plans to introduce a 1-4 star rating system, with 1 star indicating the lowest level of protection, and 4 stars the highest. Sunscreens that protect against UVB only would have no star on the label and would state "no UVA protection." The best sunscreens are resistant to being washed off by sweating or swimming—a feature that is largely determined by the product's base material. In general, the most water-resistant sunscreens are those that feel the greasiest; clear lotions and gels are the most easily washed off, while creamy lotions rank mid-way between (Epstein, 1998; Fackelmann, 1998; Napoli, 1998).

While sunscreens may indirectly increase the risk of melanoma by encouraging people to remain in the sun longer than they should, most experts continue to regard them as a last line of defense—not a pana-cea to prevent skin cancer but an important component in an overall strategy for personal protection from the sun's damaging rays.

MICROWAVES

Electromagnetic radiation comprising wavelengths ranging from approximately one millimeter to one meter (intermediate between infrared and short-wave radio wavelengths) is termed microwave radiation. Since microwave energies are so low, such radiations are typically characterized by their frequencies which, in the case of microwaves of biological interest, generally fall between 100 and 30,000 megahertz (MHz).

Humans today are continuously bombarded with microwaves from such diverse sources as military radar installations, radio and television transmitters, communications and surveillance satellites, radar and radio frequency transmitters at airports and on planes and ships, microwave ovens, telephone and TV-signal relay towers, cell phones, video display terminals, automatic garage door openers, and so on. At the low levels of exposure represented by these sources, most researchers believe that microwave radiation presents a negligible public health threat. Unlike X-rays, microwaves are non-ionizing; instead, when absorbed they cause an increased rate of vibration in the molecules of the absorbing material, resulting in the production of heat. Depending on frequency, microwaves are differentially absorbed by bodily tissues. Those of very low energy (below 150 MHz) simply pass through the body without being absorbed; those of intermediate frequency (150–1200 MHz) are absorbed by the deeper tissues without any noticeable heating of the skin. This poses a danger of serious bodily harm, since internal organs can receive highly damaging doses of microwave radiation without the victim realizing that anything is wrong. As microwave frequency increases, tissue penetration decreases and at 3500 MHz warming of the skin can be felt; above 10,000 MHz only the surface of the skin is heated and no penetration of the body occurs.

Differential absorption of microwave energy by bodily tissues is to a large degree a function of their water content. Moist tissues such as skin, muscle, and the intestines absorb more microwaves than do bones and fatty tissues. Sensitivity of specific organs to microwaves depends not only on how readily such radiation is absorbed, but also on how effectively blood circulating through the organ can dissipate the excess heat. Experiments have shown that body parts with poor circulation—the eyes, gastrointestinal tract, testes, urinary bladder, and gall bladder—are the areas most susceptible to injury from microwaves (Dalrymple, 1973).

ELECTROMAGNETIC FIELDS (EMF)

In 1979 a team of researchers at the University of Colorado Medical Center in Denver reported that children who are exposed to stronger than average magnetic fields, such as those living in the vicinity of power transmission lines, have a two to three times greater risk of developing leukemia than do children living at a distance from such sources. While this study was subsequently discredited because of methodological flaws (e.g., small size of group studied, lack of direct measurements of exposure received), the report sparked intense public alarm about an inescapable component of everyday life. The extremely low-frequency (ELF) wavelengths produced by the transmission and distribution of electric power, as well as by the plethora of electrical appliances that fill virtually every modern household, are impossible to avoid, so the suggestion that subtle but significant adverse health effects could be caused by electromagnetic fields prompted numerous scientific studies during the 1980s and 1990s.

The primary concern of researchers focused on whether exposure to the levels of low-frequency radiation typical of residential environments could, as some investigators claimed, increase the risk of childhood leukemia. The impact of EMFs in provoking birth defects, miscarriages, learning disabilities, or behavioral modifications also received attention. From the beginning, many scientists were skeptical of any cancer-EMF association, simply because the amounts of radiation emanating from power lines and appliances are so minute in comparison with the earth's own magnetic field. Numerous research efforts to verify a possible EMF-cancer connection yielded inconclusive results; some epidemiologic studies showed a slight risk of cancer with EMF exposure, while others revealed no such association. Significantly, experiments using animal models failed to demonstrate any correlation between laboratory exposure to low frequency radiation and the induction or promotion of cancer. Several major studies in the early 1990s found evidence for an association between EMF and cancer inconsistent and inconclusive. In 1995 the American Physical Society, the world's largest group of physicists, entered the fray, saying its members could find no evidence that electromagnetic fields radiating from power lines have any impact on cancer rates. The Society deplored the fact that public fears about an EMF-cancer connection were responsible for the unnecessary diversion of billions of dollars (estimated at $1–3 billion annually in the U.S.) for moving power lines and installing shielding.

The scientific debate was effectively resolved (1) when the National Academy of Sciences issued a major report stating that its review of more than 500 scientific papers failed to provide any evidence that electromagnetic fields adversely affect human health (NRC, 1997) and (2) when scientists at the National Cancer Institute convincingly demonstrated no association between electric power lines and leukemia in children (Linet et al., 1997). Although the public fears raised by more than two decades of controversy have not been altogether vanquished, the scientific community regards further investigation into the health impacts of EMF as unnecessary—sleeping under an electric blanket or living near a power line doesn't cause cancer!

The fouling of the nest which has been typical
of man's activity in the past on a local scale
now seems to be extending to the whole system.
—Kenneth Boulding

• • • • • • • Part 3 • • • • • • •

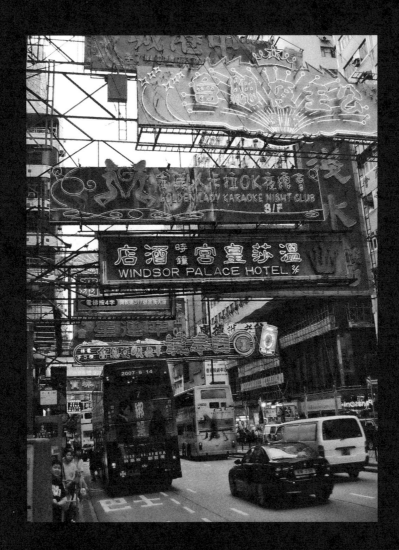

Environmental Degradation

How We Foul Our Own Nest

Air pollution, water pollution, excessive levels of noise, and the accumulation of disease-breeding refuse are not phenomena unique to the modern age. Wherever humans have congregated in appreciable numbers, the burning of fuel, the thoughtless disposal of excreta and material wastes, and the din arising from a multitude of human activities have created conditions that adversely affected the health and well-being of the very people responsible for those conditions. For most of human history, environmental degradation was primarily local in scope, concentrated in the relatively few places where humans established urban centers. The extent of pollution in these cities, however, often far exceeded the levels of filth plaguing our environmentally conscious society of today. Streets and gutters clogged with human body wastes, animal excrement, and garbage were a result of both overcrowding and a transference to the city of more casual rural practices.

By the time of the Industrial Revolution in the late 18th and early 19th centuries, belching smokestacks from thousands of factories and the noise of machinery and transport vehicles further degraded the quality of urban life. Indeed, back in the "good old days" health and sanitary conditions due to air and water pollution and to inadequate (or nonexistent) refuse collection and disposal were far worse than anything which we in the Western world are familiar with today. When repeated epidemic outbreaks of waterborne disease killed thousands of citizens or when smog-laden air caused millions to wheeze, cough, and occasionally die, the more enlightened civic leaders began to question society's shortsightedness in fouling its own nest. Many of the most important reforms in civic life that occurred late in the

19th century involved implementation of public health measures to deal with water pollution, refuse collection, and smoke abatement. However, throughout this period when urban pollution levels were rising, the countryside remained relatively uncontaminated, except for those areas where a local industry—perhaps a metal smelter or pulp mill—created noxious conditions within its own sphere of influence.

The changes that transformed local pollution problems into global concerns have occurred largely in the years since the mid-20th century, after World War II. Reverse migration from urban centers into sprawling suburbia was made possible by a quantum increase in the number of automobiles ("infernal combustion engines") whose exhaust fumes guaranteed that air pollution would no longer be restricted to areas of heavy industry. The escalating energy demands of a growing, affluent population were accompanied by construction of massive new power plants, most of them coal-burning and many located in regions previously noted for pristinely clean air. Perhaps most significant was the vast outpouring of new, synthetic chemical products, many of them toxic compounds, which do not break down readily and can be transported immense distances by air currents, water, or in the tissues of living organisms to wreak their havoc far from their place of origin. In spite of the warnings of a few farsighted individuals, several decades of experience were required before society as a whole became aware of the insidious nature and now-massive scope of environmental degradation.

During the decade of the 1970s, a national awakening in the United States regarding issues of ecology and environmental health produced a flood of federal and

278

state legislation aimed at pollution abatement. The battle has been joined and some successes have already been achieved, but it has become increasingly evident that the problem of environmental pollution is far more complex than originally perceived. Issues not even considered until fairly recently—such as acid precipitation, ozone layer depletion, contamination of groundwater with toxic organic chemicals, the fearsome dilemma of what to do about abandoned chemical waste dumps, and, overshadowing all other problems, climate change—present policy makers, scientists, and citizens with thorny technical and political problems. Solutions to older questions pertaining to community waste disposal practices, air pollution abatement measures, or stormwater runoff control are well understood but often fail to be implemented due to fiscal constraints.

The concluding chapters of this book attempt to delineate the nature of the pollution problems confronting society in the early 21st century. They also describe the legislative tools with which we are now attempting to combat the contamination of our nation's air, water, and land resources in order to prevent future generations from perpetuating the "fouling of the nest" which so endangers our health and well-being.

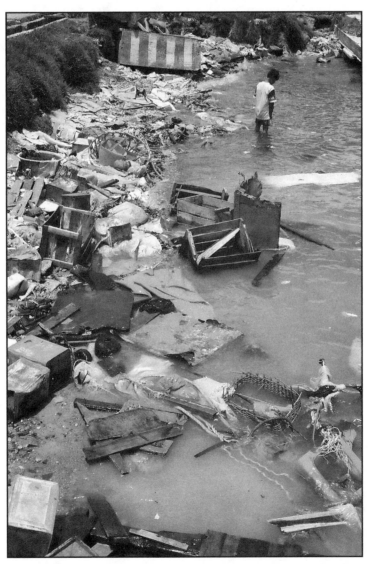

In countries where refuse collection is inadequate or nonexistent, the sad result is often indiscriminate disposal into the nearest body of water.

11

*. . . this most excellent canopy, the air, look you,
this brave o'erhanging firmament,
this majestical roof fretted with golden fire . . .*
—William Shakespeare (Hamlet)

The Atmosphere

The airy canopy above Earth which so inspires poets and painters is a physical characteristic of our planet unique in the solar system. Its existence makes possible the rich diversity of life forms found on Earth, making this globe a veritable oasis in space.

Questions regarding the origin of Earth's atmosphere have intrigued scientists for decades. It is generally assumed that Earth formed almost five billion years ago when particles in a gigantic whirling cloud of dust and gases were pulled together into an aggregate body by enormous gravitational forces. This infant planet had an atmosphere consisting primarily of light gases such as hydrogen and helium, very similar to the present-day atmosphere on the larger planets of Jupiter and Saturn. However, due to Earth's smaller size, gravitational forces were insufficient to retain these elements and they subsequently dissipated into space. This original atmosphere was gradually replaced by a secondary atmosphere produced through the outgassing of volatile materials from the interior of Earth as the once-molten orb began to cool. Modern phenomena such as volcanic eruptions provide vivid evidence that such outgassing continues right up to the present day.

While there has long been widespread agreement among scientists that the primitive Earth's atmosphere was significantly different in chemical composition from that of the present, opinions varied as to precisely which compounds were the major constituents of the early atmosphere. For many years it was widely accepted that a mixture of hydrogen, methane, ammonia, and water vapor would have provided the most congenial environment for the origin of life; these must have been the predominant gases in prebiotic times. More recently, however, this assumption has been challenged by observations that gases ejected by volcanoes consist largely of carbon dioxide and water vapor, leading to the conclusion that, unless volcanoes operated very differently in the past than they do today, the main component of Earth's early atmosphere was carbon dioxide, just as it is today on our neighboring planets of Mars and Venus. This concept of a primitive atmosphere composed primarily of carbon dioxide, water vapor, and nitrogen, with mere traces of ammonia and notably devoid of free oxygen, constitutes the consensus of scientific opinion today. The origin of our modern oxygen-rich atmosphere is traced to the evolution of green plants about two billion years ago. The photosynthetic activities of green plants resulted in the uptake of considerable quantities of atmospheric carbon dioxide and the subsequent release of free oxygen—a necessary precursor for the evolution of higher forms of life (Kasting, 1993; Budyko, 1986; Gribbin, 1982).

Although the chemical constituents of the atmosphere have existed in roughly their present proportions for at least several hundred million years, these constituents are in a constant state of flux, reacting with the continents and oceans to form our weather patterns, constantly being removed and recycled (see chapter 1 on "Geochemical Cycles") as a part of great natural processes. The intimate interrelationships between the atmosphere and land, water, and living things make it relevant to refer to such interactions as the earth-atmosphere system. This system is essentially a closed one—every material that goes into the air, though it may circulate and change in form, nevertheless remains within the earth-atmosphere system. This fact has disquieting implications for those who have always viewed the skies as a convenient garbage dump for their volatile wastes—unfortunately, the concept of a pollutant or any other substance "vanishing into thin air" is a physical impossibility.

COMPOSITION OF THE ATMOSPHERE

The modern atmosphere consists of a mixture of gases so perfectly and consistently diffused among each other that pure dry air exhibits as distinct a set of physical properties as is possessed by any single gas. By volume, the composition of dry air can be broken down as follows:

- 78% nitrogen (N_2)
- 21% oxygen (O_2)

- 0.9% argon (Ar)
- 0.03% carbon dioxide (CO_2)
- trace amounts—neon, helium, krypton, xenon, hydrogen, methane, and nitrous oxide

Of the four major atmospheric components, only two, oxygen and carbon dioxide, directly enter into biological processes. Oxygen is required by most living organisms for the production of energy, a process known as aerobic respiration; carbon dioxide constitutes the carbon source for photosynthesis—a series of photochemical reactions whereby chlorophyll molecules in green plants absorb sunlight and use its energy to synthesize simple sugars from carbon dioxide and water. Atmospheric nitrogen, on the other hand, can be utilized only by a few species of nitrogen-fixing bacteria and cyanobacteria, while argon is chemically and biologically inert and thus plays no significant role in the biosphere.

Regions of the Atmosphere

Although the composition of its component gases is uniform throughout the atmosphere from sea level to an altitude approximately 50 miles (80 km) above the earth's surface, scientists subdivide this expanse into three distinct regions based on temperature zones.

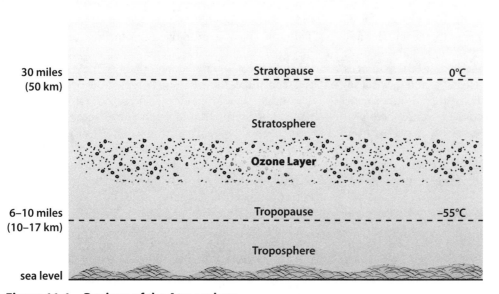

Figure 11-1   Regions of the Atmosphere

Troposphere

Extending from sea level to an altitude about 8 miles above the earth (slightly less above the poles, more above the equator) is the region known as the troposphere. Virtually all life activities occur within this region and most weather and climatic phenomena occur here. In addition to the usual gases, the troposphere also contains varying amounts of water vapor and dust particles. Within the troposphere temperature steadily falls with increasing altitude, a decrease of 5.4°F per 1,000 feet (10°C/km). The upper limit of the troposphere is known as the **tropopause**.

Stratosphere

Above the troposphere lies the stratosphere, a region distinguished by a temperature gradient reversal. Here the temperature slowly rises with increasing altitude until it reaches 32°F (0°C) at a height of about 30 miles (50 km), the upper boundary of the stratosphere known as the **stratopause**. Unlike the troposphere, the stratosphere contains almost no water vapor or dust. It is the site, however, of the **ozone layer**, a region characterized by higher-than-usual concentrations of the rare gas ozone (O_3), an isotope of oxygen (O_2). The ozone layer extends from about 8–15 miles (12–25 km) above the earth's surface, being most concentrated between 11–15 miles. Amounts of ozone vary depending on location and season of the year. Ozone concentrations are lowest above the equator, increasing toward the poles; they also increase markedly between autumn and spring (Parson, 2003).

Mesosphere

Above the stratopause is the region known as the mesosphere, where temperature once again begins to fall with increasing altitude. Since the air becomes progressively more diffuse as the altitude above the earth increases, it is difficult to say precisely where the atmosphere ends. In terms of mass, 99% of our atmosphere lies within 18 miles of the earth's surface—an astonishingly thin blanket nurturing beneath it all the life known to exist in the universe (Strahler and Strahler, 1973).

Radiation Balance

In addition to providing the major source of certain chemical elements necessary for life, the atmosphere performs a vital role in controlling the earth's surface environment by regulating both the quality and quantity of solar radiation that enters and leaves the biosphere.

The source of all energy on earth, of course, is the sun. However, solar energy can be subdivided into several categories, depending on wavelength of the various forms of radiation involved. These categories and their wavelengths are as follows:

Type of Radiation	Percent of Total Energy	Wavelength (in micrometers)
Ultraviolet rays	9	0.1–0.4
Visible light rays	38	0.4–0.7
Infrared rays (heat)	53	0.7–3000

These forms of electromagnetic radiation travel outward from the sun at a rate of 186,000 miles (300,000 km) per second, taking slightly over nine minutes to reach the earth. Although none of the sun's energy is lost as it travels through space, once it begins to penetrate earth's atmosphere both a depletion and diversion of solar radiation begin to occur.

Most of the ultraviolet radiation present in sunlight is absorbed by the ozone layer as it passes through the stratosphere, though some of the UV wavelengths longer than 0.3 micrometers (the so-called UVB region) manage to penetrate to the earth's surface where they can produce sunburn and skin cancers. The ozone layer itself is actually created by ultraviolet light, since UV radiant energy causes ordinary oxygen molecules to break apart, releasing single atoms of oxygen which then react with intact oxygen molecules to form ozone. Since, as was explained in chapter 10, ultraviolet radiation can have serious adverse effects on living organisms, the existence of the ozone layer is of great biological significance (Panofsky, 1978).

Visible light rays and infrared radiation penetrate through the upper stratosphere unaffected by the ozone layer. However, as the atmospheric gas molecules increase in density closer to the earth, these molecules cause a random scattering of the incoming visible light waves (infrared waves are not so affected and for the most part continue to stream directly toward the earth). Entering the troposphere, additional scattering and diffuse reflection of visible light waves occur due to contact with dust particles and clouds (a clear sky appears blue because the shorter blue wavelengths are scattered to a greater extent than are the longer red wavelengths and thus reach our eyes from all parts of the sky). Additional amounts of incoming solar radiation are lost by reflection from the upper surfaces of clouds, oceans, or from the land (particularly when covered with snow or ice). Energy losses also occur when carbon dioxide and water vapor absorb infrared radiation (heat waves) as sunlight enters the lower atmosphere. This heat absorption results in an increase in air temperature.

Although the carbon dioxide content of the air is constant everywhere, the amount of water vapor varies considerably and is the main factor accounting for differences in the amount of infrared absorption in various climatic regions (e.g., arid regions experience greater temperature extremes during a 24-hour period than do more humid areas at the same latitude because the low water vapor

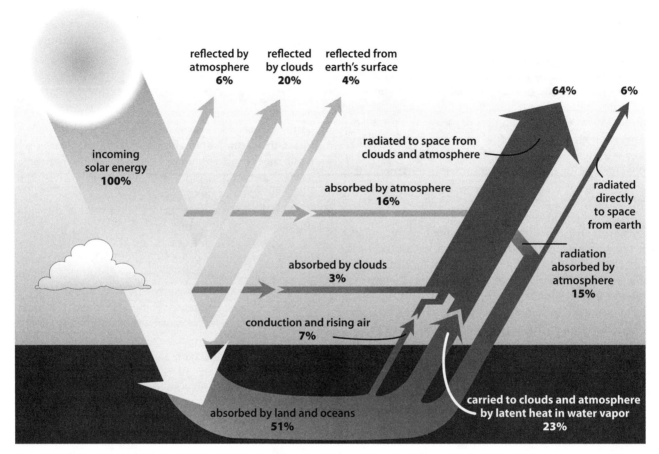

reflected by atmosphere **6%**

reflected by clouds **20%**

reflected from earth's surface **4%**

incoming solar energy **100%**

radiated to space from clouds and atmosphere

64%   **6%**

radiated directly to space from earth

absorbed by atmosphere **16%**

radiation absorbed by atmosphere **15%**

absorbed by clouds **3%**

conduction and rising air **7%**

carried to clouds and atmosphere by latent heat in water vapor **23%**

absorbed by land and oceans **51%**

Source: J. T. Kiehl and Kevin E. Trenberth, National Center for Atmospheric Research, Boulder, Colorado. Used with permission.

Figure 11-2   Energy Budget

content of desert air minimizes the absorption of the infrared waves). Altogether, scattering, reflection, and absorption of sunlight can result in the loss of as little as 20% of incoming solar radiation when skies are clear to nearly 100% under conditions of heavy cloud cover. On a global yearly average it is estimated that the earth-atmosphere system absorbs about 68% of the total incoming solar radiation, 32% being lost due to the factors just mentioned.

In order to maintain a global radiation balance, energy absorbed by the earth from incoming sunlight must be equaled by outward radiation of energy from the earth's surface. This so-called "ground radiation" occurs in the form of infrared waves longer than 3 or 4 micrometers (referred to as "long-wave radiation"), which are continually being radiated back into the atmosphere, even at night when no solar radiation is being received. Some of the infrared waves leaving the earth (those in the 5–8 and 12–20 micrometer range) are absorbed by water vapor and carbon dioxide in the atmosphere, a portion of which are reradiated back to the earth's surface, thereby keeping the earth's climate warmer than it would other-

wise be. This phenomenon, known as the **greenhouse effect**, has extremely important climatic implications that will be discussed in more detail later in this chapter.

While incoming and outgoing units of radiation are often not in balance at any one particular time and place (indeed, such imbalances provide the forces behind our constantly changing weather patterns), an equilibrium of such units for the world as a whole during any given year exists, resulting in the maintenance of annual average global temperatures that fluctuate very little from year to year (Strahler and Strahler, 1973). One of the most pressing concerns among atmospheric scientists today is that human activities may be altering the global radiation balance in ways that may have far-reaching climatic consequences.

HUMAN IMPACT ON THE EARTH-ATMOSPHERE SYSTEM

Geologic records give ample indication of drastic climatic changes at various times in Earth's long history, the most recent being four successive periods of widespread glaciation (the "Ice Ages"), the last of which ended only 10,000 years ago. Obviously humans had nothing to do with past fluctuations in the global heat balance, but our impact today may no longer be so negligible. Temperature measurements compiled over many decades clearly indicate that significant changes in climate are already underway, provoked and enhanced largely by human activities.

The major causes of human-induced atmospheric change are:

1. Introduction into the atmosphere of pollutant gases and particles not usually found there in significant amounts

2. Changes in the concentrations of natural atmospheric components

The following sections address the two most prominent issues related to the impact of human activities on the earth-atmosphere system. The first—depletion of the ozone layer—has spurred unprecedented worldwide policy initiatives to counter the threat and now promises to become a rare environmental success story. The second—global climate change, caused by excess levels of atmospheric CO_2 and other so-called "greenhouse gases"—is now widely regarded as perhaps the most serious challenge facing life on our planet, and faltering efforts to deal with the situation are only now getting underway.

Depletion of the Ozone Layer

Although ozone is one of the rarest of atmospheric gases, its presence in the stratosphere is of vital importance in protecting life on Earth from the damaging effects of solar ultraviolet radiation. As mentioned earlier, the ozone layer is created when UV energy splits the oxygen molecule and the freed atoms rejoin other oxygen molecules to form ozone (O_3). At the same time, the highly reactive ozone is being broken down again to normal oxygen (O_2); thus the ozone layer is maintained in a state of dynamic equilibrium, daytime increases being balanced by nighttime decreases.

In 1974 atmospheric chemists advanced a hypothesis that certain pollutant emissions into the atmosphere had the potential to disrupt this equilibrium, threatening the long-term integrity of the ozone layer. Initially attention focused on the damage potential of nitrous oxides emitted with jet airplane exhausts (particularly from supersonic transports such as the Anglo-French Concorde) and the use of nitrogen fertilizers. It gradually became apparent, however, that a far more serious threat to the ozone layer was posed by the widespread use at that time of a group of synthetic chemicals known as **chlorofluorocarbons (CFCs)**, one of the best known of which was the refrigerant Freon®. Utilized commercially since the 1930s for home and industrial refrigeration, freezing, and

air-conditioning, CFC applications expanded in the post-World War II period to include use as propellants in aerosol spray cans. By the 1970s the latter use constituted the single largest portion of CFC production, as hundreds of products from paints and insecticides to hair sprays and deodorants were repackaged in aerosol cans.

As new applications for CFCs were developed, world production of these chemicals soared; by the early 1970s, approximately a million tons were being produced each year. Another closely related group of chemicals, the **halons** (bromofluorocarbons), were developed in the 1950s as extremely effective fire suppressants and came into widespread commercial use in the 1960s and 1970s. Unfortunately, the very property of CFCs and halons (collectively referred to as **ozone-depleting substances**) that made them so valuable commercially—their extreme chemical stability—also made them a serious threat to the global environment. When released into the air through vaporization or leakage from enclosed systems, or when directly sprayed from aerosol containers or fire extinguishers, the chemicals don't break down. Instead, they drift upward through the troposphere into the stratosphere where the molecules are finally broken down by UV radiation, releasing atoms of chlorine (CFCs) or bromine (halons) that react with and destroy ozone. The halogen-ozone reaction is a catalytic one; in the case of CFCs, for example, the same chlorine atom can repeat the reaction with tens of thousands of ozone molecules. This, plus the fact that the chlorine atoms will remain in the atmosphere for 100 years or more, explains why CFCs' destructive impact on the ozone layer is so much greater than emission levels might suggest. Bromine is even more problematic; although its atmospheric concentrations are far lower than those of chlorine, bromine depletes stratospheric ozone 45–50 times more efficiently than CFC-derived chlorine atoms.

Depletion of the ozone layer is worrisome from a human health perspective because of stratospheric ozone's role in absorbing biologically damaging ultraviolet radiation. It is now well established that for each 1% decrease in atmospheric ozone, penetration of UV radiation to the earth's surface will increase by 2%. As scientific research on potential threats to the ozone layer intensified during the 1970s and early 1980s, concerns mounted regarding the impact such depletion might have on skin cancer incidence. Since more than 90% of nonmelanoma skin cancers are associated with exposure to UV radiation in sunlight, any increase in ultraviolet exposure could be expected to result in more skin malignancies. In 1982 the National Academy of Sciences reported that for every 1% decrease in the concentration of atmospheric ozone, cases of basal cell carcinoma would likely rise by 2–5%, squamous cell carcinomas by 4–10% (Maugh, 1982). In 1992, as efforts to do something about the problem were moving into high gear, the UN's Environment Programme underscored the urgency of the international effort by releasing estimates forecasting a 26% worldwide increase in nonmelanoma skin cancers if stratospheric ozone levels dropped by 10%.

The "Hole in the Sky"

In the United States, an intense public debate on threats to the ozone layer focused largely on aerosol propellants and resulted in a nationwide ban on such products, effective in 1978. Canada, Sweden, and Norway enacted similar bans in 1980, but aerosol products continued to be used elsewhere. This action lulled the public into assuming the problem had been solved, and for several years little more was heard about the issue. During the early 1980s, both government and many scientists downplayed the ozone depletion threat, asserting that earlier forecasts of ozone loss had been exaggerated and assuring skeptics that CFC production had leveled off and thus presented little cause for concern.

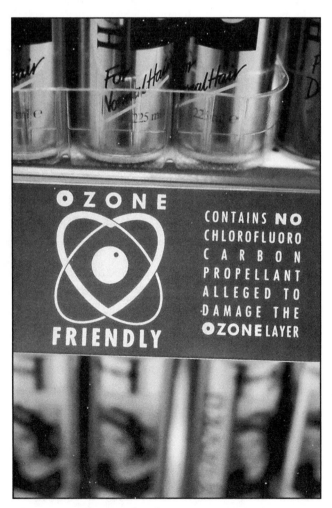

The ban on CFC use as a propellant in aerosol spray cans was one of the first steps taken to combat depletion of the ozone layer.

This sense of complacency was shattered in 1985 when members of the British Antarctic Survey announced the existence of a large hole in the ozone layer over the South Pole. Although the gap was temporary, opening in early September (Antarctic spring) and closing by mid-October as the southern atmosphere grew warmer, it had been increasing in size each year since the British researchers first noticed it in 1981; by the time of their startling revelation, the "hole" represented a 40% decline in ozone concentrations.

Subsequent confirmation by NASA that the ozone hole was real led to intensified research efforts to learn what was going wrong in the polar skies. U.S. scientists sent to McMurdo Bay in the years following discovery of the hole in the ozone layer revealed that the springtime depletion of ozone was steadily getting larger, appearing earlier, and lasting longer. In 1987, ozone losses totaled 50%; by 1991 they reached 70% over an area four times the size of the United States and measurements of UV radiation reaching the ground were the highest ever recorded in Antarctica up to that time. During the 1990s and into the early 21st century the Antarctic ozone hole grew ever larger, reaching a record 11 million square miles (28.4 million km^2) in both 2000 and 2003. During September and October of 2006, the Antarctic ozone hole reached its greatest extent ever, and on October 8 of that year NASA scientists reported the worst levels of ozone depletion yet recorded.

During the late 1980s and early 1990s conflicting theories regarding the cause of this depletion were vigorously debated by researchers. Chemical pollution, cyclical solar flares, and natural atmospheric variation were the main contenders for chief villain. Within a few years the weight of evidence tilted toward the chemical pollution theory with the discovery that concentrations of ozone-destroying chlorine molecules were 400–500 times higher within the ozone hole than outside. The presence of chlorine was widely regarded as evidence of a direct cause-and-effect link between CFC emissions and ozone layer destruction.

Throughout the 1990s, evidence continued to mount that the pace of ozone loss was accelerating, not only over the South Pole but also above the more populous regions of the Northern Hemisphere. Since 1979 the U.S. government has been collecting data on atmospheric ozone from ground-based survey stations and the Nimbus-7 satellite. By 1993 NASA scientists were reporting record low concentrations of stratospheric ozone above the middle latitudes of North America and Eurasia—down by as much as 20% from their normal levels. While this dramatic drop in ozone may be blamed, at least in part, on debris hurled into the upper atmosphere by the massive 1991 eruption of the Philippine volcano, Mt. Pinatubo, researchers pointed out that even prior to this event about 3% of the ozone layer above the United States, Europe, Russia, Japan, and China had been lost. Moreover, when the ozone dipped by 3% over the United States, it dropped by 4% over Australia and New Zealand, and 6% in Scandinavia. More ominously, this loss was occurring in the spring and summer when human exposure to sunlight is at peak levels ("Ozone Takes," 1993; WRI, 1992). While winter ozone losses over the Arctic haven't occurred as predictably year after year as they have over the South Pole, the winter of 1997 saw the highest Arctic ozone depletion yet recorded, with that of 2004–2005 close behind.

Until the 1990s, a major weakness in the claim that observed declines in stratospheric ozone levels represented a serious environmental health threat was the scarcity of data documenting an actual increase in ultraviolet light penetration anywhere except in Antarctica—where the number of exposed humans is negligible. That data gap was essentially closed in November 1993, with the publication of a five-year study conducted in Toronto by two scientists working with Environment Canada (Canadian equivalent of EPA). From 1989 to 1993, the researchers took ground-level measurements of UV radiation every hour from sunrise to sunset during winter and summer (seasons when UV levels are at their highest and lowest, respectively). They found that at wavelengths around 300 nanometers (the portion of the UV spectrum most strongly absorbed by stratospheric ozone), ultraviolet radiation increased by 35% per year in winter, 6–7% per year in summer. Since measurements of stratospheric ozone concentrations above Toronto had documented a 4% annual decrease in winter and a 2% summer decline each year during the study period, skeptics' arguments that air pollution or cloud cover will counteract the effect of ozone loss were proven wrong (Kerr and McElroy, 1993).

Policy Response—The Montreal Protocol

After years of controversy among scientists, the chemical industry, and government policy makers as to the extent of ozone depletion, the identity of the main culprits, and the most effective approach for halting—or at least slowing down—the process, consensus emerged that ozone depletion is real, that it presents a major threat to life on this planet, and that global cooperation is required to combat a phenomenon that threatens us all. A major step forward to meet this challenge was taken in September 1987, when diplomats from 29 nations, meeting in Montreal, Canada, signed an international accord aimed at controlling the chemicals most responsible for ozone layer depletion. As originally ratified, the Montreal Protocol called for the freezing of CFC consumption at 1986 levels by 1990, to be followed by a 50% reduction in the production of these chemicals by the end of the century. The treaty went into effect in January

1989, after ratification by nations representing more than two-thirds of the world's CFC production (eventually 184 nations signed the Montreal Protocol).

By the early 1990s, scientific evidence that ozone depletion was occurring much more rapidly than anticipated prompted several strengthening amendments to the international treaty. The list of chemicals targeted for controls was expanded to include halons, carbon tetrachloride, methyl chloroform, hydrochlorofluorocarbons (HCFCs), and methyl bromide; in addition, the timetable for phasing out production and use of ozone-depleting substances was advanced. For industrialized nations, the ban on domestic sale and use of CFCs took effect on January 1, 1996, and has met with near-universal compliance; developing countries, whose production and use of these chemicals rose rapidly during the 1990s, were required under the Montreal Protocol to freeze production at their 1995–1997 levels by 1999 and to halt production completely by 2010. Industrialized countries ceased manufacturing halons in 1994, an action developing nations were not required to take until 2010.

An update to the treaty negotiated in September 2007 hastened the phase-out schedule for HCFCs, once regarded as acceptable transition substances since they are less damaging to ozone than CFCs. However, a surge in production and use of HCFCs as coolants in developing countries like India and China raised concerns, especially as they are also recognized as powerful greenhouse gases. Delegates to the UN-sponsored meeting in Montreal agreed to freeze production of HCFCs in developing nations by 2013—two years earlier than previously called for—and to advance the deadline for total cessation of production from 2040 to 2030. Developed countries agreed to halt their own production of HCFCs by 2020 (Kintisch, 2007).

Unfortunately, even full implementation of the treaty's requirements will not prevent further losses of ozone. Millions of pounds of CFCs already released are gradually drifting up toward the ozone layer and will remain in the atmosphere for many decades. Nevertheless, the cutbacks in CFC production called for in the Montreal Protocol are already having an impact. In August 1993, atmospheric physicists working for the National Oceanic and Atmospheric Administration (NOAA) announced that the unexpectedly rapid drop in industrial production of CFCs even prior to the implementation deadlines set by the treaty had resulted in a substantial slowdown in the rate at which ozone-depleting chemicals were accumulating in the atmosphere. By the early 2000s, depletion of the ozone layer was measured at about 4% per decade, down from 8% in the 1980s. Although concentrations of chlorine in the upper stratosphere continue to increase, they are increasing at a slower rate than previously, an indication that the Montreal Protocol's phaseout of ozone-depleting substances is having a positive impact.

These observations have given rise to optimism in many quarters that recovery of the ozone layer is now underway. Although the transition from CFCs and halons to more environmentally benign substitutes is still incomplete, scientists and policy makers are pleased with progress to date. In reference to the Antarctic ozone hole, NASA researchers predict that statistically significant signs of ozone layer recovery should be detectable by 2024, with ozone levels recovering to their 1980 levels by about 2068 (Newman et al., 2006). The international efforts to protect the ozone layer mandated by the Montreal Protocol are extremely significant in that they represent the first time in history that the nations of the world have agreed to work together to prevent a disaster of global proportions. Initial indications of the success of this approach offer hope for similar cooperation in tackling an even more difficult environmental challenge—global climate change.

Rising Levels of Atmospheric CO_2

> Warming of the climate system is unequivocal, as is now evident from observations of increases in global average air and ocean temperatures, widespread melting of snow and ice and rising global average sea level. . . . Global atmospheric concentrations of CO_2, methane (CH_4) and nitrous oxide (N_2O) have increased markedly as a result of human activities since 1750 and now far exceed pre-industrial values determined from ice cores spanning many thousands of years.
>
> —Excerpts from *Climate Change 2007: Synthesis Report*, Intergovernmental Panel on Climate Change

Publication of the Fourth Assessment Report (AR4) of the Intergovernmental Panel on Climate Change (IPCC) in 2007 was the clearest affirmation to date that the world's scientists were convinced that momentous changes in global climate are well underway—and that we're to blame. The IPCC, a group comprising approximately 2,500 scientists from nearly 100 countries, was jointly established in 1988 by the UN Environment Programme and the World Meteorological Organization to serve as the official advisory body to governments around the world on issues pertaining to climate change. Charged with reviewing the current state of knowledge regarding the science and impacts of global warming, as well as evaluating mitigation and adaptation strategies, the IPCC conducts no research itself but draws its conclusions from thousands of peer-reviewed publications by experts in a wide range of scientific disciplines. To date, the IPCC has issued four assessment reports (1990, 1995, 2001, and 2007; a fifth is scheduled for release in 2014), each succes-

sive report affirming with increasing confidence the reality of global warming and the dire consequences of human interference with the earth-atmosphere system.

Although many in the general public are somewhat aware of climate change as an impending threat, within the scientific world it is truly the "Doomsday Issue," recognized as humanity's most serious environmental problem and the greatest long-term threat to the stability of ecosystems. Thanks to the misinformation and distortion of facts spread by a small group of so-called "greenhouse deniers," a disconcertingly large minority of Americans tends to disregard the overwhelming body of evidence supporting climatologists' warnings that something is seriously amiss with Earth's life-support systems. However, the enormous amount of data collected by researchers all over the world can no longer be ignored or discounted. A number of influential world leaders are now echoing scientists' pleas for effective action, raising hopes that humanity will, perhaps, wake up to the problem before it's too late. In the words of UN Secretary-General Ban Ki-Moon:

> The danger posed by war to all humanity—and to our planet—is at least matched by the climate crisis and global warming. I believe that the world has reached a critical stage in its efforts to exercise responsible environmental stewardship.

Nature of the Problem

The basic fact that temperatures are rising is well-documented; according to a report issued in 2009 by the U.S. Global Change Research Program, the global average temperature today is 1.5°F (0.8°C) warmer than it was at the beginning of the industrial era. In the United States, the temperature increase is higher than the world average, having risen by 2°F over the past half-century. In general, the high latitude regions of the Northern Hemisphere are experiencing the greatest increases; in Alaska and elsewhere in the Arctic, warming to date is double that experienced at lower latitudes—an increase of 4–5°F within the past 30 years.

The recording of daily temperatures began around 1850, so the temperature database, at least for some locations, extends more than 150 years. These records reveal little change in global temperatures until the early 1900s, but show a distinct upward trend since that time. The U.S. National Climatic Data Center (NCDC) documents a sustained rise in global surface temperatures from 1910 until about 1940–1945, followed by a 30-year period of slightly cooler temperatures (more about this later!), with a more pronounced warming beginning around 1976 and continuing to the present day.

The cause for this warming trend has been the subject of sometimes acrimonious debate over the past several decades, but it is now generally accepted that the main culprit since the mid-1970s is atmospheric carbon dioxide (CO_2). Concentrations of this gas have been gradually rising since the dawn of the Industrial Revolution in the late 1700s—a result of the steadily increasing use of coal, oil, and natural gas to power the world's homes, factories, and vehicles and as a by-product of cement production, since large amounts of CO_2 are released when limestone is heated. Together, fossil fuel combustion and cement production released 31 billion tons of CO_2 into the atmosphere in 2007, up from 22.6 billion in 1990 (Flavin and Engelman, 2009).

When fossil fuels are burned, one of the primary combustion products is carbon dioxide; the combustion of one ton of coal, for example, releases three tons of CO_2. In past ages, excess carbon dioxide released through volcanic outgassing was gradually absorbed into

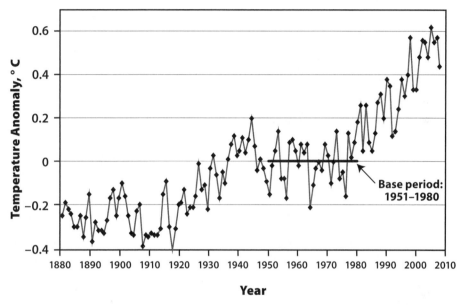

Source: Data from http://data.giss.nasa.gov/gistemp.graphs/

Figure 11-3   Global Land-Ocean Temperature Anomaly

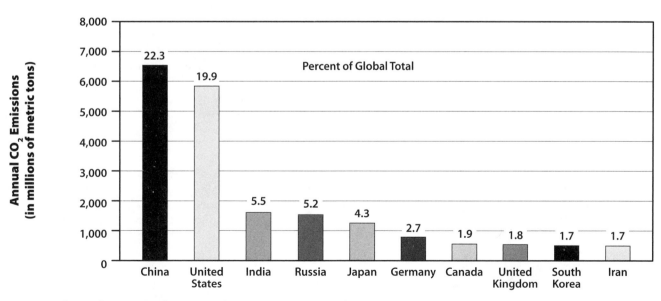

Source: Data from Carbon Dioxide Information Analysis Center, http://cdiac.ornl.gov

Figure 11-4   Top 10 CO_2 Emitters

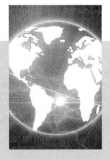

· · · · · · · **11~1** · · · · · · · ·

China's "Carbon Footprint"

Early in 2007, China surged past the United States to claim the unenviable title of world leader in CO_2 emissions—a milestone that just a few years earlier was regarded as unlikely before 2030. Since 2001, as the Chinese government eased its monetary policies and the country gained admission to the World Trade Organization, foreign investment and manufacturing in China have soared. During the past decade many Chinese cities became vast construction zones as thousands of new buildings, factories, and highways appeared almost overnight. To power their booming economy, the Chinese turned primarily to their most abundant, cheapest, and dirtiest fuel—coal; during these years of breakneck growth, two new coal-fired power plants were coming on-line in China every week, a pace that has only slowed since 2008 to just under one a week.

A few statistics will help illustrate this impact. Global emissions of CO_2 from fossil fuel burning and cement production grew by 37% between 1990 and 2007; while the increase in emissions during the 1990s was 1% each year, between 2000–2007 it shot up to 3.5% annually, largely due to China's contribution. During the period from 1990–2008, U.S. carbon emissions from fossil fuel combustion grew by 27%, but those emitted by China shot up 150%. On a *per capita* basis, Chinese greenhouse gas emissions are still much lower than those of the United States (probably because there are four times as many Chinese as there are Americans!), but its emissions are growing faster than those of any other major country and, if unchecked, could provoke disastrous climate change even if all developed countries cut their emissions to zero (Wiener, 2009). Experts struggling with international climate change treaty negotiations are convinced that unless China signs on as a full participant in mitigation strategies, there is little hope that developed countries alone will be able to stabilize atmospheric CO_2 concentrations at a level low enough to prevent damaging climate change impacts.

Are the Chinese people themselves worried enough about global warming to do something about it? An opinion survey of environmental attitudes and behavior conducted in 10 major Chinese cities in 2007 found that among the general public, climate change was near the bottom of the list of major environmental concerns. While over 20% of respondents cited health effects of pollution or poor air quality as their #1 choice, only 7% put climate change at the top of their list (Chung-En Liu and Leiserowitz, 2009).

However, a brief summary of the likely consequences of rising temperatures in that country suggests that climate change *should* be a cause for public anxiety. According to researchers there, China will be among the hardest-hit regions in the world if projections prove accurate. With many of its major cities (e.g., Beijing, Shanghai, Guangzhou, Hong Kong) and much productive farmland along the coast or near lowland areas, a sea level rise of just one meter would inundate vast expanses, severely impacting industrial and agricultural output as well as disrupting the lives of millions of people. Melting of mountain glaciers in China's Himalayan "water tower," already underway, threatens the water source feeding the Yangtze and Yellow Rivers. Environmentalists also fear that melting of permafrost in Tibet could damage the Qinghai-Tibet railway. Droughts in northern China and floods in the south are likely to become more frequent and more severe as temperatures climb, and experts estimate that by 2030 Chinese harvests could drop 5–10% below current levels. If all of this isn't enough to worry about, Chinese scientists say that ecosystem damage, including loss of tundra and mountain forests, desertification in northern China, and proliferating wildfires, could lead to the extinction of 15–20% of China's plant and animal species (Zeng et al., 2008).

Although the average Chinese citizen apparently has more immediate concerns than global warming, Chinese government leaders are well aware that climate change could seriously affect long-term political stability, just as current environmental problems due to conventional pollutants are provoking public protests and causing substantial economic losses, estimated at 6% of the nation's gross domestic product. Officials are beginning to realize that curbing fossil fuel combustion would produce double benefits, reducing health-damaging air pollutants while simultaneously lowering greenhouse gas emissions. In recent years the Chinese central government has given high priority to its fight against pollution, elevating its agency dealing with environmental protection to ministerial status in 2008 and setting ambitious targets for lowering pollution levels and increasing energy efficiency. China is also fast becoming a world leader in renewable energy technologies; it is now among the leading manufacturers of solar water heaters, solar panels, and wind turbines and in 2006 mandated renewable energy goals for China's provincial governments. The largest wind power development in the world is planned for Gansu province in north-central China, and if all the projects now on the drawing boards become reality, China will be the world's leading generator of wind energy by 2020.

Nevertheless, coal is still king and likely to remain so for the foreseeable future. In 2008 coal accounted for 67% of China's primary energy use, compared with 24% as the world average. With national energy consumption growing by about 15% each year, China's vast reserves of cheap domestic coal are essential to keep the economy booming. Thus China's leaders are faced with a daunting challenge—how to maintain the country's rapid pace of economic growth while curtailing the CO_2 emissions that are likely to provoke disastrous environmental consequences in the decades ahead.

China has been an active participant in the United Nations-sponsored negotiations aimed at averting climate change and has ratified the Kyoto Protocol. However, under the terms of this treaty developing countries like China are not subject to emissions targets and China has consistently refused to accept any mandatory limitations even as the country's greenhouse gas emissions have skyrocketed. Chinese negotiators argue that since two centuries of carbon emissions from the developed countries caused the problem in the first place, it's unfair to expect recent-industrializing nations to slow their own growth, especially when the other leading source of emissions, the United States, hasn't agreed to mandatory limits either!

While China's protests have some validity, as far as the Earth's climate is concerned, fairness scarcely matters. Unless China, the United States, and other major emitters join forces to reduce their greenhouse gas emissions as rapidly as possible, everyone will bear the consequences of inaction. But the world can't do it without China.

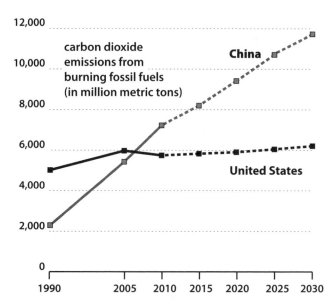

Source: Energy Information Administration, "Emissions of Greenhouse Gases Report," http://www.eia.doe.gov/oiaf/1605/ggrpt

Figure 11-5   Energy-Related CO_2 Emissions, 1990–2030

the oceans and eventually incorporated into carbonate rock or was photosynthetically "fixed" by green plants, particularly rapidly growing young forests (mature forests, by contrast, give off about the same amount of CO_2 as they take in). Scientists estimate that perhaps as much as half of the CO_2 emitted by human activities each year is currently being absorbed by the oceans and by land plants, with the latter serving as a repository for more carbon than the amount released annually by deforestation. Unfortunately, the ability of land and water to act as a "carbon sink" is reaching capacity and will decline as concentrations of atmospheric CO_2 continue to rise. As today's young forests mature, they will take up less and less excess CO_2; similarly, after more than a century of absorbing billions of tons of excess carbon, the ocean's buffering capacity is near the point of saturation and as ocean temperatures continue to rise, less carbon dioxide will be absorbed by the world's seas (the warmer the water, the less soluble is CO_2).

While fossil fuel combustion has received most of the attention—and blame—in relation to rising CO_2 concentrations, the wide-scale destruction of natural vegetation, particularly deforestation in the tropics, contributes nearly one-fourth (23%) of all global CO_2 emissions. Both forests and the organic matter in soil humus hold immense quantities of carbon that are oxidized and released as carbon dioxide when vegetation is destroyed. Space satellite monitors have revealed that the impact of forest destruction on CO_2 release may be even greater than previously realized. Data collected over the Amazon basin indicate that the thousands of fires deliberately set every year by settlers and ranchers clearing the Brazilian rain forest are generating such enormous quantities of gases and particles that they alone may account for at least one-tenth of the carbon dioxide released by human activities each year (Watson et al., 1990). The equilibrium that has prevailed for millennia has been disrupted, with the result that atmospheric CO_2 levels are now sharply increasing.

The sense of alarm felt by scientists monitoring rising levels of atmospheric CO_2 relates not to any direct adverse effect the substance might exert on human health—carbon dioxide is not a toxic pollutant—but rather is due to the impact increasing levels of the gas will have on global climate. As mentioned earlier in this chapter, atmospheric CO_2 plays a vital role in moderating the earth's temperature—a role first described in 1859 by Irish physicist John Tyndall. Working with a ratio spectrophotometer, a device he had invented to measure the absorptive properties of various gases, Tyndall found that carbon dioxide, methane, and water vapor—unlike nitrogen and oxygen—absorb infrared light waves (i.e., heat) and thus must be largely responsible for controlling the world's climate. This heat-absorbing property of certain atmospheric gases described by Tyndall eventually became known as the **greenhouse effect** (sometimes currently referred to as the "natural greenhouse effect" to distinguish it from the "enhanced greenhouse effect" caused by human activities).

Just as the glass in a greenhouse permits light to enter but prevents the escape of heat, thereby warming the air within, so the absorption of infrared ground radiation by carbon dioxide and its subsequent re-radiation back toward the earth helps to maintain an average global temperature of 59°F (15°C). Without CO_2 in the atmosphere, the earth's average surface temperature would fall to about 0°F, making the existence of life as we know it impossible. By contrast, the planet Venus, with a dense, CO_2-rich atmosphere, has a surface temperature of 890°F (hot enough to melt lead) while Mars, whose atmosphere consists primarily of CO_2 but is very diffuse and contains but a trace of water vapor, is colder than Antarctica, with an average temperature of –53°F (Revkin, 1992; Houghton, Jenkins, and Ephraums, 1990).

In 1896 Tyndall's early observations on CO_2's likely influence on climate were expanded upon by a Swedish chemist, Svante Arrhenius. Arrhenius theorized that the enormous quantities of CO_2 from fossil fuel combustion being discharged into European skies in the late 1800s were likely to result in a gradual rise in world temperatures. Arrhenius attempted to calculate what the temperature increase would be if atmospheric carbon dioxide concentrations were to double (something he thought might happen in about 3000 years!) and arrived at a figure not very different from today's advanced computer model estimates. Arrhenius' ideas attracted little notice, however, and it wasn't until the late 1950s that interest in climate science revived.

In 1957, designated by the United Nations as the International Geophysical Year, a young American chemist, Charles David Keeling, had an idea for a relevant project. Keeling had just designed and built an instrument capable of measuring extremely precise concentrations of carbon dioxide and sought to persuade the U.S. Weather Bureau to allow him to set up his equipment at its new observatory on the slope of Hawaii's Mauna Loa volcano. Keeling wanted to commence continuous readings of atmospheric CO_2 levels and reasoned that Mauna Loa, far from human-generated sources of pollution, would be the ideal location.

Regular sampling began in March 1958 and has continued to the present day, providing an invaluable record of the steady upward climb in CO_2 concentrations. Plotted on what has become an iconic graph known as "the Keeling Curve," the data show a sawtooth-like, upward sloping line documenting the inexorable rise in parts-per-million (ppm) atmospheric carbon dioxide (Kolbert, 2006; Revkin, 1992). Keeling's initial measurement of 315 ppm was already well above the 278 ppm prevailing at the onset of the industrial age—a level that scientists believe never varied more than 5 ppm throughout the previous millennium (Indermühle et al., 1999). Over the decades since Keeling's work riveted attention on the growing impact of human activities on the Earth's atmosphere, CO_2 concentrations have continued their upward trajectory, reaching 354 ppm in 1990, 366 in 1999, and 389 in 2010—about 40% higher than pre-industrial levels.

Not only are atmospheric levels of CO_2 rising, but their rate of increase is rising as well. During the decade of the 1990s, carbon dioxide concentrations grew by 1.5 ppm per year; between 2000–2007, the annual increase rose to 2 ppm (Canadell et al., 2007). Given CO_2's long-recognized heat-absorbing properties, it should probably come as no surprise that eight of the ten warmest years on record have occurred since 2001, while as of 2009, the five warmest years to date were: 2005, 1998 and 2009 (tied for second place), 2002, 2003, and 2007 (NCDC, 2009). In December 2010, NASA announced that the previous 12 months had produced the highest land and ocean temperatures ever recorded. In January 2011, NOAA scientists announced that 2010 tied with 2005 as the warmest year since detailed records have been kept (NOAA, 2011). Slowly but surely, the once-benign natural "greenhouse effect" has become a planet-threatening, man-made "greenhouse problem."

Other Greenhouse Gases

As if humanity doesn't have enough to worry about with the rise in carbon dioxide levels, climatologists warn that increasing atmospheric concentrations of several so-called **greenhouse gases (GHGs)**—particularly methane, nitrous oxide, and halocarbons—are further enhancing the greenhouse effect by capturing wavelengths of infrared radiation not readily absorbed by CO_2. Although present in concentrations far below that of carbon dioxide, these trace gases are much more efficient than CO_2 in absorbing outgoing heat waves. A molecule of methane, for example, can trap 20–30 times more infrared radiation than does a molecule of CO_2. Equally problematic is the fact that emissions of trace gases are increasing at a substantially faster rate than CO_2 and originate from sources that may be even more difficult to control. A brief look at the situation regarding the other greenhouse gases reveals the following picture.

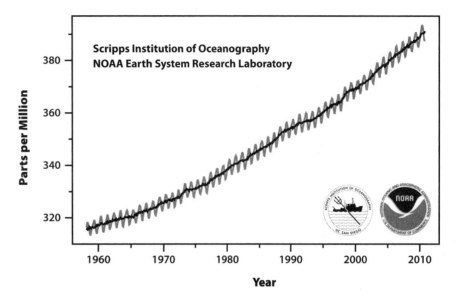

Source: http://www.esrl.noaa.gov/gmd/cccgg/trends/

Figure 11-6   Atmospheric Carbon Dioxide at Mauna Loa Observatory, Hawaii

Methane (CH_4).   Although current atmospheric concentrations of this gas are less than 2 ppm, as opposed to CO_2 levels of 389 ppm, methane is far more potent as a greenhouse gas and is increasing at a 0.6% annual rate. Curtailing methane emissions will not be easy, since over half originate from rice cultivation (due to the respiration of anaerobic bacteria in waterlogged paddy fields) and from microbial activity in the intestines of cattle and termites (it is estimated that a cow belches methane approximately twice a minute!). Other significant sources more amenable to controls include landfills, emissions from gas and coal production, flares on oil rigs, manure piles, and tropical deforestation (when vegetation is burned during clearing activities).

Nitrous oxide (N_2O).   With atmospheric concentrations up by 17% (46 ppb) since 1750 and still rising, the so-called "laughing gas" once used as a painkiller by dentists is a more efficient greenhouse gas than CO_2 but because its total atmospheric concentrations are in the parts per billion range, its overall contribution to global warming is still fairly limited. Nitrous oxide is a natural by-product of the metabolism of certain soil microbes, but the generation of this gas has been boosted significantly by the increased worldwide use of nitrogen fertilizers. It is estimated that more than a third of agricultural emissions of nitrous oxide could be eliminated by improving fertilizer application practices, incorporating fertilizers into the soil, using nitrification additives, and testing soils to determine how much fertilizer is actually needed (Siikamaki, 2008). Combustion of fossil fuels, increased land cultivation, burning of biomass, and the decomposition of agricultural wastes and sewage are additional sources of N_2O.

Halocarbons.   A group that includes the ozone-depleting chlorofluorocarbons (CFCs), as well as **perfluorocarbons** (PFCs), **sulfur hexafluoride** (SF_6), and the **hydrofluorocarbons** (HFCs), halocarbons are potent greenhouse gases, each molecule of which has a direct warming effect 12,000–20,000 times greater than that of a CO_2 molecule. It is assumed that the halt in CFC production mandated by the Montreal Protocol will result in a decrease—or slower increase—in atmospheric concentrations of these gases in the years to come. However, concentrations of PFCs, HFCs, and SF6 continue to rise due to their increasing commercial and industrial use as substitutes for CFCs and other now-banned ozone-depleting chemicals.

It should be noted that **water vapor** is one of the most powerful greenhouse gases—it's the primary contributor to the natural greenhouse effect—but because human activities have negligible impact on its atmospheric concentrations and because the amount of water in the air varies widely from place to place and day to day, levels of this atmospheric constituent are not taken into consideration when discussing global warming scenarios. It plays a key role, however, in some of the "positive feedback" scenarios regarding further enhancement of warming trends, a role that is addressed in box 11-2.

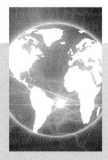

······· 11-2 ·······
Feedbacks and Tipping Points

While the conclusions of the IPCC's Fourth Assessment Report, *Climate Change 2007: The Physical Science Basis*, provide ample cause for alarm, most scientists are now convinced that it understates both the rate and extent of climate change the world will experience in the years ahead. The reasons for this understatement are several:

1. Because the panel can only consider well-established conclusions from the scientific literature, only research published before July 2006 was reviewed; thus assessments were already outdated by the time they were issued.

2. IPCC's energy economy models, developed largely in the 1990s, were not up-to-date, particularly in regards to China's GHG emissions, which began their sharp upswing around 2002.

3. Scientists themselves are reluctant to overstate anything and almost always err on the side of caution.

4. Perhaps most significant, the report fails to take **positive feedback loops** into account, even though we are already witnessing changes that could provoke more rapid and far-reaching changes than current IPCC models predict.

In the context of climate change, positive feedbacks are impacts that magnify the degree of warming beyond that provoked by the initial increase in greenhouse gases (there are some negative feedbacks as well, but their overall impact is far outweighed by the positive ones). Positive feedback loops constitute self-reinforcing trends that boost temperatures to levels higher than they would otherwise have attained, thus amplifying global warming. Among the most important positive feedback effects are the following:

Water vapor feedback. Water vapor is a powerful absorber of infrared radiation and a major contributor to the natural greenhouse effect. In the future, water vapor's role in global warming will be even greater since higher temperatures result in higher evaporation rates, further increasing atmospheric concentrations of water vapor, which then absorb even more heat waves and boost temperatures higher yet. Research published in 2009 estimates that water vapor feedback is strongly positive and likely to double the warming that would have occurred in its absence (Dessler and Sherwood, 2009).

Ice-albedo feedback. Prior to the onset of climate change, approximately one-third of incoming solar radiation was reflected back into space, largely due to Earth's **albedo** (white surfaces), particularly the snow- and ice-covered polar regions that reflect 80–90% of incident sunlight. As temperatures rise, snow and ice cover are melting, reducing Earth's albedo and exposing vast expanses of land and open water that reflect very little light—perhaps only 5–10% in the case of water. Areas now free of ice and snow are absorbing incoming sunlight and re-radiating it in the form of heat waves. As a result, seas and soils are warming, and the surrounding ice and snow melt even more—yet another self-reinforcing trend and widely regarded as the main reason the Arctic is heating up more rapidly than anywhere else on the planet (Kolbert, 2006).

Permafrost melting. Underlying most of the land in the Arctic and comprising almost 25% of the land area of the Northern Hemisphere, permafrost contains a vast repository of partially decomposed vegetation. Preserved in a frozen state for more than 120,000 years in some locations, permafrost is now beginning to thaw, with worrisome consequences for the areas involved and for the world's climate. Latest estimates suggest that 1.7 trillion tons of carbon is now sequestered in permafrost (Kintisch, 2009); as permafrost warms and bacterial decomposition of embedded plant materials accelerates, huge amounts of CO_2 and methane will be released into the atmosphere. Since methane is approximately 30 times more absorptive than CO_2 in terms of its GHG potential, thawing of permafrost constitutes another powerful feedback loop, amplifying temperature increase in the Arctic which then results in further permafrost melting and levels of GHGs released.

Warming of the oceans. Oceans constitute a major "sink" for CO_2; however, the capacity of that sink is dwindling as higher temperatures at the air-ocean interface are causing water temperatures to rise, thereby reducing their ability to absorb CO_2. As less carbon dioxide is able to dissolve into the ocean, more remains in the atmosphere, further increasing its heat-trapping capacity—and global average temperatures climb ever higher.

Collapse of the Amazon rain forest. As climate change accelerates, the Amazon region as a whole is becoming hotter and drier. Research has revealed that a substantial percentage of the rainfall in Amazonia is generated by the huge amounts of moisture transpiring from the forest canopy. As CO_2 levels increase, however, rates of transpiration decrease, leading to less cloud formation and diminishing precipitation. Warming-induced changes in weather patterns are further reducing annual rainfall from its current basin-wide average of 0.2 inch/day to a projected 0.08 inch/day in 2100. With decreasing precipitation and rising temperatures, rain forest vegetation will be stressed to the point of collapse, a process that computer models predict will become noticeable by 2040; by 2100 model projections indicate less than 10% of the Amazon basin's tree cover will remain. Higher temperatures and loss of the tree canopy will cause regional soils to heat up, spurring bacterial breakdown of organic matter and massive release of carbon currently bound in the soil. This, along with additional CO_2 released via decomposition of dead surface vegetation and drought-induced wildfires, will further ratchet up the degree of climate change.

Because feedback loops are so complex, existing climate models can't yet fully account for all the effects scientists are documenting. Nevertheless, they are real and their existence guarantees that their long-term impacts will be much greater than suggested by the projections in IPCC's Fourth Assessment Report.

Thus far climate change has proceeded at such a gradual pace that the average person feels little sense of urgency about the issue. Warnings that nations must act quickly and decisively to confront the threat meet with a "ho-hum" reaction from the vast majority, who assume the climatic response to rising GHG concentrations will be slow and linear. Those most familiar with the issue, however, argue that the opposite is more likely to be true—that climate change progresses in a nonlinear fashion, giving little evidence of increasing stress until pressure eventually reaches a critical **"tipping point"** and sudden, dramatic change occurs—at which point it's too late to prevent catastrophic damage.

There has been considerable discussion in scientific circles about what might constitute such tipping points—melting of the Greenland and West Antarctic ice sheets is the one most frequently cited, along with the unlikely but possible collapse of thermohaline circulation in the North Atlantic—and what level of greenhouse gases would trigger them. The United Nations Framework Convention on Climate Change calls on signatory nations to stabilize atmospheric greenhouse gas concentrations at a level that "would prevent dangerous anthropogenic interference with the climate system," but what *is* that level in terms of parts-per-million CO_2? While it's not yet possible to answer this question with absolute certainty, scientists' best guess, based on research published since 2007, has been steadily falling. Until a few years ago, policy makers thought serious harm could be avoided if atmospheric CO_2 concentrations could be held at about 550 ppm (double their pre-industrial level), allowing for a maximum average global temperature increase of 3°C. However, new findings indicating serious impacts at GHG levels substantially lower than those previously deemed dangerous have prompted climate change negotiators to lower the bar; they're now aiming for no greater than a 2°C rise, something they think is achievable if CO_2 concentrations aren't allowed to exceed 450 ppm.

Other researchers are less optimistic, worried that with an average temperature increase of just 1–2° above 1990 levels, unique and threatened ecosystems such as mountain glaciers, coral reefs, biodiversity hot spots, and small island nations will suffer increased damage or irreversible loss. Extreme weather events will be inevitable with additional warming of slightly less than 1°C—in fact, such events are already occurring. Averting critical tipping points is beginning to look more problematic as well; earlier projections that these would be triggered by temperature increases in the 4–5°C range have now been lowered to 1–4°C. Since the IPCC's high-end projections indicate that global average temperature could climb as high as 6.4°C by the end of this century, there's little room for complacency—especially since the projections don't fully take into account the feedback loops that are likely to amplify warming even further. The new findings are sobering and reinforce scientists' warnings that the nations of the world must forego their "business-as-usual" practices and take immediate, effective action to avert otherwise inevitable catastrophe (Smith et al., 2008).

While the lion's share of public attention regarding climate change has thus far focused on carbon dioxide emissions, it is now agreed that the cumulative effect of the other greenhouse gases will be nearly equivalent to that of CO_2. Ironically, until now air pollution has helped counteract the heat-capturing potential of greenhouse gases to some extent. Airborne sulfate particles released when fossil fuels and other organic materials are burned reflect solar radiation, thereby exerting a cooling effect on climate. Indeed, the high levels of particulate air pollution prevailing in many industrialized countries following World War II are now credited with the slight decline in average global temperature during the three decades between 1945 and 1975. Imposition of new regulations sharply limiting industrial and vehicular emissions began having an impact on air quality by the mid-1970s—and global warming rebounded.

The Latest Villain: Black Carbon

While airborne particulate pollution in general is known to counter the effects of heat-absorbing greenhouse gases, one constituent of dirty emissions has recently gained notoriety as the second-most important driver of climate change after CO_2. **Black carbon**, a component of soot, is a product of incomplete combustion of fossil fuels, biomass, and biofuels. The largest amounts are contributed by diesel engines; home cookstoves that burn wood, coal, dung, or crop residues; and open burning of fields or woodlands. Unlike carbon dioxide and other greenhouse gases, black carbon seldom remains in the atmosphere for more than two weeks, but while there it strongly absorbs infrared waves, heating the surrounding atmosphere. In addition, if it subsequently settles out on areas covered with snow or ice, darkening their surfaces, it reduces their ability to reflect light (i.e., it reduces their albedo), increasing heat absorption and speeding up the melting of glaciers and ice caps (Clare, 2009). Research indicates that black carbon is probably to blame for more than 30% of recent warming observed in the Arctic (Shindell and Faluvegi, 2009).

Black carbon content varies from one type of soot to another; higher levels are found in soot generated by fossil fuels—especially diesel—and from biofuels as opposed to soot from fuelwood burning or forest fires. This fact suggests that a vigorous effort to control emissions by retrofitting diesel buses with highly efficient diesel particulate filters (DPFs) could have a significant impact in reducing atmospheric warming caused by black carbon. DPFs have been shown to reduce emissions by 90%; however, these filters also require the use of ultra-low sulfur diesel fuel (ULSD), which is not yet widely available in developing nations where the need to curb black carbon emissions is particularly acute. (Currently, India and China together are believed responsible

for 25–35% of world black carbon emissions, while the U.S. is the source of just 6%.) Control efforts thus should include a program to increase the availability of ULSD.

Diesel particulate filters are needed not only for diesel-powered buses but also for ocean-going vessels, especially those sailing in far northern waters where black carbon emissions are particularly harmful. Other methods for reducing ship emissions, such as reducing the sulfur content of fuel and encouraging reduced sailing speeds, also are being advocated. Efforts to improve the efficiency of traditional cookstoves used in millions of developing-world homes have been underway for years in order to reduce health-damaging pollutants generated by these devices. Recent revelations about the environmental hazard posed by their black carbon emissions has added impetus for programs dedicated to helping poor women cook for their families without endangering their own health or aggravating global warming. Scientists and environmental activists are now urging governments to look more seriously at programs for sharply reducing black carbon emissions, arguing that focusing on this short-lived but powerful pollutant would be the quickest, easiest way to mitigate climate change, buying time while other, longer-term strategies are being negotiated (Clare, 2009).

EVIDENCE FOR CLIMATE CHANGE

The reality of global climate change has been vigorously debated and investigated since the late 1970s, drawing on evidence derived from such diverse sources as ice core analyses, orbiting satellites, ocean current studies, and computer modeling. As discussed earlier in this chapter, the Intergovernmental Panel on Climate Change (IPCC), a multinational group of scientists charged with assessing information related to climate change, has since 1990 released four comprehensive reports, the latest of which—*Climate Change 2007*—categorically states that "most of the observed increase in globally averaged temperatures since the mid-20th century is *very likely* (greater than 90% probability) due to the observed increase in anthropogenic greenhouse gas concentrations." The report goes on to project an increase of average global surface temperatures ranging from 2.0–11.5°F (1.1–6.4°C) by the end of this century, based on 35 different future emissions scenarios. It also describes a number of impacts likely to result from such warming. For those who, for reasons pertaining to politics or economic self-interest, still tend to dismiss climate change warnings, the following comments by Dr. John Holdren, a noted physicist and director of the Office of Science and Technology Policy in the Obama administration, aptly summarize the overwhelming weight of supporting evidence:

They are based on an immense edifice of painstaking studies published in the world's leading peer-reviewed scientific journals. They have been vetted and documented in excruciating detail by the largest, longest, costliest, most international, most interdisciplinary, and most thorough formal review of a scientific topic ever conducted.

So what *is* this evidence that has proven so persuasive to Dr. Holdren and the vast majority of his peers? Among the most compelling observations are the following.

Ice Core Analyses

Since the 1990s, scientists drilling deep into ice sheets in Greenland and Antarctica, as well as into Andean mountain glaciers, have been extracting ice cores and chemically analyzing air bubbles trapped for hundreds of thousands of years. By doing so, they have been able to construct a record of past climatic conditions, demonstrating increases and decreases of carbon dioxide and methane as warm interglacial periods alternated with colder glacial epochs. They found that even the highest concentrations of greenhouse gases in past millennia, present during the warm interglacial years, were well below present-day levels, a strong indication of human influence on today's climate (Petit et al., 1999). Ice cores dating back 670,000 years reveal that Earth's average temperature fluctuation during that period never exceeded 6°C (about 11°F) and prove that throughout past ages, CO_2 concentrations and temperatures rose and fell in tandem. They also show that warming can be surprisingly abrupt, with temperatures shifting from cold to mild over a period as brief as 1–3 years (Steffensen et al., 2008).

Melting Sea Ice and Mountain Glaciers

A break in the Wilkins ice shelf on the Antarctic Peninsula in April 2009 was just one more indication to climate researchers that the poles are heating up. While the average global surface temperature has risen by about 1.5°F (0.8°C) during the last century, it's up by 4–5°F (2.5°C) in the world's polar regions. As a result, sea ice is melting at rates more rapid than were predicted even a few years ago. In the Arctic Ocean, the extent of sea ice during late summer has plunged by 34% since 1979, reaching its lowest extent ever in the summer of 2007; 2008 set the second-lowest record and may have had an even lower total volume of sea ice than 2007 did. According to the National Snow and Ice Data Center (NSIDC) in Boulder, Colorado, sea ice extent in 2010 was reported as 1.78 million square miles, the third-lowest on record and only slightly more than that of 2008. Noting these trends, NSIDC scientists now suggest that the Arctic Ocean could be completely devoid of summertime ice within 20–30 years. Dwindling sea ice is not the only indication of substantial Arctic warming; melting of the Greenland ice sheet has been accelerating since the summer of 2004, with losses of ice along the margins exceeding additions through annual snowfall in interior regions. As a result, overall the ice sheet is losing mass and thus contributing to sea level rise (Mernild et al., 2009).

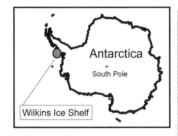

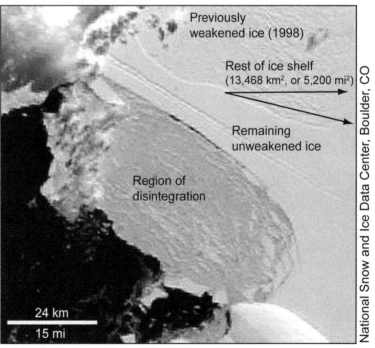

Satellite imagery shows the Wilkins Ice Shelf in Antarctica as it began to break up. [*National Snow and Ice Data Center*]

In Antarctica, the collapse of an ice bridge connecting the Wilkins ice shelf to a small island was but the most recent indication of warming at the South Pole. Since the late 1990s there have been 10 major ice shelf collapses along the West Antarctic Peninsula, the most spectacular perhaps being the breakup of the 1,250 square mile Larsen B ice shelf over a period of a few weeks in 2002. Such collapses are of concern because ice shelves function as support structures preventing the flow of land-based ice sheets into the ocean. Scientists liken the loss of these ice shelves to "pulling the cork out of a bottle," resulting in an accelerated flow of glaciers into the ocean and a corresponding rise in sea level. Until recently it was believed that while West Antarctica and the Antarctic Peninsula were warming at approximately the same rate as the northern polar regions, East Antarctica, comprising the continent's interior, had actually cooled slightly in recent decades, giving ammunition to climate change deniers. Research published in 2009, however, showed that, to the contrary, Antarctica as a whole has been warming for the past 50 years, especially in West Antarctica where temperatures over the past half-century have risen by about 0.1°C per decade. Some autumn cooling does occur in parts of East Antarctica, caused by the seasonal loss of stratospheric ozone (i.e., the Antarctic "ozone hole"). As atmospheric concentrations of ozone-depleting substances continue to decline, researchers anticipate that average Antarctic temperatures will continue to climb (Steig et al., 2009).

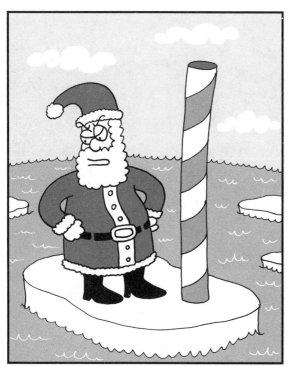

"Why did I have to give bad kids all that coal?"

Polar regions aren't the only places where ice is melting. Throughout the world's highest mountain ranges, glaciers, too, are disappearing. Switzerland's Aletsch glacier, the largest in mainland Europe, has retreated more than a mile since the mid-1800s and has shrunk by more than 300 feet in thickness. Alpine glaciers as a group have lost one-third to one-half their ice volume during the past century. On Africa's highest peak, more than 80% of the legendary "snows of Kilimanjaro" have melted since 1912; the remainder is expected to vanish by 2020. In Asia, experts predict that most glaciers in the central and eastern Himalayas could be gone well before the end of the century. Some wags suggest Americans should hold a contest to select a new name for Montana's Glacier National Park, since, at the current rate of melting, all of the park's ice sheets are expected to disappear in the next 10–20 years.

Ocean Waters Heating Up and Acidifying

It isn't just the atmosphere that's warming—ocean temperatures are rising as well. Scientists at the National Oceanographic and Atmospheric Administration (NOAA) have shown that the world's oceans as a whole have been warming for the past 50 years (Levitus and Boyer, 2005). Other observations have confirmed these reports, showing that the oceans have been warming from the surface downward to a depth of at least 9,750 feet (IPCC, 2007), indicating a transfer of heat from the atmosphere due to the enhanced greenhouse effect. Oceans are a major "sink" for excess heat, since far more energy is required to raise the temperature of a given volume of water by 1°C than for an equivalent volume of air. As a result, it's estimated that over the past half-century, more than 90% of the excess heat generated by rising greenhouse gas levels has been taken up by the oceans, while only 3% has contributed to atmospheric warming.

Ocean waters also absorb tremendous quantities of carbon dioxide, but their continued ability to do so is diminishing. Research indicates that whereas 600 kg of every metric ton of CO_2 discharged into the atmosphere 50 years ago was absorbed by the oceans, today the amount removed per metric ton has dropped to 550 kg. Two factors account for this: (1) ocean waters are warmer than in the past and CO_2 is less soluble in warm water than in cold (a fact that has been observed by anyone opening a carbonated beverage on a hot day!); and (2) as CO_2 dissolves in ocean waters it forms carbonic acid, making the ocean more acidic. Not only does ocean acidification threaten many forms of marine life, it also reduces seawater's ability to continue absorbing carbon dioxide—with the result that more greenhouse gases will remain in the atmosphere and thus further enhance global warming.

Increasing Height of the Tropopause

Satellite monitoring has revealed that between 1979 and 2001 the height of the tropopause (the upper limit of the troposphere, bordering the stratosphere) increased by 620 feet. Computer modeling studies have shown that while stratospheric cooling due to ozone depletion is responsible for 60% of this rise, anthropogenic greenhouse gas emissions can be blamed for 40% of the observed elevation of the tropopause (Santer et al., 2003).

Shifting Range of Biological Species and Temporal Advancement of Spring Events

Even the small amount of warming that has already occurred has resulted in an average 6.1 km per decade northward advance (or meters/decade upward) in the range of more than 1,700 species evaluated. For 279 species, it has also pushed forward by 2.3 days per decade the average timing of such spring events as frog breeding, bird nesting, first flowering, opening of tree buds, and the arrival of migratory birds and butterflies (Parmesan and Yohe, 2003). Both plants and animals are on the move.

In Switzerland and western Austria, nine species of alpine plants have been moving up mountainsides at a rate of about four meters per decade since the early 20th century. In the United States, a researcher at the University of Texas has documented a northward shift of about 60 miles in populations of the Edith's Checkerspot butterfly, with the insect vanishing from the southern extreme of its traditional range and expanding from its northern boundary; the butterflies are also now found at elevations 300 feet higher than in the past. Scientists attribute the shift to rising temperatures that have caused the snapdragon plants on which the Checkerspot larvae feed to dry up earlier in the season than usual, depriving the insects of a food source.

More troubling than the migration of wildflowers or butterflies has been the spread of disease-carrying mosquitoes, both northward and to higher altitudes, where temperatures formerly were too cool for them to survive. Perhaps the most dramatic example of a species shifting its range northward in response to a warming climate is the arrival several years ago of robins on a Canadian island 500 miles north of the Arctic Circle. The bemused local Inuit hunters had no word in their language for the newcomers (Kolbert, 2006).

IMPACTS OF GLOBAL WARMING

To many people, the prospect of temperatures a few degrees higher than they are at present seems little cause for dismay—particularly when they happen to be contemplating such a scenario during a January blizzard. The major impact of global warming, however, would not be felt in terms of human physical discomfort but rather in a drastic alteration of worldwide rainfall and temperature patterns. The extensive and steadily growing body of observational data described in the previous sections, along with sophisticated computer modeling studies used to predict future trends, provide a solid scientific rationale for policy initiatives aimed at mitigating climate change. Using this information, governments around the world are struggling to formulate strategies to combat climate change and to limit the most severe potential impacts of global warming, including the following.

Shifting Rainfall Patterns

As the planet warms, rates of evaporation increase, resulting in a global average rise in precipitation. However, that increase in total rainfall will not be evenly distributed. Projections based on computer modeling suggest that areas already receiving adequate rainfall—the northeastern quadrant of the United States, northwestern Europe, moist equatorial regions of Latin America, Asia, and Africa—will experience even more and heavier precipitation in the decades ahead. Heavy downpours will occur much more frequently and are expected to increase in intensity by 10–25% by the end of the century. As a result, flooding—such as that which caused mass dislocation and loss of life in Pakistan in the summer of 2010—will become a frequent occurrence in many of the world's most densely populated areas such as the Ganges Delta on the Indian subcontinent, the Pearl River Delta in southern China, the United Kingdom's Thames River basin, and the Mississippi Delta—to name but a few regions likely to make headline news due to disastrous floods in coming years.

In many already-arid regions, however, climate change will have the opposite effect—further declines in annual rainfall. In the United States, the Southwest will experience a 10–40% decrease in runoff (i.e., water appearing in streams) by 2050, as current water shortages intensify. Earlier spring snowmelts as temperatures rise are expected to result in summer droughts in parts of the American West, along with more numerous and more devastating wildfires. Other regions of the world projected to experience long-term drying conditions as climate change accelerates include lands bordering the Mediterranean, southern Africa, Central America and northeastern South America, northern Mexico, and southern Australia. According to the U.K.'s Hadley Centre for Climate Change, as the climate continues to warm in the decades ahead, moderate drought could affect 50% of the world's land area (up from 25% at present); severe drought may affect 40% of all land areas (now 8%), and extreme drought, 30% (3% today).

The human toll of increasing aridity promises to be catastrophic and is already becoming apparent. The

International Institute of Tropical Agriculture in Nigeria estimates that in 2010 approximately 300 million people in sub-Saharan Africa will suffer from malnutrition caused by worsening drought conditions. Similarly, the UN Environmental Programme reports that 450 million people in 29 countries are experiencing water shortages—a number that is projected to rise to 2.8 billion by 2025. The economic, social, and political repercussions of severe flooding or prolonged drought are likely to be enormous and will present a major challenge to governments in future decades. Unfortunately, the impacts are expected to be most severe in the poor developing-world countries least able to deal with them.

Extreme Weather Events

Flooding aside, extreme weather events are already becoming more common and are projected to increase in frequency as the climate warms. During July and August of 2010, more than 15,000 Russians died during the country's longest heat wave in at least 1,000 years (according to the Russian Meteorological Center). Elsewhere, 16 other nations, comprising 19% of the world's total land area, also experienced their hottest temperatures ever that summer.

In the United States, by the end of this century days now designated as "very hot" will be about 10°F hotter, and rather than occurring once every twenty years or so will make us miserable every other year. Aside from the discomfort they cause—and soaring energy use due to demand for air-conditioning—severe heat waves can be killers, resulting in excess deaths due primarily to heart attacks and strokes. In Chicago, 726 people died of heat stress during four days of record-high temperatures in July 1995, while an estimated 15,000 deaths in France and 18,000 in northern Italy were attributed to a blistering heat wave affecting much of western Europe in August 2003. More recently, in February 2009, a scorching heat wave in southeastern Australia killed over 200 residents of Melbourne; another 173 Australians died in that country's worst-ever wildfires, blamed on 120°F temperatures and accompanying 100 mph winds. Warmer temperatures promote the formation of additional photochemical smog, which in turn worsens air pollution and contributes to higher rates of respiratory disease (Eyles and Consitt, 2004). If pollutant emissions remain unchanged, it's estimated that by mid-century global warming will provoke a 68% increase in the number of Red Ozone Alert Days in the 50 largest U.S. cities.

Tropical storms represent another example of extreme weather events likely to become more common as sea surface temperatures rise. Along the U.S. Gulf Coast and southeast Atlantic shores, hurricanes and storm surges are predicted to become more severe. Climate change is expected to result in a gradually increasing risk of category-5 hurricanes, featuring storms with higher wind velocity and heavier rainfall than those typical of years past (Knutson and Tuleya, 2004). Considering that three-fourths of the world's people now live within 36 miles (60 km) of a coastline, such projections are not good news.

Rising Sea Levels

The most dramatic long-term consequence of global warming will be a worldwide rise in sea level. Although this development could be a boon

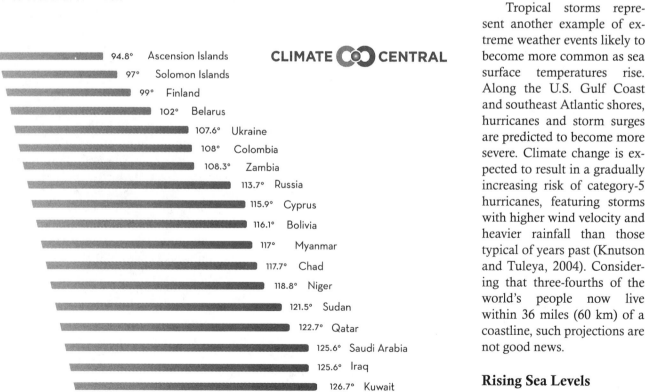

CLIMATE CENTRAL

94.8°   Ascension Islands
97°   Solomon Islands
99°   Finland
102°   Belarus
107.6°   Ukraine
108°   Colombia
108.3°   Zambia
113.7°   Russia
115.9°   Cyprus
116.1°   Bolivia
117°   Myanmar
117.7°   Chad
118.8°   Niger
121.5°   Sudan
122.7°   Qatar
125.6°   Saudi Arabia
125.6°   Iraq
126.7°   Kuwait
128.3°   Pakistan

All temperatures in degrees F.
Source: Weather Underground/Jeff Masters. Used with permission of Climate Central.

Figure 11-7   Countries That Set New Record Highs in 2010

to navigation in the Arctic (the fabled "Northwest Passage" is beginning to look like a practical alternative to the Panama Canal!), its impact on densely populated coastal regions and low-lying island nations will be devastating. In its 2007 *Fourth Assessment Report*, the IPCC projects that sea level will rise between 0.6–1.9 feet (0.2–0.6 meters) above its 1990 level by the end of the century, noting that it already has been rising by 3 mm annually since 1993. However, these estimates primarily represent the thermal expansion of water as temperatures rise, as well as a modest increase due to water runoff from melting glaciers.

In the months following publication of the IPCC's 2007 report, a number of new studies documented faster-than-expected melting of massive ice sheets in both Greenland and Antarctica. It is now believed that the IPCC significantly underestimated the extent of 21st century sea level rise and that meltwater from land-based ice sheets could contribute to a sea level rise ranging from 2.6 feet (0.8 meter) to as much as 6.6 feet (2 meters) by 2100, with a one-meter rise considered most likely (Rahmstorf et al., 2007). If atmospheric CO_2 levels and temperature continue to climb, the immense Greenland and West Antarctic ice sheets could eventually melt completely, raising sea levels by 39 feet and submerging vast areas of densely inhabited coastal lands worldwide. Although total melting of the Greenland ice sheet would require a 6°C temperature increase, even a 15% shrinkage would result in a one-meter rise in sea level (Kintisch, 2009).

The societal impacts of sea level rise will be devastating even at the low end of the projected increase. At particular risk are the inhabitants of low-lying coral atolls like the Carteret Islands northeast of Papua New Guinea, an island chain that is expected to be uninhabitable by 2015 due to rising ocean waters; the tiny Pacific nation-states of Tuvalu and Kiribati also face possible extinction in the not-too-distant future due to climate-change-induced sea level rise. Residents of other small island nations such as the Bahamas, Maldives, and Marshall Islands have been among the most vociferous advocates of international action to curb greenhouse gas emissions as they confront the prospect of their homelands disappearing beneath the waves.

Along the edges of continents, towns and cities built on barrier islands, river deltas, or low-lying shorelines can anticipate a similar scenario unless they soon embark on multi-billion dollar coastal defense construction projects. In the U.S., studies conducted by ExxonMobil researchers project that, barring massive engineering projects to build up sediments at the mouth of the Mississippi Delta, fully 10% of Louisiana will be under water by the end of the century (Perkins, 2009). In many desperately poor, densely populated regions of the world, massive expenditures are obviously impossible. It is anticipated that Egypt may lose 15% of its arable land to encroaching seas by mid-century; in Bangladesh, flooding is likely to increase up to 40% in the years ahead due to global warming. If the temperature increase under IPCC's worst-case sce-

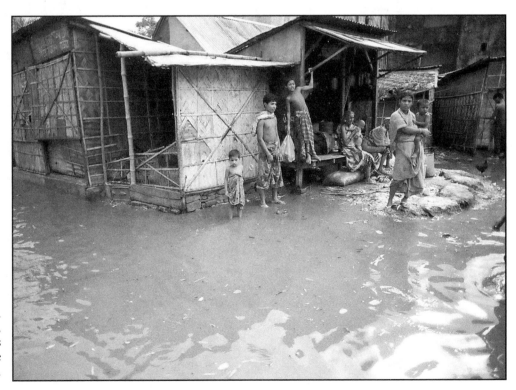

Flooding in Bangladesh, already a recurring problem, could increase by as much as 40% in the years ahead due to global warming.

nario proves correct, by 2100 slightly over half of Bangladesh will be covered by nearly 6 feet (1.8 meters) of flood water more than nine months of the year (Mirza, Warrick, and Ericksen, 2003)—a staggering prospect for a nation whose population in mid-2010 was 164.4 million, expected to rise to 222 million by 2050.

When one pauses to consider the number of major world cities located at or near sea level—New York, Washington DC, London, Shanghai, Bangkok, Sydney, Dhaka, Lagos, and Calcutta, just to name a few—the impact of sea level rise on human settlement patterns becomes clear. Although sea level will rise gradually (no one foresees the likelihood of Boston or Galveston or Miami disappearing overnight!), even a slight increase can have significant consequences. It is estimated that there could be an 8-foot horizontal retreat of sandy beach shorelines due to erosion for every one-inch rise in sea level. Some experts feel that a six-inch rise during the 20th century was responsible for much of the coastal erosion that has occurred and contend that a continuation of present trends will obliterate most beaches along the eastern coast of the U.S. by 2020.

Interestingly, two recent studies have shown that sea level rise is not uniform around the world and that the Atlantic and Pacific coasts of the United States will experience significantly higher-than-average sea level increase (Bamber et al., 2009; Yin, Schlesinger, and Stauffer, 2009). This is bad news for the insurance industry, since rising seas threaten trillions of dollars worth of coastal property, a risk not yet accurately reflected in insurance rates or in building codes. Commercial transportation will also be severely impacted by sea level rise, since each year hundreds of billions of dollars worth of goods move via highways, railroads, pipelines, airports, and seaports vulnerable to flooding. Already an estimated 60,000 miles of coastal U.S. highways experience occasional flooding due to storm surges and high waves. Rising sea levels will only exacerbate the threat (USGCRP, 2009).

Diminishing Crop Yields

The hotter, drier weather forecast for some of the world's most productive agricultural lands is bad news at a time when global food demand is steadily increasing. For farmers, climatic change could bring temporary benefits to some regions, severe hardship to others. Researchers predict that farmers in the Great Lakes region of the United States will prosper as warming temperatures extend the growing season and boost yields; by contrast, agriculture in the southeastern states is likely to be hard-hit, as a double whammy of soaring summer temperatures and decreased rainfall result in drastically reduced harvests (Siikamaki, 2008). Although some observers suggest that rising concentrations of CO_2 might actually enhance food production by increasing photosynthetic rates, recent research indicates that higher atmospheric carbon dioxide levels have a distinctly negative impact on crop production. A report submitted to Congress in 2004 stated that excess CO_2 promotes the growth of several invasive weed species far more than it stimulates crop growth; it also lowers the nutritional value of certain rangeland grasses.

Greenhouse gas-induced warming can reduce harvests, a fact demonstrated by researchers in the Philippines who documented a 10% drop in rice yields with each 1°C (1.8°F) increase in night temperatures during the growing season (Peng et al., 2004). U.S. agricultural researchers analyzing the impact of climate on corn and soybean yields came to a similar conclusion, reporting that their studies showed a 17% reduction in yields for those two crops with each degree of warming (Lobell and Asner, 2003). Real-life events corroborate the results of these experimental studies. The high temperatures that killed over 30,000 people in France and Italy during the summer heat wave of August 2003, mentioned in a previous section of this chapter, also reduced the French corn and fruit harvest by 25%; in Italy the corn harvest plummeted 36% below its level of the previous year. While this was a highly unusual event at the time, computer models indicate that by 2090 summer temperatures in France will be 3.7°C higher than the 20th century average almost every year.

Crop yield reductions will be an even more serious problem in tropical and subtropical countries, which are likely to be the first to experience unprecedented heat stress caused by global warming. By the end of the century throughout much of this region, average temperatures are anticipated to exceed the hottest recorded during the 20th century—an ominous prospect in terms of world food security. Since mid-latitude countries will likely be experiencing heat-induced shortfalls in their own harvests as temperatures continue to rise, it may prove impossible to ease world hunger problems, as now, by shipping food from areas of surplus to areas of need. Food shortages by then are likely to be global in extent, barring major agricultural advances in developing new crop varieties resistant to heat and drought (Battisti and Naylor, 2009).

Global warming could have other less obvious impacts on agricultural productivity. Livestock production will suffer due to heat-induced declines in animal fertility; pastures and rangelands can be expected to sustain heat damage. As temperatures rise, the range of plant pathogens and crop-destroying insects expand considerably; pests currently confined to southern latitudes may spread northward, causing serious agricultural losses. A shift in the balance between pest and predator species, prompted by changing environmental conditions, could also have adverse repercussions for farming by favoring the survival of more resilient pest species over that of their natural enemies. These increased pest infestations may prompt farmers to increase applications of chemical pesticides, raising the probability of more surface and groundwater pollution problems. Crop losses are likely to be further compounded by increasing levels of tropospheric ozone, a pollutant gas that forms most readily on hot, sunny days and which is responsible for about 90% of annual U.S. crop losses due to air pollution. Finally, increasing aridity in many already drought-prone areas threatens future agricultural productivity. As just one example, the EPA predicts that climate change produced by a doubling of atmospheric CO_2 will result in a 7–16% reduction in annual water supplies to California's highly productive Central Valley—a region even now beset by burgeoning water demand.

Loss of Biodiversity

While the polar bear has become the iconic symbol of the threat climate change poses to biodiversity, the golden toad (*Bufo periglenes*) has made headlines as supposedly the first species doomed to extinction by global warming. Once abundant on the upper mountain slopes of Costa Rica's Monteverde Cloud Forest Preserve, the last sighting of a golden toad—a solitary male—was in 1989; despite extensive searching, not a single specimen has been found in the years since. Scientists concluded that drier conditions on the toad's mountainside habitat, an indirect result of global warming that dissipated the mist shrouding the slopes, were the cause of the toad's demise (Pounds, Fogden, and Campbell, 1999). To date, no other species are known to have completely disappeared because of climate change, but if scientists' fears prove well-founded, as many as 37% of all terrestrial species could vanish by 2050 due to global warming (Thomas et al., 2004).

Climate change will impose even greater stresses on natural ecosystems than on domesticated plants and animals because many nonagricultural species have gradually become adapted to life in a specific habitat and have a rather narrow range of tolerance to changing environmental conditions. According to the World Conservation Union's *Red List of Threatened Species*, those most at risk as temperatures climb are (1) warm-water reef-forming coral species (71% of which are potentially susceptible to climate change), (2) amphibians (52%), and (3) birds (35%). Plants and animals, particularly those living in temperate regions, will be forced to move hundreds of miles toward the poles (or thousands of feet up mountainsides) in order to maintain the temperature conditions to which they have become adapted. For many species such migration will be virtually impossible. Plants, for example, can shift location only as far as their seeds are dispersed. A gradual poleward migration might be conceivable if the rate of climate change is very slow,

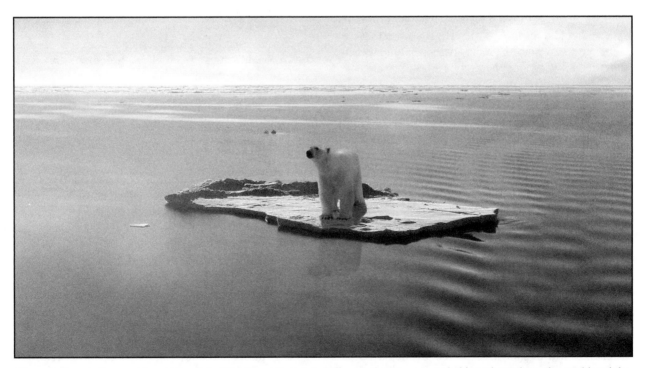

The polar bear is the most iconic symbol of the threat that global climate change poses to habitats throughout the world and the biodiversity which they support.

but if warming is so rapid that the present habitat becomes unsuitable before a new area can be colonized, then the species will die out.

One might assume that animals, capable of moving under their own power, would find migration relatively easy. In today's world, however, barriers to migration in the form of cities, highways, dams, and so on make large-scale movements of many species highly problematic (visualize the challenges faced by a group of alligators heading north out of Okefenokee Swamp as they attempt to traverse Atlanta!). While some animal species migrate easily, others are genetically programmed to be highly territorial and wouldn't even try to move as their environment became uninhabitable. Others might be capable of migrating, but if the plant species on which they feed don't move also, they would perish of starvation. The plight of Europe's pied flycatchers (*Ficedula hypoleuca*) illustrates the problems faced by species whose existence is threatened by warming-induced life cycle changes in a major food source. Populations of pied flycatchers have declined by 90% in recent years because the insects they feed to their young are now reaching peak levels much earlier than in the past; the birds' breeding time is now too late for offspring to have an adequate food supply and, as a result, the species is gradually dying out (Ehrlich and Ehrlich, 2008).

Prevalence of infectious diseases among plant and animal populations is likely to increase as the climate warms, presenting another threat to species survival. Pathogens already have been implicated in the rapid die-off of frogs in Australia and Central America, birds in Hawaii, and wild dogs in Africa. Scientists warn that climate change could exacerbate host-pathogen interactions in numerous ways, among them:

1. warmer winters are likely to permit the survival of many pathogens currently killed by low temperatures (more than 99% of pathogens responsible for plant diseases typically die over winter)

2. warmer summers may promote pathogen development, increase rates of disease transmission, and increase the number of generations per year

3. a pathogen's plant or animal host may become more susceptible to infection as temperatures rise

Researchers report that plant diseases like Dutch elm disease and wheat stripe rust are more severe following mild winters. Among wildlife populations, rising incidence of vectorborne disease is expected as their insect carriers respond to higher temperatures by expanding their geographic range and experience increased rates of reproduction, population growth, and biting. Animal parasites also will exhibit faster development rates and increased infectivity as the world grows steadily hotter (Harvell et al., 2002). Biodiversity, already suffering severely from pressures imposed by overhunting, pollution, and habitat destruction, may find greenhouse warming the most devastating blow of all.

Human Illness

Although climate change is primarily an environmental problem rather than a human health issue, the increasing frequency of heat waves is already having an impact on morbidity and mortality rates, as mentioned previously. However, the most significant public health concern associated with global warming is the spread of certain mosquito-borne tropical diseases such as malaria and dengue fever (see chapter 8) into regions where they are currently unknown. As a possible indication of things to come, unusually hot, humid weather during the mid-1990s sparked a dengue epidemic in Mexico and Central America when virus-carrying mosquitoes moved from endemic coastal areas into the usually cool and previously mosquito-free highlands. Warmer temperatures (1) cause mosquitoes to develop faster, (2) induce females to bite more frequently, (3) extend the length of the transmission season in temperate regions, and (4) enable adults to survive winters in areas that formerly were too cold. They also hasten development of the virus inside the mosquito. Since the 1950s, climate change has resulted in a 30-fold increase in the incidence of dengue fever, with the disease spreading beyond the tropics to more than 100 countries worldwide. Outbreaks in the United States to date have been restricted to the U.S.-Mexico border region and Hawaii, but the mosquito vectors of this disease, *Aedes aegypti* and *A. albopictus*, are now established in 28 states and represent a serious future health threat (Knowlton, Solomon, and Rotkin-Ellman, 2009).

Collapse of Thermohaline Circulation in North Atlantic

While currently regarded as highly unlikely during the 21st century, if ever, weakening thermohaline circulation concerns some scientists. They reason that as rising temperatures cause increased precipitation and melting of ice in the far North, the increased flow of freshwater into polar seas could shut down the thermal conveyor belt responsible for carrying heat from the equator to the polar regions of the North Atlantic. The warm, salty surface waters of the Gulf Stream gradually cool as they flow northward, becoming more dense and sinking deeper into the ocean as they release heat to the atmosphere. In doing so, they help to keep Europe nearly 10°F warmer than it would otherwise be. If fresh water from melting ice should dilute the salt content of ocean water, it would become less dense and hence too light to sink. Should this happen, Gulf Stream flow could weaken or halt entirely and average temperatures over Europe might drop by as much as 9°F. While IPCC climate models show a weakening of thermohaline circulation and some resultant reduction of heat transport to high latitude areas of the Northern Hemisphere, they nevertheless predict a net temperature increase in Europe until at least until 2100, due to rising greenhouse gas concentrations. They do not, however, rule out a complete, and possibly irreversible shutdown in thermohaline circulation if CO_2 levels continue to rise indefinitely.

National Security Concerns

While IPCC projections indicate that most regions of the world will experience some adverse effects due to climate change, the impacts will obviously be more severe in some areas than in others. The United States is likely to experience a significantly higher-than-average increase in temperature, frequency and intensity of severe weather events, and sea level rise than many other countries. However, the U.S. and other technologically advanced nations will be better able to adapt and cope with climate change challenges than will many developing nations, particularly those in equatorial regions. In poor and densely populated countries, even a slight increase in temperature can trigger or worsen food shortages, water scarcity, and resource conflict. Like so many other environmental problems, global warming is likely to have its greatest impact on those already living a marginal existence.

In today's interconnected world, however, a climate change-induced crisis in one place inevitably will have repercussions elsewhere—and national security planners in both Europe and the United States are beginning to take notice of projected trends. In 2007 the Center for Naval Analysis Corporation issued a report stating that the chaos resulting from climate change impacts "can be an incubator of civil strife, genocide, and the growth of terrorism" and went on to warn that such developments could cause security problems requiring a response from already overburdened American military forces. Concerns focus primarily on "environmental refugees," those forced to leave their homelands due to prolonged drought or sea level rise. Such migration will be both within countries (e.g. the dispersal of New Orleans' residents following Hurricane Katrina) or across international borders. For the United States, this scenario is most likely to involve desperate migrants from drought-stricken areas of Central America and northern Mexico or refugees from hurricane-ravaged Caribbean islands. India is bracing itself for waves of migrants from Bangladesh and the Sundarbans in the Bay of Bengal as increasingly severe cyclones, storm surges, and sea level rise render much of the delta area uninhabitable. Europeans are already troubled by the prospect of a flood of new migrants from North Africa, the Middle East, and South Asia, further exacerbating ethnic and religious tensions in societies where existing immigrant communities have as yet been poorly assimilated.

Competition over increasingly scarce water resources and pasturelands is provoking conflict between rival groups in areas where the impacts of climate change are already being felt. Years of warfare in Sudan's Darfur region, referred to by some as "the first genocide of the 21st century," is generally portrayed as an ethnic conflict but in actuality represents a clash between camel herders and agriculturalists over dwindling resources as desertification forces pastoralists to move southward into farming areas. Such strife is likely to increase exponentially in a warming world. As Harvard archaeologist Steven LeBlanc remarked when commenting on the connection between the environment's carrying capacity and warfare, "Every time there is a choice between starving and raiding, humans raid" (Flannery, 2005). As water shortages give rise to food shortages and hunger leads to conflict over resources, migration of one group into another's territory is likely to result in food shortages there as well; these problems are interconnected and self-perpetuating and will threaten political stability and national sovereignty as warming accelerates (Campbell, 2008).

Rate of Global Warming

As mentioned earlier, the rate at which global temperatures rise will be extremely important in determining how serious the impacts of climate change will be. Humanity may be able to adjust reasonably well to a very gradual warming trend, whereas a more rapid change could be catastrophic. Which of these two scenarios is more likely? Columbia University geochemist Wallace Broecker, in testimony submitted to a congressional hearing, remarked that:

> Earth's climate does not respond in a smooth and gradual way; rather it responds in sharp jumps. If this reading of the natural record is correct, then we must consider the possibility that the major responses of the system to our greenhouse provocation will come in jumps whose timing and magnitude are unpredictable. Coping with this type of change is clearly a far more serious matter than coping with a gradual warming.

In this context, reports from scientists working in Greenland provide considerable cause for alarm. Analysis of air bubbles in layers of ice from cores drilled deep into the island's massive ice cap provides evidence for the rate of climate change in the distant past. University of Rhode Island researchers have found that the end of the last ice age, slightly over 11,000 years ago, occurred much more rapidly than previously thought possible. In just a few decades or less, average temperatures in Greenland suddenly rose 9–18°F. A similarly abrupt, though less extreme, warming trend occurred over much of the Northern Hemisphere at this time (Severinghaus et al., 1998).

Another study conducted by researchers from Columbia University's Lamont Doherty Earth Observatory focused on Atlantic Ocean sediments for clues to how quickly climate change might occur. Working off the northwestern coast of Africa, researchers discovered that since the end of the last ice age, ocean temperatures there have experienced wide, abrupt fluctuations roughly every 1,500 years. These changes, and their consequent impact on regional climate, occurred within a period of about 50 years. Converging lines of evidence from these and similar investigations suggest that the relatively stable climate of the past 10,000 years, the period during which human civilizations developed and flourished, is an anomaly— an exception to the rule of frequent and sudden change throughout much of geologic time.

THE GREENHOUSE POLICY DEBATE

> Few challenges facing America—and the world—
> are more urgent than combating climate change.
> —Barack Obama

Since the early 1970s, climatologists have been raising increasingly strident warnings about the impending greenhouse warming, urging policy makers to take action to forestall this so-called "doomsday issue." While the general public until recently tended either to ignore such predictions or to regard them as plot material for a science fiction novel, opinion polls now show a majority of those questioned accept scientists' near-unanimous declaration that the world's climate is indeed heating up. Unlike his predecessor, President Obama, too, is convinced of the need for urgent action by the United States to mitigate climate change, pledging at the time of his inauguration to push for legislation and programs to reduce greenhouse gas emissions and to join the international community's effort to limit further warming. This represented a significant policy shift for the federal government, since even now many legislators, acutely aware of intense opposition by the politically influential fossil fuel industry, are reluctant to endorse any meaningful policy actions to reduce carbon emissions.

Calling for action is easier than implementing such changes, however. Delegates to the United Nations' Earth Summit, held in Rio de Janeiro in 1992, took the first substantive steps when they endorsed the **Framework Convention on Climate Control (FCCC)**. Calling for a voluntary reduction in signatory nations' greenhouse gas emissions to 1990 levels by 2000, the treaty was quickly ratified by the U.S. Senate and equivalent legislative bodies in Canada and Australia. By 1995, 186 countries had signed on to the FCCC, agreeing in concept with the treaty's ultimate objective—"stabilization of the greenhouse gas concentrations in the atmosphere at a level that would prevent dangerous anthropogenic interference with the climate system." Negotiators at the Rio Conference agreed that the rich developed nations whose greenhouse gas emissions are largely responsible for the present state of affairs must take the lead in emissions reductions. Although it was assumed that at some future time the developing countries would need to curb their emissions as well, no specific timetable for their doing so was established.

By the mid-1990s, as emissions continued their upward trajectory in most of the countries party to the UNFCCC, it became obvious that a voluntary approach to curbing greenhouse gases wasn't working. Consequently, after a series of preliminary meetings in 1995 and 1996, representatives of 117 nations met in December 1997 in Kyoto, Japan, to hammer out an agreement that would establish mandatory emissions reductions for 38 industrialized countries, while imposing no such restrictions on developing nations. The prevailing philosophy at the time was that the rich countries were primarily responsible for the problem, so they should bear the burden and expense of solving it. The **Kyoto Protocol** was signed by 84 countries, including the United States (then under the Clinton administration), but could not become legally binding until ratified by the legislatures of 55 countries representing 55% of the world's 1990-level greenhouse gas emissions.

The treaty quickly encountered strong opposition in the United States because of concerns that compliance would seriously damage the U.S. economy and because it exempted rapidly developing nations like China and India from any emissions restrictions. In spite of pleas from European allies who feared treaty efforts would collapse without U.S. participation, President George W. Bush in March 2001 declared the Kyoto Protocol "dead" and announced that the United States was withdrawing from the treaty. While this action provoked outrage in the international community, it didn't derail ratification efforts. By late autumn of 2004, Russia became the 127th country and the last major emitter (17.4% of world GHG emissions in 1990) to ratify the Kyoto Protocol. The treaty's provisions took effect in February 2005, 90 days after Russia delivered its signed papers to the United Nations.

After treaty ratification, the European Union nations subject to the treaty's emissions reduction goals initiated an international Emissions Trading Scheme covering about half of all EU carbon dioxide emissions. In addition, through the Protocol's Clean Development Mechanism, they have financed "green development" projects in poor countries in an effort to help those nations reduce their "carbon footprint." Several years into the program, however, the emissions reductions achieved by participating countries remained quite modest. Advocates of urgent action to deal with climate change agreed that some fundamental changes in the treaty needed to be negotiated when representatives of 193 countries, including 119 heads of state, gathered in Copenhagen, Denmark, in December 2009 for the largest-ever UN Climate Change Conference.

Originally, the intent of this much-heralded gathering had been to finalize negotiations initiated two years earlier at a conference in Bali, Indonesia, for a new international agreement on climate change that would take effect after the Kyoto Protocol's first commitment period expires in 2012. Even before the delegates gathered, however, it was obvious that achieving a legally binding commitment to which all countries could agree would be nearly impossible. Representatives of developing nations—most notably China and India—declared that responsibility for solving the climate crisis rested with those who had caused it (i.e., the United States, Europe, and other industrialized countries) and indicated that they expected those governments to lead the way before the developing world took action. They also argued that even though their own emissions are now increasing rapidly, they are still much lower on a per capita basis than those of wealthy nations and that they are far poorer and thus less able to deal with the problem (Bradley, 2009). Nevertheless, by this time it had also become abundantly clear that unless developing countries undertake meaningful steps to reduce their own green-

house gas emissions, atmospheric carbon levels will be so high as to make catastrophic climate change inevitable— even if the industrialized world should succeed in meeting strict emissions reduction targets (Aldy and Stavins, 2008).

As the 12-day conference headed into its final day, negotiations were deadlocked and on the point of collapse when U.S. President Obama personally intervened and, in a series of head-to-head meetings with the leaders of China, India, Brazil, and South Africa, managed to craft a document, subsequently called the Copenhagen Accord, that established a politically feasible approach that most—though not all—of the participating countries were able to accept. Although the terms of the Accord are not legally binding like those of the Kyoto Protocol, they were hailed by President Obama and many environmental groups as an important step forward, not least because all 188 countries signing on to the Accord acknowledged that climate change is a problem they must individually address, either by national legislation, regulations, or via multi-year development plans, with the aim of restricting the increase in global average temperature to no more than 2°C. Signatory countries pledged to submit their specific plans for mitigating GHG emissions to the United Nation's FCCC Secretariat by the end of January 2010, and agreed that emissions reductions will be measured, reported, and verified according to vigorous and transparent guidelines. Recognizing that a major deficiency of the Kyoto Protocol had been its failure to address tropical deforestation, the Copenhagen Accord includes funding to help developing

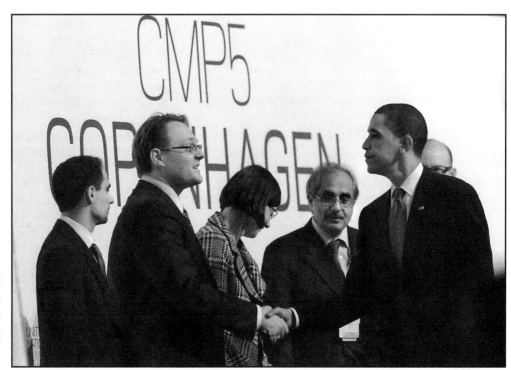

President Barack Obama led the U.S. delegation to the United Nations Climate Change Conference in Copenhagen, Denmark in December 2009. [*AP Photo/ Susan Walsh*]

countries reduce emissions caused by deforestation. It also calls for wealthy countries collectively to provide $30 billion to poor countries over the 2010–2012 time frame, while setting a goal of $100 billion annually from both private and public sources by 2020. This money is to be targeted toward poor countries most vulnerable to the adverse impacts of climate change and is to be used for both adaptation and emissions mitigation strategies.

While many observers were deeply disappointed that the terms of the Copenhagen Accord are aspirational rather than binding and that the announced short-term (i.e., by 2020) emissions reduction goals are well below what many scientists consider necessary, the general consensus seemed to be that, given the domestic political realities of the major countries involved, this was the best agreement that could be achieved at the time. Unlike the Kyoto Protocol which exempted the so-called "emerging economies" from emissions reduction requirements, the Copenhagen Accord greatly expands the number of countries agreeing to participate (17 nations that, collectively, are responsible for 90% of global GHG emissions have signed the Accord); it also extends the time frame for action well beyond the limited 5-year period set at Kyoto. An evaluation of how well the Copenhagen Accord is achieving its aims is to be completed by 2015, at which time the international community will have to determine whether science and climatic developments suggest the Accord needs to be strengthened. Robert Stavins, Director of the Harvard Environmental Economics Program, aptly summarized the results of the Copenhagen Conference:

> The climate change policy progress is best viewed as a marathon, not a sprint. . . . We may look back upon Copenhagen as an important moment—both because global leaders took the reins of the procedures and brought the negotiations to a fruitful conclusion, and because the foundation was laid for a broad-based coalition of the willing to address effectively the threat of global climate change. Only time will tell. (Stavins, 2009)

Mitigation Strategies

Efforts to mitigate climate change focus largely on three complementary strategies:

1. improving energy efficiency
2. transitioning from a fossil fuel-dependent energy economy to one powered by clean, renewable energy sources
3. putting a price on carbon emissions

The first two strategies cited here will be discussed at length in chapter 12. The third, mandating some form of market-based cost to encourage significant reductions in GHG emissions, is regarded as essential to spur the energy transition so vital to combating climate change.

The major policy alternatives within this strategy include the following:

Cap and Trade

The approach adopted by the European Union and advocated by the Obama administration is modeled after the highly successful U.S. program introduced in the 1990s to combat acid rain. Under cap and trade, the government sets an upper limit (a cap) for the total amount of CO_2 emissions that could be released into the atmosphere during a given period. The government would then allocate specific reduction levels among targeted segments of the nation's economy—manufacturing plants, utilities, transportation, and so forth. Tradable allowances, equivalent to their maximum allowable emissions, would be sold or given free to these industries, who will then be allowed to achieve the mandated reductions in any way they choose. With the establishment of a nationwide (or worldwide) emissions trading program, innovative, proactive companies whose energy-efficient technologies or adoption of alternative fuels have enabled them to exceed their mandated emissions-reduction goals will be able to sell credits for those excess emissions to other emitters unable or unwilling to make the changes necessary to meet their assigned targets. These tradable allowances provide a strong incentive for all parties involved to find the most effective, least-costly route to a low-carbon future.

Currently, under the Kyoto Protocol's Joint Implementation provision, a company can also earn credits toward its emissions reduction cap by investing in specific emissions-lowering projects in another developed country (usually one of the former Soviet republics) or, under the Protocol's Clean Development Mechanism, can similarly meet a portion of its assigned target by engaging in developing-world projects—activities such as tree-planting or installing low-emission technologies in factories—that will help developing countries reduce their emissions.

Advocates for a cap-and-trade system argue that such a mechanism provides certainty that the government-established emissions ceilings won't be exceeded and that such a program is more politically palatable than a direct tax. Critics worry about the difficulty of creating what would be an extremely complex regulatory framework and of ensuring that no CO_2-emitting facilities evade obtaining permits.

Carbon Tax

Under this approach, the production of gasoline, heating oil, coal, natural gas, and electricity generated from fossil fuels would be taxed incrementally according to the carbon content of those fuels. This would provide a direct motivation for energy purchasers to use less-polluting fuels. It would incorporate the environmental costs of energy use into energy prices, thereby encouraging consumers to shift to alternative energy sources such as solar or wind power, since these emit no carbon and hence would be tax-free.

Carbon tax proponents point out several advantages to this approach over cap-and-trade: it's much simpler, easy to calculate, and readily understood by the average person. Since the tax would be paid by the oil and coal companies who are the primary producers, its impact would extend throughout the entire fossil fuel energy economy and be directly felt by the end user, providing a strong incentive for cost-conscious consumers to make environmentally friendly choices. Alternatively, opponents contend that a carbon tax would make a country's exports less competitive due to higher costs and that it isn't guaranteed to cut pollution because some buyers will simply opt to pay the tax in order to purchase the less energy-efficient, more-polluting products they desire. Undoubtedly the major obstacle to adopting a carbon tax in today's political environment, however, is that it is a tax and hence anathema to many policy makers.

Technological Approaches

While the strategies described above have attracted the most attention and debate, other mitigation options involve various technological approaches to prevent carbon dioxide and other greenhouse gases from getting into the air in the first place. As mentioned in a previous section of this chapter, a number of experts are advocating measures to reduce emissions of black carbon as one of the quickest and easiest ways of slowing climate change. Representatives of the coal industry and politicians from states where mining is an important component of the economy are touting "clean coal" technologies, advocating a still-experimental process known as **carbon capture and sequestration** (see box 11-3) to remove CO_2 prior to release of combustion gases at coal-fired power plants and industrial facilities.

Yet another "technological fix" advanced by some scientists while regarded by others as dangerously unwise is so-called **geoengineering** (sometimes referred to as "climate engineering"). Inspired by observations of the temporary slight cooling of global climate in the aftermath of the 1991 eruption of Mount Pinatubo in the Philippines, the concept of geoengineering basically involves an attempt to cool the surface of the Earth by blocking some of the incoming sunlight. Of the various schemes advanced to achieve this objective, the one being most seriously considered is a proposal to employ a small fleet of jet planes or high-altitude balloons to inject a stream of sulfur dioxide into the stratosphere to deflect

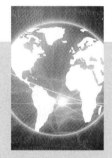

· · · · · · · 11-3 · · · · · · ·

Is "Clean Coal" Possible? The CCS Debate

The term "clean coal" strikes many environmentalists as an oxymoron. Coal has long been acknowledged as the dirtiest, most-polluting of fuels and the single largest contributor to carbon dioxide emissions—about 40% of the world total. In most industrialized countries, as well as in rapidly-developing China and India, coal is the leading source of power generation because it's both plentiful and considerably cheaper than the alternatives. Although a number of promising renewable sources offer the potential for a clean energy revolution in the decades ahead (see chapter 12), in the near-term coal is likely to retain its position as the world's primary source of electrical power. If nations are seriously committed to confronting the threat of climate change by limiting greenhouse gas emissions, yet unwilling to abandon coal as a major power source, then there's no choice but to pursue so-called "clean coal technologies." With this imperative in mind, President Obama in 2009 earmarked $3.4 billion of federal economic stimulus dollars for this purpose, citing its importance in America's quest for energy independence.

Burning coal without releasing CO_2 into the atmosphere could, in theory, be accomplished through an approach known as **carbon capture and sequestration (CCS)**, in which CO_2 is captured at the source of combustion, converted to a quasi-liquid, and then injected under pressure deep underground. CCS technologies require a complex infrastructure and are very expensive, thus limiting their application to large centralized power plants or cement kilns.

The most promising of several CCS technologies currently being developed is known as the *oxyfuel process*, in which coal is burned in 95% pure oxygen rather than air, resulting in CO_2-rich flue gas emissions that can be captured at the stack with 99.5% efficiency. An alternative approach, *pre-combustion capture*, is restricted to power plants built to use integrated gasification combined cycle technology (IGCC); currently there are only four IGCC plants in the world, two of these in the U.S.—and none of them now sequester CO_2. An IGCC power plant uses heat to convert coal to a gaseous mixture of carbon dioxide and hydrogen, burning the hydrogen gas to run a turbine to produce electricity, while the exhaust produces steam to power a second turbine. During the gasification process, CO_2 can be removed relatively easily, but the method hasn't yet been successfully demonstrated on a commercial scale. *Post-combustion capture*, in which CO_2 is removed from flue gases in conventional power plants, is already available but requires a very large energy input and, like the pre-combustion process, is somewhat less efficient than the oxyfuel process and has yet to be proven viable on a large scale.

In spite of the optimism expressed by CCS proponents—most of whom represent fossil fuel interests or hail from regions where coal mining is an important part of the local economy—several factors raise serious doubts that CCS will ever evolve much beyond the demonstration or pilot-plant stage. Among the constraints on full-scale development are the following:

Time frame. CCS technologies are unlikely to become commercially available before 2020–2030, but the big increase in anticipated coal-fired plant construction will occur within the next few years. Retrofitting the new CCS technologies onto existing power plants is both more expensive and less efficient than installing them at the time of new construction.

Sequestration siting concerns. Prospective underground sites for liquefied carbon sequestration, including depleted oil and gas fields, saline aquifers, non-exploitable coal seams, or geologic formations deep under the ocean, will require time-consuming, case-by-case analyses to ensure against leakage and long-term safety. Local opposition is likely to create additional siting headaches, as exemplified by the Dutch town of Barendrecht, where citizens have been fighting plans by Royal Dutch Shell to pump CO_2 from a nearby oil refinery into nearly empty gas fields underlying the community. Residents expressed fears of a catastrophic gas leak or explosion and protested that such an experiment shouldn't be conducted in an urban environment.

CCS energy use. The energy and environmental impacts of CCS are considerable; carbon sequestration technologies consume 24–40% of the power plant's total output, thus requiring additional fuel consumption—resulting in additional GHG emissions—in order to generate the same amount of power the plant would have produced without CCS. What's more, the technology only captures the CO_2 going up the smokestack; it does nothing to minimize other greenhouse gases associated with mining or transporting fossil fuels nor does it have any potential for reducing emissions from small stationary sources or from the transportation sector. Another major environmental concern associated with large-scale deployment of CCS is water supply, since the technology requires the use of 90% more water than do conventional coal-fired plants. Hazardous waste generation would increase, due to chemical reactions associated with scrubbing agents, as would other local environmental problems related to coal mining and transport: habitat destruction, degradation of waterways, and air pollution among them.

High costs. High investment and energy penalty costs are further deterrents to adoption of CCS; it is estimated that consumers' utility bills would rise at least 25–30% for electricity generated at plants using CCS, assuming that coal prices remain constant.

Infrastructure requirements. Extensive infrastructure requirements provoke second thoughts about the feasibility of CCS projects. Since power plants are unlikely to be situated in areas where appropriate conditions for deep geologic storage prevail, a new pipeline system would have to be installed to carry the liquefied CO_2 from point of capture to distant sequestration sites. Alternatively, power-generating facilities could be built adjacent to underground repositories and the electricity transported to centers of demand.

Assessing all of these challenges inherent in turning the dream of "clean coal" into reality, a growing number of energy experts argue that there's a better, less-expensive way to reduce carbon emissions while still meeting future energy demands. They advocate a three-part strategy: (1) improvements in energy efficiency; (2) rapid development and deployment of renewable energy technologies; and (3) more widespread use of natural gas-fired combined cycle power plants. If ambitious efforts to implement these goals were to get underway immediately, they say, there would be no need for expensive CCS technologies when they're finally ready for large-scale deployment sometime after 2020 (Viebahn, Fischedick, and Vallentin, 2009).

incoming solar radiation (SO_2 combines with O_2 to form reflective sulfate particles). Sulfate injection could be carried out with existing technology and would be less expensive than other proposed geoengineering strategies. However, critics point out that, as happened following the Mount Pinatubo event, it would likely cause an overall decrease in precipitation, especially in the tropics, and could aggravate ozone layer depletion over polar regions. It also would do nothing to counter increasing acidification of the oceans, since atmospheric CO_2 concentrations would continue to rise.

Another approach being seriously considered is the use of specially designed ships to pump seawater thousands of feet into the lower atmosphere to promote the formation of clouds, as well as thickening existing ones, to reflect more incoming sunlight. While predicted to have fewer environmental side-effects than sulfate injection, cloud brightening is likely to have a similarly powerful influence on world rainfall patterns, provoking heavy rains in some areas, droughts in others. Geoengineering advocates concede that the technologies they propose represent only short-term solutions, since temperatures would rebound and even accelerate if they were discontinued. However, they argue that, despite the risks, in the absence of effective international cooperation to reduce GHG emissions drastically, they represent the only hope for averting imminent climate disaster and might buy time for implementing essential carbon reduction strategies. Nevertheless, the international political ramifications of geoengineering could be extremely problematic, since the entire world would feel the impacts of any attempt at climate manipulation. Who would have the right to decide whether, when, and how such an experiment should be conducted? Such questions remain unanswered and although the pros and cons of geoengineering continue to be debated, most of the discussion regarding mitigation efforts continues to focus on curtailing emissions (Caldeira, 2009; Cascio, 2009).

It should be mentioned that land-use alterations contribute an estimated 17% of GHG emissions; thus, national policies to curb deforestation, promote afforestation, and improve agricultural practices can have a significant impact on minimizing climate change. These issues are discussed at greater length in chapter 5.

ADAPTING TO CLIMATE CHANGE

In the early years of climate change negotiations, many environmental groups were reluctant to advocate adaptation strategies, fearing that doing so would reduce pressure for ambitious emissions reduction measures. It is now apparent, however, that a certain degree of climate change is inevitable and that the impacts will be dis-

proportional, affecting most severely poor nations that have contributed least to the problem. As a result, the need for wealthy countries to finance adaptation strategies aimed at limiting loss of life, livelihood, and property associated with climate change-induced calamities in developing countries is now a major topic of debate for international negotiators.

Examples of proposed adaptation measures are numerous and include relocation of vulnerable populations living at or near sea level; construction of sea walls and storm surge barriers; creation of wetlands as a buffer against flooding; relocation of transportation routes; expanded rainwater harvesting; improvements in water storage and conservation practices; improvements in irrigation efficiency; development of drought-resistant crop varieties and new cultivation practices; upgraded systems of disease surveillance and control; improvements in water and wastewater treatment; and improved infrastructure standards to cope with climate change-induced damage (Dodman, Ayers, and Huq, 2009). Undoubtedly, rich and poor nations alike will need to take adaptive measures, but the latter are far more vulnerable and less able to meet the challenge. Within the United Nations a coalition of 130 developing countries, led by China, has called for the industrial nations to provide a level of funding equivalent to 0.5–1.0% of their cumulative gross national product to provide developing nations with grants for adaptation and mitigation programs. Political realities make funding of this magnitude unlikely, but without rapid deployment of adaptive strategies, climate change will make life increasingly precarious for many of the world's most vulnerable people.

Averting Catastrophe

As atmospheric CO_2 levels and temperature continue to rise, the need for effective, immediate action to implement the long-term strategies outlined above becomes increasingly urgent. Many scientists warn of catastrophic consequences if Earth's climate warms by more than 2°C—a temperature increase likely to occur if CO_2 concentrations rise from their current 389 ppm to 550 ppm, a figure roughly double that of pre-industrial levels. Some scientists, like Dr. James Hansen, Director of NASA's Goddard Institute of Space Studies, are convinced that even current levels of CO_2 are too high, arguing that only below 350 ppm can humanity hope to avoid damaging effects of climate change. In a business-as-usual world with no efforts made to curtail emissions, CO_2 levels could reach 450 ppm by 2030, 800–1000 ppm by the end of the 21st century.

Because carbon dioxide persists in the atmosphere for centuries, global average surface temperatures will continue to rise even after their concentrations have stabilized. The general assumption that climate conditions will return to their pre-21st century status is woefully misguided. Researchers at the National Oceanic and Atmospheric Administration contend that the CO_2-induced temperature increases now occurring will persist for 1,000 years after emissions cease—and the longer we delay effective GHG mitigation, the hotter the next millennium is likely to be. As a result, some once-hypothetical climate impacts are now regarded as inevitable, some sooner rather than later. Among these are a sharp decrease in dry-season precipitation in several already-arid subtropical regions (most notably the U.S. Southwest and the Mediterranean basin) and a rise in sea level—trends that are already becoming apparent (Solomon et al., 2009).

The modest initiatives just now getting underway are encouraging, but they won't succeed in reversing global warming unless all countries enlist in the effort. Even if the United States joins the other industrialized nations in taking action, rapid economic growth in developing countries such as China and India—currently exempt from Kyoto Protocol-mandated emissions cuts—will result in a further increase in atmospheric CO_2. Today almost 80% of global GHG emissions are produced by just 14 countries plus the European Union; of these, nine are rapidly industrializing developing nations. As the economies and populations of the latter continue to grow, their emissions will soar to 2–3 times the level of those in developed countries. Mustering worldwide cooperation to combat what is still perceived by many as a distant threat is extremely difficult, since the basic problem stems from the desire for a better life by billions of individuals throughout the world and the determination of their governments to provide them with a Western standard of living as rapidly as possible.

Unfortunately for those Americans who care deeply about the fate of the planet, initial optimism following the 2008 presidential election that the U.S. Congress was finally poised to impose significant curbs on GHG emissions has now given way to the pessimistic realization that climate change legislation is dead for the foreseeable future. Although the House passed the American Clean Energy and Security Act in June 2009, establishing national GHG emissions limits along with cap-and-trade provisions, the Senate failed to take similar action. Fierce opposition by the fossil fuel industry and by conservative politicians opposed to any expansion of governmental

regulatory authority stymied efforts to bring the bill to a vote in the Senate. Federal climate change legislation thus died a quiet death prior to the 2010 mid-term elections and is unlikely to be reintroduced in Washington any time soon.

At the regional level, however, 23 states and four Canadian provinces have been engaged in their own emissions reduction initiatives for several years, implementing cap-and-trade programs that generate revenues for energy efficiency and renewable energy programs.

While legislators continue to debate the issue, the U.S. Environmental Protection Agency has moved ahead on the regulatory front, declaring that GHGs pose a threat to public health and welfare and proposing new standards for GHG emissions from motor vehicles and large industrial sources under the Clean Air Act. In the absence of federal legislation, which all parties agree would be the preferred approach to mitigating climate change, EPA emissions limitations on greenhouse gases are likely to be imposed on polluters. Elsewhere, the world's largest GHG emitter, China, has promised to cut its "carbon intensity" (i.e., the amount of CO_2 emitted per unit of GDP) by at least 40% below 2005 levels by 2020. China has already made significant progress in this regard through improvements in energy efficiency, but its carbon emissions have continued to rise, albeit at a slower rate. India, Japan, Brazil, South Africa, Korea, and Mexico have also indicated they have set their own emissions reduction targets and plan to take action. All of this is welcome news, provided that good intentions are followed by effective action.

The challenges and opportunities confronting the international community in the decades ahead—as well as the consequences of inaction—are aptly described by Rajendra Pachauri, Chairman of the Intergovernmental Panel on Climate Change:

> If the world does not take action early and in adequate measure, the impacts of climate change could prove extremely harmful and overwhelm our capacity to adapt. At the same time, the costs and feasibility of mitigation of GHG emissions are well within our reach and carry a wealth of substantial benefits for many sections of society. Hence, it is essential for the world to look beyond business as usual and stave off the crisis that faces us if we fail to act. (Pachauri, 2009)

12

And each day brings further evidence that the ways we use energy strengthen our adversaries and threaten our planet.
—President Barack Obama, Inaugural Address
January 20, 2009

Clean Energy Alternatives

As the threat of global climate change becomes increasingly obvious, government leaders, corporations, and ordinary citizens worldwide are beginning to acknowledge that reducing heat-trapping carbon emissions will necessitate a radical shift in the way we produce and use energy. Since the early years of the Industrial Revolution, economic growth and rising living standards have been driven by carbon-based fuels, first by coal, then oil, and, more recently, natural gas. Fossil fuels have powered our factories, heated our homes, generated most of our electricity, and fueled the millions of cars, trucks, buses, planes, ships, and railroads that comprise our transportation system. In recent decades the rapidly growing economies of India, China, Brazil, and other developing countries have similarly been powered by carbon-intensive fuels, as people everywhere strive to attain the affluent lifestyles long enjoyed by Western nations and Japan. Fossil fuels have enjoyed their preeminent status because, historically, they have been both abundant and cheap, since the "externalities" of their use were never, until quite recently, reflected in their cost. As a result, in the first decade of the 21st century, fossil fuels provided 86% of world energy use; substantially reducing this amount by shifting to alternative clean energy sources as global energy demand continues to soar will be a major challenge in the years ahead.

That challenge will be especially daunting for the United States, long accustomed to profligate energy use.

Although Americans comprise slightly less than 5% of the world's total population, we currently consume 25% of its energy resources. Aside from issues of equity, this situation is troubling in terms of national security. Oil now constitutes 39% of total energy use in the United States—a larger share than any other source—but domestic oil production peaked in 1970 and has been basically flat since the late 1980s. Demand has continued to rise, however, so the growing gap between supply and demand has been filled by imports, which now constitute two-thirds of our total supply. Although significant amounts of imported oil come from friendly neighbors (Canada and Mexico), we've also become dangerously reliant on purchases from countries in politically unstable parts of the world where a sudden cut-off in shipments could have disastrous consequences. Add to this concern the fact that oil is a nonrenewable resource, supplies of which are expected to peak within the next few decades. Although experts disagree as to exactly when this will happen, most concede that "crunch time" is coming in regards to world oil resources, with soaring prices and intense competition for dwindling supplies the likely consequence (Wolfson, 2008).

It should be noted that one bright spot in terms of America's fossil fuel supply is the situation regarding natural gas. As recently as 2006 it was widely believed that the United States was running out of domestic supplies of the fuel that heats half of all U.S. homes and generates

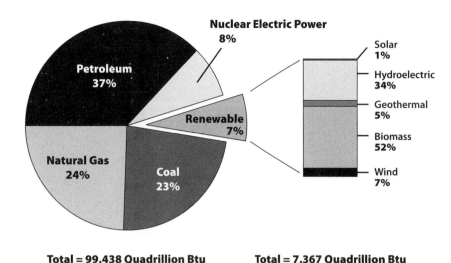

Total = 99.438 Quadrillion Btu   **Total = 7.367 Quadrillion Btu**

Source: U.S. Energy Information Administration, "Renewable Energy Trends," August 2010.
www.eia.doe.gov

Figure 12-1   U.S. Energy Consumption, 2008

20% of our electricity. However, since 2007 major new reserves have been discovered in shale formations across Appalachia from West Virginia to upstate New York, as well as in northern Texas, Arkansas, and, especially, northern Louisiana. Industry experts now estimate the United States has enough natural gas to meet the current level of demand for the next 100 years. That's very good news, because carbon emissions from natural gas combustion are about 50% less than those from coal. While environmentalists and many policy makers are looking to clean renewable energy sources such as solar and wind power to meet our long-term power needs, they view natural gas as an interim solution—a "bridge fuel" that can help meet energy demands until renewables are in a position to provide a larger share of our energy. Falling natural gas prices resulting from increased supply are prompting utilities to favor gas over coal for generating electricity, with the majority of new power plants expected to come on-line within the next few years slated to be gas-fired. Natural gas is even making inroads as a transportation fuel, with some municipal governments and corporations converting their bus or truck fleets to natural gas (Casselman, 2009).

The energy challenges confronting the United States and the world community are enormous:

1. preserving a habitable planet by slashing carbon emissions

2. enhancing national security by reducing dependence on foreign oil supplies

3. avoiding major economic disruption when oil reserves peak and ultimately decline.

It's imperative that we abandon our "business-as-usual" energy practices by using existing technologies more efficiently while beginning the transition to clean, renewable fuels without delay. The remainder of this chapter will examine some of the more promising options for doing so.

ENERGY EFFICIENCY

While breakthroughs in the development of wind power, solar and geothermal energy, biomass, and other renewable energy technologies offer tremendous long-term potential for an environmentally sustainable future, in the short term our most promising option lies simply in improving the efficiency of current energy production and use. This is so because existing energy efficiency technologies are performing at a level far below what is theoretically achievable, thus providing enormous opportunities for improvement (Wolfson, 2008).

Improvements in U.S. energy efficiency have been ongoing since early in the twentieth century but especially after the mid-1970s, when the shock of the 1973–1974 Arab oil embargo highlighted the dangers inherent in our ever-increasing reliance on foreign oil. That wake-up call stimulated entrepreneurial efforts to improve energy efficiency, efforts that produced an estimated $700 billion in energy savings over the following decades (Randolph and Masters, 2008). Unfortunately, such investments slowed considerably from the mid-1980s until relatively recently because low energy prices discouraged innovation. The election of Barack Obama in 2008 gave a boost to programs aimed at increasing U.S. energy efficiency, touted, along with renewable clean energy initiatives, as a linchpin of economic development in the years ahead. Passage in 2009 of the American Recovery and Reinvestment Act (ARRA) directed billions of federal dollars to energy efficiency research, programs to increase energy efficiency in low-income housing, tax credits encouraging consumers to purchase new energy-efficient appliances, and funding for state and local governments to make investments in energy efficiency and to purchase energy-efficient alternative fuel trucks and buses. Due to such initiatives, it's likely that in the years immediately ahead, improvements in the way Americans use energy will provide the quickest, easiest, and least-expensive opportunity for sustaining economic productivity and high standards of living while simultaneously curtailing carbon emissions.

Before examining some of the strategies and policy initiatives for promoting greater energy *efficiency*, we need to highlight the distinction between this concept and energy *conservation*, a term that the general public often assumes to mean the same thing. **Energy efficiency** basically means getting "the most bang for the buck" out of the technologies we're using now, while **energy conservation** involves curtailing normal or desired activities in order to reduce energy consumption. Examples of the former include replacing an old refrigerator with a new Energy Star-rated model or weather-stripping an older home, while the latter involves actions such as putting on a sweater and turning down the thermostat on a cold winter day. Both are eco-friendly options and reduce energy consumption, but energy conservation entails some degree of thought, commitment, and personal sacrifice—although usually at no financial cost—while energy efficiency initiatives may require an initial expenditure of money, but little follow-up thought or action. Interestingly, while most people assume that the greatest energy savings will be reaped by changes in personal behavior (changes many are unwilling to make!), energy experts insist that investments to improve energy efficiency can yield far greater energy savings without the need to forego desired services (Gardner and Stern, 2008).

The following paragraphs discuss the readily available options for improving energy efficiency—the "low-hanging fruit" represented by new, or not-so-new, technologies that reduce energy demand while simultaneously cutting carbon emissions.

Lighting

Worldwide, keeping our homes and buildings illuminated accounts for approximately 20% of total electricity demand—and much of this energy is wasted in the form of heat from standard incandescent lightbulbs. Energy experts at the National Renewable Energy Laboratory claim that the quickest, easiest, and cheapest way to reduce power demand is to transition from traditional inefficient incandescent bulbs to newer lighting technologies that do the same job using far less electricity. New **compact fluorescent (CFL)** bulbs use approximately ¾ less energy than standard incandescents and, although they cost more, typically last 10 times as long, significantly reducing utility bills over their lifetime. Another rapidly evolving lighting technology, **light-emitting diode (LED)** lamps are now revolutionizing lighting in commercial establishments where they are gradually replacing conventional fluorescent lights. LEDs use only

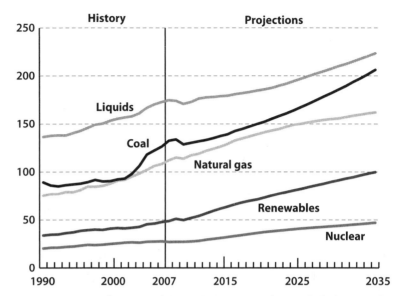

Source: U.S. Energy Information Administration, *International Energy Outlook 2010: Highlights,* July 2010. www.eia.doe.gov/oiaf/ieo/emissions.html.

Figure 12-2   World Marketed Energy Use, 1990–2035 (quadrillion Btu)

10% as much energy as standard fluorescents and last more than 30 times longer—approximately 3,000 hours for a fluorescent bulb compared to more than 100,000 hours for a LED fixture. LEDs are more than twice as efficient as CFLs and they contain no mercury, thus minimizing disposal concerns (since they last so long, disposal is seldom a concern anyhow); in addition, they turn on quickly and are compatible with dimmer switches.

Another advantage of LED bulbs is that they don't emit ultraviolet radiation and hence don't attract insects. Lighting quality of LEDs is more pleasing than that of fluorescents and they can be manufactured in a wide variety of shapes and sizes, including tiny chandelier lights that last 25,000 hours, compared to just 1,500 hours for an incandescent chandelier bulb. Although replacing conventional fixtures with LEDs is still quite expensive—over $20 for a 40-watt equivalent bulb—the payback time in energy savings can be as little as two years. Price considerations have thus far dampened serious consideration of LEDs for residential lighting, but this could change within a few years as rapid advances in research promise to lower costs dramatically. One famous residence has already begun making the switch—Buckingham Palace recently installed LEDs in chandeliers and on the exterior façade of the building; palace officials claim this lighting uses less electricity than that consumed by a standard electric teakettle! Currently the most common use of LEDs is for outdoor lighting; such cities as Los Angeles, San Jose, San Francisco, Ann Arbor, Anchorage, Raleigh, and Toronto have installed

LEDs for street and/or parking garage lighting, while New York City employs LEDs for traffic lights (Taub, 2009; Rosenthal and Barringer, 2009).

Energy efficiency considerations have prompted a number of countries to mandate a phase-out of incandescent bulbs; a ban on sales of incandescents took effect in Australia in 2010; Canada and the European Union will impose a similar restriction in 2012. China has announced its intention to eliminate incandescent bulbs before 2020, Brazil has already replaced about half its incandescents with CFLs, and residents of Moscow are being urged by their municipal authorities to make the switch as well (Brown, 2008).

In the United States, the 2007 Energy Independence and Security Act, while not specifically banning incandescents, requires that all common lightbulbs achieve a 30% energy savings over the conventional incandescents between 2012–2014, starting with a phase-out of 100-watt bulbs in January of 2012 and ending with 40-watt bulbs in January 2014. The legislation also set Tier 2 standards requiring all incandescent bulbs to be 70% more efficient—essentially equivalent to current CFLs—by 2020. Recently introduced advanced incandescent bulbs using halogen capsules with infrared reflective coatings should make it possible to meet the 2012–2014 target (these Halogen Energy Saver bulbs are considerably more expensive than the traditional incandescents they're replacing, but are also 30% more efficient), while the longer-term goal will probably be met by CFLs, LEDs, halogens, and much-improved incandescents still in the developmental stage. Hopes are high that these new technologies will result in improved performance and lower costs within the next few years.

In addition to efficiency improvements in lighting technology, further savings in public buildings can be achieved through the use of motion sensors that turn lights off when spaces such as restrooms, stairwells, or hallways aren't occupied. Similarly, on bright, sunny days dimmers can be employed to reduce the intensity of interior lighting; for outdoor monuments or public areas, timers can be installed to turn off lights during hours when people are typically asleep and not frequenting such places (Brown, 2008).

Appliances

Household appliances such as refrigerators, freezers, washing machines, water heaters, furnaces, and air conditioners are energy hogs—especially if they are more than 10 years old, since their efficiency tends to diminish over time. In recent years, thanks to federal government regulations that set minimum energy efficiency standards for a range of products, newer models of major appliances waste significantly less energy than their older predecessors. In 2009 President Obama instructed the U.S. Depart-

ment of Energy to begin drafting updated, more stringent efficiency standards for 30 product categories, ranging from ovens to vending machines to industrial boilers. Laws calling for such standards have been on the books for years, but past administrations refrained from writing regulations to carry out the intent of such legislation.

In 1992 the U.S. EPA introduced its widely acclaimed **Energy Star** program, intended to create public awareness of how much energy is consumed by commonplace devices used around the home and office and to inform consumers as to how their purchasing decisions can reduce utility bills while protecting the environment. (Several years later the Department of Energy joined EPA to make the Energy Star program a joint venture.) First applied in 1993 for personal computer equipment, the Energy Star label now appears on more than 50 product categories, from dishwashers to televisions to commercial air-conditioning systems. In recent years EPA has expanded the program to include Energy Star labeling for commercial and industrial buildings, and for new homes.

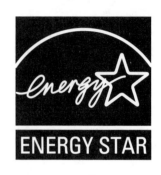

For conscientious shoppers, the Energy Star label assures that the item exceeds the government's minimum energy efficiency standard by 10–50%, depending on the particular product category. For example, while virtually any new refrigerator uses about 75% less energy than a 1970s model, a buyer who opts for an Energy Star-rated refrigerator will reap an additional 15% or more in energy savings due to the superior insulation, better compressors, and more precise temperature control. Like many energy efficiency options, appliances bearing the Energy Star label cost a bit more, but they soon recoup the difference through reduced utility bills. (Note: When shopping for a new appliance, customers should be aware of the difference between the Energy <u>Star</u> and Energy <u>Guide</u> labels. The former, as described above, indicates that the product in question is the most energy-efficient in its category; the latter, required on all new appliances, simply provides information allowing prospective buyers to compare the annual energy consumption and operating cost of that appliance with other models in the same category. *All* new appliances bear the Energy Guide label—only the *best* are labeled Energy Star.)

Aside from purchasing Energy Star-rated models, additional opportunities for enhancing the energy efficiency of appliances abound:

- Whenever possible, opt for gas-powered rather than electric appliances, since it's more energy-efficient to burn natural gas at its point of use than to transmit electricity long distances over wires to your home.

- Choose a refrigerator with a freezer on top rather than a side-by-side model of similar capacity, since the former consumes 10–15% less energy.

- When doing laundry, select cold or warm water wash and cold rinse, as 90% of the energy used by a standard washer is for heating water.

- Choose a washer with a faster spin speed; this feature results in more water removal from clothes, thereby reducing dryer time—with corresponding lower energy consumption.

- When running your dishwasher, use the "air-dry" option, which employs circulation fans instead of a heating coil to dry the dishes.

- Whenever possible, use a microwave oven rather than a conventional oven, since the former requires less energy and radiates less heat into the kitchen.

- Unplug extra refrigerators or freezers that are rarely used.

- Be aware that ink-jet printers are more energy efficient than laser printers and that liquid crystal display (LCD) televisions and monitors consume less power than cathode-ray tube (CRT) or plasma screens (Natural Resources Defense Council, 2004; Union of Concerned Scientists, 2001).

For detailed information on Energy Star appliance models and where they can be purchased, go to EPA's Energy Star Web site at http://www.energystar.gov.

Home Weatherization Programs

While growing numbers of visionary architects are already working diligently to design the "zero emission green homes" of the future, hundreds of millions of existing structures offer ample opportunities for improved energy efficiency. In general, homes built prior to 1939 require approximately 50% more energy per square foot for heating and cooling than do those constructed after 2000, thanks largely to air leakage caused by tiny cracks and crevices. Weatherization programs aimed at caulking the leaks around doors, walls, and windows, along with installation of better insulation and double-pane windows, can go a long way toward improving the energy efficiency of older buildings. The 2009 American Recovery and Reinvestment Act allocated almost $8 billion in federal grants to state and local governments for home weatherization projects targeting low-income households. Other efforts are underway at both the state and federal level to boost subsidies and rebates that would help ordinary homeowners offset the up-front costs of expensive retrofits (Walsh, 2009). Recognizing the impact that older structures have on both energy consumption and carbon emissions, some municipal govern-

ments, most notably New York City and Seattle, are actively promoting energy efficiency upgrades of existing buildings while simultaneously tightening energy standards for new construction and renovations.

Building "Green"

Energy retrofit and weatherization programs for existing homes and commercial buildings are having a significant impact on energy savings, reducing power use by 20–50%. However, the energy-saving potential for new construction is far greater, as far-sighted architects, builders, and real estate executives anticipate a future generation of "green buildings" that will revolutionize the construction industry. At the forefront of groups committed to environmentally responsible, sustainable building practices is the U.S. Green Building Council (USGBC), a private nonprofit organization headquartered in Washington, DC, whose stated mission is "to transform the way buildings and communities are designed, built, and operated." The USGBC is probably best known for its **LEED**® (Leadership in Energy and Environmental Design) **Green Building Rating System**, a voluntary certification system that initially focused on new construction—generally large commercial or government buildings—but today has expanded to include renovations of existing buildings, neighborhood development, schools, and private homes.

The current LEED rating system, USGBC 2009 (v3), addresses numerous issues in six major categories pertaining to the development and construction process. Depending on the number of points earned out of a possible 100, a building winning certification may qualify for one of four levels: certified (40–49 points); silver (50–59 points); gold (60–79 points); or platinum (80 points or more). Points are awarded for features such as sustainable siting (e.g., good access to public transportation, pollution prevention measures taken during construction, protecting or restoring critical habitat, maximizing open space); water conservation (e.g., reducing overall water consumption through use of water-efficient landscaping and innovative wastewater management technologies); energy use (e.g., maximizing energy savings, utilizing on-site renewable energy sources such as photovoltaic panels or rooftop solar water and space heaters); reusing and recycling construction materials; selecting construction materials that are rapidly renewable or choosing certified wood products; and providing a high quality indoor environment (e.g., control of environmental tobacco smoke, increased ventilation, maximized exposure to daylight, use of low-emitting materials for flooring, paints, sealants, composite wood products).

To obtain LEED certification, a builder must request and pay for it, submitting an application to USGBC documenting compliance with the rating criteria. By late 2008, ten years after the inception of the program, over 14,000 projects in all 50 U.S. states as well as in 30 other countries had earned LEED certification. Internationally, the growing popularity of the LEED concept prompted the Canada Green Building Council in 2003 to establish its own LEED program, called LEED Canada. A number of other nations are also working to develop assessment methods appropriate for their countries.

Although the up-front costs of designing and constructing a building that meets LEED certification standards are higher than those for structures that simply comply with existing codes, LEED buildings have lower operating costs and provide a healthier environment for those who live or work in them. As a result, demand for LEED-certified buildings has been steadily growing, especially for commercial construction in metropolitan areas. Many municipal and state governments are encouraging this trend, either through mandates that new construction meet LEED standards or by offering incentives to those who voluntarily choose to do so. The town of Normal, Illinois, in 2002 became the first community in the United States to require that new construction within the town's business district be LEED-certified; Cincinnati, Ohio, opting for the voluntary approach, provides a 100% property tax exemption for residential or commercial properties that meet minimal LEED standards; the state of Nevada waives local taxes on construction materials used for LEED buildings. Other incentives adopted by local governments across the country include tax credits or tax breaks, grants and low-interest loans, reduced fees, faster permitting, and free or low-cost technical assistance.

The LEED program has been so successful and its rating system so rigorous that it has largely supplanted the federal government's Energy Star certification system for buildings. LEED continues to evolve, incorporating new standards as green building technologies advance. Its latest version for new construction, LEED-NC 3.0, includes a requirement for reductions in a building's carbon footprint and greenhouse gas emissions. The USGBC is also supporting the 2030 Challenge initiated by architect Edward Magria, who has appealed to his colleagues across the country to be designing buildings with zero carbon emissions by 2030. Green buildings are rapidly entering the mainstream and will make a significant contribution to increasing energy efficiency in the years ahead (Brown, 2008; Wikipedia, "Leadership in Energy and Environmental Design").

Transportation

As indicated in box 12-1, there are a number of simple actions that individuals can take to increase energy efficiency as they travel via automobile: buying a more fuel-efficient car; purchasing low-rolling resistance tires and keeping them properly inflated (mileage improves 2–3% when tires are properly inflated); and getting frequent tune-ups and air filter changes. Of course bicycling or walking to one's destination, when feasible, would save even more energy! Beyond individual actions, however, there are a number of policies that governments could adopt that would have a significant impact on the energy efficiency of transportation: promoting the development of hybrid-electric, plug-in electric, and flex-fuel cars; lowering the highway speed limit to 55 mph (fuel savings can be as high as 15% when the 55-mph speed limit is enforced); prohibit excessive idling of vehicles—a practice that not only wastes large amounts of fuel but also negatively impacts air quality (Black, 2008).

A major step in improving the energy efficiency of motor vehicles was taken in 2009 when the Obama administration announced that, beginning in 2012, it would gradually increase the federal fuel economy standard from slightly over 25 mpg to a national car fleet average of 35.5 mpg by 2016 (39 mpg for cars, 30 mpg for light trucks)—a 30% improvement. The 2007 Energy Independence and Security Act mandates a 40% improvement in fuel economy by 2020, and by mid-2009 EPA and the Department of Transportation had begun working together to write regulations for enforcing this standard. Environmentalists are pleased that, after years of inaction on the fuel economy front, the United States has finally begun to move in the right direction. However, many feel that mileage standards should be set even higher and point out that other countries, most notably Japan, are far outpacing the U.S. in producing energy-efficient vehicles. They also point out that as the percentage of people living in large metropolitan areas continues to grow, various forms of mass transportation promise greater energy efficiency and less driver frustration than the private auto gridlock that now so often characterizes the urban commute.

The greatest potential for energy savings in transportation, however, would be the development of high-speed rail lines. Japan and several European countries already boast efficient high-speed passenger rail lines, but it is in China where the largest, fastest, and most high-tech rail system in the world is currently under construction. Expected to cost $300 billion, the project was launched in 2005 and should be completed by 2020, at which time almost 16,000 miles of new track will have been laid. The effort dwarfs anything currently envisioned by U.S. transportation planners and serves as a model for what is technologically possible with strong government commitment and funding. Electrified high-speed trains, with operating speeds up to 200 mph, offer a level of comfort and convenience that would persuade many travelers to choose rail

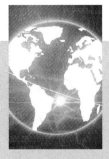

· · · · · · · · 12-1 · · · · · · · ·

Household Energy Savings—the "Short List"

According to the Department of Energy, American households and individuals account for 39% of all U.S. energy consumption through in-house use and nonbusiness-related travel. Energy efficiency experts insist that existing technologies, along with some modest lifestyle changes, could reduce that amount by approximately 30% (about 11% of total U.S. energy use)—and simultaneously curtail overall carbon emissions by an equivalent amount. Since a majority of us now believe that we, personally, can lessen our own carbon footprint by reducing energy consumption, why do so many individuals fail to take meaningful action? Undoubtedly a number of factors are involved, including the often high up-front costs of energy-saving home improvements, the fact that renters have little or no control over their landlord's energy-use decisions, and simply lack of time to dwell on the issue. Behavioral scientists, however, are convinced that a more fundamental reason for our unrealized potential for improving household energy efficiency is the fact that most people lack clear, concise information on what personal actions yield the greatest energy savings. Publications outlining "*101 Ways You Can Save the Planet*" and offering well-meaning advice are legion, but their suggestions are typically too numerous, nonprioritized, and, in some cases, just plain silly ("*. . . if all else fails, buy a camel!*"). Little wonder that their intended audience is left with scant guidance on a meaningful course of action. As a result, those who want to do their part but have limited time and resources are likely to choose whichever option sounds easiest and then feel satisfied that they've done something that "made a difference."

Experts insist that what is really needed is a wide-ranging public education effort promulgating a prioritized "Short List" of the most meaningful steps individuals can take to reduce household energy use. Research has shown that the five top-ranked actions on such a list (and % energy saved) would be:

1. buy a more fuel-efficient automobile (13.5%)
2. install/upgrade attic insulation and ventilation (up to 7.0%)
3. carpool with at least one other person (up to 4.2%)
4. replace 85% of all incandescent bulbs with compact fluorescent bulbs (4.0%)
5. get frequent car tune-ups, including air filter changes (3.9%)

Of course many other actions, cumulatively, can have a significant energy-savings impact as well: turning down the thermostat in winter and up in summer; avoiding sudden starts and stops while driving; installing a more efficient furnace, A/C unit, or water heater; combining errands to reduce trips into town; caulking/weather-stripping the house; reducing highway driving speed; maintaining correct tire pressure; and using only warm or cold water with cold rinse when doing laundry.

By focusing on just a few of these high-ranked opportunities for energy savings, concerned individuals can transform good intentions into a meaningful environmental impact. Where high up-front costs pose an obstacle to carrying out such actions, public-private partnerships that offer financial incentives such as rebates for home retrofits of energy-efficient appliances, deferred-payment loans, or loan subsidies can motivate householders to act. Equally important are programs aimed at overcoming nonfinancial barriers to action, programs such as those that provide households with free home energy audits to identify opportunities for energy savings, along with lists of approved contractors, help in securing low-cost financing, and inspection of completed work. Active promotion and marketing of such programs is also essential for informing householders of the available opportunities.

As public awareness of the link between climate change and energy continues to grow (and as utility bills continue to rise!), increasing numbers are becoming convinced that "Saving the Planet" begins at home. This "Short List" of household energy-saving options provides a guide to steer us in the right direction (Gardner and Stern, 2008).

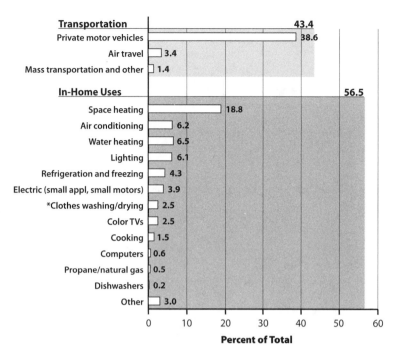

* Hot water for clothes washing is included under water heating.

Source: Data from Gardner, G., and P. Stern, "The Short List: The Most Effective Actions U.S. Households Can Take to Curb Climate Change." *Environment* 50 (Sept. /Oct.), 2008.

Figure 12-3   Total U.S. Individual/Household Energy Consumed, 2005

over airplanes or private cars, particularly for trips of 500 miles or less. By doing so, passengers would be saving both time and energy, while simultaneously reducing greenhouse gas emissions (Brown, 2008). With $8 billion in federal funds from ARRA allocated for development of high speed rail, the United States is finally beginning to take steps toward the transportation system of the future.

Smart Grid

In order to maximize the potential for energy savings by households and businesses, widespread deployment of emerging "smart-grid" technologies is of primary importance. According to the Energy Future Coalition, a nonpartisan alliance of business, labor, and environmental groups working to speed the transition to a new energy economy, modernizing the 50-year-old technology that characterizes the U.S. electricity grid would yield numerous benefits. These include helping to reduce greenhouse gas emissions by bringing renewable energy sources from distant sites of generation to the urban centers that need them and making the transmission and distribution of power throughout the system more reliable and secure. A smart grid, accompanied by the installation of smart meters, smart appliances, automated control systems, and digital sensors would also have a revolutionary impact on

energy efficiency by enabling two-way communication between utility companies and energy consumers.

Under the current 20th-century one-way communication system, a consumer, in essence, tells the utility "I need X amount of power" and the utility responds by producing a corresponding amount. If demand exceeds capacity, blackouts or brownouts can result. To forestall such an eventuality, power companies historically have built in excess capacity, designed to handle unusually heavy loads that may occur only a few days each year. Development of a smart grid would transform this scenario, changing the way electricity is used by balancing supply and demand, leveling out peaks and valleys, involving customers in decisions regarding power delivery, facilitating end-use energy efficiency—and reducing consumers' utility bills in the process.

To visualize how this might work in your own home, imagine that you request your power company to install a "smart meter" that will integrate the controls of all your appliances, lights, heating and air conditioning devices, communications systems, television—even your plug-in hybrid electric car and battery! Your smart meter can be programmed in various ways, causing it to reduce or shut off power to specified appliances when not needed (e.g., during working hours when no one is at home) or when the price of electricity rises above a certain specified level. Although the current flat rate pricing system doesn't reflect hour-to-hour variability, in fact the cost of producing electricity fluctuates constantly throughout the day, depending on supply and demand. For example, if you choose a pricing option designed to shift power usage from peak daytime or evening hours to off-peak hours in the middle of the night (e.g., programming your dishwasher to run at 3:00 AM or allowing your refrigerator to shut off briefly during periods of high power demand), you'll receive a monthly deduction on your utility bill. Alternatively, you could opt for a scheme in which your appliances are programmed to run only when the kilowatt-hour cost drops below a certain agreed-upon point or to cycle down when it rises above a specified level. Under this option, for example, your furnace, air conditioner, hot water heater, and so forth would only operate when the price of electricity is below a certain point; when it's higher, they automatically shut off and you adjust by donning a sweater, opening a window, or postponing your shower—with a lower monthly power bill as your reward. By controlling power demand, smart grid technology will also facilitate wider use of renewable energy sources, particularly wind and solar power, supplies of which are variable, depending upon whether the wind is blowing or the sun is shining.

As the smart grid shifts power demand to off-peak nighttime hours when wind velocity is often the greatest, wind energy can be utilized cost-effectively; during daytime when the sun is shining brightly, solar energy can be tapped to lower electricity costs. For consumers who have installed rooftop photovoltaic panels or own plug-in hybrid electric cars, the smart grid also makes it possible to sell any excess electricity they generate back into the grid, again lowering overall energy costs and helping to avoid the need for new power plant construction (Friedman, 2008).

Although the smart grid is still evolving, with full development a decade or more in the future, pilot programs in California and elsewhere have demonstrated the potential for significant energy and cost savings. With $11 billion in federal stimulus funding allocated for development of an electric smart grid, hopes are high that energy efficiency initiatives will receive a major boost as these new smart grid technologies go mainstream.

Gains in energy efficiency such as those discussed above will undoubtedly accelerate during the coming years, as new technologies move from the drawing boards into the marketplace. Such advances will make a significant contribution to resolving our current energy problems, reducing the need for new power plants, and thereby lowering both greenhouse gas emissions and utility bills. However, energy efficiency alone cannot solve all the problems associated with soaring worldwide energy demand. Meeting long-term energy needs without precipitating disastrous CO_2-induced climate change while reducing dependence on foreign oil requires a paradigm-shift in how we produce energy—a shift that is now underway as several promising clean, renewable energy technologies take center stage.

ALTERNATIVE ENERGY TECHNOLOGIES

We will harness the sun and the winds and the soil to fuel our cars and run our factories.
—President Barack Obama, Inaugural Address
January 20, 2009

Humans have utilized renewable energy resources such as fuelwood, wind, and flowing water for millennia, yet in terms of modern-day commercial energy production, such sources contribute only 6–7% of the total, both in the United States and internationally, with a few exceptions that will be cited later. (Note: this figure doesn't include the non-commercial use of firewood, animal dung, and other biofuels used for cooking and home

heating by families in many developing countries; these fuels are estimated to account for as much as 10% of world energy use.) Of the renewable energy sources being utilized commercially during the first decade of the 21st century, fully 80% comes from hydropower and wood wastes (Randolph and Masters, 2008).

Recently, however, concerns about rising oil prices and carbon emissions have prompted a new look at some renewable fuel technologies that have been talked about for years but remained more dream than reality due to high developmental costs and cheap fossil fuels. That situation is now changing. Three renewable sources—wind, solar photovoltaics, and biofuels—by 2008 were experiencing annual growth rates of 20–40%, the fastest growth rates for any energy source. Despite the economic slowdown that began by late 2008, hopes remain high that government incentives included in the 2009 federal economic stimulus package will provide the price signal to spur a fundamental transition in the American energy economy. Before examining what the future may hold regarding several of the most promising clean energy alternatives, however, a few words need to be said about nuclear energy, a topic discussed in much greater detail in chapter 10.

Although some in the environmental community automatically relegate increased reliance on nuclear power to the same "unacceptable" category as coal, tar sands, and oil shale, many others believe it has a legitimate role to play in the world's emerging clean energy economy. In comparison with carbon-intensive, highly polluting coal and oil, nuclear power does not generate CO_2 emissions, health-damaging particulates, or acid-rain precursors such as SO_2 or nitrogen oxides. As a result, around the world today, especially in rapidly developing nations like China and India, interest in nuclear power has soared as governments look for carbon-free methods of meeting the exploding energy demands of industrial and residential consumers. In 2010, according to the World Nuclear Association, 58 new nuclear power plants were under construction in 15 countries, with many more on the drawing boards.

Although replacing coal-fired power plants with nuclear facilities would, indeed, slash greenhouse gas emissions and thus boost efforts to combat climate change, many observers—while not necessarily averse to expansion of nuclear power—doubt that nuclear can provide the "magic bullet" needed to halt global warming or to solve energy supply problems. The exorbitantly high construction costs of new nuclear plants, the many years required to build a new facility, and the lack of any permanent high-level radioactive waste disposal site are all seen as factors inhibiting a significant expansion of nuclear power production. The Nuclear Energy Agency at the Organization for Economic Cooperation and

Development estimates that, on average, 12 new reactors worldwide would have to become operational each year from now until 2030 in order to have a significant impact on reducing greenhouse gas emissions. At present, however, the number of new reactors under construction isn't sufficient even to replace the number about to be decommissioned. While "nuclear optimists" contend that nuclear capacity can be tripled by 2050 if challenges facing the industry can be overcome, achievement of this goal would still represent no more than 20% of world electricity and would have a similarly modest impact in reducing world carbon emissions. Thus most analysts agree that in the years ahead, nuclear power will represent only one among several contributors to our clean energy technology mix; some of the other promising alternatives include the following.

Wind Power

Today's most rapidly growing source of clean, renewable energy, wind power has been utilized by humans since antiquity; sailing ships began plying the seas more than 5,000 years ago and windmills for grinding grain and pumping water were in widespread use in many parts of the world for centuries. The modern wind electricity industry is much more recent, however, rising to prominence in the late 1970s. Spurred by the "energy crisis" that temporarily shut off oil exports from the Middle East, commercial wind power generators began erecting turbines in California. Initially, the United States led the world in wind electricity-generating capacity, but high costs, lack of market incentives, and cheap fossil fuel stalled development of wind power in the U.S. throughout most of the 1980s and early 1990s. During this period, technology development shifted to Europe, with Germany, Denmark, and Spain taking the lead in world wind power generation. By the mid-1990s, larger, more efficient, more reliable, and less-costly European-manufactured turbines entered the marketplace, spurring a global sales boom that has persisted to the present day. As a result, interest in wind electricity revived in the United States and wind power development soared. By the end of 2008, with wind power capacity exceeding 25,300 megawatts, the United States surpassed Germany to regain its position as the world leader for installed wind power capacity.

Further gains were made in 2009, with U.S. installed wind capacity rising to 35,100 megawatts. Growth in China was even faster, thanks in part to that country's 2005 Renewable Energy law requiring all large power companies to generate at least 3% of their power from renewable sources by 2010; by 2020 that figure rises to 8%, excluding hydropower. As a result, wind projects in China are being installed at a rate three times faster than in the U.S., and by the end of 2009 China had overtaken

Germany to rank as the world's second largest generator of electricity from wind. Rounding out the top five in 2009 after the U.S. and China were Germany, Spain, and India. France and Canada are also experiencing large increases in wind electricity. Although wind currently generates just 1% of Canada's electricity supply, it now represents that country's fastest-growing source of energy. In terms of the percentage of total electricity supply generated by wind power, tiny Denmark (pop. 5.5 million) is the champion, currently meeting slightly over 20% of its electricity demand with wind energy and aiming for 50% when anticipated offshore wind farms become a reality (Brown, 2008).

Although the total percentage of electricity produced by wind in the United States is still miniscule—just 1.8% by the end of 2010—the potential for future growth is huge. According to the American Wind Energy Association, 46 states have adequate winds for commercial power production, with 36 states now hosting utility-scale wind power installations. Obviously, some regions of the country have greater wind energy potential than others. A study conducted by the Department of Energy (DOE) in 1991 concluded that just three states—North Dakota, Kansas, and Texas—have enough harnessable wind energy to meet the electricity demands of the entire nation. Since then, the advent of new technologies has led some experts to insist that these three states could supply not just all the *electricity* the country needs, but could also meet the entire U.S. energy demand. The High Plains region as a whole, from Montana and Minnesota in the north to Texas in the south, are referred to by some as America's "Saudi Arabia of wind" (Randolph and Masters, 2008).

The potential is high in other regions of the nation as well; a DOE assessment in 2005 stated that wind turbines installed offshore out to a distance of 50 miles could provide 70% of U.S. electricity demand. Contrary to the situation in Europe, where eight countries (Denmark, Belgium, Sweden, Finland, Germany, the United Kingdom, the Netherlands, and Ireland) now have offshore wind turbines, the United States currently has no such facilities. However, in October 2010 U.S. Secretary of the Interior Ken Salazar signed a lease authorizing the long-stalled Cape Wind project off the coast of Massachusetts. Terms of the lease give Cape Wind developers authority to construct 130 offshore wind turbines on Horseshoe Shoal in Nantucket Sound and to operate the wind farm for a 25-year period. When complete, Cape Wind is expected to provide three-fourths of the electricity demand for Cape Cod, Nantucket, and Martha's Vineyard. Cape Wind is likely to be but the first of many offshore wind farms in the U.S. In September 2010, the DOE released a draft plan calling for the nation to install 54,000 MW of offshore wind power capacity by 2030;

achieving this goal would require construction of more than 100 Cape Wind-sized projects. While currently in its early developmental stage, offshore wind power installations offer greater power-generation potential than on-land turbines, due to steadier winds and higher wind speeds in such locations. In addition, because they can generate power in close proximity to population centers, transmission lines carrying the electricity to customers can be shorter, thus alleviating transmission bottlenecks. In some densely populated areas near coastal waters like New England and parts of western Europe, limited space for on-land wind farms, combined with extensive offshore wind resources, make the latter an obvious choice for wind power development (AWEA, 2009).

Although the economic recession slowed installation of new wind energy facilities below the record-breaking 2008 level, by the end of 2009 total wind power generating capacity in the United States exceeded 35,100 MW—enough to provide electricity for more than 9 million American homes. Wind developers have high hopes that

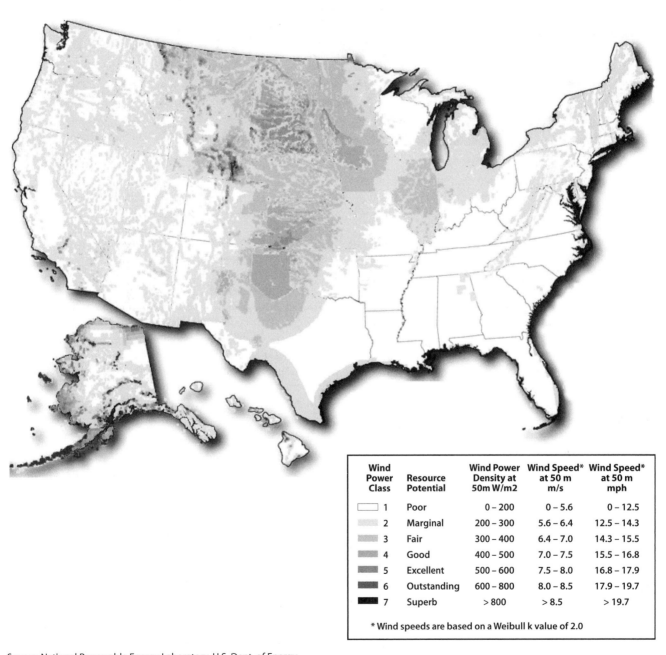

Wind Power Class	Resource Potential	Wind Power Density at 50m W/m2	Wind Speed* at 50 m m/s	Wind Speed* at 50 m mph
1	Poor	0 – 200	0 – 5.6	0 – 12.5
2	Marginal	200 – 300	5.6 – 6.4	12.5 – 14.3
3	Fair	300 – 400	6.4 – 7.0	14.3 – 15.5
4	Good	400 – 500	7.0 – 7.5	15.5 – 16.8
5	Excellent	500 – 600	7.5 – 8.0	16.8 – 17.9
6	Outstanding	600 – 800	8.0 – 8.5	17.9 – 19.7
7	Superb	> 800	> 8.5	> 19.7

*Wind speeds are based on a Weibull k value of 2.0

Source: National Renewable Energy Laboratory, U.S. Dept. of Energy.

Figure 12-4   U.S. Wind Resource Potential

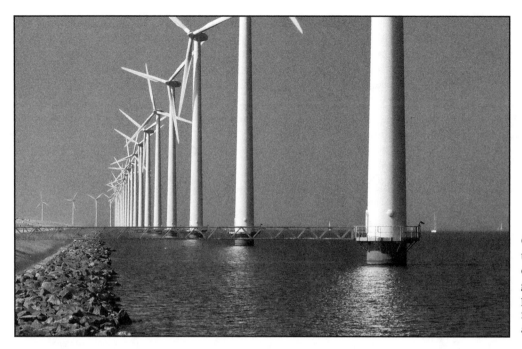

Offshore wind farms, like this installation off the coast of The Netherlands, offer greater power-generating potential than on-land wind farms due to steadier winds and higher wind speeds.

renewable energy incentives included in ARRA will promote continued rapid development of the nation's wind energy potential. It is evident that the federal government expects this to happen; in a report issued in May 2008—*Wind Energy by 2030 Technical Report*—the Department of Energy concluded that wind power is capable of meeting 20% of America's electricity demand by 2030, thereby reducing projected carbon emissions by 25%.

Unlike the situation a few decades ago, in good locations wind energy is now cost-competitive with conventional energy sources. It also boasts one of the shortest energy payback times (i.e., the time a power plant or, in this case, a wind turbine, has to operate to produce the same amount of energy used in its manufacture and installation) of any energy technology—in most cases just 3–8 months, depending on average wind speed at the site in question. Wind energy can also bring significant economic benefits to local communities and to landowners living in the vicinity of wind farms. Wind project developers typically negotiate with farmers or ranchers for the right to install turbines on their land. Since each turbine occupies only a small plot of land and is spaced quite a distance from other turbines, "harvesting the wind" can easily coexist with crops or livestock. Farmers and ranchers can thus earn considerable supplemental income by agreeing to the installation and operation of wind turbines on their land—extra income that can make the difference between prosperity and bankruptcy in years when commodity prices are low. Wind development thus offers a major boost to rural economic development, providing well-paid construction jobs, local tax revenues, and annual royalties to landowners.

However, there remain some developmental constraints that need to be overcome in order for wind energy to achieve its full potential.

Getting Power from Where It's Generated to Where It's Needed

The nation's current power distribution system is in drastic need of overhaul. Many of the best sites for capturing wind power are far from urban centers of high demand, necessitating major construction projects to install collection lines, extra-high voltage transmission facilities, and a distribution grid that is more reliable, resilient, and secure. To achieve this goal, groups like the Energy Future Coalition call for a "national clean energy smart grid," recommending that Congress replace the existing geographically fragmented state-by-state approach for planning, developing, and financing the transmission infrastructure with a consolidated certification and siting authority that can expedite construction of new regional or inter-regional grid facilities. They also call on the federal government to provide strong financial incentives for rapid deployment of smart grid distribution and metering technologies and new policies to make electric grid security a priority.

"Plan B" for Times When the Wind Isn't Blowing

Unlike the situation with coal-fired or nuclear power plants, utilities that rely on wind power must contend with the natural variability of this resource. While critics of wind energy question the reliability of wind electricity for providing uninterrupted power, in the context of large utility companies for which wind power is but one of several sources of supply, such variability poses little problem. When wind energy output decreases, electric utilities simply switch to natural gas-fired facilities or hydroelectric generators (or, in future years, solar power plants!), maintaining reliable electrical service by dispatching generators up and down as wind generation and electrical demand vary from hour to hour. While many people assume that expensive batteries or other costly means of energy storage are essential for the viability of wind power, this is not the case for electric generating systems where backup power sources are readily available. It should also be noted that wind farms supplying power to a utility typically comprise many—sometimes hundreds—of turbines spread out over a wide area and even with a rapid drop in wind speed it generally takes more than an hour for overall power production to drop significantly. Practical experience in places such as Denmark, where over 20% of the nation's electricity is wind generated, demonstrates that integrated power systems function quite reliably without expensive energy storage technologies (AWEA, 2008).

The environmental benefits of wind energy are obvious and compelling: a source of power that is carbon-free, nonpolluting, and infinitely renewable. The Department of Energy estimates that if the United States succeeds in meeting the federal agency's goal of generating 20% of U.S. electricity from wind power by 2030, yearly CO_2 emissions from the utility sector could be reduced by 825 million metric tons annually. Doing so would also displace 18% of the electricity now generated by coal, forestalling the need to construct more than 80 gigawatts of new coal capacity—and would also reduce overall electricity sector water consumption by 4 trillion gallons (8%), nearly 30% of this amount in water-stressed western states where water shortages are already stymieing new construction of coal-fired plants.

Other Concerns

While environmentalists have long been among the most enthusiastic advocates for clean energy technologies such as wind power, the prospect of wind farms sprouting on the horizon doesn't please everyone. Some environmentalists, in fact, have been among the most vocal critics of such development, complaining that wind turbines are noisy, ugly, a threat to birds and bats, and a deterrent to tourism. Energy companies have worked diligently to minimize each of these concerns and a closer look at the facts reveals none to be a serious threat to future development.

Noise.   Sounds emitted from whirling turbines are of two types: (1) mechanical, produced by internal equipment, and (2) aerodynamic, the "whooshing" sound produced as the turbine blades displace surrounding air. The former has now effectively been eliminated through improved sound-proofing, while the latter, at a distance of 350 meters (about 1100 feet), ranges from 35–45 decibels—about the same as background noise in a typical home. Since wind farms are typically located in areas of low population density and must comply with local sound ordinances, noise issues associated with wind energy today are minimal.

Aesthetics.   As the old adage goes, "beauty is in the eye of the beholder"; while some object to wind turbines as unsightly blights on the landscape and a detraction to local tourism, others find them awe-inspiring. And attitudes can change; in Palm Springs, California, residents were initially irate when a large wind farm was constructed in nearby San Gorgonio Pass, fearing that this "eyesore" would discourage tourists from visiting—and spending money—in their community. When they subsequently discovered that the whirling turbines were *attracting* visitors, local boosters began promoting bus tours to the site, producing advertisements and picture postcards encouraging outsiders to come and see the magnificent sight (Randolph and Masters, 2008)!

Wildlife impacts.   Bird mortality due to collision with turbine blades emerged as a troublesome issue in the early 1990s as reports surfaced of the deaths of nearly 200 golden eagles, hawks, California condors, and other raptor species between 1989–1991 at Altamont Pass, a 7,000-turbine wind farm located 50 miles east of San Francisco. Subsequent investigations revealed that the situation at Altamont Pass is quite different from that at other wind farms, where bird mortality has been considerably lower. The unique combination of topography, old turbine technology, and high raptor populations made this wind farm significantly more hazardous to birds, but even at Altamont the toll was relatively low. The outcry by environmental groups and negative media coverage prompted a quick response from the wind power industry to alleviate the problem by making equipment adjustments—installing perch guards to prevent birds' attempts to perch on turbine towers, insulating wires, covering exposed electric components on poles, and relocating overhead power lines. New wind-farm projects are now being constructed with power lines located underground in an effort to further reduce bird kills. These efforts have been largely successful and objective observers are in general agreement that while wind farms still kill *some* birds, they don't kill very many and, by comparison, represent a miniscule percentage of the bird death toll from collision with buildings and windows, house cats, moving vehicles, pesticide poisoning, and flying into high tension lines or communication towers (Erickson, Johnson, and Young, 2005). Overall, it is estimated that for every 10,000 birds killed by human activities, less than one is killed by colliding with a wind turbine.

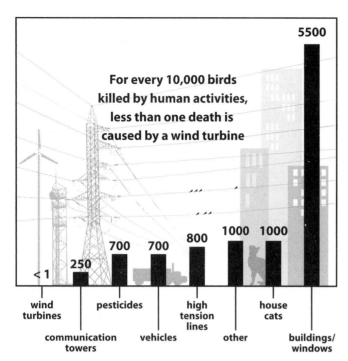

For every 10,000 birds killed by human activities, less than one death is caused by a wind turbine

5500

< 1   250   700   700   800   1000   1000

wind turbines   communication towers   pesticides   vehicles   high tension lines   other   house cats   buildings/ windows

Source: Adapted from American Wind Energy Assoc. (www.awea.org); source data from Erickson et al., "Summary of Anthropogenic Causes of Bird Mortality," U.S. Forest Service Tech. Report PSW-GTR-101 (2005).

Figure 12-5   Wind Turbine Contribution to Bird Deaths

More recently, bat deaths associated with wind farms have emerged as a concern as well. Large kills, especially of migratory tree bats such as the hoary bat (*Lasiurus cinerius),* have been reported at facilities in West Virginia, Pennsylvania, and Tennessee, raising fears among environmentalists already worried about declining bat populations due to disease. Since most of these fatalities occur over a relatively short time period during the late summer when bats are migrating, research has been conducted at several locations to ascertain whether curtailing turbine operations at such times might reduce the frequency of bat-turbine collisions. Studies carried out at a wind farm in Pennsylvania show that bat fatalities can be reduced significantly by changing the speed at which wind-generated electricity enters the power grid (i.e., the "cut-in speed") and that turning off the turbines during periods of low wind velocity resulted in bat mortality reductions of more than 70%—with minimal impact on annual power production. Such findings suggest that minor adjustments in operational procedures offer a practical approach for reducing wind energy's impact on bats (Arnett et al., 2009).

While the wind energy industry takes the above-mentioned issues seriously and continues efforts to mitigate any adverse effects associated with wind turbines, it's widely acknowledged that any environmental con-

cerns associated with wind energy are minor compared to its environmental benefits.

Solar Energy Technologies

Energy from the sun represents the ultimate in clean, renewable power—a source of supply that is essentially limitless and which many energy experts conclude is the only source capable of meeting the modern world's long-term energy needs. As in the case of wind energy, interest in harnessing solar power, both for heating and for electricity generation, grew out of the oil supply crises of the 1970s, but for many of the same reasons that wind power failed to take off until the late 1990s, solar energy remained a marginal player in terms of world and U.S. energy supply until recently. Although solar energy today supplies less than 1% of U.S. electricity, its growth rate is second only to that of wind power. Worldwide, the same trends are evident, as solar technologies attract billions of investment dollars. Business analysts see enormous growth in the years ahead, particularly for photovoltaic systems, predicting that "solar power generation is in the early stage of a 30–50 year run, serving an unquenchable demand for clean, renewable energy" (Martin, 2009). Among the several solar technologies experiencing rapid growth are the following:

Rooftop Photovoltaic (PV) Systems

Based on semiconductor technology that creates an electron flow by capturing the energy of solar photons, photovoltaic cells were first used for powering equipment on space satellites. They subsequently proved useful for providing electricity to homes or equipment in remote areas not served by high voltage electric cables. More recently, the focus of interest in PV systems has shifted to their potential for providing electricity to homes and businesses anywhere by installing ground-mounted or, most commonly, rooftop panels of photovoltaic cells aligned in an array oriented to capture the maximum amount of solar radiation and convert it to electrons. Although theoretically it might be possible to generate all the electricity needed by a household via a rooftop PV system, doing so is currently impractical due to the high cost of energy storage (this situation may change in the years ahead as battery technology advances rapidly). Instead, approximately 90% of all PV systems today are connected to the electricity grid via an inverter box installed on the house to convert the direct current (DC) generated by the solar cells to the alternating current (AC) flowing through the utility lines. As a result, when the sun isn't shining, power from the grid provides an uninterrupted flow of electricity; on bright sunny days, when the PV system is generating more electricity than householders are using, the excess flows back into the grid. In essence, the home-

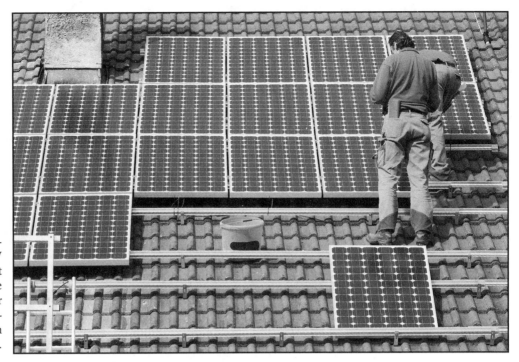

Rooftop photovoltaic systems feature panels of PV cells aligned in a way that allows them to capture the maximum amount of solar radiation. Such systems generally pay for themselves in about 5–10 years.

owner is selling surplus energy back to the power company, with a corresponding deduction from his/her monthly utility bill. Although the up-front cost of a PV system is still relatively high, once it's in place, electricity is essentially free. Depending on the size of the house, its location, and prevailing power company rates, rooftop PV systems generally pay for themselves in about 5–10 years. Emerging new technologies utilizing materials such as cadmium telluride and amorphous silicon applied to a supporting substrate as a thin film (as opposed to the now-dominant crystalline technologies used for flat panels) could significantly reduce costs by reducing material mass. They also promise higher conversion efficiencies and cheaper production costs. Experts are convinced that PV development will be very rapid in the years immediately ahead, with costs steadily declining and productivity improving (Martin, 2009).

With sales doubling every two years, use of solar cells worldwide is now expanding rapidly, although PV systems still represent a very small percentage of total electricity generation. Germany currently leads the world in sales of PV systems, even though it enjoys only about half the amount of solar radiation as California! Japan, the U.S., and Spain are among other world leaders in PV installations, but many other countries are now witnessing rapid growth as well (Brown, 2008). Thanks to government incentives, PV production and installation are taking off in China, India, Qatar, Abu Dhabi, and Korea, with the latter predicted to become Asia's largest solar market by 2012 (Martin, 2009). In the United States,

state rebates and federal tax credits are helping to make PV systems more affordable. Perhaps in the not-too-distant future, rooftop PV systems will become a standard feature on every home!

Solar Thermal Collectors (Active Solar Heating)

Most solar thermal collectors in use today serve primarily to heat water, but they have potential for space heating as well. These systems utilize flat plate solar collectors to absorb energy from the sun and then employ pumps or fans, depending on whether the system is water- or air-based, to transfer it to an energy-storing medium and from there to wherever it's needed within a building. Active solar systems fit in better with the architecture of conventionally built homes than do passive solar systems—structures in which the orientation and design of the building maximizes the capture of heat energy and ensures its even distribution. Active systems also are capable of achieving significantly higher temperatures than are passive systems, thus making them feasible for heating water, the second-largest consumer of energy (about 20%) in a typical home, after space heating (Wolfson, 2008).

Although at present rooftop solar water heaters in the United States are used almost exclusively for heating swimming pools, a famous couple is hoping to change that situation by setting a good example. In October 2010 it was announced that in the spring of 2011 solar panels will be installed on the White House above the president's living quarters. The solar power thus generated will be

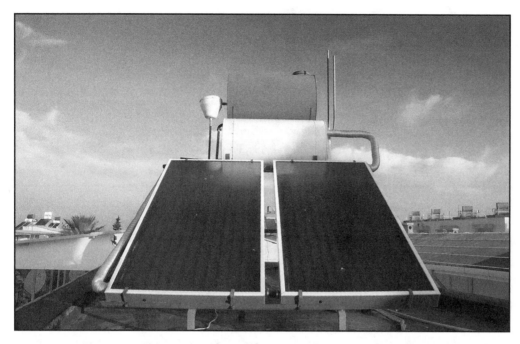

Rooftop solar water heaters are widespread in Europe, Israel, and throughout China, where it is estimated that 60% of the world's solar water heaters have been installed.

used to heat water for the first family, in addition to supplying some electricity (Cappiello, 2010). Elsewhere in the world, solar water heating is making far more rapid gains. In Austria 15% of homes heat their water with solar power, as do 3% of those in Australia; two million Germans live in homes where both water and space heating are provided by rooftop solar collectors; Spain requires solar hot water heaters for all new construction and renovation, while in Israel *all* homes must have solar water heaters. Growth of rooftop solar water heaters is exploding in China, where 2000 Chinese companies are now manufacturing these devices and their use is growing at an annual rate of 15–20%. By early 2009 it was estimated that 60% of the world's solar water heaters were sitting on Chinese rooftops, with 10% of Chinese households possessing one. In the city of Kunming (pop. 5 million), fully half the residents have solar water heaters and the city of Shenzhen recently mandated that they be installed on all buildings less than 12 stories high. Obviously, such popularity suggests there are significant advantages to capturing the sun's energy to heat water: (1) the technology is simple and straightforward; (2) solar water heaters are easy to retrofit onto existing homes and once the installation costs are paid, hot water is essentially free; and, perhaps of greatest importance in developing countries, (3) solar heaters provide householders in rural areas with access to hot water even when they are not connected to a power grid (Wolfson, 2008; Brown, 2008).

Concentrating Solar Power (CSP) Technologies

In contrast to the on-site electricity-generating systems represented by rooftop PV systems and solar thermal collectors, centralized facilities operated by large utility companies are today attracting renewed attention and investments as a potential major power source for wholesale markets. It is hoped that as the technology improves, it will be possible to produce commercial solar electricity for less than 10 cents a kilowatt-hour, a price that is cost-competitive with natural gas. Several CSP technologies, all capable of converting sunlight into electricity with efficiencies ranging from 10–20%, equivalent to that of most PV systems, are now already on the market or in advanced developmental stages.

All of these technologies, while different in design, basically operate by using large arrays of reflectors with automated tracking systems to concentrate sunlight on a closed vessel containing water or some other liquid, raising the temperature as high as 750°F to produce steam that powers an electric generator. By mid-2010 there were two commercial solar power plants operating in the United States, both of the parabolic trough type that employs curved mirrors to focus sunlight on a fluid-filled receiver tube that runs the length of the trough (100 meters); the heated fluid then carries thermal energy to a "power block" where a turbine converts it to steam and then electricity. The older of these two plants, Solar Energy Generating Systems (SEGS), located in the Mojave Desert near Barstow, California, has been in operation since 1991 and is currently the world's largest commercial solar facility, featuring 9 plants with an installed capacity of 354 MW. The second CSP now operating in the U.S., Nevada Solar One, went on-line for commercial use in mid-2007 on the outskirts of Boulder City. Though smaller than SEGS (64 MW generating

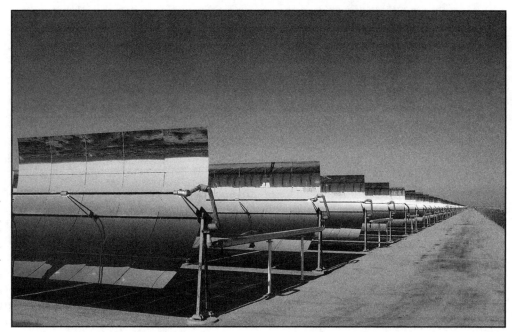

Commercial solar power plants, like this operation in the Mojave Desert, employ curved mirrors to focus sunlight on a fluid-filled receiver tube, raising the temperature of the fluid high enough to produce steam that powers an electric generator.

capacity), Nevada Solar One nevertheless ranks as the world's second-largest CSP.

Two additional parabolic trough-type commercial solar power plants are now operating in Spain and several more are under construction in that country. Spain also boasts Europe's first commercial "power tower"—a CSP plant near Seville featuring a high tower containing a heat-absorbing receiver, surrounded by a field of hundreds of mirrors ("heliostats") that track the sun as it moves across the sky and focus the sunlight onto the top of the tower. Energy absorbed by the receiver is then utilized to generate steam and produce electricity. Similar "power tower" technology will be employed by solar developer BrightSource Energy at a 370-megawatt CSP plant that broke ground in October 2010 at Ivanpah in the Mojave National Preserve in southeastern California. The Ivanpah Solar Electric Generating System (ISEGS), currently the world's largest CSP under construction, will include three "power towers" surrounded by 347 large mirrors on 3,500 acres of federal land. The project is scheduled for completion in 2013, with the electricity it generates contracted to two utility companies. Other emerging CSP technologies include linear Fresnel reflectors and dish-Stirling systems, with several new facilities featuring these designs coming on line, under construction, or announced both in the United States and elsewhere around the world (Moran and McKinnon, 2008).

Concentrating solar power has the advantage of producing electricity from steam with no emissions and, because facilities utilize back-up natural-gas storage systems to ease output variations on cloudy days and at night, they don't require storage batteries. On the down-side, they are expensive to build and, depending on the specific technology employed for cooling and condensing generator steam, they can require very large amounts of water—a serious drawback in the sunny, arid regions that offer the greatest potential CSP development. A proposed solar farm in Nevada's Amargosa Valley ran into serious public opposition when area residents learned that the cooling technology chosen would consume about 20% of the valley's available water supply.

In California, solar developer BrightSource Energy plans to install a dry-cooling process using fans and heat exchangers in place of the more common and less expensive wet-cooling technology, thereby reducing total water demand for its "power tower" facilities by 90%. The relatively small remaining water requirement is primarily for washing the heliostats (i.e., mirrors) that focus sunlight onto the boiler atop the central tower. The other prerequisite for CSP development is open space—such facilities require extensive land areas featuring strong, direct sunlight for the installation of reflector fields. Geography is thus a limiting factor for siting large CSPs, unlike the situation with on-site PV systems that can be installed on any sunny rooftop. In the United States, commercial power generation from solar energy is likely to be restricted to the Southwest, across a broad expanse from southern California to Texas. Elsewhere around the world, regions where solar intensity is sufficient to operate CSPs profitably include areas of southern Europe bordering the Mediterranean; North Africa, where Algeria has expressed intentions to construct a solar power facility and export electricity via undersea cable to Europe; Israel; the Arabian peninsula; desert regions of

Pakistan and northwestern India; and areas in northern and western China (Brown, 2008).

Such development isn't always welcomed by the locals, however. Just as proposed wind farms often generate opposition from those living in close proximity to such facilities, solar electric plants can also rouse conflicting emotions. The controversy in California illustrates the challenges and trade-offs involved in making concentrated solar power a major energy alternative. While theoretically supporting renewable energy technologies as a means for mitigating greenhouse gas emissions, some California environmentalists adamantly oppose plans to locate CSPs in desert areas that are home to endangered species like the desert tortoise or that have unique ecological value. To resolve this dilemma, groups like the Sierra Club and the Natural Resources Defense Council have been working with industry representatives in an advisory group helping California state regulators decide on the most appropriate sites for renewable energy development.

Even more contentious than site selection, however, has been the issue of building high-voltage power lines to connect desert power plants with urban centers of demand. Angry opposition to running such lines through the numerous national parks, wilderness areas, military bases, and communities that share this part of the Golden State has slowed project development and aroused local ire. In December 2009, California Senator Diane Feinstein introduced legislation to create two new national monument areas in the Mojave Desert in an attempt to thwart proposed solar and wind development projects in an area prized by environmentalists for its natural beauty and unique desert habitat. In response to Senator Feinstein's expressed concerns, the state agency in charge of planning the energy transmission grid has agreed to re-route proposed power lines to avoid passing through monument areas (Woody, 2009). As an indication that such conflicts can be satisfactorily resolved, in late 2010 Interior Secretary Salazar gave final approval to several proposals for large solar power plants in the California desert, remarking to reporters that "it's our expectation we will see thousands of megawatts of solar energy sprouting on public lands" (Barringer, 2010).

Geothermal Energy

In a number of volcanically active regions of the world, heat flowing upward from the interior of the earth is of sufficiently high temperature to constitute a source of marketable energy that is relatively clean and cost-competitive with conventional fuels. Virtually all geothermal systems now being exploited involve those in which cracks in the rock allow water to penetrate downward into regions where the earth is hot, thereby raising the temperature of the water. In the most valuable of these hydrothermal systems, the spaces between rock particles become saturated with high-pressure steam that can be used directly to power a turbine-driven generator. In other systems, hot water under pressure can be brought to the surface, at which point some of it converts to steam that can be used to power a generator. In some locations where the geothermally heated water isn't hot enough to produce electricity, it can still be used for such direct applications as heating buildings, greenhouses, swimming pools, and fish farms.

Geothermal currently ranks third among renewable energy sources worldwide (though not all geothermal resources are used in a renewable manner), after hydropower and biomass, but it still comprises a very small percentage of total world energy use. Growth of commercial geothermal energy in recent years has been slow— only about 3% annually. Although the United States produces more geothermal electricity than any other country, geothermal accounts for only 0.4% of domestic electricity generation (but 5% of that produced in California). Currently 24 countries have facilities for converting geothermal energy into electricity; the United States and the Philippines generate approximately half the total amount (by the end of 2009, the Philippines was generating 17% of its electricity from geothermal power), while Mexico, Indonesia, Italy, and Japan produce the bulk of the remainder.

Geothermal energy comprises more than just electricity, however. In fact, geothermal sources provide 10 times more thermal energy than they do electricity, their heat being used directly to warm homes, greenhouses, and swimming pools and for industrial process heat. Almost 90% of Iceland's homes are now heated by this nonpolluting energy source, replacing the country's former reliance on coal for home heating; altogether, geothermal supplies more than 50% of Iceland's total energy demand, more than in any other country (Wolfson, 2008).

The chief advantage of geothermal power is that, unlike wind or solar, it represents a steady, uninterruptible energy flow, 24 hours a day, 7 days a week. It's not quite as clean, since CO_2 and other dissolved gases such as SO_2, NO_x, and H_2S escape into the atmosphere when pressurized geothermal fluids are brought to the surface. However, the amounts involved are minimal compared with the levels of pollutants released by fossil-fuel plants. Perhaps the major downside of geothermal in terms of electricity generation is the limited number of sites with high energy-producing potential; in the United States these are located primarily in the more geologically active western states.

Since geothermal energy is most commonly extracted in the form of pressurized steam or hot water, power production over time may decline unless water is reinjected into the ground to recharge the depleted supply; in this sense, without recharge geothermal energy is not always renewable as is power from the sun or wind. Environmental concerns are that: (1) geothermal plants are noisy; (2) extraction of steam or hot water may cause land subsidence; and (3) the pumping of recharge water back into the ground may trigger small earthquakes (Wolfson, 2008). The latter concern was responsible for the cancellation in 2009 of two major geothermal projects, one in Basel, Switzerland, where several small earthquakes had resulted from preliminary drilling, and the other at The Geysers, near San Francisco. Nevertheless, energy experts agree that the advantages of geothermal energy far outweigh any disadvantages, a fact that has led oil giant Chevron to make big investments in this field, becoming the world's leading private producer of geothermal electricity (Friedman, 2008).

Perhaps the most widespread application of geothermal energy, practical even for regions that are not geologically active, is the use of **ground source heat pumps** (also referred to as **geothermal pumps**) to provide home heating, cooling, and hot water. The operating principle behind these systems is the fact that soil temperatures at depths greater than three feet remain fairly constant year-round at the mean temperature for that region (at six feet underground, soil temperatures in the United States range from 45–75°F, depending on the latitude). Geothermal heat pumps can be installed as either closed-loop or open-loop systems, depending on site characteristics, but all function in basically the same way.

The most cost-effective configuration is one in which an antifreeze solution or water circulates through a parallel series of high-density polyethylene plastic pipes laid in trenches 3–6 feet deep, connected with the house in a horizontal closed loop. In winter, the circulating liquid absorbs heat from the earth and carries it to the house where an electric-powered compressor concentrates the heat energy and a heat exchanger releases it at a higher temperature inside the home. In the summer the process is reversed, with the house being cooled when excess indoor heat is absorbed by the fluid in the pipes and is carried away via the underground loop where it dissipates into the ground. When the system is equipped with an additional device called a "desuperheater," heat absorbed by the fluid circulating through the house during hot summer months first passes through the home's hot water tank, heating the water at no extra cost before flowing to the underground portion of the closed loop. Studies have shown that approximately 70% of the energy powering ground-source heat pumps is carbon-free, renewable energy from the earth, while the remainder is supplied by household electricity. Although geothermal heat pump systems are not cheap, they typically reduce household energy bills by 30–40% and pay for themselves in 5–10 years through savings on utility bills (California Energy Commission, 2006).

Biofuels

The need to end our current dependence on fossil fuels by shifting to clean, renewable energy sources is now widely acknowledged. The technologies previously described, especially wind and solar power, are now experiencing a worldwide surge in research, development, and investment. As government incentives authorized in 2009 kick in, many experts are confident that the contribution of renewable energy sources to meeting U.S. energy demand will grow rapidly, as is happening already in Europe and elsewhere. That said, these sources will have little, if any, short-term impact on our fastest-growing use of energy—transportation.

By 2008, there were an estimated 800 million vehicles cruising the world's roads and highways—a number that, if present trends continue, is likely to climb to 3.25 *billion* by 2050. Currently, transportation consumes over 20% of the

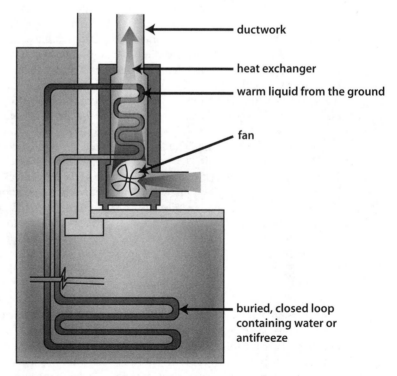

ductwork
heat exchanger
warm liquid from the ground
fan
buried, closed loop containing water or antifreeze

Source: California Energy Commission.

Figure 12-6   Geothermal (or Ground Source) Heat Pump

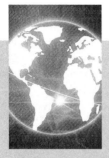

···· **12-2** ····

Beyond Corn and Soybeans—The Next Generation of Biofuels

The food-versus-fuel controversy currently bedeviling biofuels development may be resolved in the not-too-distant future by the recent emergence of several weedy plants and microscopic algae as unlikely stars in the contest to replace gasoline and diesel as transportation fuels. Sometimes referred to as "third-generation biofuels," these new energy crops are characterized by a superior energy-yielding feedstock, as opposed to the improved fuel-making process represented by second-generation biofuels like cellulosic ethanol.

Among potential oilseed crops that promise high yields without diverting land from food crop production, the one being promoted most aggressively today is jatropha (*J. curcas*), a tropical shrub/small tree native to the Caribbean but now grown in parts of Asia and Africa as well. Unlike the soybeans, rapeseed, and palm oil that now provide most of the world's biodiesel, jatropha grows vigorously on wastelands unsuitable for food crop production, making it particularly appealing for fuel-short developing countries where good land is in short supply. An acre of jatropha can yield four times as much oil as an acre of soybeans and the plant itself is considerably lower-maintenance. Jatropha grows rapidly, reaching maturity three years after planting, and continues to produce at optimal levels for 30 years or more. The plant needs little or no fertilizer (though fertilization improves growth and oil production), is relatively resistant to pests and disease, and can survive up to three years of drought. Excessive water-logging is about the only thing that seems to kill jatropha—plants can't survive two or more successive days of flooding (Schill, 2009).

A major effort to propel jatropha to the forefront of biofuels production is now underway in India, where a private company, Mission New Energy, plans to develop a million acres of jatropha. Enlisting over 100,000 small farmers to grow company-provided trees on degraded lands unsuited for food crops, Mission New Energy claims to have planted more than 300 million jatropha trees by mid-2009; later that year commercial jatropha oil production commenced in India. Some observers caution that expectations for jatropha oil to supply all of India's future biodiesel demand are unrealistic, warning that domestication of a wild plant is fraught with unknowns and that projected yields may be inflated. Nevertheless, proponents see a bright future, predicting that production will increase rapidly in the years immediately ahead. The Indian government, too, is betting on jatropha, mandating a floor price for jatropha biodiesel and requiring that fuel suppliers buy this home-grown fuel source to reduce dependence on imported diesel supplies.

Elsewhere in the world, several other countries are now pursuing jatropha oil production as well: Australia, Kenya, Brazil, and China are all excited about jatropha's biofuels potential. Interest is growing in the United States as well. In 2006, a company based in Ft. Myers, Florida—appropriately named MyDreamFuel—began cultivating jatropha trees in southwestern Florida. By 2009 over 1.5 million trees had been planted; a cloning facility set up by the company will produce about a million more plants per month. Roy Beckford, a researcher at the University of Florida, contends that jatropha is so well suited for growing conditions in the Sunshine State that oilseed yields there are likely to far surpass those in India and Africa.

As a tropical plant species, jatropha's potential for U.S. growers is sharply limited by geography, with southern Florida being one of the few suitable locations for its cultivation. Farmers in America's Midwest are focused on a more cold-tolerant species, **field pennycress** (*Thlaspi arvense*), an invasive weed in the mustard family (Cruciferae), now found throughout much of North America. Pennycress appears to be an ideal candidate for biodiesel production; not only do its tiny seeds have a 36–40% oil content (double that of soybeans and about equivalent to that of rapeseed) it also produces these seeds in great abundance, close to 2000 pounds per acre (however, since a typical soybean harvest is 4000 pounds per acre, per acre oil yields are about the same for the two crops). Equally important, since field pennycress is a winter annual, germinating in the fall and reaching maturity at a height of about 30 inches in late spring, it doesn't compete for space with other crops. Farmers can plant pennycress in September or October after their main-season crops have been harvested. The newly germinating pennycress will then form a low cover over the field during the winter, helping to prevent soil erosion, and is ready to harvest by June, after which another crop such as soybeans can be planted on the same land. While more research is needed, preliminary studies suggest that pennycress requires little fertilizer or herbicide use to obtain high yields and it can be harvested with existing types of farm equipment.

Studies on pennycress' potential as a biofuel and on optimal cultivation practices will continue at the USDA Agricultural Research Service laboratory in Peoria, Illinois, but commercialization efforts are already underway. An entrepreneur in the Peoria area has launched a start-up company, Biofuels Manufacturers of Illinois (BMI), to begin producing 60 million gallons of biodiesel per year from pennycress oil at a plant that developers hope will break ground in late 2011. BMI has enlisted several progressive local farmers from a group called the AgGuild of Illinois to cultivate test plots of pennycress, since previous research had focused exclusively on wild stands of the weed. In 2009 the total harvest consisted of about 200 acres, expanding to 1,000 acres in 2010 and expected to reach 500,000 acres within 5 to 10 years. BMI hopes to begin commercial biodiesel production by 2012 and is optimistic that within a few years field pennycress will completely replace soybeans as a biodiesel feedstock (Schill, 2008; Rao, 2010).

Another group of researchers and entrepreneurs, however, is betting that the #1 biofuels source in future decades will be neither jatropha nor pennycress but rather microalgae (i.e., microscopic unicellular algae), of which a number of species appear to be suitable candidates for producing biodiesel, bioethanol, biobutanol, and several other biofuels. Whereas acre-for-acre pennycress yields the same amount of oil as soybeans, and jatropha four times as much, according to the U.S. Department of Energy, algae are believed capable of producing up to 100 times the oil yield of soybeans—and the only inputs they need are sunlight, CO_2, and water. Because algae grow 20–30 times faster than land-based crops, they can be harvested much more frequently, thus increasing their commercial value. Although at the present time most farmed algae are grown in open ponds, in theory no land is required for cultivation—another advantage of algae over its biofuels competitors. More advanced cultivation methods that provide significantly higher yields rely on "bioreactors"—plastic tubes exposed to sunlight, containing algal cells growing in nutrient-enriched water (to conserve freshwater supplies, sea water or municipal wastewater can be employed as the growth medium). NASA has recently been experimenting with growing algae in wastewater-filled, semi-permeable plastic bags floating on the ocean. Preliminary results indicate that this approach not only yields large quantities of harvestable algae, but also provides an efficient method of sewage treatment, purifying the wastewater to the point that it can be safely discharged into the ocean; to make this process even more eco-friendly, the bags can then be recycled! In May 2009, NASA won agreement from officials in Santa Cruz, California, to allow the agency to use city wastewater for a pilot-scale demonstration project in the Pacific Ocean.

Elsewhere, other efforts to commercialize algae for biofuels production are moving ahead. In mid-2009, several promising new initiatives were launched by U.S. companies: Dow Chemical announced a deal with Algenol Biofuels Inc. to build a pilot plant in Freeport, Texas, to produce bioethanol from algae, utilizing CO_2 captured from industrial sources to grow hybrid algae in seawater enclosed in clear plastic bioreactors. Another corporate giant, Exxon Mobil, is also investing in algae biofuels research, partnering with Synthetic Genomics in a joint venture that company executives agree won't be ready to go commercial for at least 5–10 years. Yet another company, Ag-Oil in Delray Beach, Florida, made public its plans to open a state-of-the-art integrated oilseed processing and biofuels refinery in 2011, utilizing both jatropha seeds and algae to produce biodiesel. Ag-Oil has high expectations that their patented technology represents a major advance in biofuels production, yielding significantly higher amounts of biodiesel for the same amount of oilseed input as compared with other processing methods.

Admittedly, much more research and development is needed before the optimistic claims advanced by boosters of these new alternative biofuels can be verified. In the meantime, the lower-cost and more widely available first-generation biofuels—corn ethanol and soy biodiesel—are likely to retain their preeminent status for the near-term. Nevertheless, the recent surge of interest and investment in "third-generation biofuels," as well as continuing concerns about the environmental and food supply impacts of corn- and soy-based biofuels, makes it likely we'll be hearing much more about jatropha, pennycress, and microalgae in the years ahead (Tournemille, 2009).

world's energy (almost all of this amount from petroleum), and demand is expected to grow by 2.5% annually through 2025. In developing countries, growth rates for petroleum consumption are even higher than the world average—about 4.4% per year (Randolph and Masters, 2008).

Since motor vehicle emissions are a major source of both greenhouse gas emissions and conventional air pollutants and because of national security concerns regarding our dependence on foreign oil, clean, renewable, domestically produced biofuels have been rapidly gaining favor. On a global basis, biofuels have seen production increases of more than 20% annually until the economic crisis that began in late 2008 caused a marked slowdown in production and investment. Biofuels are touted as being carbon-neutral, since the carbon they contain recently came from the atmosphere and, when emitted during combustion, will be reabsorbed by vegetation; they also emit fewer harmful pollutants than does gasoline. However, they have a lower energy content than gasoline, so vehicles powered by biofuels get fewer miles per gallon than do those running on gasoline. Of the various types of biofuels, the lion's share of attention has focused on ethanol, with biodiesel a distant second.

Ethanol

Ethanol, or ethyl alcohol (C_2H_5OH), is produced through the biological fermentation of plant sugars or other plant substances such as starch or cellulose that can be converted to sugars. As a potential substitute for gasoline, ethanol has several advantages: it can be produced domestically and it has far lower greenhouse gas emissions than gasoline. The two most common forms of ethanol now available in the U.S. as motor vehicle fuels are:

- *E 10 ("gasohol")*, a blend containing 10% ethanol and 90% gasoline, constituted 87% of all alternative fuels in 2005. First used as an oxygenate additive to reduce wintertime carbon monoxide emissions, more recently *E 10* has been added to gasoline simply to stretch supplies.

- *E 85*, consisting of 85% ethanol and 15% gasoline, is considered the alcohol fuel with the greatest future potential, provided there is an increase in production levels of *E 85* and in the number of flex-fuel vehicles capable of using this ethanol blend. At present, most U.S. drivers have no access to the fuel because it is sold almost exclusively in the upper Midwest where most of it is produced. In 2007, there were only 11,000 filling stations selling *E 85*; in Minnesota, the nation's leader in *E 85* sales, *E 85* was available at just 6% of service stations and only 5% of Minnesota's cars were flex-fuel and thus capable of using it.

Biodiesel

Produced from vegetable oils and animal fats, biodiesel can be substituted for conventional petroleum-based diesel fuel without the necessity of engine modification. The primary sources of biodiesel in the United States today are soybeans and other oilseeds, as well as waste cooking oil from restaurants and fast-food chains. In Europe, the world's leading producer and consumer of biodiesel, rapeseed oil (canola) is the main feedstock (Randolph and Masters, 2008).

Biodiesel is frequently blended with standard diesel in various proportions, though pure biodiesel is also used by many car owners. Although world biodiesel production is rising, it still accounts for a substantially smaller proportion of biofuels production than does ethanol, in large part because a much smaller portion of the entire plant can be used for biodiesel production as compared with ethanol. As in the case of ethanol, the main benefits of biodiesel center on reduced greenhouse gas emissions and other air pollutants as compared to conventional diesel and reduced dependence on foreign oil. There are concerns, however, that large-scale biodiesel production in some ecologically sensitive regions of the world could have an adverse environmental impact. This is particularly an issue in regard to Indonesia, where vast areas of tropical rain forest on Borneo are being burned to clear the land for expanded palm oil cultivation in order to meet a growing demand for biodiesel.

In the United States, the rapid expansion of biofuels production has sparked considerable controversy in recent years, primarily because at the present time the main feedstock for U.S. ethanol is corn. Objections to corn ethanol center around the adverse impact diverting corn from food to fuel has on world food prices, with particularly severe impacts on the world's poor. In 2007 food riots broke out in several countries in response to a near-doubling of world corn prices when close to one-third of the U.S. corn harvest was diverted to ethanol production. Corn ethanol opponents have also long insisted that boosters greatly overstate the energy-saving benefits of corn ethanol. When all the energy inputs required to grow, harvest, and process the corn to produce ethanol are taken into account, gains are minimal—only 1.1 unit of energy output for 1.0 unit of input (Wolfson, 2008).

Researchers also argue that large-scale ethanol or biodiesel production from corn or other food crops will increase, rather than reduce, world greenhouse gas emissions because of land use changes. An indirect, yet ecologically significant, impact of biofuels production will occur if farmers elsewhere convert forests or pastures to cornfields or palm oil plantations in response to rising commodity prices. Net annual carbon emissions will rise significantly—many times more than the amount reduced by substituting biofuels for gasoline—due to the loss of carbon-sequestration services provided by natural habitats. Only if the biofuels crops are grown on wastelands or abandoned farmland are greenhouse gas reduc-

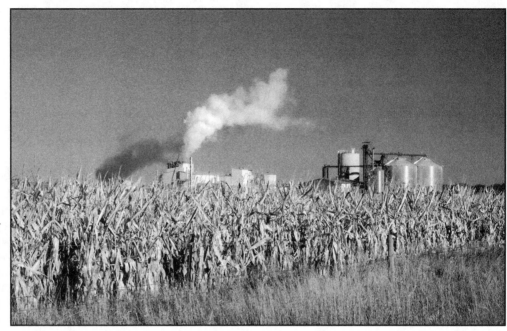

An ethanol plant in South Dakota rises behind acres of corn fields. Corn is the main feedstock for ethanol production in the U.S., sparking considerable controversy over the diversion of corn from food to fuel.

tions achieved through the use of biofuels (Fargione et al., 2008; Searchinger et al., 2008). The main benefit of corn ethanol over conventional gasoline fuels is that it somewhat reduces U.S. dependence on foreign oil. Politically, corn ethanol is a controversial issue in the United States and has been detrimental to harmonious international relations.

A better approach that reaps the benefits of ethanol without the disadvantages of corn ethanol is now being promoted by clean energy advocates of so-called "second-generation biofuels" produced from cellulose, hemicellulose, or lignin. Exemplifying the advantages of second-generation biofuels is **cellulosic ethanol**, particularly ethanol derived from certain native perennial grasses as well as wood chips, corn stalks, and wheat straw. Cellulosic ethanol has a far superior energy balance than corn ethanol, as well as greater net carbon emissions reductions. The Natural Resources Defense Council estimates that by 2050 half the fuel used to power American vehicles could be supplied by cellulosic ethanol if vigorous efforts to move in this direction get underway now. Unfortunately, high developmental costs have hindered research on advanced biofuels. Converting cellulose into sugars requires hydrolysis of woody lignins using expensive enzymes, and to date progress has been slow. As an energy expert at Cambridge Energy Research Associates remarked, "Cellulosic ethanol is something that is always five years away and five years later you get to the point where it's still five years away" (Krauss, 2009).

Tropical countries have an even better option—**cane ethanol**. For over 30 years, Brazil has been the pacesetter in producing ethanol-based transportation fuels from sugar cane, a crop with a far-superior energy input-output ratio than either corn or grasses. Because there's no need for the additional fuel-intensive steps required to transform starch or cellulose into sugar for fermentation, at least 4–10 times as much energy can be derived from cane ethanol as the amount used to produce it. By law, the gasoline sold today in Brazil must contain at least 25% ethanol and a large portion of that country's car fleet is made up of flex-fuel vehicles powered by pure ethanol or various ethanol-gasoline blends. Approximately half of all the sugar now grown in Brazil is destined for production of ethanol, which is now cost-competitive with gasoline. As an extra energy benefit, the waste left over from sugar cane processing can be burned at ethanol conversion plants to generate electricity on-site, with any surplus being funneled into the power grid (Wolfson, 2008).

Until the onset of a worldwide economic recession in late 2008, growth in biofuels production had been very rapid, yet its use was still miniscule in comparison with that of gasoline—in the U.S. about 3.5% of total motor fuel consumption. In hopes of increasing production and use of biofuels by guaranteeing investors and producers an assured market, Congress established a **Renewable Fuels Standard** under the 2007 Energy Policy Act, mandating a doubling of corn ethanol use—15 billion gallons per year by 2015—while setting a longer-term goal of producing 21 billion gallons of cellulosic ethanol annually by 2022. Incremental gains were also required in the near-term; the 2007 legislation requires the production of 100 million gallons of cellulosic ethanol by 2010 and 250 million gallons by 2011—goals unlikely to be met, since by 2010 virtually no cellulosic ethanol was being produced on a commercial scale. Nevertheless, ethanol producers are optimistic that they will soon overcome the technological challenges and insist the government's mandates will be met, albeit a few years late (Krauss, 2009). Elsewhere, other governments are mandating standards for renewable fuels use as well; by 2010 refiners in Canada will be required to produce gasoline blends with a minimum 5% ethanol content, while the European Union has pledged to get 5.75% of its diesel fuel from biodiesel by the same year—a target achieved by Germany in 2006.

While ethanol and biodiesel are likely to provide an increasing percentage of U.S. transportation fuel in the years ahead, some groups like the Union of Concerned Scientists (UCS) strike a cautionary note. UCS points out that producing the 21 billion gallons of advanced ethanol per year mandated by the Renewable Fuels Standard will require 300 million tons of biomass. While attaining this goal is achievable through utilization of agricultural and forestry residues, as well as municipal and construction wastes, the group warns that attempts to produce even larger amounts of biofuels in the future could conflict with other biomass demands such as food, fodder, generation of electricity, and biogas production. Citing the numerous ecological services provided by the forests and grasslands eyed for exploitation by some biofuels boosters, UCS reminds society that there are limits to sustainable biofuels production; exceeding such limits could create major problems for food supplies and ecological stability.

Other Possibilities

While the emerging clean energy technologies already discussed are attracting the major share of attention from researchers and investors and offer the greatest potential for transforming our energy economy, a number of other renewable energy options are also generating interest.

Methane Recovery

Methane, the major component of natural gas, is a vastly underexploited resource, even though the technologies for its capture and use are well-understood, widely available, and relatively cheap. That they haven't been utilized to a greater extent is due in part to a general lack of awareness about the magnitude of methane emissions and the amount of profit foregone in not capturing them, although the difficulty in obtaining access to the electricity grid in order to market the power generated at sites of methane capture is also a deterrent.

Sources with the greatest potential for methane recovery include **underground coal mines**, where drilling prior to mining can release methane, facilitating its capture and conversion to energy while at the same time reducing the risk of mine explosions; **oil and gas drilling operations**, where further measures to reduce leaks and

losses of methane could increase companies' profitability; **sanitary landfills**, many of which are already benefiting financially from methane recovery operations; and **manure piles** at cattle feedlots, where "biogas" digesting tanks can transform odorous wastes into a source of renewable energy. Such operations have acquired added importance in recent years as their potential for reducing levels of the second-most important greenhouse gas has become more widely recognized. Since methane, unlike CO_2, has a relatively short atmospheric lifetime, aggressive efforts to reduce methane emissions could have an immediate impact in slowing the pace of climate change, buying time for implementing longer-term strategies for dealing with carbon dioxide emissions.

Recognizing that no country yet has a comprehensive methane recovery and use policy in place, the U.S. EPA in 2004 created an international **Methane to Markets (M2M) Partnership** to help countries fight climate change and make the transition to a clean energy economy. By 2010, the number of M2M partner governments had grown from 14 to 38, collaborating on more than 300 projects that promote cost-effective, near-term recovery of methane while providing clean energy to markets around the world. Building on M2M's success and existing structure, the EPA in October 2010 launched a new Global Methane Initiative to fight climate change. Working in partnership with Mexico's Ministry of Environment and 36 other countries, as well as the European Union, the Asian Development Bank, and the Inter-American Bank, EPA hopes to enhance and expand efforts to implement methane-reduction projects and technologies and to encourage new financial commitments from both private and public sector donors. EPA estimates that increasing worldwide efforts to reduce methane emissions could achieve greenhouse gas reductions equivalent to the annual emissions of 280 million cars.

Tidal and Wave Power

These technologies, which harness the mechanical power of incoming and outgoing tides, can be utilized by power plants located on coastlines where the tidal flow is concentrated in narrow inlets, bays, or estuaries and is at least several meters high. The oldest and largest of such plants, the La Rance barrage in northwestern France, has been operating since the late 1960s, relying on an impoundment dam to capture incoming waters at high tide and then using the outgoing flow to turn a water wheel powering a generator. Within the past few years renewed interest in tidal power has been growing in some Asian (e.g., India, China, South Korea) and European (e.g., U.K., Russia) countries where several large facilities are being constructed or are under consideration. In the United States, a few small tidal facilities have been proposed for San Francisco Bay, Puget Sound, and New

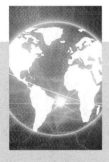

· · · · · · · 12-3 · · · · · · ·

Delivering Renewable Power—Controversy and Innovation

Is a massive expansion and upgrading of America's electricity grid essential in order to exploit the nation's vast wind and solar energy potential? Many renewable energy advocates, utility companies, and business executives like Texas oilman T. Boone Pickens would reply with a resounding "Yes!," arguing that the country's present infrastructure of long-distance transmission lines are incapable of handling the envisioned power load. This situation, they contend, makes transmission capacity the most serious short- and mid-term obstacle to continued growth of commercial-scale wind and solar electricity production. They see no alternative to big power line projects that can bring energy generated at remote locations on the High Plains or desert Southwest to distant metropolitan areas.

Agreeing with these arguments, President Obama ranked the upgrading and expansion of the U.S. power grid among the top priorities of his economic recovery plan, and federal legislation passed in 2009 allocated approximately $17 billion for grid and transmission spending, according to the Center for American Progress. In response, ITC, the largest independent transmission company in the United States, immediately proposed a "Green Power Express" plan—a $10–12 billion project that would bring wind electricity from the Dakotas, Minnesota, and Iowa to major population centers in the Chicago/northwest Indiana region. If this plan overcomes numerous regulatory hurdles and comes to fruition (ITC's target date for project completion is 2020), it would represent the world's largest clean-energy transmission network, consisting of 3000 miles of power lines capable of handling up to 12,000 megawatts of electricity (Makower, Pernick, and Wilder, 2009).

However, not everyone is convinced that a national power grid for renewable energy is a good idea, or even necessary. As plans for massive grid expansion gather momentum, a growing chorus of dissenters advocates a very different approach. **Distributed generation (DG)**—the production of electricity from numerous small sources close to its point of use—would represent a radical departure from the large centralized power plants that most industrialized countries, including the United States, traditionally have relied upon for electrical power generation and distribution. In contrast to the giant wind farms and concentrated solar power technologies now moving from the drawing board to commercial production, DG proponents contend that it would be more cost-effective to install solar panels on millions of rooftops and develop numerous small (10–40 MW) local wind farms that could tap into the existing power grid without the need for new, long-distance transmission lines. The DG concept is especially well-suited for promoting rooftop PV systems, since the generation of electricity on-site precludes the need for any expensive new lines.

In addition to being less costly, distributed generation eliminates several environmental problems related to impending transmission line mega-projects. Bitter controversies over threatened disruption of high-value natural habitats or rural communities situated in the path of proposed transmission lines would be avoided, as would be fears that the new extra-high voltage lines also could be used for transmitting electricity generated by dirty nonrenewable sources. Add to these arguments the fact that energy losses during transmission and distribution are significantly lower when the source of power generation is located close to the user, and the benefits of DG are even more apparent.

The potential for distributed generation is greater than commonly recognized. A study conducted in 2008 by the Institute for Local Self-Reliance concluded that half the states in the U.S. could become energy self-sufficient through harnessing the solar, wind, and biomass resources within their borders, while most of the remainder could meet a sizeable portion of their energy needs in this way. Picking up on this theme, a California engineer recently published a study contending the $2 billion that San Diego Gas & Electric plans to spend on Sunrise Powerlink—a new 150-mile transmission line to bring solar electricity from the desert to the city—could have provided 1,300 MW of electricity from PV panels with negligible transmission costs. Other California researchers have concluded that widespread installation of rooftop PV systems in San Diego could generate 5000 MW of power, supplying all the electricity the city needs at noon on a hot day (Rose, 2009).

So why is there not yet a rush to install solar PV systems or wind turbines on every rooftop in the national quest for energy self-sufficiency? While there has indeed been an upswing in such installations in the past few years, especially in states like California and New Jersey that offer attractive financial incentives to homeowners or businesses that purchase renewable energy systems, the still-hefty up-front costs, typically ranging from $15,000 to $50,000 for residential installations, remain a major deterrent to widespread adoption. So long as the prevailing system compels energy users to buy their own renewable energy production technology, the market for such devices will remain severely limited. Alternative approaches are needed to make small-scale renewable energy technologies economically feasible for interested homeowners who acknowledge their long-term payback potential in terms of reduced utility bills but simply can't afford to wait the 15 years or so before such investments "break even." Illinois has instituted one such approach, termed "net metering," whereby excess power generated during peak hours is fed back into the grid, with the value of that electricity being deducted from the homeowner's monthly utility bill.

This challenge has been tackled quite successfully in Germany through national legislation establishing a **feed-in tariff (FIT)** that requires German utilities to buy electricity generated by homeowners or corporations from renewable sources, such as rooftop PV systems or wind turbines, at above-market rates set by the government. German utilities must sign 20-year contracts with would-be participants to purchase the power they produce, providing a significant financial incentive for ordinary citizens to install renewable energy systems. Germany's FIT program has been widely acclaimed as the best approach yet devised for encouraging adoption of renewable energy technologies; a majority of European Union countries are now following Germany's example and are experiencing a corresponding surge in residential solar and wind power. In the spring of 2009, Gainesville, Florida, became the first U.S. city to adopt a feed-in-tariff system similar to those in Europe, though its municipally owned utility has limited the number allowed to sign up for the program. FIT proposals have also been floated by the governor of Oregon and the mayor of Los Angeles, but the concept has yet to generate widespread interest in this country, perhaps because the FIT represents a sizeable subsidy—often 2–4 times the retail rate—for those who install the systems, and that subsidy is ultimately paid by other consumers.

A "made in the USA" approach to motivating homeowners and businesses to invest in renewable technologies has met with considerable success in recent years and is responsible for a surge in PV installations. The concept of **Purchasing Power Agreements**, or **PPAs**, originated in 2003 when Jigar Shah, a young MBA entrepreneur, realized that the solar PV industry needed financial innovation more than technological improvement; he founded a new company, SunEdison, now North America's leading provider of solar energy, and proceeded to change the industry's game rules. Targeting his sales pitch to large corporate customers like Kohl's, Walmart, and Costco, as well as to smaller businesses, universities, and municipal governments, Shah convinced his clients to sign on with a company that is essentially an independent solar electric utility. Customers sign a PPA, agreeing to buy power generated by a rooftop array of solar panels provided by SunEdison at a fixed monthly rate for at least 10 years. Throughout this time period, SunEdison owns, maintains, and earns profits from the system while the client is charged for the solar electricity produced by the panels—a fee that is lower than the prevailing local utility rate and thus represents a win-win situation for both SunEdison and its customers.

The PPA business model has proven so persuasive that in 2008, according to the AltaTerra Research Network, it accounted for about 72% of all nonresidential solar market sales. That model is now being introduced in somewhat modified form to the residential PV market in California, where state tax credits, rebates, and high utility prices make the concept particularly attractive. The leading programs at present include a residential PPA offered by San Francisco-based SunRun, in which customers must make a modest pre-payment for 18 years worth of electricity, as well as the SolarLease concept offered by Solar City, involving little or no up-front costs. Both companies are doing a brisk business and expect even better times ahead, as federal economic stimulus dollars further energize the solar industry. If such programs expand to include the remaining 49 states, the promise of distributed power generation will brighten considerably (Behar, 2009).

In all likelihood, the United States needs both the "bigger, better, smarter grid" called for by President Obama, as well as further development of distributed generation in areas where local resources make this a feasible option. The revolutionary transformation now underway in how we produce, distribute, and use energy will, by necessity, involve many players.

York's East River. Wave power, too, is raising interest, with ambitious futuristic plans for offshore wave power development now envisioned for Ireland, the southwestern coast of England, and northern California (Brown, 2008). Nevertheless, it is highly doubtful that tidal or wave power will ever provide more than a locally significant source of alternative energy due to the limited number of sites suitable for such development (Wolfson, 2008).

Wood and Other Biomass

As noted earlier in this chapter, on a worldwide basis, wood and other biofuels provide approximately 10% of the energy used by humans, primarily in poor societies where firewood, other plant materials, and animal dung are routinely used for home cooking and heating. In terms of commercial energy use in the United States, about 2–3% of the total is supplied by biomass, a figure that the Energy Information Administration predicts will rise to 4.5% by 2030. Half of this comes from the forest products industry that burns its own wood wastes and pulping liquors to generate in-house process steam, heat, and electricity. In recent years there has been a growing interest, especially in the forest-rich Southeast and New England states, for wood-generated electric power. A wood-burning public utility in Burlington, Vermont, now supplies that city with one-third of its electricity (Randolph and Masters, 2008; Wolfson, 2008). Energy from municipal solid wastes is yet another option currently being exploited in numerous communities and will be discussed in greater detail in chapter 17.

In passing, it should be mentioned that one previously touted alternative energy source, hydrogen fuel cells for cars, is no longer regarded as a viable option. Due to technical problems in developing the cells, concerns about transporting hydrogen, and the fact that producing the fuel cells generates carbon emissions, most experts now consider flex-fuel or plug-in hybrid electric vehicles a better, cheaper, "greener" alternative. As a result, in 2009 funds previously allocated by the Bush administration for hydrogen fuel cell development were cut from the federal budget.

FUTURE OUTLOOK

The fact that these emerging alternative energy technologies will eventually transform the way we produce electricity, heat our homes and workplaces, and power our transportation system seems indisputable—especially since the fate of our planet depends upon making the necessary, though difficult, transition. The big, as-yet unanswered, question is *when* will clean, renewable energy sources play more than a peripheral role in powering the world economy? Estimates range from the 2020

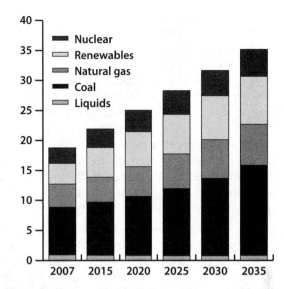

Source: Energy Information Administration, *International Energy Outlook 2010: Highlights.* July 2010. www.eia.doe.gov/oiaf/ieo/emissions.html.

Figure 12-7   Outlook for Renewables: World Electricity Generation, 2007–2035 (trillion kilowatt hours)

target date advocated by the Worldwatch Institute to 2050 or beyond by pessimists who insist that fossil fuels will continue to dominate the world energy picture for decades to come. The rapidity—or slowness—of our anticipated energy transition will depend on a number of factors, including:

- *World oil prices.* A sharp rise, such as occurred in the summer of 2008, would provide a major market incentive for biofuels, hybrid and electric cars, high-speed rail, and so forth.

- *A price on carbon emissions.* The ultimate fate of ongoing congressional debates over cap-and-trade policies (see chapter 11) versus a carbon tax or other approaches for putting a price on carbon emissions (e.g., raising the gasoline tax or putting a floor on the price of natural gas, crude oil, and gasoline to keep prices from falling below a set level) will have an enormous impact on making alternative energy sources economically viable.

- *Government financial incentives.* The federal government's renewable energy production tax credit (PTC) has been a primary motivator for the rapid growth of solar and wind energy; in 2009 a new program offered renewable energy developers a 30% investment tax credit (ITC) in lieu of the PTC, an option that was deemed critical for enabling wind and solar power to continue growing in spite of the economic downturn. For those interested in purchasing solar panels or wind turbines but deterred by the high purchase price, federal investment tax credits as well as state rebates help to make the cost more affordable, thereby promoting sales and stimulating further growth and development. Similar customer rebates have been helping to boost sales of energy-efficient appliances and home-weatherization projects. Government investment in alternative energy research and development programs is also essential as clean energy technologies strive to become economically competitive with fossil fuels. Billions of dollars made available through the 2009 American Recovery and Reinvestment Act will provide crucial funding for such efforts and help hasten America's energy transition.

• *Renewable electricity standards (RES).* Much of the growth already witnessed in renewable electricity generation has occurred because of state government mandates requiring their utilities to meet specified renewable energy goals. By 2010, 29 states and the District of Columbia had adopted renewable electricity standards, with target levels and deadline dates varying from state to state. Although progress in meeting the designated targets has been spotty (utilities in about half the states are falling short of their goals and may be penalized by fines), some states have made impressive gains since mandates were enacted.

Texas provides a dramatic example of the positive impact such laws can have on spurring growth of renewable energy. In 1999 the Lone Star State passed the Texas Renewable Portfolio Mandate, requiring that utilities generate 2,000 new megawatts of electricity from renewables by 2009. Choosing wind as their most viable option, Texas utilities installed so many wind turbines that the 2,000 MW goal was achieved four years ahead of schedule, in 2005—whereupon the Texas legislature raised the bar, requiring they achieve 5,000 MW by 2015. By the end of 2008, wind power generated 4.5% of Texans' electricity supply, a figure well above the national average (Friedman, 2008).

In California as well, mandates have been spurring the growth of renewables. Recent proposals for numerous solar and wind-energy facilities are not motivated by an altruistic urge to stop global warming but by California's strict mandate requiring utilities in that state to generate 20% of their power from renewable sources by 2010—and 33% by 2030 (skeptics have serious doubts that either of these goals will be met, however). Important as such mandates have been in spurring growth in renewable energy technologies, many clean energy advocates and policy makers are convinced that a state-by-state approach is insufficient, saying that a *national* RES is essential to create a long-term and stable market for capital investment. A national standard would ensure that all states reap the benefits of renewable energy development, including more than 185,000 jobs the Union of Concerned Scientists estimates would be created within the coming decade if a 20% national RES is enacted.

Despite continuing technological challenges and economic uncertainties, the ultimate future of clean, renewable energy sources looks brighter today than ever before. As nations around the world search for ways to reduce greenhouse gas emissions, improve air quality, and ensure future energy supplies, a shift to increased reliance on renewables seem inevitable. A quote from *Atlas World Press Review* more than 30 years ago seems prescient today:

> Alternative energy is a future idea whose time is past. Renewable energy is a future idea whose time has come.
>
> —Bill Penden, April 1977

········ 13 ········

> ...why, it appears no other thing to me
> but a foul and pestilent congregation of vapors.
> —William Shakespeare (*Hamlet*)

Air Pollution

Humans have undoubtedly been coping with a certain amount of polluted air ever since primitive *Homo sapiens* sat crouched by the warmth of a smoky fire in their Paleolithic caves. An inevitable consequence of fuel combustion, air pollution mounted as a source of human discomfort as soon as people began to live in towns and cities. More recently it has become an extremely serious problem on a worldwide basis for two primary reasons: (1) there has been an enormous increase in world population, particularly in urban areas, and (2) since the early 1800s the rapid growth of energy-intensive industries and rising levels of affluence, first in the industrialized nations and recently in the large developing countries as well, have led to record levels of fossil fuel combustion.

Prior to the 20th century, problems related to air pollution were primarily associated, in the public mind at least, with the city of London. As early as the 13th century, coal from Newcastle was shipped into London for fuel. As the population and manufacturing enterprises grew, wood supplies diminished and coal burning increased, in spite of the protests of both monarchs and private citizens who objected to the odor of coal smoke. One petitioner to King Charles II in 1661 complained that due to the greed of manufacturers, inhabitants of London were forced to "breathe nothing but an impure and thick Mist, accompanied by a fuliginous (sooty) and filthy vapour, which renders them obnoxious to a thousand inconveniences, the Lungs, and disordering the entire habit of their Bodies. . . ." (Evelyn, 1661).

In spite of such railings, English coal consumption increased even faster than the rate of population growth and by the 19th century London's thick, "pea-soup" fogs had become a notorious trademark of the city. Numerous well-meaning attempts at smoke abatement were largely ignored during the heyday of laissez-faire capitalism, epitomized by the industrialists' slogan, "Where there's muck, there's money."

The same conditions that had made London the air pollution capital of the world began to prevail in the United States as well during the 19th and early 20th centuries. St. Louis, plagued by smoky conditions, passed an ordinance as early as 1867 mandating that smokestacks be at least 20 feet higher than adjacent buildings. The Chicago City Council in 1881 passed the nation's first smoke abatement ordinance. Pittsburgh, once one of the smokiest cities in the United States, was the site of pioneer work at the Mellon Institute on the harmful impact of smoke both on property and human health.

In spite of gradually increasing public awareness of the problem, levels of air pollution and the geographical extent of the areas affected continued to increase. Although by the late 1950s and 1960s large-scale fuel-switching from coal to natural gas and oil had significantly reduced smoky conditions in many American cities, other newer pollutants—products of the now-ubiquitous automobile—had assumed worrisome levels. Today foul air has become a problem of global proportions; no longer does one have to travel to London or

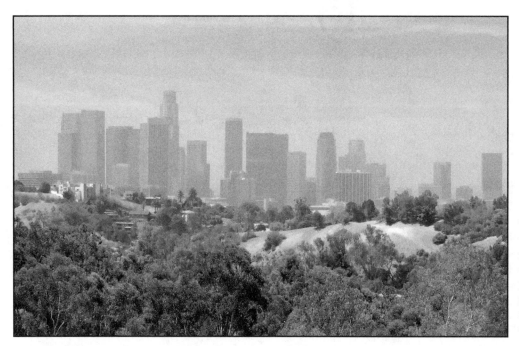

The bright sunlight, warm temperatures, and heavy traffic of southern California often combine to produce a photochemical smog that gives the Los Angeles skyline its characteristic hazy appearance.

Pittsburgh or Los Angeles to experience the respiratory irritation or the aesthetic distress that a hazy, contaminated atmosphere can provoke. In the early 21st century, virtually every metropolitan area in the world, from Beijing to Bangkok, Delhi, Tokyo, Athens, Moscow, and Mexico City—all are grappling with the problem of how to halt further deterioration of air quality without impeding industrial productivity and development.

SOURCES OF AIR POLLUTION

Where is all this dirty air coming from? Not surprisingly, the sources of air pollution are quite diverse and vary in importance from one region to another. Some air contaminants are of natural origin; volcanic eruptions, forest fires, and dust storms periodically contribute large quantities of pollutant gases and particles to the atmosphere. In June 1991, immense quantities of volcanic ash and an estimated 18 million metric tons of sulfur dioxide (roughly equivalent to U.S. emissions of this pollutant gas during an entire year) were spewed into the atmosphere during a single massive eruption of Mt. Pinatubo in the Philippines. For several months during the fall of 1997, fires deliberately set by farmers and loggers to clear land on the Indonesian island of Sumatra burned out of control, creating a pall of pollution over much of Southeast Asia. Covering an area inhabited by 200 million people, the smoke provoked acute respiratory problems throughout the region, caused transportation accidents that killed hundreds, devastated the tourist trade, and severely damaged the economies of the nations affected. British experts estimate that the burning forests released more

greenhouse gases than were emitted in an entire year by all the cars in Europe.

Less dramatic but worthy of note, considerable amounts of methane gas are released into the air when organic matter decays in the absence of oxygen, and some plant species produce volatile hydrocarbons that are thought to be responsible for the blue haze observed in the Smoky Mountains and other forest regions. However, most of the pollutants befouling outdoor air are products of fossil fuel combustion, generated as humans seek to extract energy from coal, oil, natural gas, and diesel fuel—emission sources that have proliferated with the development of industries and transportation networks.

At present in the industrialized world the largest sources of air pollution, in order of importance, are (1) transportation, primarily automobiles and trucks; (2) electric power plants that burn coal or oil; and (3) industry, the major offenders being steel mills, metal smelters, oil refineries, and pulp and paper mills. Of less importance now than in past decades is the contribution made from heating homes and buildings and burning refuse, though the latter still remains a problem in developing world cities that lack adequate municipal waste disposal. In the industrialized nations, a general trend toward heating with oil, gas, or electricity instead of with coal has greatly reduced pollution from space heating. At the same time, increasingly common municipal bans on home refuse burning, along with the utilization of sanitary landfills or incinerators equipped with pollution control devices for community solid waste disposal, have accounted for a marked decline in emissions from trash combustion. Within any one region or community, of course, the relative importance of various emission sources may differ from the overall national rankings noted here. In most metropolitan areas, automobiles contribute by far the largest amount of air pollutants; in small towns, by contrast, significant levels of contamination may be caused by just one polluting factory.

Criteria Air Pollutants

Air pollution, of course, is no single entity; thousands of gaseous, liquid, and solid compounds contribute to the atmospheric mess. The nature of some of these substances is well known while others are only now being studied and their threat to human health assessed. The most common and widespread air pollutants include six that the federal government has designated **criteria pollutants**, requiring the Environmental Protection Agency to gather scientific and medical information on their environmental and human health effects. These are the pollutants for which **National Ambient Air Quality Standards (NAAQS**—familiarly referred to as "nax") have been set, specifying the maximum levels of concentration of these pollutants allowable in the outdoor air. The six criteria air pollutants are discussed in the following sections (it should be noted that most industrialized countries, and some developing nations as well, now have regulations controlling these same air contaminants).

Particulate Matter (PM_{10} and $PM_{2.5}$)

All airborne pollutants that occur in either liquid or solid form, including pollen, dust, soot, smoke, acid condensates, and sulfate and nitrate particles are referred to as particulate matter. Particulates range in size from pieces of fly ash as large as a thumbnail to tiny aerosols, known as "ultrafines," less than 0.1 micrometers (100 nanometers) in diameter—so small that they remain suspended in the air and are transported on wind currents as easily as are gases. Originating from a multiplicity of different sources, particulates consist of hundreds of different compounds and may undergo various chemical and physical transformations after entering the atmosphere. Ultrafine particles often act as nuclei to attract other hazardous particles and gases that adhere to them and are inhaled. Not surprisingly, their impact on human health is related both to their size and to their chemical composition (Russell and Brunekreef, 2009). To many people, particulate matter and "air pollution" are synonymous, since easily visible dark plumes of smoke and soot or clouds of dust are the only forms of air pollution of which they are aware. Marked reductions in particulate levels in a number of urban areas in recent years have led many citizens to conclude erroneously that air quality is no longer a problem, since most other air pollutants are invisible.

Particulate matter is generated by a wide variety of activities—fuel combustion, road traffic, agricultural activities, certain industrial processes, and natural abrasion. The most visible damage caused by particulate matter is the layer of grime deposited on buildings, streets, clothing, and so on. Prior to pollution-control efforts launched during the 1970s, it was estimated that in the most polluted areas of big cities as much as 50–100 tons of particulate matter per square mile fell each month (Air Pollution Primer, 1969).

Particulate matter can obscure visibility and corrode metals; more important is the fact that when inhaled, particulates irritate the respiratory tract. Most dangerous in this regard are the tiny aerosols that, because of their very small size, can evade the body's natural defense mechanisms and penetrate deeply into the lungs (in most cities, these very small particles comprise 50–60% of suspended particulates). In recognition of this fact, the EPA in 1987 replaced the original standard for total particulates with a revised standard that applies to those particles with a diameter of 10 micrometers or less (PM_{10}) that are small enough to penetrate to the highly sensitive alveolar region of the lungs. In 1997, EPA again revised the standards for particulate matter, adding new requirements for so-called "fine" particles smaller than 2.5 micrometers in diameter. This action was taken in response to studies indicating that the characteristics, sources, and health effects of these smaller particles are substantially different from those in the PM_{10} category. Although it is now recognized that ultrafines, the smallest particles in the $PM_{2.5}$ category, are the most damaging in terms of their health impact, there is as yet no separate regulatory standard for these because current filtering technology is incapable of capturing such tiny particles, making them virtually impossible to measure (Russell and Brunekreef, 2009).

Sulfur Dioxide (SO_2)

The major source of this colorless pollutant gas is fuel combustion, inasmuch as sulfur is present to a greater or lesser degree as an impurity in coal and fuel oil. When these sulfur-containing fuels are burned, the sulfur is oxidized to form SO_2. By itself sulfur dioxide is not particularly harmful, but it readily reacts with water vapor in the atmosphere to form other sulfur compounds such as sulfuric acid, sulfates, and sulfites that irritate the respiratory system, corrode metals and statuary, harm textiles, impair visibility, and kill or stunt the growth of plants. Sulfur dioxide is also one of the main precursors of acid precipitation, a subject that will be dealt with in greater detail later in this chapter.

Carbon Monoxide (CO)

No other pollutant gas is found at such high concentrations in the urban atmosphere as is carbon monoxide—extremely toxic, odorless, and colorless. Any type of incomplete combustion produces CO, but the most significant source in terms of urban air pollution is automobile emissions; according to EPA, in 2005 on-road vehicles and non-road equipment together accounted for 84% of all CO emissions to the ambient air (in indoor situations, cigarette smoking is a major source of carbon monoxide).

When inhaled, CO binds to hemoglobin in the blood, displacing oxygen and thereby reducing the amount of oxygen carried in the bloodstream to the various body tissues. For this reason, carbon monoxide can provoke severe reactions among heart patients. Studies have shown that more deaths among heart attack victims occur during periods of high CO concentrations than at other times. Patients suffering from angina pectoris, a coronary disease in which there is an insufficient supply of oxygen to the heart during exercise, experience a much more rapid onset of pain during periods of increased carbon monoxide pollution. Depending on the concentration of CO in the air and the length of exposure, inhalation of carbon monoxide can result in adverse health effects ranging from mild headaches or dizziness at relatively low levels of exposure to death at high levels. Fortunately, the health effects of short-term carbon monoxide exposure are reversible, but people who work for many hours in areas of heavy traffic (e.g., police officers, toll collectors, parking garage attendants) are obviously receiving substantial doses. Some evidence indicates that blood absorption of CO slows down mental processes and reaction time, raising the suspicion that many rush-hour traffic accidents can be at least partially attributed to low-level carbon monoxide poisoning.

Nitrogen Oxides (NO_x)

Consisting primarily of nitric oxide (NO) and nitrogen dioxide (NO_2), oxides of nitrogen are formed when combustion occurs at very high temperatures. Nitrogen oxides enter the atmosphere in approximately equal amounts from auto emissions and power plants (in urban areas, cars are generally the predominant source of NO_x emissions). Nitrogen dioxide is the only criteria pollutant gas that is colored. The yellow-brown "smoggy" appearance typical of southern California on bad days is due to the high concentrations of NO_2 in the air. At high levels of pollution, nitrogen dioxide has a pungent, sweetish odor. When present in the high concentrations that sometimes occur indoors in the vicinity of gas stoves or other sources of combustion, NO_2 can provoke shortness of breath or coughing; children living in such environments suffer an enhanced risk of respiratory disease. Nitrogen dioxide also stunts plant growth and visibly damages leaves. It reduces visibility and, like sulfur dioxide, contributes to the formation of acid rain.

Ozone (O_3)

The main constituent of a group of chemical compounds known as **photochemical oxidants**, ozone and such fellow travelers as peroxyacetylnitrate (PAN) and various aldehydes are considered to be auto-associated pollutants even though they are not emitted directly from the tailpipe into the atmosphere. Instead, these substances form in a complex series of chemical reactions when nitrogen dioxide and **volatile organic compounds (VOCs)**, especially certain hydrocarbons from both auto exhausts and a variety of stationary sources, react with oxygen and sunlight to produce a witch's brew of chemicals dubbed **photochemical smog**. First observed in the Los Angeles area in the 1940s (the bright sunlight, warm temperatures, frequent atmospheric inversions, and heavy traffic make southern California particularly well-suited for photochemical smog formation), photochemical smog is now often observed in other cities as well, especially on bright summer days ("ozone season" is considered to extend from May 1 through September 30). Ground-level ozone, an early and continuing product of the photochemical smog reaction, is the chemical whose presence is used to measure the oxidant level of the atmosphere at any given time. This pungent, colorless gas irritates the mucous membranes of the respiratory system, causing coughing, choking, and reduced lung capacity. Heart patients, asthmatics, and those suffering from bronchitis or emphysema are at special risk during periods of high O_3 levels; research results also suggest that

Table 13-1   Change in Annual Emissions per Source Category (1990 vs. 2008) (thousand tons)

Source Category	$PM_{2.5}$	PM_{10}	SO_2	NO_x	VOC	CO	Pb
Stationary Fuel Combustion	−773	−813	−10,490	−5,323	+445	−228	−0.42
Industrial and Other Processes	−343	−217	−731	−144	−3,150	−442	−2.80
Highway Vehicles	−213	−216	−439	−4,386	−5,970	−71,389	−0.42
Non-road Mobile	−17	−24	+85	+474	−76	−3,411	−0.27
Total Change (thousand tons)	−1,346	−1,270	−11,575	−9,379	−8,751	−75,470	−3.91
Percent Change (1990 vs. 2008)	−58%	−39%	−50%	−36%	−35%	−53%	−79%

Source: *Our Nation's Air: Status and Trends Through 2008*. EPA-454/R-09-002, February 2010.

ozone exposure may contribute to the growing incidence of type 1 diabetes (Dahlquist and Hustonen, 1994).

Ozone also cracks rubber, deteriorates fabrics, and causes paint to fade. The eye irritation and watery eyes frequently experienced during smog episodes is caused both by ozone and by PAN. Plant growth is severely impacted by ground-level ozone; either alone or in combination with SO_2 and NO_2, ozone accounts for about 90% of annual U.S. crop losses due to air pollution. Symptoms of ozone damage are most visible between the veins on the upper surface of leaves, exemplified by tiny flecks (irregular light tan spots) or small stipples (darkly pigmented areas); alternatively, in some plant species a bronzing or reddening of the leaf surface is characteristic of ozone injury. Among evergreen species such as pine, needle tips turn yellow and die. Premature leaf or needle drop is a typical consequence of such damage. Less visible but equally harmful, ground-level ozone interferes with a plant's ability to photosynthesize, thereby reducing plant biomass and lowering crop yields.

Lead (Pb)

The adverse impact of this toxic metal on the intellectual development of children (see chapter 7) caused it to be added to the list of criteria pollutants when the Clean Air Act was reauthorized in 1977. Since most airborne lead can be traced to automobile emissions, the major control strategy for this pollutant was to phase out the use of leaded gasoline, a process completed in the United States by the end of 1995. Today the vast majority of the world's nations have similarly banned the use of leaded gasoline and levels of this pollutant in the ambient air have correspondingly plummeted.

Hazardous Air Pollutants (HAPs)

In addition to the criteria air pollutants, a large number of less common, but much more hazardous, chemicals are released into the atmosphere from a wide range of industries and manufacturing processes, as well as from motor vehicles. Although the sources of these emissions are more localized than are those of the criteria pollutants, the fact that many of them are either toxic or carcinogenic suggests that they deserve special attention. In 1970 Congress directed the EPA to develop a list of industrial air pollutants that can cause serious health damage even at relatively low concentrations and to establish protective emission standards for those so listed. No deadline date for listing substances as hazardous was mandated, however, and implementation of the congressional directive was exceedingly slow.

By 1990, twenty years after the original congressional mandate, only eight toxic air pollutants had been listed—**asbestos, mercury, beryllium, benzene, vinyl chloride, arsenic, radionuclides, and coke oven emissions**—and standards had been set only for the first seven (a standard for coke oven emissions was finally promulgated in 1993). Frustrated with this snail's pace, environmentalists for years had prodded EPA to speed up the evaluation process, urging the agency to list and set standards for additional toxic air pollutants that pose a special hazard to public health. In 1986, congressional passage of the Emergency Planning and Community Right-to-Know Act (Superfund Amendments and Reauthorization Act, commonly referred to as SARA Title III), prompted by a tragic chemical accident in Bhopal, India two years earlier, led to heightened public awareness of the toxic threats lurking in hundreds of communities across the nation. By requiring that manufacturers disclose information on the kinds and amounts of toxic pollutants they discharge into the local environment each year, this law prompted demands from community activists and the media for tighter controls on health-threatening emissions. In turn, the necessity of revealing data that might alarm previously complacent local residents prompted voluntary emissions reductions by a number of firms eager to maintain a positive corporate image. In 1990 Congress responded to the mounting pressure to "do something" about air toxics by identifying 189 chemicals that it ordered EPA to regulate as hazardous air pollutants and by establishing comprehensive, technology-based controls for dealing with this largely ignored public health threat; two of the original air toxics have now been delisted—caprolactam in 1996 and ethylene glycol mono-butyl ether (EGBE) in 2004—leaving 187 regulated HAPs. The current regulatory approach to controlling air toxics will be discussed in greater detail later in this chapter.

IMPACT OF AIR POLLUTION ON HUMAN HEALTH

If dirty skyscrapers or impaired views were the only consequence of polluted air, concern about the phenomenon would undoubtedly be considerably less than it is today. The unfortunate fact is, however, that over the years there has been a steadily growing mass of evidence indicating that the quality of the air we breathe has a measurable impact on human health.

Some of the ill effects of air pollution have, of course, been known for a long time: Los Angelenos knowingly curse the smog as they wipe tears from their burning eyes; motorists roll up their car windows in heavy traffic, trying to avert a carbon monoxide-induced headache; and asthmatics brace for an attack when the weather forecaster proclaims an ozone alert. For many years, discomforts such as these were shrugged off as necessary consequences of economic growth. Only after several air pollution disasters made world headlines did the general public begin to realize the extent of the threat. In each case, already-bad air quality was made much worse by an atmospheric anomaly known as an **inversion**—a condition where a layer of cool surface air is trapped by an overlying layer of warmer air. This situation is a reversal of normal conditions in which the air is in a constant state of flux, with air near the earth's surface rising as it warms, carrying with it pollutant particles and gases that are gradually dispersed. During an inversion the cool air, being heavier than the air above, is unable to rise and mix, remaining atypically stable. If the inversion layer remains in place for several days, pollutant emissions within the affected area have nowhere to escape and can accumulate to health-threatening concentrations.

This is precisely what happened in Belgium's heavily industrialized Meuse River Valley in 1934 when 60 people died of the foul air during a three-day inversion; thousands of others fell seriously ill, coughing and gasping for breath. In the fall of 1948, the small Pennsylvania town of Donora, near Pittsburgh, similarly fell victim to a five-day inversion. Situated in a valley characterized by smokestack industries, Donora was enveloped in a cold, damp blanket of murky air permeated with the smell of sulfur. During this time, fully 42% of the town's population suffered eye, nose, and throat irritation; chest pains; coughing; difficulty in breathing; headaches; nausea; and vomiting. When the inversion finally lifted, it was found that 20 people had died during the period (Waldbott, 1978). Most notorious of all was London's famous killer smog of 1952. For a period of five days shortly before Christmas, emissions from coal-burning home fireplaces, factories, and motor vehicles accumulated to 10 times their usual levels. Even at noon the pervading gloom was so thick that car-train collisions were common and cine-

mas were forced to close because the projector beam from the back of the theater couldn't reach the screen. When the inversion layer finally lifted, officials were shocked to discover the grim health toll of this episode— 4,000 excess deaths, most of them among elderly sufferers of heart or respiratory diseases (Goldstein and Goldstein, 2002).

These dramatic examples of pollution-induced death and disease were all associated with levels of air contamination considerably worse than those experienced by urban residents in developed countries today, even those living in visibly smoggy cities (the same cannot be said, however, for residents of rapidly industrializing areas of China, India, and elsewhere in the developing world where chokingly high levels of air pollution are taking a deadly toll on human health). For many years researchers have been trying to determine whether air pollution at levels typically encountered in metropolitan areas of Europe and North America can, by itself, increase mortality and morbidity rates and, if so, which specific pollutants pose the greatest hazard. Results obtained from a number of studies now confirm fears long suspected—air pollution kills, and at levels of pollutant concentration well within the legally allowable limits established by the NAAQS.

The Air Pollution-Health Connection

Investigations aimed at determining precise cause-and-effect relationships linking given levels of pollution with specific health responses have encountered numerous difficulties. One such problem relates to scientific ethics: it simply isn't acceptable to expose the most vulnerable members of society—children, the elderly, asthmatics, etc.—to high levels of air pollution and then watch to see what happens to them. In addition, because urban air contains so many different pollutants, deter-

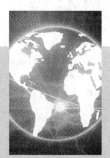

· · · · · · · 13–1 · · · · · · ·

Childhood Asthma and Air Pollution

Concerned parents have reason to be alarmed; since 1980 the prevalence of childhood asthma in the United States has risen by over 75%, making it the most prevalent chronic ailment among young people in this country. CDC reports that 13% of all American children under the age of 18 have been diagnosed with the disease, with African-American children experiencing disproportionately high rates. Prevalence of asthma is even higher elsewhere in the world, with Australia, New Zealand, Ireland, and the United Kingdom all experiencing rates of asthma that exceed those in the U.S. (IOM, 2000). Nor is the condition a health threat only to children; the elderly are also considered a high-risk group for asthma. The National Center for Health Statistics estimates that over 31 million Americans will be diagnosed with asthma at some point during their lifetime. In the majority of cases, however, symptoms of asthma first become manifest during early childhood, with diagnosis of the disease dependent on the frequent recurrence of symptoms over a period of time.

Asthma is a chronic, incurable lung disorder in which the muscles surrounding the airways constrict and become inflamed. The condition is characterized by reduced airflow to the alveoli, resulting in breathing problems. Persons suffering from asthma typically experience a tightness in the chest, accompanied by coughing, wheezing, and an inability to catch breath. In very severe cases, death may result; close to 200,000 American children are hospitalized each year due to asthma attacks and approximately 2 million emergency room visits annually are attributed to asthma. CDC estimates that childhood asthma can be blamed for 14 million lost school days each year (as well as 12 million lost work days by asthmatic adults) and for restrictions on physical activities of young sufferers.

The causes of asthma are complex and remain the focus of scientific study. Research has shown that a number of environmental factors, either alone or through synergistic interactions, can precipitate asthma attacks in persons who are genetically predisposed to the disease. Since the genetic makeup of the population obviously hasn't changed radically during the past 40 years of rising asthma rates, it is assumed that the increasing prevalence of the disorder must be due to some as-yet unidentified environmental change (IOM, 2000). Among the environmental factors known to provoke asthma attacks are cigarette smoke, pollen and other allergens, household dust mites, cockroach droppings, mold, wood smoke, and cold weather. Outdoor air pollution also has a significant impact on childhood asthma; studies have shown that air pollution increases both the frequency and severity of asthma attacks and reveal that asthmatic children are 40% more likely to have an attack on days when the levels of ambient air contaminants are high.

Particulates are among the most problematic of the criteria pollutants for those afflicted with asthma. As outdoor concentrations of particulates rise, both the prevalence and the severity of asthma increase. Studies have shown that brief periods of exposure to high particulate levels are more likely to bring on an attack of asthma in children than is more prolonged exposure to moderately elevated levels. Asthmatic children exposed to air contaminated with high levels of fine particulates tend to use more medications and have an increased frequency of emergency room visits, hospital admissions, and premature death. Ground-level ozone also aggravates the symptoms of asthma in children and is, in fact, the criteria pollutant most frequently linked to newly diagnosed cases of the disease. Sulfur dioxide also poses a risk to those with asthma; one study that exposed strenuously exercising asthmatics to SO_2 for a period of ten minutes revealed that the volunteers' symptoms became more severe than usual.

Indoor air pollution may be an even more important factor in triggering asthma attacks than outdoor pollution, in part because people today spend 85–90% of their time inside their homes, schools, workplaces, shopping centers, or vehicles—and because indoor air is often more contaminated than that outside. Among indoor air pollutants with the greatest impact on asthmatic children is tobacco smoke, which not only increases the severity of childhood asthma, but also may cause the disease. The impact is greatest if a child's mother smokes; research has shown that the more a mother smokes, the more likely it is that her child will become asthmatic, a risk that more than doubles for children of heavy smokers. Medical researchers have demonstrated that asthmatic children exposed to significant levels of second-hand smoke suffer 70–80% more attacks and hospital admissions than children subjected to little or no such exposure, and often experience marked improvement if their parents stop smoking. Unfortunately, the U.S. Surgeon General reported in 2007 that close to 60% of American children ages 3–11 were regularly exposed to second-hand tobacco smoke in their homes.

Indoor emissions of volatile organic compounds such as paint fumes, fragrances added to various products, and formaldehyde can all contribute to asthma-like symptoms, especially when tobacco smoke is also present. Nitrogen dioxide, if not properly vented from gas stoves, has been shown to cause respiratory problems and reduced lung function among asthmatic and healthy children alike.

Aside from asthma's grievous toll in terms of human suffering, death, and disability, still-rising rates of the disease represent an enormous financial burden. A study conducted in 2002 estimated the costs of childhood asthma caused by environmental contaminants at $2 billion per year. The enormous—and growing—health and economic consequences of pollution-induced asthma make ongoing efforts to reduce both indoor and outdoor levels of air pollution an environmental health priority (Wargo, 2009).

mining with certainty *which* pollutant at *what level* is causing an observed health effect has been problematic. The likelihood that synergistic effects play a role in determining the response to polluted air is a further complicating factor, as is the possibility of contributory occupational exposure. Particularly vexing to researchers has been the overwhelming influence of cigarette smoking—i.e., how much is due to the pollutants in city air and how much is due to self-inflicted tobacco pollutants? In spite of these challenges, a substantial body of evidence documenting the health effects of air pollutants has been compiled by researchers in many parts of the world. Epidemiological data collected in the United States since the 1970s supports environmentalists' contention that air pollution can be deadly. An estimated 2–3% of all deaths in the U.S. each year are attributed to air pollution-induced respiratory or cardiovascular disease. In Europe, according to a World Health Organization (WHO) report released in 2003, urban air pollution reduces life expectancy more than any other environmental risk factor. WHO estimates that long-term exposure to air contaminants from road traffic alone is responsible for 80,000 European deaths each year.

Mortality due to foul air is even higher in cities of the developing world, where soaring rates of urbanization, rapid industrial development, proliferation of motor vehicles, and lack of effective pollution control programs combine to produce far worse air quality than anything experienced by the industrialized nations. Air pollution is thought to be the primary cause of nearly half of all respiratory ailments in China (Brunekreef and Holgate, 2002) and some researchers estimate that every year as many as 1 million premature deaths in that country are the result of airborne particulate pollutants (Wang et al., 2009). Very few developing countries possess the data required to evaluate air pollution's public health impact, but observers have no doubt the toll is significant. Worldwide, WHO estimates that approximately 2 million deaths each year can be attributed to air contaminants, both indoors and outdoors, providing ample justification for government regulation of air pollution in order to protect human health.

Major Health Effects

Not surprisingly, air pollution's major impact on health is the result of irritants acting on the respiratory tract. Not all air pollutants are equally harmful, however. Research indicates that the most serious health effects can be attributed to elevated levels of very fine particulates—those with an aerodynamic diameter of 2.5 micrometers or less—and especially to ultrafines, particles so tiny that when they are inhaled deeply into the lungs they may pass directly into the bloodstream. While

the exact mechanism by which they increase the risk of heart attack and stroke is still under investigation, ultrafine particles are thought to provoke systemic inflammation and oxidative stress, leading to plaque buildup and clogged arteries. These tiniest aerosols have no threshold level below which they don't present a health risk; in recent years numerous studies have implicated ultrafine particles in hundreds of thousands of premature deaths, even in places where their concentrations don't violate air quality standards (Raloff, 2009). Particulate pollutants, along with ozone and sulfate particles, have been more directly associated with heightened risk of death and disease than have any other contaminants in the ambient air; since the mid-1990s as concentrations of the other criteria air pollutants—CO, NO_x, SO_2, and Pb—steadily declined, particulates and ozone have become the prime focus regarding health impacts of air pollution. Elevated levels of particulates alone are now said to cause as many premature deaths worldwide as overweight and obesity. In Europe, researchers estimate that exposure to airborne fine particulates has reduced life expectancy by an average of 9 months (Russell and Brunekreef, 2009), while some U.S. studies suggest a 1–2 year shortening of life expectancy at prevalent levels of $PM_{2.5}$ exposure (Brunekreef and Holgate, 2002).

In regards to lung cancer specifically, mortality risk has been shown to rise by 8% for every 10 $\mu g/m^3$ increase in concentrations of fine particulate pollution (Pope et al., 2002). Epidemiologic studies conducted from 1975–1988 in six U.S. cities convincingly demonstrated the link between high levels of particulate air pollution and death due to lung cancer, respiratory disease, and heart ailments—even after controlling for individual risk factors such as smoking, occupational exposure, excessive weight gain, and so on. The correlation was most dramatically evident in Steubenville, Ohio, the most polluted city in the survey group, where adjusted mortality rates were 26% higher than in Portage, Wisconsin, the least polluted of the six communities studied. Interestingly, the link between pollution levels and increased risk of premature death was statistically significant only in relation to concentrations of fine, inhalable particles; varying levels of total suspended particulates, NO_x, SO_2, or ozone appeared to have no measurable impact on death rates—an indication that fine particulates constitute the most dangerous form of air pollution (Pope et al., 2002; Dockery et al., 1993).

Although it was long assumed that the observed premature mortality caused by both short-term and long-term exposure to particulates was due primarily to adverse respiratory effects, recent studies have shown that the impact of fine particulates on the cardiovascular system may be even more significant. California researchers demonstrated that the condition of elderly retirement home residents suffering from cardiovascular disease became noticeably worse on days when ultrafine particulate levels, generated by nearby traffic, were high. Even though the subjects of the study spent most of their time inside, with doors and windows closed, fine particulates were detected seeping into their rooms, provoking increases in blood pressure, inflammation, and cellular stress caused by oxidation. A similar study conducted in Germany that measured calcification of coronary arteries in a group of 4,500 middle-aged and elderly individuals found that the closer the subjects lived to a major road, the worse their arterial blockage. Diabetics seem to be a special risk group for cardiovascular problems associated with $PM_{2.5}$; epidemiologic studies have shown that diabetic adults exposed to traffic-generated fine particulates are at increased risk of heart attack due to impaired ability of their arteries to control blood flow (O'Neill et al., 2005).

Ground-level ozone can also be a killer. Scientists studying the impact of short-term outdoor ozone exposure in 95 U.S. metropolitan areas, home to 40% of all Americans, found that a 10-ppb increase in the previous week's ozone concentrations resulted in a statistically significant (0.52%) increase in daily mortality rates, primarily involving deaths due to cardiovascular or respiratory disease. The researchers calculated that for the 95 communities studied, ground-level ozone was responsible for an estimated 3,767 excess deaths each year—clear evidence that this common air pollutant is negatively affecting public health (Bell et al., 2004). Another study that tracked nearly 450,000 people in 96 U.S. metropolitan areas over a 20-year period found that people residing in cities with the highest ozone levels had a 25–30% greater risk of dying from respiratory disease than did those living in test areas with the lowest ozone concentrations (Jerrett et al., 2009).

Without question, air pollution can be deadly, especially for young children, the elderly, and persons with chronic cardiopulmonary disease. Despite notable improvements in air quality in recent decades, research has consistently shown that even current levels of air pollution increase the risk of premature death and hospitalization due to cardiovascular and respiratory ailments. These studies demonstrate a distinctly linear concentration-response relationship, with adverse health effects increasing in direct proportion to increasing concentrations of air contaminant, with no threshold of safety below which pollutants don't wreak some degree of health damage. Such findings make it imperative that we continue efforts to strengthen air quality standards, and assure that doing so will result in corresponding improvements in public health (Pope and Dockery, 2006).

POLLUTION CONTROL EFFORTS— THE CLEAN AIR ACT

As air quality in the United States steadily deteriorated during the 1950s and 1960s, it became increasingly evident that a broad-based, concerted effort was needed to deal with what was increasingly perceived as a problem of national scope. Until 1955 any attempts to regulate pollutant emissions were based solely at the local or state level; in that year the first federal law dealing exclusively with air pollution offered research and technical support to states and municipalities, thereby initiating a policy of federal-state-local partnership in the pollution control effort. By 1963, worsening levels of air pollution generated pressure for more effective action and led to passage of the first Clean Air Act, which gave the federal government a modest degree of authority to attack interstate air pollution problems and further increased the flow of federal dollars to state and local pollution control agencies.

By 1965 recognition of the automobile's contribution to air quality problems precipitated the first emission standards for automobiles (these standards, set for carbon monoxide and hydrocarbon emissions, took effect with 1968 model year cars). In 1967 the comprehensive Air Quality Act established a regional approach for establishing and enforcing air quality standards, though the main responsibility for control of emission sources (except for automobiles) remained at the state and local levels. This gradual transition from total reliance on state and local authorities to an increasing federal involvement grew out of general recognition that the problems of air pollution were so immense, diverse, and complex that environmental improvement could be achieved only through intergovernmental cooperation at all levels.

Although such laws were well-intentioned, they relied on voluntary compliance by states, many of which were reluctant to adopt strict controls for fear of driving away industry, thereby forfeiting jobs and tax revenues. As a result, pollutant levels continued to rise and public outcry mounted. By 1970, spurred by a grassroots demand that something be done about the environmental crisis facing the nation (a public outcry that culminated in the first national observance of "Earth Day" on April 22, 1970), an historic turning point was reached with congressional passage of the **Clean Air Act Amendments of 1970** (henceforth referred to here simply as the Clean Air Act). This landmark piece of environmental legislation provided the first comprehensive program for attacking air pollution on an effective nationwide basis.

The 1970 Clean Air Act established a number of legal precedents that form the basis of U.S. air quality control regulations in effect today—and, coincidentally, served as a model subsequently adopted by many other nations. Some minor modifications to the law, primarily in the form of deadline extensions for meeting stringent new auto emission requirements, were made in 1977. However, by the early 1980s, continuing problems with high levels of certain auto-related pollutants, complaints that portions of the act had not been implemented with sufficient vigor, and the emergence of acid rain as a troublesome new issue not even addressed by the 1970 mandate, gave rise to demands from the environmental community for changes that would make the Clean Air Act both stronger and more comprehensive. At the same time, the new Reagan administration viewed its mission as one of dismantling many of the environmental programs enacted during the 1970s. Although Congress refused to approve most of the changes proposed, decisions by the Reagan EPA to waive implementation of certain regulations deemed burdensome to industry resulted in a gradual reversal of air quality improvements. On the most contentious issue of all—what to do about acid rain—the Reagan White House adamantly opposed any new initiatives other than further study, remaining steadfastly unconvinced that the phenomenon posed any real problems.

As a result of this impasse, efforts to reauthorize the Clean Air Act as required by law languished throughout the 1980s, in spite of continued public support for improving air quality. The legislative logjam remained unbroken until 1988 when newly elected President George H. W. Bush, citing his desire to be remembered as the "environmental president," threw his active support behind efforts to resolve the clean air controversy. Within Congress the clash among regional interests and competing ideologies frequently threatened to derail negotiations, but eventually, the differences were resolved. Passage of the Clean Air Act Amendments of 1990, signed into law by President Bush in November of that year, marked a significant strengthening of U.S. air quality legislation. The amendments expanded the scope of regulatory requirements, addressed new issues ignored by the 1970 act, and made the law more consistent with other environmental mandates. Some of the most significant provisions of the Clean Air Act are discussed in the following paragraphs.

National Ambient Air Quality Standards (NAAQS)

In setting national ambient air quality standards for the six criteria air pollutants, the EPA reviews the existing medical and scientific literature to establish **primary standards** at levels intended to safeguard human health, allowing a margin of safety to protect more vulnerable segments of the population such as young children, asthmatics, and the elderly. These standards are subject to periodic revision as new data become available. The Clean Air Act differs from other major environmental laws in requiring that primary standards be set solely on the basis of protecting health, without regard for the costs of pollution control.

The primary standards were originally mandated to be attained by 1975, with penalties (e.g., bans on the construction of new sources of pollution, cut-off of federal highway construction funds, etc.) to be imposed on those **nonattainment areas** that failed to bring their pollution levels into conformance with the NAAQS. Twenty years after passage of the original legislation, numerous urban areas were still in violation of the primary standard for ozone, historically the most difficult-to-control pollutant, and many cities also exceeded the standard for carbon monoxide as well. Therefore, with the enactment of the 1990 amendments, Congress revised its approach for dealing with nonattainment areas. Under the current program, regions still in violation of any of the air quality standards are classified according to the seriousness of their pollution problems (categories range from "marginal" to "extreme"), and are given varying amounts of time—anywhere from 3 to 20 years, depending on the severity of nonattainment—to comply with the standards. The higher the pollution levels, the more regulatory steps states must take in dealing with the problem. The 1990 amendments further require specified annual emission reduction goals to ensure steady progress toward full compliance, lest affected areas postpone action until deadlines are imminent.

The specific numerical standard set for each of the criteria air pollutants is, of course, subject to change as new scientific findings clarify their human health and environmental impacts. In June 2010, for the first time in almost 40 years, EPA issued revised SO_2 emissions standards. Citing the link between elevated concentrations of sulfur dioxide and a wide range of human health problems, the agency changed its previous SO_2 standard of no more than 140 parts per billion (ppb) averaged over a 24-hour period to a maximum of 75 ppb, measured hourly (the one-hour measuring period is regarded as more significant in terms of protecting sensitive individuals against spikes in short-term exposure). As this book goes to press, the EPA is reviewing public comments on a proposed strengthening of the primary standard for ground-level ozone, from the 0.075 ppm standard set in 2008 (a standard that had been lowered from 0.084 ppm set in 1997) to no more than 0.060–0.070 ppm. EPA contends that the present limit on ozone is insufficiently protective of human health and bolsters its arguments with recent research suggesting that stricter standards could prevent as many as 12,000 premature deaths each year, as well as thousands of cases of respiratory ailments and nonfatal heart attacks. The agency is expected to issue its final rule by January 2011, with the new requirements to be phased in over the next 20 years. If the proposed new standard is finalized, as expected, hundreds of counties that were in compliance with the 0.075 ppm standard will find themselves scrambling to meet—and pay for—the more stringent requirements. Of the 675 counties that currently monitor ozone levels, 322 fail to meet the 0.075 ppm standard; if 0.070 ppm were the standard, 515 counties would be in violation of the limit; and fully 650 of the 675 would fail to meet a standard of 0.060 ppm! Tighter limits for fine particulates are also under review as a result of a federal appeals court ruling that levels set by the EPA in 2006 were insufficiently protective.

In addition to the primary standards, EPA was told to set more stringent **secondary standards** that would promote human welfare by protecting agricultural crops, livestock, property, and the environment in general. No timetable for compliance with secondary standards has been set. However, since the secondary standards set by the EPA are, in most cases, identical to the primary standards, the lack of a deadline date is largely irrelevant.

It is difficult to overemphasize the importance of national (as opposed to state or local) air quality standards. As experience prior to 1970 amply demonstrated, drifting air pollutants pay little heed to political boundaries, a fact that largely nullified feeble state attempts to improve air quality within their own borders. States or cities that tried to impose emission controls on polluters within their jurisdictions found that air quality gains were minimal due to airborne pollutants arriving from less concerned states upwind. Threats by polluting industries to leave a particular state and relocate in a more lenient regulatory environment made many state legislatures extremely reluctant to get tough with polluters.

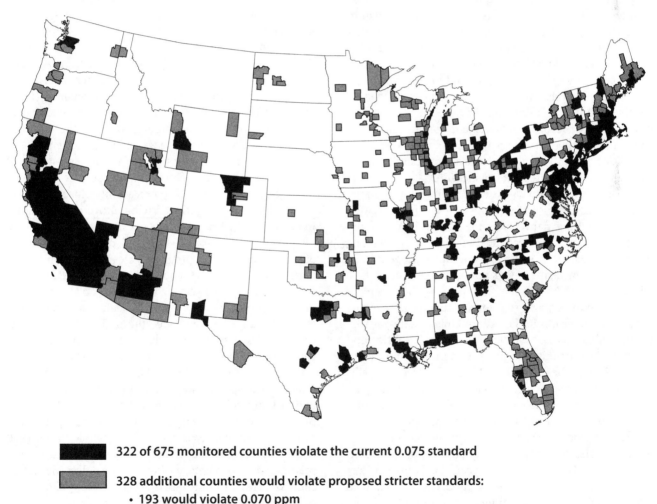

■ 322 of 675 monitored counties violate the current 0.075 standard

▨ 328 additional counties would violate proposed stricter standards:
- 193 would violate 0.070 ppm
- 93 would violate 0.065 ppm
- 42 would violate 0.060 ppm

Source: EPA, "Ground-Level Ozone Standards," http://www.epa.gov/air/ozonepollution/pdfs/20100104maps.pdf.

Figure 13-1   Current and Projected Counties Violating Ground-Level Ozone Standards

Thus, establishing uniform nationwide standards has been a key element in improving air quality since 1970.

Emission Limitations for New Stationary Sources of Pollution

The intent in establishing **new source performance standards (NSPS)** for factories and power plants is to reduce pollutants at their point of origin by ensuring that pollution controls are built in when factories and plants are newly constructed or substantially modified. Note that this requirement is not retroactive; that is, polluting power plants or factories already in operation at the time the Clean Air Act was passed are not affected by the NSPS guidelines. However, if "grandfathered" facilities are expanded or rebuilt in ways that increase their total output of pollutants, under its **new source review (NSR)** program the Clean Air Act requires they obtain a permit specifying what emission levels must be met and requiring installation of modern pollution controls. The new source performance standards are set on an industry-by-industry basis, taking into account such factors as economic costs, energy requirements, and total environmental impacts such as waste generation and water quality considerations. The 1990 amendments strengthened this provision by adding a requirement for all stationary sources to obtain operating permits from the state regulatory agency, specifying allowable levels of pollutant emissions as well as required control measures.

In an effort to help 28 eastern and midwestern states, as well as the District of Columbia, meet their NAAQS for ozone and fine particulates, the EPA in 2005 promulgated its Clean Air Interstate Rule (CAIR), mandating drastic reductions in sulfur dioxide and nitrogen oxide emissions from coal-burning power plants. Set to take effect in 2009 for NO_x and in 2010 for SO_2, the new regulations were touted as a step toward substantially reducing premature deaths in the eastern United States, as well as providing marked visibility benefits by 2015 and beyond. This optimistic scenario was thrown into doubt in July 2008, when the U.S. District Court of Appeals ruled that EPA had exceeded its authority in setting up an emissions-trading system to reduce the pollutants in question and ordered the agency to rewrite the rules. Environmentalists criticized the Court's decision as a significant reversal of efforts to improve air quality in populous eastern states. In December of that year, the Court partially reversed its earlier ruling, allowing CAIR to remain in effect while EPA made program modifications to address the objections raised earlier. As a result, utilities in the 28 states subject to the Clean Air Interstate Rule are still required to achieve sizeable emissions reductions to meet the designated standards—at least until EPA finalizes a replacement rule, expected in July 2011.

Strict Emission Standards for Automobiles

Emission standards for automobiles and other mobile sources form an integral part of Clean Air Act requirements, inasmuch as motor vehicles spew more pollutant emissions into the outdoor air than any other single source. In the U.S., on-road vehicles contribute 51% of all CO emissions, 34% of NO_x, and 29% of VOCs in the ambient air; in traffic-congested metropolitan areas, the percentage of these pollutants originating from mobile sources often exceeds 90% (EPA, 2001; WRI, 1996). Detroit eventually settled upon modified engine design plus installation of catalytic converters as the chief means by which American car manufacturers would reduce emissions, and by 1981 new cars for the first time were able to meet Clean Air Act standards. According to the EPA, automobiles coming off the assembly lines today emit 90% less carbon monoxide, 80–90% fewer hydrocarbons, and 70% less nitrogen oxides than did cars manufactured prior to passage of the Clean Air Act.

To ensure that in-use vehicles continue to achieve these emission reductions, the 1990 Clean Air Act Amendments required that all nonattainment areas in the U.S. institute auto **inspection and maintenance (I/M)** programs to detect those vehicles whose emissions control systems are malfunctioning and to require that they be repaired. Since surveys have shown that the majority of mobile source emissions come from the worst 10% of vehicles on the road, such programs represent one of the most effective and least costly means of combating urban smog, short of prohibiting driving altogether. EPA estimates that a well-run I/M program can reduce levels of air pollution in a traffic-congested city by as much as 30%. Currently I/M programs are operating in all or parts of 39 states, some requiring annual inspections, others testing every two years.

Improvements in urban air quality resulting from reduced auto emissions since the mid-1970s have been dramatic, but a shift in vehicle preference among American motorists has, at least temporarily, slowed progress toward clean air goals. Since the late 1990s, the growing popularity of sports utility vehicles (SUVs), midsize vans, and pickup trucks has accounted for a steadily increasing proportion of vehicle miles traveled. This fact poses serious air quality concerns because a loophole in the 1970 Clean Air Act, enacted when these types of vehicles comprised a small percentage of the nation's fleet, permitted such vehicles to emit 2–3 times as much pollution as ordinary passenger cars. That situation is now being rectified; during the 1990s, emissions requirements for SUVs were gradually tightened and in 2004 the phase-in of even more stringent "Tier 2" standards began. Today, all new passenger cars, SUVs, and light trucks are subject to the same emissions requirements. Nevertheless, the

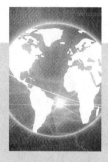

· · · · · · · 13-2 · · · · · · ·

Traffic-Related Air Pollution—An Insidious Killer

Although air quality in the United States has improved markedly since passage of the Clean Air Act, surveys have shown that almost every large American city continues to struggle with air pollution problems. In the developing world, conditions today are far worse, with chokingly high levels of smog, particulates, and other airborne contaminants an inescapable part of daily life in scores of megacities from Cairo to Beijing. As discussed elsewhere in this chapter, the sources of air pollutants are extremely diverse, but as decades of increasingly stringent controls in the U.S. and other industrialized nations have reduced emissions levels from stationary sources, the health-damaging impact of mobile sources has been attracting growing attention and research. So-called "traffic-related air pollution"—or TRAP—is now recognized as an insidious killer in many urban areas, as well as an exponentially growing threat in rapidly industrializing countries like India and China. Throughout the developing world, rising levels of affluence have resulted in an explosive increase in the number of passenger cars, heavy trucks, buses, and motorcycles, all spewing toxic emissions into the urban air. Observers in India shudder to imagine what traffic conditions will be like when the Tata Nano, billed as the world's cheapest car, begins full production and millions of current motorcycle owners trade in their two-wheelers for a new car!

Closer to home, the millions of vehicles traversing American streets and highways—as well as off-road equipment—continue to impact the health, and in some cases shorten the lives, of those who work in areas of heavy traffic or live near busy highways. During the 2000 Summer Olympics in Atlanta when auto traffic was restricted in the city center, hospital admissions for heart and respiratory problems declined sharply (Wargo, 2009). A time-series study conducted in the Netherlands revealed that residents along the main roads in Amsterdam have a significantly higher relative risk of death than do those living at some distance from these busy roadways; numerous other studies have shown a similar association between close-up exposure to traffic pollutants and enhanced risk of death or disease. Although the emergence of TRAP as a significant public health concern may seem paradoxical as levels of auto-related pollutants such as CO, PM_{10} and, to a lesser extent, NO_x have declined, a closer look reveals that the nature of vehicular air contaminants is changing.

Thanks to growing traffic volumes, ozone concentrations continue to rise in many cities, particularly on warm, sunny days. Moreover, ultrafine particulates—difficult to measure but increasingly recognized as a major health hazard—are taking a fearsome toll, especially for those living adjacent to busy roadways (Brunekreef and Holgate, 2002). Fine particulates present several challenges to those striving to reduce emissions further. Among these is the fact that a not-inconsiderable amount of $PM_{2.5}$ originates from non-tailpipe sources such as particles generated by wear and tear on brakes and tires, as well as from re-suspended dust. There are no regulatory controls on sources such as these and their volumes are likely to increase as the worldwide car fleet continues to grow and distances driven increase.

Diesel emissions constitute a much larger, and growing, part of the problem. Emitted by trucks, buses, ships, construction equipment, and some models of passenger cars, diesel exhaust is now associated with increased incidence of several respiratory diseases, allergies, heart attacks, diabetes, lung cancer, and premature death. In 1990 California designated diesel exhaust "a known human carcinogen" and, in 1998, an "air toxic." Scientists in California and elsewhere estimate that diesel emissions constitute close to 70% of the public's cumulative health risk due to toxic air pollutants. Although diesel provides more energy per gallon than gasoline, it is less refined and burns less efficiently, emitting a complex mixture of chemicals. These include hazardous VOCs such as benzene, formaldehyde, 1,3-butadiene, and polycyclic aromatic hydrocarbons, as well as high concentrations of ultrafine particles. Measurements of diesel exhaust particulates have shown that 94% are in the $PM_{2.5}$ category, while 92% are smaller than 1 micron in diameter.

Among vehicles, heavy engines pollute more than lighter ones and older vehicles are dirtier than newer models. Certain driving practices also cause an increase in diesel emissions; studies have shown that acceleration or deceleration releases more emissions than does maintenance of a steady speed, while driving uphill or downhill or carrying a heavy vehicle load increases the level of pollutant emissions. Idling of vehicles is particularly bad in terms of excess emissions (it also wastes fuel; a study conducted by the Department of Energy found that every year in the U.S., long-haul trucks that idle overnight consume over 838 million gallons of fuel). Fumes can be dangerously high when vehicles or equipment powered by diesel engines are used inside enclosed structures such as warehouses or sports arenas. In addition, diesel exhaust can be drawn inside buildings located near highways, posing an indoor air hazard. Similar problems can occur inside vehicles moving through heavy traffic. A study conducted by the California Air Resources Board found that levels of pollutants such as benzene, formaldehyde, toluene, and carbon monoxide frequently measured 2–10 times higher inside cars than at nearby outdoor fixed monitoring stations. The more congested the traffic, the higher the levels of air contaminants inside vehicles were; in cars directly behind diesel-powered trucks and buses, pollutant concentrations were double those recorded by roadside monitors.

An interesting study with special relevance to parents of the approximately 24 million American children who daily ride to and from home on diesel-powered school buses was conducted in Connecticut recently by Environment and Human Health, Inc. (EHHI), a nonprofit research group based in that state. Seeking to identify the cause for rising rates of childhood respiratory diseases, especially asthma, EHHI researchers fitted child participants with various pieces of monitoring equipment designed to measure air quality in their immediate vicinity every 10 seconds after leaving home in the morning until their return home in late afternoon. Expecting to find that children attending older schools were being subjected to such indoor air pollutants as molds, pesticides, or fumes from cleaning supplies, they were quite surprised to discover that none of these potential sources of exposure were present in troublesome amounts. To the contrary, the only time during the school day when the children were subjected to high concentrations of fine particulates, carbon, or VOCs was during the time they were riding on school buses; as soon as the bus engine started, the level of contaminants began to rise sharply.

That these pollutants were traffic-related was clearly demonstrated by the fact that particulate levels were higher when the buses were driving through heavy traffic than when they were traveling on roads with no other diesel vehicles. Similarly, particulate levels quickly shot up when the bus followed close behind another diesel vehicle, such as it routinely did at the end of the school day when a caravan of buses pulled away from the building. At such times when buses are queued, their engines idling as they pick up or drop off students, their tailpipes may be only 6 feet away from the open door of the next bus in line. Monitors showed that in these situations, particulates inside the bus can quickly soar 10–15 times above background levels, with exhaust fumes readily detectable by odor and a burning sensation in the throat. In some locations, these exhaust fumes may also be pulled into the adjacent school building through air-intake vents. These findings are disquieting because high levels of exposure to these pollutants present a serious health risk to children, especially to those already predisposed to respiratory ailments. Transportation via bus is a regular, unavoidable, and lengthy part of the school day for millions of children—one hour/day, 180 days/year on average, with even lengthier transportation times for rural children or those with disabilities who must attend regional schools.

While the problem is real, the solutions aren't cheap. In 2006 California approved spending $200 million to replace or retrofit older buses; the EPA has provided some state grants to do the same thing. Fines collected from several major corporations for federal air quality violations have been spent on programs to retrofit school buses. Mandates to end unnecessary idling could have a major impact on curtailing emissions; at least 21 states have now passed laws limiting school bus idling to 3 minutes. Stringent rules limiting the sulfur content of diesel fuel that went into effect in 2010 will bring significant public health benefits, as did federal standards requiring that trucks and buses manufactured since 2006 have engines that reduce PM emissions by 90% below those of earlier models; NO_x emissions must be slashed 95% below their previous levels by 2010. Welcome as these requirements are, the long lifespan of existing diesel engines means it could be several decades before all the older, more-polluting vehicles are retired. The problem is even more acute, of course, in countries where traffic volume is booming and where, thanks to the higher price of gasoline, diesel-powered vehicles comprise an even larger proportion of the car fleet. Traffic-related air pollution will undoubtedly remain a public health issue for the foreseeable future (Wargo, 2009).

legacy of past discrepancies in allowable emissions will persist for many years until most of the current SUV fleet is no longer on the road (Plotkin, 2004).

While reducing tailpipe emissions has been a key component of efforts to curb mobile source pollution, other approaches are being pursued as well. Altering the relative proportions of the ingredients used in making gasoline can have a major impact in reducing emissions of ozone-forming chemicals and toxic air pollutants such as benzene. Recognizing the pollution-reducing potential of such reconfigured fuels, the 1990 amendments to the Clean Air Act mandated the use of so-called **reformulated gasoline** in the major metropolitan areas experiencing the most severe ozone problems. In addition, service stations in such areas were told to install vapor recovery systems on gasoline pumps to capture hydrocarbons that would otherwise be released during refueling. Cities in violation of carbon monoxide standards were required to use reformulated gasoline containing oxygen additives ("oxygenates") during winter months to increase the combustion efficiency of gasoline, thereby reducing tailpipe emissions of CO.

A major step forward in improving urban air quality was taken in May 2004, with the adoption of tough new regulations on diesel fuel. Prompted by the recognition that emissions from diesel-powered bulldozers, tractors, locomotives, barges, and other off-road vehicles emit more particulates than all the cars, trucks, and buses on American streets and highways, EPA mandated drastic reductions in the sulfur content of diesel fuel, from 3,400 ppm in 2004 to 15 ppm in 2010, for all off-road diesel vehicles except boats and locomotives, which have two additional years to comply with the new standard. Strict regulations for diesel-fueled trucks and buses were adopted in 2000 and took effect in 2007. Health experts, heralding EPA's action, estimate that the new rules curbing diesel emissions will prevent thousands of premature deaths and heart attacks every year.

Unfortunately, even with extremely tight standards for tailpipe emissions and improved fuel economy, the sheer increase in the number of cars on the road will pose an enormous air quality challenge in the years ahead. In 2007 the Federal Highway Administration reported that the U.S. car fleet that year exceeded 246 million, and numbers continue to climb; worldwide, the total is close to one billion—and growing rapidly. Thanks to suburban sprawl, individual cars are being driven more miles than in decades past and their owners now tend to drive them longer before purchasing new, less-polluting models (Wargo, 2009). All these factors virtually guarantee a reversal of air quality gains in the years ahead unless a radically different approach to curbing emissions is adopted. All the more reason to root for a swift transition to electric cars—powered by solar and wind energy!

Regulation of Hazardous Air Pollutants through Technology-Based Controls

Under the 1990 Clean Air Act Amendments, EPA was told to adopt a technology- and performance-based approach to reducing air toxics emissions. In response, the agency developed **maximum achievable control technology (MACT)** standards for each group of industrial emitter (source category). These standards are based on levels of control already being accomplished by the best-performing, most proactive industrial plants within that source category. In most cases, MACT standards take the form of a specified percent reduction in emissions or a concentration limit that regulated sources must achieve. Facilities are not mandated to use any specific type of pollution control equipment to achieve the required reductions but rather are allowed to employ whatever methods they find most cost-effective. Such methods might include redesigning industrial processes, installing new pollution control technologies, changing work practices, or capturing and recycling emissions.

It should be pointed out that the regulatory program described above pertains solely to stationary sources (e.g., refineries, power plants, factories, gas stations, dry cleaners), which collectively contribute close to 60% of all human-generated *toxic* air emissions. The remainder comes from mobile sources, including both on-road and off-road vehicles. EPA currently has programs in place that are expected to reduce 1996 levels of mobile source air toxics by more than a million tons by 2010. The new diesel fuel standards, emissions reduction requirements for off-road equipment, reformulated gasoline programs, and further progress in controlling standard tailpipe emissions should all contribute to a further lowering of ambient air toxics concentrations.

Acid Deposition Controls

Perhaps the most bitterly debated issue during the Clean Air Act reauthorization process was acid rain controls. Such controls became a part of federal clean air legislation only after passage of the 1990 amendments. The main focus of the Acid Rain Program has been to reduce 1980 levels of SO_2 emissions from electric power plants by approximately one-half; the current goal is to cap such emissions at 8.95 million tons annually, starting in 2010. NO_x, the other major contributor to acid rain formation, is also a target of emissions reduction efforts. The market-based cap-and-trade approach for reducing SO_2 emissions under the Acid Rain Program proved so successful that European signatories to the Kyoto Protocol have employed a similar strategy for reducing greenhouse gas emissions in an effort to mitigate climate change (see chapter 11).

The Clean Air Act provisions described here represent only the highlights of this extremely complex piece of legislation. Responsibility for implementing and enforcing the federal mandate falls primarily on the environmental agencies of state government, which must develop **State Implementation Plans (SIPs)** that detail strategies for compliance with Clean Air Act requirements. SIPs must list all the pollution sources within the state, estimating the quantities of each pollutant emitted annually, including both mobile and stationary sources. They must issue operating permits for stationary sources, as well as timetables for compliance, and must include some kind of transportation control strategy for dealing with auto-related pollutants in areas of heavy traffic. States must have their SIPs approved by the federal EPA or be working with the agency to improve a conditionally approved plan before they can issue a construction permit for any new polluting facility.

Enforcement provisions under the Clean Air Act, and the civil and criminal penalties for violation of the law, were significantly strengthened under the 1990 amendments. EPA can levy large financial penalties against facilities in violation of air quality requirements—penalties sufficiently stiff to cancel any economic benefits a firm might derive from delaying compliance. Criminal liability, which may be imposed on people *knowingly* violating the law, can result in fines, imprisonment, or both. The Clean Air Act gives citizens the right to file suit against polluters if the EPA fails to take action. To encourage "whistle-blowing" by people aware of Clean Air Act violations, Congress has authorized EPA to pay informants up to $10,000 for information leading to a civil penalty or criminal conviction (Bryner, 1993; "Easy Guide," 1993; Environmental Law Handbook, 1993).

GLOBAL AIR QUALITY TRENDS

Deadline dates have come and gone, hot summers are punctuated with ozone alerts, and a haze of smog still hovers over many of our cities. Nevertheless, 40 years after the Clean Air Act ushered in a "get tough" approach regarding air pollution control, overall trends in American skies are favorable. Elsewhere in the world, progress in cleaning up dirty air varies considerably from one country to another.

A comprehensive assessment of international air quality trends is complicated by the fact that little routine monitoring has been conducted in the developing nations that comprise the bulk of world population. Anecdotal information suggests that pollution levels in many developing world cities are far higher than in most industrialized countries—and getting steadily worse. In fact, according to the World Bank, in terms of particulate pol-

lutant levels, the ten worst cities in the world are all in developing countries. Many of their urban areas—Cairo, Delhi, Beijing, Shanghai, Mumbai, Hong Kong, Mexico City, to cite just a few—currently experience air pollution levels far higher than those considered "healthy" under World Health Organization guidelines. Some experts fear that air pollution is likely to take a heavier public health toll in the developing countries than it does in the industrialized world, even at similar levels of pollutant concentrations, simply because exposed populations in developing countries include a higher percentage of citizens living in poverty and suffering from malnutrition, both factors that increase the risk of ill health; they also include a much larger proportion of the very young—the most vulnerable age group in any population. As developing nations strive for rapid economic growth, environmental protection may be regarded as a luxury they can't yet afford, while air pollution is but one of many public health issues clamoring for attention (Romieu and Hernandez-Avila, 2003).

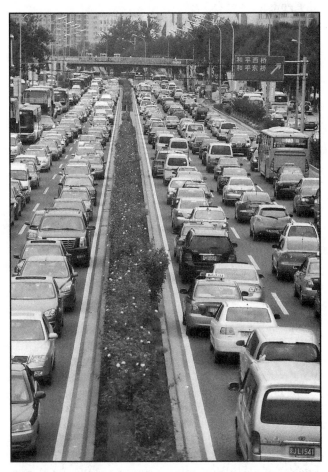

Rising affluence and an exponential increase in car ownership are producing legendary traffic jams in China, including one in August 2010 that lasted 10 days and stretched for 60 miles. [*Imaginechina via AP Images*]

Air quality problems originate from many sources, but are due primarily to exhaust fumes from the developing world's rapidly growing fleet of motor vehicles, as car ownership becomes synonymous with "the good life" for increasing millions of the newly affluent. In most developing countries, and particularly in Asia, the number of cars on the road is increasing exponentially and the fact that many are old, poorly maintained, and frequently fueled with adulterated gasoline ensures choking levels of pollutant emissions. Diesel-fueled heavy trucks are major contributors to street-level pollution, especially fine particles of lung-penetrating, sulfur-laden soot. Motorcycles and scooters also are proliferating at a record pace, especially in Asia where their highly polluting two-stroke engines further degrade the quality of urban air. Particulate pollution is an especially serious problem in developing world cities, with levels of PM_{10} regularly exceeding WHO guidelines. In Lanzhou, China—ranked among the world's 15 most polluted cities in terms of airborne particulates—the air is so foul that simply breathing is the equivalent of smoking a pack of cigarettes daily. In developing world cities characterized by heavy traffic and bright sunshine, ground-level ozone (a constituent of photochemical smog) is increasingly associated with an upswing in asthma attacks and respiratory problems. Ozone levels in Mexico City exceed WHO air quality guidelines as many as 300 days in a year. Concentrations of sulfur dioxide, another pollutant known as a respiratory irritant and a precursor of acid rain, are increasing in some developing countries, most notably China, as well as in Russia and eastern Europe, where plentiful supplies of high-sulfur coal are burned without pollution controls.

Some positive developments have become evident in recent years, however, as governments in developing countries begin to take the air pollution/health threat seriously. As mentioned previously, numerous Asian and Latin American nations have joined the developed countries in outlawing the use of leaded gasoline. Moreover, Brazil, Thailand, China, India, South Korea, Taiwan, Hong Kong, Singapore, and the Philippines now require all new cars to be equipped with catalytic converters. The entire bus fleet in India's capital city, Delhi, now runs on low-emission compressed natural gas (CNG), as do the city's thousands of three-wheeled auto-rickshaws. Taiwan has implemented an aggressive program to curb motorcycle emissions, inspiring several of its Asian neighbors to adopt similar programs (Walsh, 2003).

A less-successful approach to reducing auto-related pollutants imposed by Mexico City authorities in 1989 and subsequently adopted in Bogotá, Santiago, and Sao Paulo—as well as in Beijing prior to the 2008 Summer Olympics—has been to prohibit drivers from using their vehicles on certain days during the work week, depend-

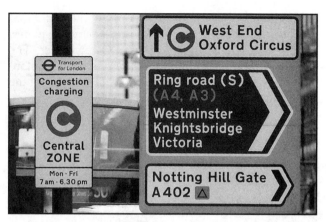

Megacities around the world are seeking ways to reduce the volume of traffic and auto-related pollutants in congested downtown areas; London's approach is to charge a fee to private motorists for entering central London and several surrounding neighborhoods. [*AP Photo/Alastair Grant*]

ing on the last digit of the car's license plate. In Mexico City, for example, automobiles whose license plate ends with a 5 or 6 can't be driven on Mondays. Although in theory the program should have resulted in nearly half a million fewer passenger cars on crowded Mexico City streets each day, monitoring stations around the city reported virtually no improvement in air quality. Subsequent investigations found that many drivers, rather than using mass transit on their car's "day off" as municipal authorities had assumed they would do, instead purchased a second car and made sure the last number on its license plate differed from that on the first car—thus giving owners the ability to drive their private vehicle each day of the week. Further undermining the program's pollution-reduction goal was the fact that most of these second cars were older, higher-polluting models brought into the city from other parts of the country; little wonder that air pollution continues to be a serious problem in Mexico City. In spite of growing evidence that policies to restrict driving have minimal impact in terms of improving air quality, in 2008 Mexico City expanded its driving restrictions to include Saturdays as well (Davis, 2008).

In contrast with the downward trends in air quality evident in many developing countries, in parts of the industrialized world emission levels from both stationary sources and motor vehicles have been drastically cut in recent years. While the United States was the pacesetter in air pollution control initiatives until the early 1980s, since then several European nations and Japan have equaled or surpassed the American record. Prompted by international treaty obligations, the European nations reduced sulfur dioxide emissions by 32% between 1980 and 1990 (McDonald, 1999). Japan requires state-of-the-art controls on automobiles, incinerators, power plants, and steel mills and is the only country in the world that compensates victims of air pollution—deriving monies for those so injured from a tax on SO_2 emissions. The Canadian province of Ontario has an ambient air standard for SO_2 considerably more stringent than that of the United States.

Germany, jolted out of complacency in the early 1980s by reports of widespread forest damage due to acid rain, has since implemented one of the world's most vigorous air quality control programs. Unlike the situation in the United States, where power plants in operation prior to promulgation of new source performance stan-

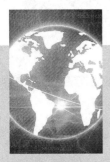

········ 13-3 ········

Measuring Air Pollution—How Representative Are the Data?

EPA's reported air quality trends in the United States present a reassuringly positive account of sharp reductions in pollution levels since 1980. According to the federal agency, by 2008 emissions of the six criteria air pollutants had declined by 54%, thanks to regulatory controls imposed under the Clean Air Act. The Agency derives this information from measurements collected from a network of monitoring sites across the country, most of them located in major metropolitan areas. However, while the nation's air is undeniably cleaner than it was three decades ago, flaws in the monitoring system itself suggest that actual air quality in some places may not be quite as good as the existing data suggest.

One reason for skepticism is the fact that the federal EPA requires states to monitor only a relative handful of pollutants at a very limited number of locations. In the entire United States, for example, there were just 64 sites that monitored for lead concentrations between 1990 and 2008, 151 for NO_2, 206 for CO, 266 for SO_2, 325 for PM_{10}, and 547 for ozone (EPA, 2010). Presumably these are the locations where the regulatory agency assumes those pollutants are likely to be problematic, but certainly the possibility exists of their presence elsewhere; in the absence of monitoring stations, it's unknown whether non-monitored areas are in compliance with the NAAQS or not. Aside from the six criteria air pollutants, few other known air toxics are subject to regulation or monitoring. There exists very limited monitoring data for most hazardous air pollutants—and virtually none for the 40% of HAPs from mobile sources. Currently only 27 sites nationwide monitor for a small number of air toxics, with sampling conducted over a 24-hour period, once every six days. Readings are taken of individual chemicals only, with no consideration of possible synergistic effects.

Although it's generally recognized that brief but intense levels of air pollution can cause severe health problems among certain segments of the population, such episodes can be masked by the common practice of averaging pollution levels over a 24-hour period and across urban/rural areas. In this way short-term or localized pollution episodes that violate existing standards become hidden in the data, resulting in the area's being listed as in compliance whereas the reality may be more ambiguous. In general, as the length of the averaging period increases, apparent pollution concentrations decline, thus conveying a sometimes misleading impression of safety.

A final qualification is that indoor air quality is not subject to regulation and hence is seldom monitored at all, yet the vast majority of people spend most of their time in buildings or vehicles where levels of air contamination may be far higher than they are outdoors—and far higher than they are in the vicinity of pollution monitoring devices. Data indicating substantial ambient air quality gains are totally irrelevant in terms of indoor air pollution (Wargo, 2009).

In spite of these data shortcomings, significant progress in cleaning up the nation's air has been made and is ongoing. Nevertheless, EPA admits that, as of 2008, more than 126 million people lived in counties that failed to meet the NAAQS for all 6 criteria air pollutants. If, as expected in early 2011, the O_3 standard is made more stringent, many more counties will be in violation. Achieving full compliance with national clean air goals remains a work in progress.

dards were exempted from the requirement for the best available technological controls, Germany has mandated the retrofitting of all its medium and large-size power plants, regardless of age, with state-of-the-art pollution control devices. The Swiss and Austrians, similarly concerned about dying forests, have adopted what may be the most stringent air quality regulations in the world, like Taiwan setting emission standards even for motorcycles.

In the United States, air quality in most parts of the country has improved significantly since passage of the Clean Air Act. In 2009 the EPA reported that total emissions of the six criteria air pollutants had dropped by 54% since 1980, in spite of the fact that during that same period U.S. population grew by 34%, energy consumption was up 29%, vehicle miles traveled rose 91%, and the nation's GDP increased by 126%. Progress in cleaning up the nation's air has not been uniform—concentrations of some pollutants have declined more than others and some regions of the country have experienced air quality trends better or worse than national averages would indicate. Of the criteria air pollutants, since 1980 ambient levels of lead have dropped by 92%, carbon monoxide by 79%, sulfur dioxide 71%, nitrogen dioxide 46%, and ozone (8-hour average) 25%. Trend data for particulate pollutants are more recent, showing that from 1990–2008 the 24-hour average for PM_{10} is down by 31% while that for $PM_{2.5}$ has declined by 20% since 2000.

Nevertheless, levels of the criteria pollutants in a number of urban areas still remain high enough to endanger the health of their residents. EPA, which gathers information on air concentrations of the various criteria pollutants from over 4,000 monitoring stations across the United States, reports that in 2008 over 126 million people lived in areas that still exceeded the NAAQS for at least one pollutant.

Ozone remains by far our most troublesome pollutant in terms of numbers of people affected. Concentrations of this pollutant have changed little since the mid-1990s and are now beginning to increase slightly in some areas. Air monitoring in national parks and federal lands outside urban areas shows that ozone pollution there hasn't declined since 1990 and has actually increased in six national

parks. Since emission levels of the major ozone precursors, NO_x and VOCs, are now tightly regulated and continue to decline, why ambient ozone levels haven't shown comparable reductions is puzzling, but is thought to be due to several factors. Among these is the fact that while NO_x and VOCs from auto tailpipes have been reduced significantly, emissions from unregulated sources such as off-road vehicles and equipment have been increasing; it's estimated that off-road equipment currently emits as much NO_x as all the nation's power plants. While recently imposed regulations promise to reduce emissions of ozone precursors from new equipment, enormous numbers of existing older machines will remain in use for many years before being replaced by cleaner models. As a result, new EPA emissions regulations won't achieve their full impact until 2030.

Other contributors to problematic ozone levels that are virtually impossible to regulate include long-distance transport of pollution across international borders, including China and Mexico, as well as biogenic emissions of VOCs from forests. Ironically, the latter seems to be a growing problem in some regions of the U.S., especially in the Southeast where plantation forests of loblolly pine and sweet gum are releasing quantities of natural VOCs that more than compensate for the anthropogenic emissions captured by pollution control devices! Global warming could further complicate ozone reduction efforts, since heat waves are known to increase ozone concentrations (Bernstein and Whitman, 2005). It is likely that in the years immediately ahead there will also

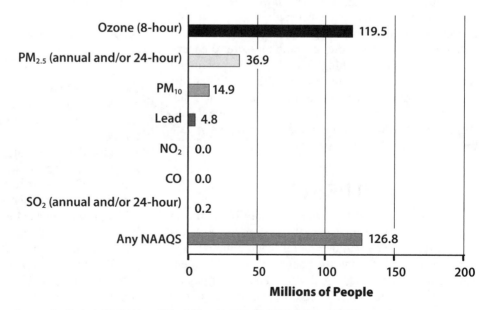

Source: *Our Nation's Air: Status and Trends Through 2008: Highlights.* EPA-454/R-09-002, February 2010.

Figure 13-2   Number of People Living in Monitored Counties that Exceeded National Ambient Air Quality Standards (NAAQS) in 2008

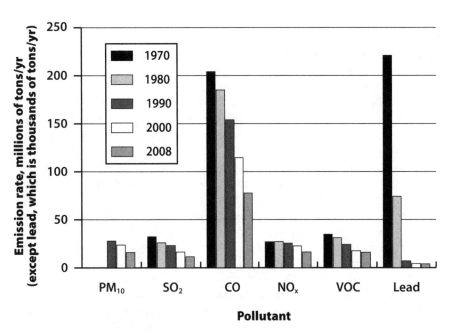

Source data from U.S. EPA, "National Emissions Inventory (NEI)," n.d.

Figure 13-3   U.S. Trends in Emission Rates, 1970 through 2008

be much more aggressive efforts to tighten controls for nitrogen oxides, which appear to be more important contributors to ozone formation than previously realized. Controls are likely to expand over a wide range of formerly unregulated sources of VOCs such as dry cleaning establishments, furniture refinishers, auto body shops—and possibly even consumer items such as charcoal lighter fuel, spray starch, and power lawn mowers!

In spite of remaining challenges, U.S. air quality trends overall are encouraging. While declining levels of pollutant emissions are due in some measure to energy conservation, fuel-switching, and the demise of many smokestack industries, a large share of the credit must be given to the regulatory programs that have mandated significant investment in pollution control technologies. Although the battle is by no means over, progress to date proves that the Clean Air Act is working.

ACID DEPOSITION

An air quality problem virtually unrecognized and unmentioned at the time the 1970 Clean Air Act was passed, the issue of acid deposition (commonly referred to as "acid rain," though the phenomenon includes not only rain but also snow, fog, dry SO_2 and NO_2 gas, and sulfate and nitrate aerosols) became political dynamite during the 1980s, pitting region against region, nation against nation. Although the domestic policy battles generated by the debate over acid rain controls were largely

resolved by key provisions of the 1990 Clean Air Act Amendments and by the Canada-United States Air Quality Agreement of 1991, acid deposition remains an important air quality concern both in the United States and internationally.

What Is Acid Deposition?

On a pH scale, distilled water has a pH of 7.0, considered "neutral" because the number of hydrogen (H+) and hydroxyl (OH-) ions is equal, making the solution neither acidic nor basic. However, since atmospheric CO_2 tends to dissolve in water, forming a weak solution of carbonic acid, rainfall is slightly acidic by nature. Measurements of the pH of precipitation in many parts of the world have led researchers to conclude that natural, unpolluted rain has a pH around 5.0. Thus, by definition, any precipitation measuring **less than 5.0** on the pH scale is considered acid deposition. Since the pH scale is logarithmic, rainfall with a pH of 4.0 is ten times more acid than precipitation with a pH of 5.0 and 100 times more acid than that of pH 6. A reading below 2.0, such as that recorded during a three-day drizzle in the fall of 1978 at Wheeling, West Virginia, represented a level 10,000 times more acid than unpolluted rainfall.

Extent of the Problem

Acid precipitation had been observed as a local phenomenon in the vicinity of coal-burning facilities since the 19th century. In fact, the term "acid rain" was first coined by an English chemist, Robert Angus Smith, to describe the corrosive brew falling on industrial Manchester more than 100 years ago. In the early 1960s Canadian ecologist Eville Graham, a pioneer of acid rain research in North America, described the acidification of lakes in northern Ontario in the vicinity of the huge Sudbury smelting complex, then the world's largest single source of sulfur emissions (Munton, 1998). Not until the 1970s, however, did acid rain emerge as a regional problem, affecting areas far from the source of pollutant emissions.

The alarm was first raised in 1972 by Swedish delegates attending the UN Conference on the Human Environment in Stockholm. After initial disbelief by many national governments, Swedish views about the extent and seriousness of this newly recognized environmental threat became widely accepted. On the basis of measurements taken during the past few decades, scientists have shown that until the late 1990s, when government-mandated controls began to take effect, the pH of rainfall steadily dropped throughout large areas of North America and Europe. Not only did rainfall become more acid in the affected areas, but the geographical extent of the problem widened also. Early measurements of rainfall pH indicated that in the years 1955–1956 only 12 northeastern states were experiencing acid precipitation. By 1972–1973 the number of states experiencing excessive rainfall acidity extended over the entire eastern portion of North America, except for the southern tip of Florida and the far northern regions of Canada. In addition, acid rain was detected in several of the major urban areas of California and in the Rocky Mountain region of Colorado.

Today the pH of rainfall averages 4.4 throughout the United States east of the Mississippi River, with substantially lower readings being obtained during some individual storm episodes. However, encouraging news has been reported by scientists working for the U.S. Geological Survey who documented a steady drop in the concentrations of acid-forming sulfates in precipitation since the 1990 Clean Air Act imposed strict SO_2 reductions on coal-burning power plants. Between the 1989–1991 and 2005–2007 time periods, the Northeast and Midwest regions of the United States experienced a 30% decrease in deposition of sulfates; during that same interval, nitrate deposition fell by about 30% in the Northeast and mid-Atlantic regions and by 20% in the Midwest. As a result, in many of the affected regions, the average pH of rainfall has gradually been rising and water quality in lakes and streams has improved. Such field data are hailed as evidence that pollution control technologies are having the intended impact.

Beyond North America, acid deposition today also affects most countries of Europe, although on that continent, as in North America, increasingly stringent controls on sulfur dioxide emissions have reduced the seriousness of the problem. By contrast, acid rain has emerged as a growing environmental threat in Asia, particularly in the rapidly industrializing provinces of southeastern China, a country where acid precipitation now affects approximately one-third of the total land area. Japan and South Korea are reporting acidification problems, largely due to transboundary air pollution wafting eastward from China, and high levels of acid precipitation are now being experienced in northeastern India and in northern and central Thailand (Economy, 2004; WRI, 1998).

Mystery of the Dying Lakes

During the 1960s and 1970s anglers, campers, and resort owners raised the first alarms concerning what was to become a major environmental tragedy. From the spar-

kling lakes of the remote Adirondacks, to the popular vacationlands of Ontario and Quebec, to the waterways of Scandinavia, reports of the mysterious disappearance of once-abundant fish, amphibians, and aquatic insects began to generate public concern. The fact that such lakes and streams were far from any of the usual sources of water pollution that have traditionally been associated with fish kills only increased the bewilderment. To a casual observer the water remained blue and clear; beneath the surface, however, the affected lakes had become watery deserts, devoid of life. By 2003, surveys showed that in New York's Adirondack Mountains approximately 41% of the lakes had become too acidic for fish and other aquatic life; the same situation applied to 15% of lakes in the New England states (Driscoll et al., 2003). In New Jersey's Pine Barrens, fully 90% of all streams are acidic—the highest percentage in the nation. In eastern Canada the toll is even higher—acidified lakes total 14,000, with approximately 150 now fishless. Such lakes are acid dead, poisoned by pollutants falling from the sky in the form of sulfuric and nitric acid.

Formation of Acid Rain

Acid precipitation forms when its major precursors, sulfur dioxide and nitrogen dioxide, are chemically converted through a complex series of reactions involving certain reactive hydrocarbons and oxidizing agents such as ozone to become sulfuric or nitric acid. The reactions involved can take place either within clouds or rain droplets, in the gas phase, on the surface of fine particulates in the air, or on soil or water surfaces after deposition (Rhodes and Middleton, 1983).

In 2008, 11 million tons of SO_2 were discharged into the atmosphere in the United States, down sharply from the 26 million tons emitted in 1980. Of this amount, approximately two-thirds originate from coal- and oil-burning power plants; the remainder is primarily from smelters and industrial boilers. A certain amount of SO_2 enters the atmosphere from natural sources such as volcanoes or mud flats, but such emissions contribute relatively little to the problem of acid rain; it is estimated that in the northeastern U.S., 90% of the sulfur in the air comes from human sources of pollution.

Nitrogen oxides, of which about 16 million tons were emitted in the U.S. in 2008, come predominantly from auto emissions, power plants, and industry. Until recently, SO_2 emissions have widely been perceived as posing a more serious problem than NO_x in terms of acid rain formation; however, as technological controls are increasingly successful at reducing levels of airborne sulfur compounds, the role of nitrogen oxides as acid rain precursors has grown in importance. Clean Air Act requirements have been less successful in reducing airborne emissions of NO_x than they have been in controlling SO_2 and most observers agree that additional measures to cut nitrogen emissions will be needed to protect sensitive ecosystems.

Long-Distance Transport

The aspect of acid rainfall that makes it such a politically charged issue is the fact that the pollutant emissions that are the precursors of acid rain formation may be produced hundreds of miles from the regions suffering the effects of acid deposition. Because some pollutants can remain in the air for a relatively long period of time, they can be carried on the prevailing winds across geographical and political boundaries far from their place of ori-

gin—a phenomenon known as **long-distance transport**. There are documented examples of acid rain-forming pollutants being carried more than 600 miles before being deposited on the earth's surface.

Ironically, pollution control technologies adopted early in the 1970s to reduce local levels of ambient air pollution had the unintended effect of increasing the long-distance transport problem. The approach adopted most often by utilities striving to lower SO_2 concentrations in the vicinity of their plants was to pursue a **tall stack strategy**; that is, to build extremely tall "superstacks" that discharged pollutant gases into the persistent air currents more than 500 feet above the ground. This approach was indeed effective in reducing local pollution levels, but it

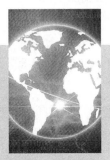

········ 13-4 ········

Air Quality Aloft

Prohibitions on in-flight smoking imposed during the 1980s and now enforced by the vast majority of domestic and international airlines were expected to resolve the most serious concerns voiced by passengers and flight attendants regarding the quality of aircraft cabin air. Certainly such restrictions made air travel more pleasant for the majority of the population who were nonsmokers, but they didn't end complaints, most of them rather broad, about what many travelers and crew members feared were health-threatening levels of airborne contaminants aloft.

While maintenance of good air quality is important in any indoor space, aircraft cabins present a more challenging situation than most, since occupants are in extremely close proximity to one another and are unable to leave if they find conditions oppressive. The steadily increasing number of people traveling by air each year—currently about 1.5 billion worldwide and growing by 6% annually—means that cabin air quality affects a significant portion of the population. In addition, those flying today include an increasing percentage of passengers with preexisting medical conditions such as respiratory or cardiovascular disease, as well as the very young and the elderly, both age groups known to be more vulnerable to environmental stress.

To prevent problems and maintain acceptable cabin air quality, commercial airliners rely on an **environmental control system (ECS)** designed to control cabin pressure, ventilation, temperature, and humidity and to prevent entry of harmful airborne contaminants into the cabin. A typical jetliner uses a mixture of outdoor air, brought in through the engines, and cabin air that is filtered and then recirculated, the portion of recirculated air in the total mix varying from 30% to 55%.

Although the ECS in general does a good job in maintaining safe, comfortable in-flight conditions, the potential exists for a number of airborne contaminants to enter the aircraft cabin. Entry of stratospheric ozone into the cabins of high-flying aircraft could pose a possible health threat to those aboard. At high altitudes, when outside air is drawn into the ventilation system, ozone—a known respiratory irritant—can be present at concentrations that exceed FAA limits on O_3 for cabin air. To avoid this problem, most large commercial airliners now employ O_3 converters which, when new, remove 90–98% of the ozone in the air passing through them. Some concerns have been expressed, however, that there is no process in place to ensure that converters are operating at a high level of efficiency (the useful lifespan of a converter ranges from 10,000–20,000 flight hours); this, plus the fact that some aircraft are still not equipped with O_3 converters, means that on some flights ozone concentrations could exceed existing standards.

Another air quality issue of concern on some international flights involves in-cabin **disinsection**—whereby employees spray insecticides prior to passengers disembarking. Numerous airline passengers have protested this practice, claiming adverse reactions to contact with pesticidal chemicals, but several countries insist it is necessary to rid in-bound flights of any unwelcome insect pests the planes might be harboring. The U.S. Centers for Disease Control and Prevention agrees with those calling for a discontinuation of the practice, asserting that disinsection is both ineffective for its intended purpose and poses a potential health risk for passengers and crew. Nevertheless, India, Uruguay, Grenada, Trinidad, and a few other countries continue to treat all in-bound aircraft while passengers are still on board; the Czech Republic, Switzerland, and the U.K., among others, treat planes arriving from specified areas where malaria is a problem; and Australia, New Zealand, and some Caribbean nations require treatment of aircraft with a residual insecticide when passengers are not on board. The most commonly used pesticides for disinsection are pyrethroid chemicals recommended by WHO for this purpose as effective contact poisons with low human toxicity. Few, if any, studies have been conducted on the amount of pesticide exposure to those on board as a result of disinsection; nevertheless, when on-board spraying is conducted both inhalation and skin (dermal) exposure is inevitable.

The most worrisome in-flight air contaminants are infectious bacteria and viruses, introduced into the aircraft cabin not through the ventilation system but by other passengers or members of the flight crew. Reports regarding transmission of infectious organisms during air travel abound, not surprisingly since such trips involve close contact with a large number of people, in some cases for long periods of time. When such travel involves international flights to tropical destinations, the opportunity for exposure to exotic disease organisms is substantially higher for air travelers than it is for the general public. In addition, with the longer nonstop flights that now characterize much international air travel, passengers are together for more prolonged periods of time than was the case in years past, further increasing opportunities for disease transmission.

Some of the infections known or strongly suspected to have been transmitted in-flight include influenza, measles, and tuberculosis; transmission of acute respiratory infections and meningococcal disease is also considered possible. Contrary to the commonly held belief that germs are spread throughout the aircraft cabin via recirculated air, studies show no difference in infection rates whether or not recirculated air is used. The credit for this is undoubtedly due to the fact that the vast majority of aircraft now employ HEPA filters, capable of removing over 99% of particles and pathogens in the airstream. In-flight sampling studies have shown that concentrations of bacteria are significantly higher near floor vents than in the passenger breathing zone—an indication that airborne microbes are effectively entrained and removed from the cabin with exhaust air. Only in situations where the ventilation system has been shut off, as sometimes happens when ground delays keep a plane sitting on the runway for several hours, are infectious agents likely to spread throughout the cabin. It should be mentioned that air from restrooms is *not* recirculated, in order to avoid the possibility of introducing infectious organisms or odors from sewage disposal systems into the passenger cabin.

The risk of contracting an infectious disease during air travel, therefore, is determined almost entirely by seat assignment; only people sitting (or working, in the case of flight crew) in close proximity to an infected source are exposed to a sufficient number of pathogen-laden droplet nuclei to become infected themselves. The number of source cases and the occupant load of the aircraft are significant factors in determining how many passengers will contract an infection during the flight. Investigations involving suspected cases of disease transmission on aircraft suggest that unless the ventilation system is inoperable, one source case on a plane seldom results in any but adjacent passengers subsequently becoming infected. Clearly, keeping aircraft cabin air free of infectious organisms depends less on equipment (though a properly functioning ventilation system is essential) than it does on common sense and personal responsibility among air travelers. People knowingly suffering from an infectious respiratory disease should postpone flying until they are no longer contagious or, at a minimum, practice good personal hygiene, move around the cabin as little as possible, and cover their mouth and nose while coughing or sneezing. Assuming that many are unlikely to heed such pleas, other travelers are advised to take advantage of immunization against such vaccine-preventable diseases as influenza, measles, and pneumonia (for elderly passengers) as a precautionary measure.

Although current data do not indicate serious air quality-related problems among passengers or cabin crew now that in-flight smoking is no longer permitted, the almost complete lack of detailed studies on contaminant exposure and related health effects, both short- and long-term, make it impossible to state categorically that anecdotal reports of problems are unfounded. Until a systematic effort is launched to collect, analyze, and report health data relating to aircraft cabin air quality, that uncertainty will persist.

promoted long-distance transport and thereby increased the range and severity of acid deposition in regions downwind. Until the 1990 Clean Air Act Amendments committed the United States to aggressive acid rain control efforts, relations between Canada and the United States were seriously strained because half of the corrosive rain falling over southeastern Canada originates in the heavily industrialized Ohio River Valley and upper Midwest. New York and the New England states harbored a similar grudge against Illinois, Indiana, and Ohio—the source of fully one-fourth of all U.S. sulfur emissions.

In the same way, much of the acid rain now damaging vegetation and aquatic environments in Japan originated in China, whose sulfur emissions in 1990 were 40–45 times higher than those during Japan's worst air pollution years in the mid-1970s. Prior to the 1980s, acid rain provoked harsh words among neighboring European countries as well, since the corrosive precipitation wreaking havoc on lakes and forests in Norway and Sweden was produced primarily in central Europe and Great Britain. Such circumstances make the formulation of acid rain control policies politically difficult because those bearing the cost of pollution abatement strategies and those reaping the benefits are not one and the same.

Effective action toward resolving this dilemma was taken first in Europe in 1979 when 35 countries signed the **Convention on Long-Range Transboundary Air Pollution**, an agreement requiring the signatory nations to achieve a 30% reduction in SO_2 emissions from 1980 levels by 1993. Targets have subsequently been set for reducing NO_x and VOC emissions as well. In the United States, the acid rain debate raged in Congress for years. Legislators from the Midwest were nearly unanimous in their opposition to federal rules that would impose more stringent sulfur emission controls on coal-burning power plants in their region. Citing the financial burden that would be passed along to electric consumers and the inherent threat controls would pose to coal-mining interests in states like Illinois and West Virginia, midwestern representatives were acutely aware that the environmental gains achieved by tougher regulations would be enjoyed by citizens outside their own constituencies. Conversely, legislators from such states as New Hampshire and Maine, areas that had few large sources of emissions yet were suffering severe economic and ecological damage due to acid rain, were among the most vocal in demanding regulatory action.

Regional Vulnerability to Acid Rain

Although the entire eastern United States is now experiencing acid rainfall, not all areas are suffering adverse ecological effects. An ecosystem's sensitivity to acid precipitation is determined primarily by the chemical composition of the soil and bedrock—an attribute referred to as the **buffering capacity** of that environment.

Buffering capacity refers to an ability to neutralize acids, the buffer acting to maintain the natural pH of an environment by tying up the excess hydrogen ions introduced by acid rain. Regions such as New England, the Mid-Atlantic states, the Southeast, northern Minnesota and Wisconsin, the Rocky Mountain states, and parts of the Pacific Northwest are characterized by soils that are naturally already acidic or underlain by granitic bedrock; these areas are said to have a low buffering capacity and hence are very sensitive to acid rain. By contrast, most parts of the Midwest, the Great Plains, and portions of the Southwest have predominantly alkaline soils and bedrock of limestone, giving them a high buffering capacity. This fact explains why a state such as Illinois, which is currently experiencing rainfall almost as acid as that falling in New York or New England, is not suffering comparable ecological damage. Nevertheless, such apparent invulnerability is not guaranteed to last forever. Over time, a given soil's buffering capacity can be overwhelmed by continual acid inputs, a phenomenon that seems to be occurring already in parts of the upper Midwest. It seems a cruel twist of fate that prevailing wind currents are transporting acid rain-forming pollutants to precisely those regions that are most sensitive to their harmful effects.

Environmental Effects of Acid Rain

Acid precipitation can cause a number of adverse environmental changes, the best-understood of which include the following.

Damage to Aquatic Ecosystems

That acid rain can decimate the biotic communities inhabiting lakes, ponds, and streams in those regions where natural buffering capacity is low has been well documented in numerous studies. Most freshwater organisms do best in waters that are slightly alkaline—about pH 8. As lakes gradually become acidified due to steady inputs of acid rain, one aquatic species after another disappears. The first affected are the tiny invertebrates that constitute a vital link in aquatic food chains; at pH 6.0 the freshwater shrimp are eliminated; at pH 5.5 the bacterial decomposers at the lake bottom begin to die off, as do the phytoplankton, the producer organisms in aquatic ecosystems. Fish populations, the subject of most human attention, are somewhat more tolerant to increasing acidity; little change in their numbers is noticed until the pH drops below 5.5. Under pH 4.5 all fish species disappear, as do most frogs, salamanders, and aquatic insects ("Acid Rain," 1982).

Interestingly, falling pH levels seldom kill adult fish directly. The primary cause of fish de-population is acid-induced reproductive failure; pH values below 5.5 can prevent female fish from laying their eggs, and those eggs which are laid frequently fail to hatch or result in the production of deformed fry. (Just as the early developmental stages of humans are the most vulnerable to of environmental contaminants, the same holds true for the larval stages of lower organisms.) Interference with hatching is accentuated by the fact that the most critical developmental period usually coincides with the time of the annual snow melt when several months' accumulation of acid suddenly inundates the spawning areas in one massive dose, a situation known as **shock loading** or **episodic acidification**. This sort of periodic drop in pH, due either to snow melt or heavy downpours, is much more common than chronic acidification of lakes and streams. While the abrupt drop in pH levels during such events is generally of short duration, the ecological impact on young fish or fish eggs can be as devastating as chronic exposure. Large-scale reproductive failure leads to a situation in some lakes where the older fish grow larger and larger, thanks to decreased competition for food, and anglers boast of their excellent catches until, with further increases in acidity, all the fish disappear. As a professor at the University of Toronto stated: "There is no muss, there is no fuss, there is no smell. The fish quietly go extinct . . . They simply fail to reproduce and become less and less abundant, and older and older, until they die out" (Weller, 1980).

At one time it was assumed that acid rain's impact on aquatic environments was limited to freshwater ecosystems. It is now recognized, however, that acid precipitation contributes 30–40% of all the nitrates entering Chesapeake Bay. Studies have shown that these airborne nutrients are as important as farmland fertilizer runoff in stimulating the algal blooms that are degrading water quality in that important saltwater estuary.

Mobilization of Toxic Metals

Contact with acidified water can cause tightly bound toxic metals such as aluminum, manganese, lead, zinc, mercury, and cadmium to dissolve out of bottom sediments or soils and leach into the aquatic environment. Such metals, especially aluminum, can kill fish by damaging their gills, thereby causing asphyxiation. Acid-induced release of aluminum, even at concentrations as low as 0.2 mg/L, has resulted in fish kills at water pH levels that wouldn't have been lethal in the absence of the toxic metal. Toxic metals in the water also can bioaccumulate in fish tissues, making them dangerous for humans to eat.

Mobilization of poisonous metals also presents a direct threat to human health if the acidified lakes are a source of drinking water supplies. A resort owner from the Adirondacks testified before a congressional committee that, in response to his children's complaints about the taste of water piped to their lodge, he had the water

tested and found it contained five times the safe level for lead and 10 times that for copper. In other communities, acidified water that was originally free of toxic metals became contaminated upon passing through lead or copper plumbing systems—the low pH of the water caused corrosion of the pipes, resulting in leaching of toxic metals into the water. Homeowners who obtain their drinking water from roof catchments in areas affected by acid rain are also at special risk (Boyle and Boyle, 1983).

Deterioration of Buildings, Statuary, and Metals

While it is extremely difficult to assign a precise monetary value to the impact of acid rain on materials, it is nevertheless acknowledged that the scope of the damage is large indeed. Most pronounced are the effects of acid deposition on stone and metal buildings and statues, on textiles, leather, and paint, and to some extent on paper and glass. Many monuments of great historic and cultural significance are today slowly disintegrating under the impact of airborne pollutants, of which various sulfur compounds are by far the most important. Corroding surfaces of the Statue of Liberty, the Washington Monument, the Capitol Building in Washington, D.C., Canada's Parliament buildings in Ottawa, and the Field Museum in Chicago all give evidence of the ravages produced by acid rain. In India, the Supreme Court ordered nearly 300 coal-burning facilities near Agra to close by the end of 1997 because their SO_2 emissions were severely corroding the beautiful marble façade of the Taj Mahal (Brown et al., 1997). On a more mundane level, EPA estimates that acid rain increases the cost of each new car by $5.00 due to the necessity of using more expensive acid-resistant paint on vehicles sold in regions where acid rain is a problem.

Reduction of Crop Yields

The extent of acid rain damage to field crops is less clear-cut than with other types of acid-induced environmental damage. Yields of some species appear to be diminished by acid rain, some are stimulated, while others show no change as pH levels of rainfall drop (Cohen, Grothaus, and Perrigan, 1982). Chinese officials report that approximately 30% of their country's agricultural land is affected by acid precipitation. Some authorities estimate that by 2002 acid rain was causing over $13 billion in damage each year to Chinese farms, forests, and human health (Economy, 2004). In northeastern India, steep reductions in wheat yields in fields downwind of a coal-burning power plant are attributed to acid rain damage (WRI, 1998).

Damage to Forest Productivity

From the wooded slopes of the Adirondacks to the forests of central Europe and Scandinavia, acid-laden rain and fog are contributing to death and reduced

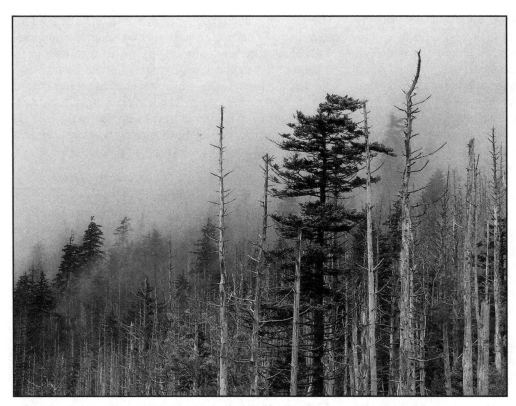

Acid rain damage is evident in this forest in Great Smoky Mountains National Park.

growth rates among an ever-increasing number of important tree species. Most affected are conifer forests at high elevations, frequently shrouded in acid fog or mist. At many sites above 850 meters in the White Mountains of New Hampshire or the Green Mountains of Vermont, over half the red spruce have died since the early 1960s. In Germany, the rate at which wide areas of forest have been similarly affected just since the early 1980s has been so dramatic that distraught German scientists have coined a word for the phenomenon—*waldsterben* ("forest death"). By 1989 German scientists were estimating that more than half the trees in the country were suffering some degree of defoliation. Fortunately, the rate of forest decline in Germany now appears to be slackening, possibly in response to the aggressive pollution control policies enacted specifically for that purpose in 1983.

The extent to which acid rain can be blamed for the decline of forests on two continents is currently a subject of intensive investigation by scientists in Europe and North America. In some cases acid rain causes direct damage to leaves, resulting in the leaching of nutrients such as calcium from foliage. Such loss in certain evergreen species decreases resistance to foliar freezing and is thought to account for the dieback of large expanses of red spruce in mountain areas of the northeast (Driscoll et al., 2003). This phenomenon is particularly associated with the acid fog that commonly occurs on ridgetops and is further enhanced by the presence of ozone.

For the most part, however, it appears that acid rain's role in the forest decline drama is less direct. Acid precipitation increases the solubility and migration of soil-bound aluminum ions, which act as a poison to the delicate root hairs responsible for nutrient uptake. Acid rain also causes the loss of essential plant nutrients—calcium, potassium, magnesium—from forest soils. Calcium depletion in particular is emerging as one of the most significant factors explaining forest decline in eastern North America. An essential element for plant growth, calcium is leached out of forest soils into waterways as precipitation becomes increasingly acidic. Research during the 1990s revealed a marked drop in the calcium content of soils in both the northeastern and southeastern United States since the 1960s—a decline linked to acid rain. This trend is worrisome because calcium loss undermines a tree's ability to resist insect attack, disease, and extreme temperatures. Field investigations have documented a distinct correlation between reduced stress tolerance in ailing red spruce and sugar maple forests to soil calcium deficiencies. Unfortunately, calcium that is leached out of soils by acid precipitation is no longer being replaced at the rate it once was. Studies have shown that rainfall today contains approximately 80% less calcium than it did in the 1950s. As a result, even if the problem of acidification were to vanish overnight, forest recovery would require many decades before the damage is repaired. Researchers working at the Hubbard Brook Experimental Forest in New Hampshire's White Mountains have discovered that the acid-impacted forest essentially stopped growing in 1987, with virtually no new biomass added since that time. Such observations may help to explain why natural ecosystems damaged by past acidification fail to show signs of recovery in spite of recent reductions in acid-rain-forming pollutants (Driscoll et al., 2003; Lawrence and Huntington, 1999; Likens, Driscoll, and Buso, 1996).

Acid Rain Controls

Throughout the 1980s a growing awareness of the extent and severity of the acid rain problem led to increasingly vociferous public demands for regulatory action, primarily in the form of laws requiring stringent pollution controls on coal-burning power plants. Passage of the 1990 Clean Air Act Amendments, containing the strong acid rain control provisions previously discussed, ended nearly a decade of vituperative debate. An innovative cap-and-trade market-based approach was devised to make the requirements more financially feasible by allowing the regulated utilities to choose among numerous options for meeting mandated emission limits.

Observers of the acid rain saga are in unanimous agreement that the control program mandated by the 1990 Clean Air Act Amendments has been resoundingly successful in meeting the Phase I goal of a 10-million-ton reduction in SO_2 emissions. All 110 power plants targeted under this phase of the program met the EPA deadline for both sulfur and nitrogen oxide reduction. By 2007, power plant emissions of SO_2 had been reduced by 48% below their 1990 levels; NO_x emissions during that same period had declined by about 3 million tons, with total emissions in 2007 less than half of what they would have been in the absence of controls. The biggest surprise was that these reductions were achieved at a far lower financial cost than even the most optimistic analysts had predicted—approximately $1 billion per year as opposed to the $3–7 billion cited by industry lobbyists fighting enactment of the legislation. Although market-based allowance trading is frequently credited for this remarkable accomplishment, several other factors were equally, if not more, instrumental. The unusual degree of flexibility built into the program made it possible for power plant managers to take advantage of unexpected opportunities to cut emissions in the most cost-effective manner. EPA's "just do it" directive—setting limits but not specifying the means for achieving them—prompted most of the affected utilities to meet the designated goal by switching to relatively cheap low-sulfur coal rather than by installing expensive flue gas desulfurization systems ("scrubbers"). The small percentage that did opt for scrubbers were pleasantly surprised to discover that, due to new, more efficient technology and manufacturers' need to keep the purchase price competitive, the equipment was both cheaper and more reliable than originally expected. Finally, the availability of a market-based pollution credit system gave plant operators additional leeway in choosing the most economical way of getting the job done.

Successful as the current approach has been in measurably reducing the acidity of precipitation, however, there is growing doubt that sensitive ecosystems will recover without the imposition of even more stringent controls. Just as particulate pollutants and ozone-laden smog continue to bedevil regulators, so the problem of acid rain promises to remain a challenge for the foreseeable future (Munton, 1998; Kerr, 1998).

INDOOR AIR POLLUTION

While the attention of scientists, citizens, and government regulators has until recently been focused almost exclusively on problems of ambient air pollution, it is now apparent that contaminants within private dwellings may pose a greater risk to human health than do outdoor air pollutants. In fact, with the exception of ozone and sulfur dioxide, all the air pollutants regulated under U.S. laws occur at higher concentrations indoors than out, prompting the EPA to rank indoor air pollution among the top five environmental risks to public health. This is particularly troubling because the majority of people spend considerably more time indoors than outside; thus their exposure to indoor air pollutants is nearly continuous. Such pollutants pose a special threat to the very young, the ill, and the elderly—those most susceptible and also the ones most likely to spend long periods of time inside. Justifiable concerns about energy conservation may have worsened the indoor air pollution problem because thick insulation, triple-glazed windows, and magnetically sealed doors greatly reduce air exchange with the outside, effectively retaining and accumulating contaminants inside the home.

While most people tend to equate the risk of harm they might suffer from toxic pollutants to the total amount and toxicity of such substances, in fact the main determinant of danger is the *dose* actually received by the individual. Thus, large amounts of toxic pollutants such as benzene, formaldehyde, or carbon monoxide, for example, when emitted from a factory smokestack or the tailpipe of a car, pose minimal risk to the average citizen because they break down or are diluted in concentration before individuals are directly exposed to them. By contrast, much smaller amounts of the same chemicals, released in close proximity to people inside their homes or offices, have a quick, direct route into the body and hence pose a much greater overall risk. Studies demonstrate that personal exposures and concentrations of indoor air pollutants exceed those occurring outdoors for all of the 15 most prevalent chemicals studied (Wallace, 1987). In addition, peak pollutant concentrations, as well as overall averages, are generally higher indoors than in the ambient air.

Some of the more common air pollutants known to be present in the home environment include the following.

Radon Gas

When Stanley Watras started radiation-detection alarms ringing at the Limerick nuclear power plant near Philadelphia one December morning in 1984, he didn't realize that he was about to become a national celebrity, alerting Americans to a hitherto unsuspected menace within their own homes. The radioactive contamination that was detected by Watras when he arrived for work that morning had obviously come from outside the nuclear facility, so Watras requested Philadelphia Electric, the utility company that owned the plant, to check his home. To everyone's amazement, tests revealed that the Watras home had levels of radon gas approximately 1,000 times higher than normal. Investigators estimated that Watras, his wife, and two young sons were receiving radiation exposure equivalent to 455,000 chest X-rays a year simply by living in their house. As Pennsylvania officials hastened to determine the extent of the indoor radon threat, it quickly became apparent that the Watras family was not alone in its predicament. Throughout sections of eastern Pennsylvania, New Jersey, and New York, underlain by a uranium-rich geological formation known as the Reading Prong, thousands of homes exhibit elevated levels of radon. Nor is the problem limited to a few mid-Atlantic states. EPA surveys reveal that indoor radon contamination problems span the country and agency officials, as well as the U.S. Surgeon General, urge that all homes be tested for the radioactive gas that is now widely recognized as a serious health hazard.

Radon originates from the natural radioactive decay of uranium. It is present in high concentrations in certain types of soil and rocks (e.g., granite, shale, phosphate, pitchblende), but most soils contain amounts high enough to pose a potential health hazard. Radon dilutes to harmless concentrations in the open air, but when it enters the confined space inside a structure it can accumulate to potentially hazardous levels. Since radon is a gas, it readily moves upward through the soil; small differences in air pressure between indoors and outdoors (very slight negative air pressure inside a heated building results from the "stack effect," created by air's tendency to rise whenever it is warmer than the surrounding atmosphere) cause the gas to seep into homes through dirt floors or crawl spaces, through cracks in cement floors and walls, through floor drains, sump holes, joints, or pores in cinder-block walls. Occasionally, radon gets into well water supplies and enters homes when water is used, particularly for showers or baths.

Radon is dangerous because it is radioactive, undergoing decay to produce a series of "radon daughters," the most troublesome of which are alpha-emitters polonium-218 and 214. These can be inhaled and deposited in the lungs where they constitute an internal

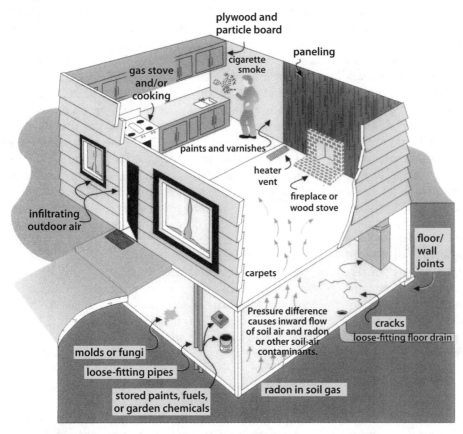

Courtesy of DOE/NREL, Lawrence Berkeley National Laboratory.

Figure 13-4   Factors Affecting Indoor Air Quality

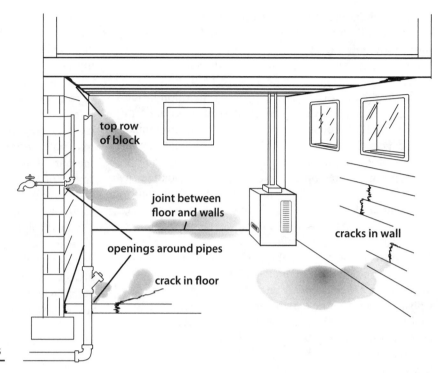

Figure 13-5 (a)
Points Where Radon Can Enter Homes

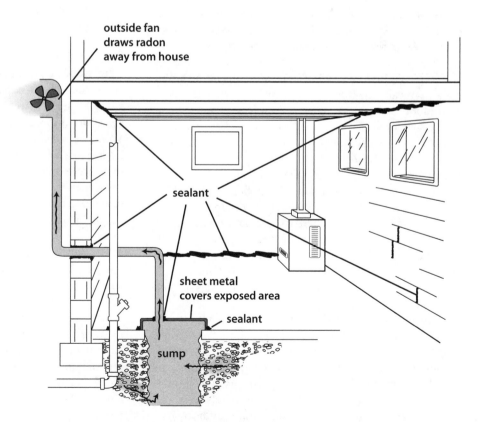

Figure 13-5 (b)
Radiation Reduction Methods

source of alpha radiation exposure, increasing the risk of lung cancer. Radon's contribution to overall human exposure to ionizing radiation is considerable. The National Council on Radiation Protection and Measurement estimates that the average individual receives fully 55% of his or her yearly dose of ionizing radiation from radon inside homes. The health consequences of such exposure, according to EPA's updated "best estimate," is an annual lung cancer death toll of 21,000—a number that would make radon the second-leading cause of lung cancer deaths in the United States, behind cigarette smoking. In parts of the country where radon levels are unusually high, hundreds of thousands of Americans are receiving as much radiation exposure from radon in their homes as that received by the Ukrainian citizens who lived near Chernobyl at the time of the nuclear accident there in 1986. An individual's chances of developing radon-induced lung cancer depend on radon concentrations inside the home and the length of time one is exposed. It is thought that long-term exposure to slightly elevated levels of radon poses a greater cancer threat than does short-term exposure to much higher levels. Cigarette smoking has a synergistic effect in enhancing the radon/lung cancer risk by a factor of 10.

Until the 1980s, radon was regarded as a health hazard only to uranium miners, so estimates of risk to residents of radon-contaminated homes have simply been extrapolated from standards set for occupational exposure in the mines. Indoor radon concentrations are measured as the number of picocuries of radiation per liter of air (pCi/L). Outdoors, radon concentrations in the ambient air typically measure about 0.4 pCi/L, while the average indoor level approximates 1.3 pCi/L. Acknowledging that any amount of exposure to ionizing radiation entails some degree of risk, for practical reasons EPA regards 4 pCi/L as the **action level**—the point at or above which homeowners are advised to take some kind of remedial action. It is estimated that about 6% of homes in the U.S. exceed this action level, the vast majority of them located in geographical regions where the soil and rocks have a high uranium content (Goldstein and Goldstein, 2002). Readings above 20 pCi/L are considered cause for serious concern and may require significant abatement measures (as a basis for comparison, radon levels in the Watras home measured 2,700 pCi/L).

Since it is impossible to predict with certainty which structures are likely to have elevated radon levels (some homes in the Watras neighborhood were essentially radon-free), the need for radon reduction measures can only be determined by actual measurements, which often can be done by the homeowner with relatively inexpensive devices (see box 13-5). If test results indicate the need for some sort of radon remediation efforts, a variety of options are available. Most require the services of a professional contractor, though some can be as simple as covering sump holes or improving ventilation. More extensive—and expensive—possibilities include installing fans or air-to-air heat exchangers to replace radon-contaminated indoor air with outdoor air; covering any exposed earth inside homes with concrete, gas-proof liner, or sheet metal; sealing all cracks and openings with mortar, polyurethane sealants, or other impermeable materials; installing a drain tile suction system around the outer foundation walls of a house; or by installing a series of exhaust pipes inside hollowblock basement walls or baseboard to draw radon out of the voids within such walls before it can enter the living space. In structures with significantly elevated levels of radon, it may be necessary to utilize several methods to achieve sufficient reductions. For people planning to build a new home in areas with known radon problems, use of radon-resistant construction techniques is far more cost-effective than installing a radon reduction system after the fact.

Products of Combustion

Carbon monoxide, nitrogen oxides, and particulates can reach very high levels inside homes where gas stoves or other gas appliances are used, where kerosene heaters or wood-burning stoves are operating, where auto emissions from a garage can enter the house, or where there are cigarette smokers. In homes with gas ranges, for example, nitrogen oxide levels are frequently twice as high as those outdoors. Carbon monoxide emissions from wood, coal, or gas stoves often exceed Clean Air Act standards for outside air. The growing popularity of wood-burning stoves is a particular cause for concern, since wood is a much dirtier fuel than either oil or gas. Wood smoke contains approximately 100 different chemicals, at least 14 of which are the same carcinogens found in cigarette smoke.

Cigarette smoking (the by-product of which is now referred to technically as **ETS** or "Environmental Tobacco Smoke") may constitute the most significant source of indoor air pollution in many homes; particulate levels may go as high as 700 micrograms/m³, far above the primary ambient air quality standard of 50, when there are smokers in a house. A study conducted by researchers at Harvard University found that household tobacco smoke is the main source of exposure to particulate pollutants for most children. It also demonstrated that whereas typical particulate levels in a home without smokers is 10–20 micrograms/m³, each smoker contributes an additional 25–30 micrograms/m³, more than doubling the base level amount (Ware et al., 1984). That parental smoking could be considered another form of child abuse has been amply documented in numerous studies. EPA reports that children exposed to environmental tobacco smoke are at

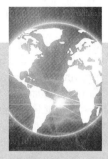

· · · · · · · · 13-5 · · · · · · · ·

Assessing Home Radon Risk

Radon detection businesses have proliferated rapidly following EPA's announcement advising that homes nationwide be tested for the presence of this apparently ubiquitous indoor air pollutant. Since 1985, millions of homeowners have heeded the agency's advice, but many others have yet to follow through, deterred by the hefty fee charged by many professionals offering radon-monitoring services. Such individuals should be heartened to learn that they can purchase relatively inexpensive devices that will give a reasonably accurate indication of the extent of radon problems in the user's home.

The two most popular do-it-yourself home radon detectors are (1) short-term tests using charcoal canisters—small containers of activated charcoal that should be opened and left in place for three to seven days, then sealed and returned to the manufacturer for analysis and (2) longer-term alpha track detectors that are left in place for several weeks to as long as one year. Since radon levels can fluctuate considerably from day to day and season to season, alpha track detectors are good for determining yearly averages; charcoal canisters are useful for short-term screening tests, but since their results are indicative only of radon levels during the few days when the test was performed, they may over- or underrepresent the actual extent of hazard. Both devices, however, can be effectively used by nonprofessionals to give a rough approximation of radon pollution. If laboratory analysis reveals that radon levels are high, consultation with a radon abatement specialist would be advisable, but if the screening test indicates negligible amounts of the gas, the homeowner is saved the expense of contracting for a radon survey that might cost several hundred dollars.

Those interested in doing their own radon monitoring can improve the accuracy and relevance of the results by understanding a few basic concepts about radon. Because radon infiltrates into homes through the ground, basements are likely to exhibit the highest radon levels. For this reason, if residents want to know the peak concentrations to which they may be exposed, a monitoring device should be located in the basement (or lowest level of the dwelling), placed about 3–6 feet above the floor and away from walls, doors, or windows. However, if occupants spend little time in the basement and want a measurement more representative of the exposure they are receiving, monitors can be placed in living areas of the next highest floor. Another likely spot for monitor placement is near suspected sources of radon entry, such as sump holes or crawl spaces (however, don't use charcoal canisters in humid environments such as bathrooms and kitchens; the charcoal absorbs moisture and test results will not be accurate). All windows and outside doors should be closed at least 12 hours before beginning the test; avoid conducting short-term tests during periods of severe storms or strong winds. Since monitoring devices are relatively inexpensive, it may be advisable to use two or three simultaneously in different areas of the house. Radon concentrations in most states tend to be highest in winter, so this is the best time for using short-term monitoring devices.

Home radon detectors are available for purchase online, at hardware stores, supermarkets, or other retail establishments; local public health departments may also be a source of monitoring devices or information on where they can be obtained. Until October 1998, manufacturers could voluntarily submit their products to EPA for evaluation; that program has since been terminated, so any "EPA-Approved" designation on products or services currently on the market is no longer valid.

In situations where preliminary monitoring indicates a need for radon mitigation (i.e., where the radon level measures 4 pCi/L or higher), homeowners would be well advised to consult a remediation professional. Currently two private groups—the National Environmental Health Association (NEHA) and the National Radon Safety Board (NRSB)—offer accreditation/certification for radon testing and mitigation. Anyone planning to contract for radon-related work in a state where licensing of radon professionals is not required by law should first inquire whether the contractor in question has met the certification requirements of one of these organizations.

increased risk for lower respiratory tract infections, bronchitis, and pneumonia, with those under 18 months of age more susceptible than older children. Fluid in the middle ear, wheezing, and asthma all occur more frequently among children whose parents smoke. Maternal smoking can even affect the unborn; studies have shown that tobacco use by a pregnant mother can interfere with the normal lung development of her fetus (Wargo, 2009).

Particulates are but one of several indoor air pollutants generated by smokers; carbon monoxide is another, as is benzene, a known carcinogen and a listed toxic air pollutant. Researchers calculate that fully 45% of Americans' total exposure to benzene comes from inhaling tobacco smoke, while a mere 3% is due to industrial emissions (Ott and Roberts, 1998). Such findings have provided scientific justification for the proliferation of smoking bans in restaurants and other public facilities. Even in the absence of enforceable federal standards, ETS has become a socially unacceptable indoor air pollutant.

Formaldehyde

Known to cause skin and respiratory irritation, formaldehyde was classified by the EPA in 1987 as a probable human carcinogen in situations where exposure is unusually high or prolonged. More recently, in response to studies that have shown an association between formaldehyde and certain types of cancer (e.g. nasopharyngeal cancers, leukemia, and lymphatic system malignancies), the International Agency for Research on Cancer bypassed the "probable" terminology and designated formaldehyde as a human carcinogen. A wide variety of household products contain formaldehyde, most notably particleboard, plywood, and some floor coverings and textiles. Levels of formaldehyde are particularly likely to be high in mobile homes, where residents frequently complain of rashes, respiratory irritation, nausea, headaches, dizziness, lethargy, or aggravation of bronchial asthma. A scandal involving 120,000 mobile homes provided to homeless Gulf Coast evacuees by the Federal Emergency and Management Agency (FEMA) after Hurricane Katrina focused on widespread complaints of respiratory problems by residents. A subsequent investigation by CDC found elevated formaldehyde levels in 42% of the FEMA-supplied trailers whose walls and cabinets were made of particleboard.

Within the same home, formaldehyde levels can fluctuate dramatically, depending on environmental conditions. A 15°F increase in temperature can result in a doubling of formaldehyde levels, while the lowest formaldehyde concentrations have been recorded on cold winter days; similarly, increases in relative humidity cause a corresponding rise in formaldehyde emissions; in all likelihood, the hot, humid weather typical of Louisiana and Mississippi contributed to the toxic emissions problem with the FEMA trailers.

In terms of its effect as an irritant, there does not appear to be a threshold level for formaldehyde exposure, though few people experience symptoms when concentrations are below 0.1 ppm. The National Academy of Sciences estimates that as many as 10–20% of the population experiences some form of irritation due to formaldehyde exposure even at very low concentrations. Since formaldehyde is so ubiquitous in the modern environment, avoiding exposure entirely is almost impossible. Nevertheless, sensitive individuals can reduce exposure and thereby minimize symptoms by substituting metal or lumber products for those containing pressed wood or selectively purchasing low formaldehyde-releasing pressed wood construction materials, cabinets, or furniture. Similarly, those allergic to the chemical should always launder permanent-press fabrics prior to use to remove the formaldehyde finish, since a single wash can reduce textile formaldehyde emissions up to 60% (unfortunately, this approach won't work for draperies, which also are large formaldehyde emitters).

Chemical Fumes and Particles

Numerous household products (including furniture polish, hair sprays, air fresheners, oven-cleaners, paints, carpeting, pesticides, disinfectants, solvents, etc.), release chemical fumes and particles that can reach very high levels indoors. While relatively little research has been done on the health impact of inhaling these substances on a regular basis, it is known that several commonly used household chemicals cause cancer in laboratory animals. Paradichlorobenzene, the active ingredient in moth crystals and many air fresheners and room deodorants, as well as limonene, another odorant, present perhaps the highest cancer risk among indoor organic chemicals. Tetrachloroethylene, a solvent used in dry cleaning, is another carcinogen to which household residents may receive significant exposure when wearing freshly dry-cleaned garments or by breathing emissions from closets in which such articles were stored (Smith, 1988).

When used in accordance with instructions, most household chemicals are not known to provoke acute health effects. However, use of pesticides inside homes has occasionally resulted in a wide range of health complaints, including headaches, nausea, vertigo, skin rashes, and emotional disorders. Chlordane, which for almost 40 years was the most widely used insecticide for controlling termites, was taken off the market in 1988 in response to hundreds of complaints about alleged chlordane-induced illnesses among residents following pesticidal applications in homes. Inappropriate pesticide use inside homes can result in long-term exposure to toxic residues and

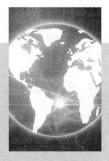

· · · · · · · 13-6 · · · · · · · ·
Cleaner Cookstoves, Healthier Cooks

When India's Ministry of New and Renewable Energy (MNRE) announced its National Biomass Cookstoves Initiative in December 2009, it took a major step toward simultaneously reducing air pollution, improving public health, and combating climate change. Within 10 years, if all goes according to plans, India will sell 150 million improved biomass cookstoves to rural households where today the simple task of preparing dinner is undermining the health of women and their children. Unfortunately, India is but one of more than 100 countries where widespread reliance on firewood, animal dung, crop residues, or coal as the main domestic fuel source is creating serious indoor air pollution problems that the World Health Organization in 2004 blamed for close to 2 million premature deaths worldwide, almost half of them due to pneumonia in children under 5 years old. As they stoke fires and stir pots in small, poorly ventilated kitchens, housewives throughout the developing world daily work in a smoke-laden environment that exposes them to levels of pollution the WHO equates to consuming two packs of cigarettes per day. As a result, they and the small children who spend most of their time close to mother are falling ill and often dying from diseases provoked by indoor air pollution.

Of the various ailments associated with cookstove emissions, acute respiratory infections affect the largest number of people, with infants and toddlers the most frequent victims. Studies of Zulu children in South Africa found that youngsters living in homes with wood cookstoves were five times more likely to be hospitalized with severe respiratory infections. In Nepal, a significant correlation was found between the incidence of moderate to severe respiratory infections among 2-year-olds and the number of hours they spent near a fire. In Gambia, researchers found that babies whose mothers carried them on their backs while cooking over an open wood fire inside a smoky hut were six times more likely to contract acute respiratory infections than were children not exposed to wood smoke. Adult women experiencing long-term smoke exposure are themselves at high risk of developing chronic lung diseases such as emphysema, bronchitis, and asthma. A study conducted in Mexico among women who had been exposed to wood smoke for many years found their risk of lung disease was equivalent to that of heavy smokers and 75 times that of women not exposed. Cancer is another health threat associated with this form of indoor air pollution, as are reproductive problems such as stillbirths, low-birth-weight babies, and difficulties during delivery for women who inhale cookstove emissions during pregnancy (WRI, 1998).

The types of pollutants emitted from cookstoves vary, depending on the type of fuel burned. Biomass fuels—wood, charcoal, crop residues, animal dung—are the dirtiest. Used by over two billion of the world's poorest people, wood and other biofuels emit levels of carbon monoxide, benzene, and particulate matter many times higher than WHO limits and significantly add to the haze of pollution blanketing virtually every developing world city today. This problem is particularly acute in the skies over India and other south and southeast Asian countries where the so-called "Asian Brown Cloud" hovers over the landscape. This two-mile thick haze is an omnipresent reminder that air pollution has become one of the region's most serious environmental problems. Although a variety of sources contribute to the blanket of smog, researchers have concluded that smoke from millions of inefficient home cookstoves bears a large share of the blame for the witches' brew of ash, black soot, sulfate particles, NO_x, CO, acids, and toxic aerosols that comprise the pervasive haze (Gustafsson et al., 2009).

Coal, though considered a step up the energy ladder from biofuels in terms of pollutant emissions, is nevertheless a dirty fuel as well, emitting prodigious amounts of $PM_{2.5}$, the most dangerous form of particulate matter. In China, where close to 400 million people rely on coal as their chief domestic fuel, the problem of indoor air pollution has assumed major proportions in both rural and urban areas. The coal used in Chinese cookstoves is, for the most part, mined from deposits containing excessive traces of toxic elements such as arsenic, mercury, fluorine, and antimony. Used directly without washing, these coals release toxic emissions when burned. Millions of Chinese homemakers are also affected by volatile organic compounds released by coal-burning cookstoves. Polycyclic aromatic hydrocarbons (PAHs) from unvented coal stoves are believed to be the main cause for the high incidence of lung cancer in China. In homes where smoky coal is burned, the lung cancer death rate is five times above the national average. Studies conducted in China by EPA researchers found a strong association between lung cancer incidence in women and the length of time they had spent cooking indoors. Blood samples taken from the women, along with indoor air analyses, demonstrated that indoor coal-burning was to blame for the observed cancers (Finkelman et al., 1999).

The solution to these problems is perfectly straightforward: replace wood and coal-burning stoves with those fueled by solar panels, natural gas, or electricity. Even liquid fuels such as kerosene and liquefied petroleum gas (LPG) would be far preferable to the dirty fuels so widely used today. Unfortunately, a rapid changeover is scarcely conceivable, given the widespread poverty in the countries affected and the sheer numbers of households still dependent on biofuels or coal. In the short term, efforts to improve the health of women and children have focused on designing a better cookstove. Over the past 25 years, hundreds of projects have been launched throughout the developing world to introduce appropriate cookstove technologies using locally available materials to produce improved stoves at a price poor people can afford. To date, however, for a variety of reasons, very few of these programs have been successful. Fortunately, within the past several years cookstove technology has advanced rapidly, with even more improvements in the pipeline.

Following a failed attempt in the early 1980s, India is basing its new clean cookstove initiative on a completely new strategy intended to increase the availability of clean and efficient energy for the poorer segments of Indian society. The government's intent is to start with a series of pilot projects using several existing, commercially available brands of improved cookstoves, as well as different grades of processed biomass fuels, in order to evaluate a range of technologies. Simultaneously, a number of activities, including a multi-million dollar "innovation prize" (young inventors, take notice!), will be launched to encourage the development of new, improved cookstove designs. As part of its initiative, India is setting up state-of-the-art testing, certification, and monitoring facilities and plans to strengthen research and development programs at its leading technical institutions. These activities will be independently monitored, evaluated, and fine-tuned on a continuous basis.

Essential to the ultimate success of this effort is ensuring that low-income families can afford to buy the new stoves. One promising solution is to encourage the involvement of microfinance organizations—entities that loan money to poor people unable to borrow from regular banks. Eager to make the cookstove initiative a viable public-private partnership, India is urging private businesses and organizations to participate. As soon as the Initiative was announced, several of these entities, including a company that manufactures stoves, began conferring with the Indian government on approaches to raise public awareness about indoor air pollution—and how improved cookstoves can alleviate the problem. A lesson learned from past failures is that focusing on health issues is not a very effective way of persuading potential acceptors to switch to biomass stoves; when told that their traditional cooking methods were making them sick, women's first response was to ask for medicines! A more successful approach has been to stress how these new devices save both time and fuel and don't befoul the kitchen with soot. Finally, an ongoing customer support effort is critical to ensuring that families continue to use the improved stoves—and to urge their neighbors to buy one as well. Previous cookstove programs in India and elsewhere ultimately failed because housewives weren't taught how to use them or because their use necessitated a change in familiar cooking methods. As a consequence, several cookstove manufacturers now not only train women in how to use their stoves, but also provide manuals and follow-up visits to check on customer satisfaction with the product.

As its new project gets underway, Indian officials are hopeful that the new cookstove technologies and delivery models developed through the country's Biomass Cookstove Initiative will prove useful in many other regions of the developing world as well. Since experts estimate that 600–800 million homes worldwide need improved cookstoves to reduce the burden of illness imposed by smoky kitchens, India's ambitious experiment could bring far-reaching health and environmental benefits (Adler, 2010).

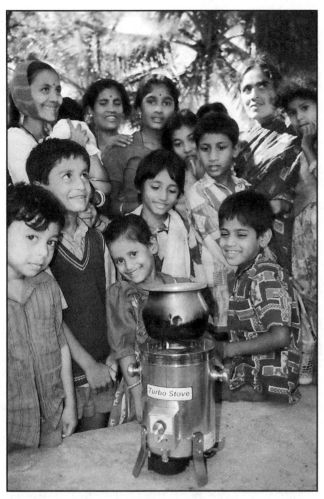

Villagers in India admire a new biomass cookstove. Initiatives to design and market cleaner-burning cookstoves at a price poor people can afford have been launched throughout the developing world to reduce indoor air pollution and rates of respiratory ailments and premature death among women and children. [*Courtesy of DOE/NREL; Community Power Corporation*]

vapors. Chemicals that break down quickly outdoors in the presence of sunlight and bacteria can persist for years in carpets, presenting an ongoing threat to residents (Ott and Roberts, 1998). Currently, over a hundred pesticidal active ingredients are registered for indoor use and there is no legal requirement to inform building occupants about the chemicals that have been applied or their possible health effects (Wargo, 2009).

Biological Pollutants

A diverse group of living organisms, most of them too small to be seen with the naked eye, also can pose serious indoor air quality problems. Bacteria and fungal spores can enter structures via air-handling systems and occasionally cause disease outbreaks (the Legionnaires'

disease episode in Philadelphia in 1976 is the classic example of this). Many allergies are associated with exposure to household dust that may contain fungal spores, bacteria, animal dander, and feces of roaches or mites. Perhaps most significant in stimulating allergic reactions are live dust mites, tiny arthropods less than 1 millimeter in size that are found in enormous numbers on bedsheets and blankets where they feed on sloughed-off scales of skin. Humid conditions or the presence of stagnant water seem to favor buildup of large populations of these unwanted guests and their dissemination has sometimes been associated with the use of humidifiers or vaporizers that harbored fungal or bacterial growth.

Flooding problems or other water damage to homes can result in an indoor air quality problem that was largely unrecognized until the mid-1990s. Growth of the toxin-producing mold, *Stachybotrys chartarum*, on damp wallpaper, ceiling tiles, carpeting made of natural fibers, cardboard boxes, bundles of newspapers, and, especially, the paper covering sheetrock can cause serious illness among residents of affected structures. Symptoms include headaches, respiratory distress, recurring colds, heart palpitations, fatigue, skin rashes, and general malaise.

Detecting the presence of *S. chartarum* requires careful inspection of areas that may not be readily visible—in wall voids, above false ceilings, in basements—any place where leaks, condensation, or sustained flooding could occur. The fungal mass is black in appearance, slightly shiny when fresh and powdery when dry. Although the mold won't continue to grow once it dries out, spores can be sucked up by the furnace fan and spread throughout a dwelling. If mold growth is found in a structure, the situation requires prompt action, first to correct the water problem and then to clean up the mold. The latter step usually requires professional help, since householders are not advised to tackle any mold-contaminated area larger than two square feet. The surface of small areas can be disinfected using one cup of chlorine bleach in a gallon of water (rubber gloves and a dust mask should be worn while working). However, the fungal mycelium within the contaminated material often survives surface disinfection and may subsequently resume growth. Thus most experts advise that while smooth, hard-surface materials such as ceramic tile, glass, or metal can be effectively cleaned and salvaged, it is virtually impossible to remove all fungal contamination from soft porous materials like paper, textiles, cellulose ceiling tiles, or paper-covered gypsum board; if these types of materials sustain water damage, they should, in most cases, be discarded and replaced (Nelson, 1999; IOM, 2004).

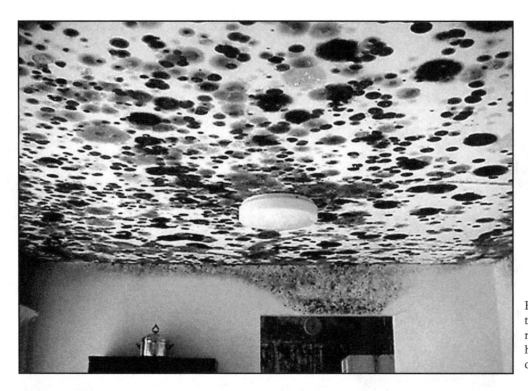

Extensive mold growth on the ceiling and walls of this room represents a significant health threat to the home's occupants. [*U.S. EPA*]

Sick Building Syndrome

Some indoor air pollutants can provoke complaints among building occupants of problems such as chest tightness, muscle aches, cough, fever, and chills. These symptoms of what is now termed **building related illness (BRI)** may persist for an extended time period after affected people leave the building, but they have clearly identifiable causes and can be clinically diagnosed. By contrast, a somewhat more mysterious malady reported with increased frequency since the mid-1970s is a condition described as **sick building syndrome (SBS)**. SBS refers to situations where building occupants experience various forms of acute discomfort—eye irritation, scratchiness in the throat, dry cough, headache, itchy skin, fatigue, difficulty in concentrating, nausea and dizziness—but no causative agent can be found. Furthermore, these symptoms generally vanish soon after sufferers leave the building (sometimes the complaints are associated with only one part of the building or even with a single room).

This situation has become so widespread in recent years that a committee of the World Health Organization has suggested that as many as 30% of the world's new and remodeled buildings may be generating complaints. While some of the symptoms reported may, in fact, be caused by illnesses contracted somewhere else, by preexisting allergies, or by job-related stress, in many cases poor indoor air quality is the major culprit. Although some of the reported outbreaks of sick building syn-drome are eventually traced to specific pollutants—e.g., microorganisms spread through ventilation systems, vehicle exhausts entering intake vents, ozone emissions from photocopying machines, VOCs outgassing from new carpeting—in most cases these contaminants aren't present in concentrations high enough to provoke the reported symptoms. Synthetic mineral fibers released into the air from acoustical ceiling tile and insulating material have been identified by researchers at Cornell University as the prime cause of many SBS situations. Most often, however, SBS has been traced to inadequate ventilation and its rise in frequency parallels efforts since the 1973 Arab oil embargo to incorporate energy conservation features into building design.

Unlike the situation in homes, most new nonresidential structures are equipped with mechanical heating, ventilation, and air conditioning (HVAC) systems and feature windows tightly sealed to restrict air infiltration from outside. These HVAC systems recirculate air throughout the building, with a significant portion of the air being reused several times prior to being exhausted, the purpose of such reuse being to lessen energy costs for heating or cooling incoming fresh air. Building codes require that a specified minimum amount of outside air be provided in order to establish an acceptable balance between oxygen and CO_2 indoors, to dilute odors, and to remove contaminants generated within the structure. Prior to 1973 that specified minimum was approximately 15 cubic feet per minute (cfm) per building occupant;

after 1973 the standard was reduced to just 5 cfm, an amount which, in a number of situations, proved inadequate for maintaining healthy, comfortable conditions. In some situations HVAC systems were improperly installed, had defective equipment, or functioned poorly because of improper vent placement. When errors such as these occur, an insufficient amount of ventilation air will be supplied. Once such problems are identified, they can generally be corrected by repairing or adjusting the air-handling system to provide additional outside air; in some cases, however, building design itself may be at fault, requiring much more extensive renovations (Turiel, 1985; Beek, 1994).

In general, the public has been slow to demand action on this problem because access to information about indoor air pollutants has been very limited and possibly because people don't want to believe that pollution problems have invaded the home. Nevertheless, an increasing awareness of the threat posed by indoor air pollutants has stimulated thinking on new ways to deal with this problem. Monitoring and enforcing air quality standards inside millions of American homes is obviously impossible. However, standards could be set to control pollutant emissions by modifying product design or manufacture. For example, the United States and a number of other countries have set standards regulating emissions of formaldehyde from plywood. In the future, updated building codes that incorporate design features and materials which minimize release and retention of indoor air pollutants could ensure that most new structures have acceptable air quality. In the meantime, efforts must be made to educate homeowners and occupants on the impact personal behavior and consumer choices can have on the quality of the indoor environment. Decisions as to which products we buy, how we use certain appliances, our consideration for the health of others as reflected in personal smoking habits—all have a profound impact on indoor air quality.

······· 14 ·······

Noise, n. A stench in the ear. . . .
The chief product and authenticating sign of civilization.
—*Devil's Dictionary* (1911)

Noise Pollution

An ever-increasing cacophony of sound is today grudgingly accepted as an inescapable component of the modern urban environment. From the traffic-clogged streets of New York and Paris to the bustling bazaars of Baghdad and the crowded sidewalks of Hong Kong, the blessings of "the quiet life," extolled by poets of yesteryear, are increasingly difficult to procure. Unfortunately, public and policy makers alike tend to regard noise as an inevitable by-product of modern life, sometimes unpleasant but largely unavoidable. At the same time, polls taken among urban residents in both the United States and Europe reveal that most city dwellers certainly are bothered by noise. According to EPA, every day over 138 million Americans are exposed to noise levels they find annoying and disruptive; among those living in big cities, 87% endure levels of noise that could, over time, impair their hearing ability (Wolkomir and Wolkomir, 2001).

In 2004 when Mayor Michael Bloomberg proposed the first complete overhaul of New York City's Noise Code in 30 years, noise ranked as the number one quality-of-life complaint in that city, prompting nearly 1,000 calls daily to its 311 citizen service hotline. Similarly, a poll conducted by a research group in the United Kingdom found that one out of every three Britons felt their enjoyment of life was diminished by noisy neighbors or the din of traffic (Bond, 1996). In Greece, reputedly the noisiest nation in Europe, a senior member of the Association for the Quality of Life remarked that "noise pollution is becoming the country's greatest health threat. If effective measures are not taken, Greeks will either turn mad or deaf."

SOURCES OF NOISE

Most concerns about noise as a pollutant have focused on the occupational environment where high levels of noise associated with machinery, equipment, and general work practices have long been recognized as a serious threat to both the physical and psychological health of workers. However, the sources of noise that torment the general public are far more diverse than those that constitute an occupational hazard. Around the world, rapidly growing numbers of cars, trucks, and motorcycles have been boosting noise levels on crowded streets and highways, while the skies above metropolitan neighborhoods are regularly deafened by the roar of jets taking off or landing at urban airports. Even once-quiet residential areas are losing their tranquility as noise-generating home appliances and motorized yard tools are increasingly regarded as essential components of the good life. Within the last few years a growing avalanche of complaints from communities large and small has been aimed at the cell-phone chatter encountered virtually everywhere, from commuter trains, buses, and planes to restaurants, theaters, and other public places.

While most people perceive community noise as a general din, originating from a multiplicity of sources, vehicular noise—particularly that from motorcycles and large trucks—seems to be regarded as the most annoying by community residents. Unfortunately, overall noise levels are growing steadily worse, in part because modern lifestyles and transportation habits are changing in ways that inevitably result in more noise generation. We also are carrying noise with us to places that formerly were havens of peace and quiet. The advent of snowmobiles, trail bikes, and powerful motorboats have brought noise pollution to once-silent wilderness areas (witness the current controversy regarding curbs on the use of snowmobiles in Yellowstone National Park), as have overflights of helicopters and small planes catering to the tourist trade in places like Arizona's Grand Canyon and Hawaii's Volcanoes National Park. Amplified music now jars city parks when partying crowds forget that not everyone finds loud rock bands pleasurable, and the desert air occasionally reverberates to a similar beat, thanks to "boom car" sound-offs where enthusiasts compete to see whose car stereos are the most ear splitting.

Beyond the technological and lifestyle changes that have made contemporary life noisier than in days gone by, there are simply more of us on the planet, adding to the din. For the most part, levels of outdoor noise are directly related to population density—the more populous the city, the noisier it is likely to be. Predicted trends in noise levels are not particularly encouraging. One of the most important sources of community noise, urban traffic, is expected to increase considerably in the years immediately ahead, with the U.S. Department of Transportation estimating that the number of automobiles on the road will increase by 0.6–0.7% annually.

Overseas, a study on noise control strategies revealed that efforts taken to reduce traffic noise in several western European countries (e.g., screens along main highways) helped to offset the increase in traffic noise but didn't result in an overall lowering of noise exposure—simply because of the rapid increase in size of the car fleet. Europeans have been experimenting with rerouting traffic, prohibiting vehicles entirely in certain areas, and constructing noise screens, a combination of which has resulted in some lowering of noise levels in central cities. However, the spread of residential suburbs into rural areas is resulting in a steady expansion of noise exposure into areas formerly undisturbed by such problems (OECD, 1991).

NOISE AS A NUISANCE

More than 2,000 years ago, the Roman Emperor Julius Caesar grappled with the issue of noise as a public nuisance when he attempted to ban chariot racing on the Eternal City's cobblestone streets due to the racket it created. History doesn't record whether or not he was suc-

cessful, but as the clamor of urban life continued to increase during the ensuing centuries, the irritant value of noise grew apace and has occasionally caused frayed tempers to snap, sometimes with fatal results. An elderly Greek farmer was given two life sentences in a maximum-security prison for shooting two residents of a neighboring apartment who ignored his repeated complaints about the loud music blasting from their residence. When taken into custody, the old man said that all he wanted was to listen to the evening news in peace ("Mad about the Noise," 1998). Disputes over noise can also be bad for business. Parisian bars and concert halls have been reeling under fines and closures due to an onslaught of noise complaints after the imposition of a tobacco ban in 2008 forced swarms of late-night revelers onto the sidewalks outside. Nearby residents, furious at the disturbance to neighborhood peace and quiet, regularly summon the police, demanding the bars and clubs be closed. Sometimes neighbors take matters into their own hands; patrons at one bar in an otherwise quiet section of the city have been pelted with eggs, had water dumped on their heads from overhanging balconies, and were once doused by a man wielding a garden hose who subsequently commented to a reporter, "At 3 in the morning when you can't sleep, you just want to destroy them" (Sayare and de la Baume, 2010).

Just as beauty is in the eye of the beholder, the perception of a sound as "noise" (arbitrarily defined by one writer as "sound at the wrong time and in the wrong place") depends on the point of view of the individual listener. A case in point is the furor that erupted in Hamtramck, Michigan, near Detroit, in the spring of 2004 when the city council amended its noise ordinance to allow a local mosque to broadcast a call to prayer from outdoor loudspeakers five times daily. Many non-Muslim residents vehemently objected to the council's decision, insisting that one group's right to religious freedom shouldn't impinge on another group's right to peace and quiet. Unfortunately for those attempting to set standards regulating noise exposure, loudness of a noise and the annoyance it causes are not always directly correlated. As any college student partying near a residential neighborhood well knows, people generating loud sounds may enjoy them, while those forced to listen usually find the same noise profoundly objectionable. In general, people most easily tolerate noise when (1) they are causing it, (2) they feel it is necessary or useful to them, or (3) they know where it is coming from. As the old French proverb aptly puts it, "I do not like noise unless I make it myself."

While most people are well acquainted with the feelings of annoyance and irritation that unwanted sounds can arouse, it is becoming increasingly evident that noise levels commonly encountered in thousands of cities, factories, places of recreation, and even inside homes represent far

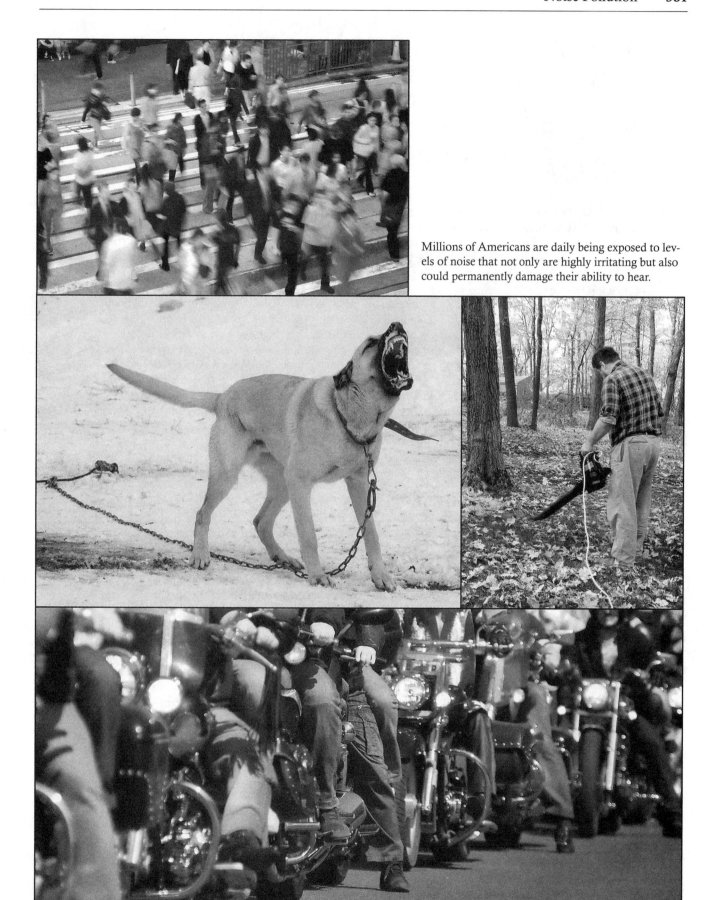

Millions of Americans are daily being exposed to levels of noise that not only are highly irritating but also could permanently damage their ability to hear.

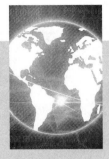

· · · · · · · 14-1 · · · · · · ·

The Not-So-Friendly Skies

Motor vehicles still top the public's noise complaint list, but aircraft din is a rapidly growing contender for first place, as millions of people worldwide suffer the environmental impacts of airport construction and expansion. In the United States, air travel is the fastest-growing form of transportation, with the number of annual passenger boardings expected to increase from their current 650 million to one billion by 2011. In Europe, the increase in air passenger loads has been even greater than in the U.S., while total world demand is now approaching two billion passengers each year. Growth in air cargo is also increasing dramatically. To meet the burgeoning demand, airports in the U.S. and abroad are expanding operations, building new runways or runway extensions to accommodate a steadily growing number of daily flights.

All of this means a greater noise burden for communities located near these facilities. Of the numerous environmental problems posed by modern airports—air pollution, odorous fumes, toxic releases, contaminated runoff—noise is by far the most frequent complaint. Concerns expressed by affected residents go well beyond mere annoyance and fear of declining property values; studies demonstrate significant health problems among people subjected to the constant roar of planes overhead. Research conducted in the Netherlands near Amsterdam's Schiphol International Airport revealed that incidence of heart disease had doubled and the use of sleeping pills increased 20–50% during a 10-year period after the addition of a new runway. One resident of the area who keeps a decibel meter on his balcony reports regular readings of 100 dB or higher as aircraft roar overhead every 90 seconds during peak hours. Researchers in Sweden found that people living near the Stockholm airport were more likely to have high blood pressure than were those living slightly farther away ("Mad about the Noise," 1998). The opening of a new international airport in a rural area outside Munich, Germany, provided researchers from Cornell University an opportunity to observe the impact of noise on a group of elementary school children residing within the airport's noise impact zone. By testing the children both before and after operations at the facility commenced, the Cornell scientists demonstrated that exposure to chronic airport noise caused children to exhibit such stress-related responses as increased blood pressure and elevated adrenaline levels. Nor were the children's adverse reactions restricted to physical symptoms; researchers also found that the youngsters' reading skills and long-term memory were impaired as a result of their noisy surroundings (Evans, Bullinger, and Hygge, 1998). In the United States, similar reports of reading problems among children in a New York school impacted by aircraft noise constitute persuasive evidence of its harmful effects and bolster efforts by groups pressing for stronger noise pollution controls.

Airport authorities, often prodded by citizen complaints or municipal lawsuits, have attempted to alleviate noise problems by altering flight patterns to avoid nighttime jet overflights of residential areas. While providing relief to noise-stressed airport neighbors, however, this practice can pose safety risks to air travelers when weather conditions make landing on the designated runway dangerous. In 1997 a jetliner landing at Schiphol swerved off the assigned runway after being denied use of a safer one due to noise pollution concerns ("Mad about the Noise," 1998).

In many cases airports can tap federal funds to soundproof nearby homes and schools or even buy out homeowners whose residences are excessively impacted by airport noise. Effective zoning laws also can help forestall citizen complaints about aircraft noise. The FAA strongly urges local governments to prohibit residential development or other noise-sensitive land uses from locating close to airports. However, FAA's admonitions are all-too-frequently ignored and the agency has no authority to overturn local land-use decisions.

The most significant initiative taken to alleviate airport noise, both in the U.S. and abroad, has been the introduction of the quieter planes required by stricter certification standards of the International Civil Aviation Organization (ICAO). This new generation of jet aircraft has had a major impact in reducing aircraft noise. In 1976, before stringent noise-reduction standards were imposed, an estimated 6–7 million Americans were exposed to objectionable levels of aircraft noise. By 2000, when the new Chapter Three standards took effect in the U.S. for all civil turbojet planes heavier than 75,000 pounds, FAA estimated the numbers of Americans exposed to significant aircraft noise levels had dropped to 500,000—in spite of rapid growth in the national aviation system during the intervening quarter-century. In addition to these efforts to reduce noise by improving aircraft design, FAA touts other new tools such as Global Positioning Systems (GPS) technology that can help mitigate noise by keeping planes from straying outside designated noise corridors (Baliles, 2001).

The success or failure of these noise abatement initiatives has profound long-term economic, as well as environmental, implications. At a time of rapidly increasing demand for air transportation, numerous aviation construction projects around the world have been delayed or abandoned in recent years due to public opposition to the noise such facilities generate. If aircraft noise problems are not adequately resolved, the ability of the global aviation industry to expand services to meet steadily growing consumer demand will be jeopardized. Further progress in reducing aircraft noise is thus critical not only for human health and quality of life, but for the health of the aviation industry as well.

more than a simple nuisance. Noise today has become a public health hazard; more insidious than easily recognized air and water pollution, noise is invisibly undermining the physical and psychological well-being of millions of people around the world. The remainder of this chapter will describe the ways in which noise affects human health, but first it is necessary to take a brief look at the physical nature of sound and how noise levels are measured.

NATURE OF SOUND

Sound is produced by the compression and expansion of air created when an object vibrates. The positive and negative pressure waves thus formed travel outward longitudinally from the vibrating source. Two basic characteristics of sound, **frequency** (or **pitch**) and **amplitude**, are related to how loud and annoying a sound will be perceived.

Frequency describes the rate of vibration—how fast the object is moving back and forth. The more rapid the movement, the higher the frequency of the sound pressure waves created. The standard unit used today for measuring frequency is the **hertz (Hz)**, equivalent to one wave per second passing a given point. Most people can hear sounds within a frequency range of 20–20,000 Hz, though there exists a great deal of individual variation in ability to perceive very low or very high frequency sounds. Because low-frequency sounds (e.g., bass sounds from amplified music, traffic noise) are more penetrating than those of high frequency, they are more difficult to control by shielding and thus are often the main source of irritation related to community noise.

Amplitude refers to the intensity of sound—how much energy is behind the sound wave. Sound waves of the same frequency can be heard as very loud or very soft, depending on the force with which they strike the ear. In technical terms, amplitude measures the maxi-

mum displacement of a sound wave from its resting, or equilibrium, position, but it is perceived psychologically as **loudness**, measured with a sound level meter in units called **decibels (dB)**. This system allows comparison of a measured sound's intensity to the level just detectable by normal, healthy ears, with a decibel level of zero representing the threshold of hearing. The decibel scale is logarithmic rather than linear; hence even a small rise in decibel values can make a significant difference in noise intensity. For example, to a pedestrian standing on a subway platform, the noise of the passing train, measured at 90 dB, sounds twice as loud as does street traffic registering 80 dB. It should be noted in passing that this discussion relates to sound measurements in *air*, where the point of reference is the human ear. The decibel scale also is used to measure sound level intensity in water, but a different reference point is employed in making such calculations. For this reason, a sound level intensity of, say, 100 dB in water is not the same as 100 dB in air.

A listener's perception of a sound as loud does not depend entirely on its amplitude, being affected to some extent by its frequency as well. Although hearing ability ranges from 20–20,000 Hz, not all of these frequencies sound equally loud to the human ear. Maximum sensitivity to sound occurs in the 1,000–5,000 Hz range. For reference, normal human speech frequencies can vary from 500–2,000 Hz. However, sounds at the very low or very high ends of the full audible range seem much fainter to our ears than do those in the middle frequencies. Thus, for example, an extremely low-pitched sound must have an amplitude many times greater than a sound of medium pitch in order for both to be heard as equally loud. For this reason, decibel values are sometimes weighted to take into account the frequency response of the human ear. When this is done, the unit measurement designation may be written as dB(A). Table 14-1 indi-

Table 14-1   Sound Levels and Human Response

Common Sounds	Noise Level (dB)	Effect
Fireworks, gunshot	140	Painfully loud
Air raid siren	140	
Jet takeoff	130	
Nightclubs	120	Maximum vocal effort
Rock concert	120	
Pile driver	110	
Stereo headphones (with volume turned up)	105	
Garbage truck	100	
City traffic	90	Very annoying, hearing damage
Alarm clock	80	Annoying
Freeway traffic	70	Phone use difficult
Air conditioning	60	Intrusive
Light auto traffic	50	Quiet
Living room	40	
Library	30	Very quiet
Broadcasting studio	20	
	10	Just audible
	0	Hearing begins

Source: Environmental Protection Agency.

cates approximate decibel values for a number of commonly encountered sounds.

NOISE AND HEARING LOSS

. . . I've shot my hearing; it hurts and it's painful, and it's frustrating when little children talk to you and you can't hear them.

—Pete Townshend

While everyone has experienced irritation due to noise, many people are unaware that the sounds that annoy them may also be affecting their hearing. Pete Townshend's confession during a 1989 press conference that his career as a rock musician had irreversibly damaged his hearing may not have dampened fans' enthusiasm for ear-splitting concerts, but it did serve as a warning to the general public that loud music may produce long-lasting effects. Unfortunately, Townshend is joined by an estimated 10 million Americans who have already suffered full or partial hearing loss due to excessive noise exposure; according to EPA, at least 20 million people in the U.S. are daily being exposed to noise levels that will permanently damage their ability to hear.

Most people are familiar with the temporary deafness and ringing in the ears that occurs after sudden exposure to a very loud noise such as a cap gun or firecracker exploding close to one's head. This type of partial hearing loss generally lasts a few hours at the most and is referred to as **temporary threshold shift (TTS)**. In addition to the obvious impact of sudden, high-intensity sounds, noise research has found that TTS also can result from longer-term exposure (16–48 hours) to noise and that recovery to normal hearing may take as long as two days, depending on both the intensity and duration of noise exposure (Melrick, 1991). The type of short-term hearing loss typified by TTS is an accepted fact of life among workers in noisy occupations, performers and patrons at rock concerts, wildly cheering spectators at sporting events, and many others. However, most people don't realize that regular, prolonged exposure to noise, even at levels commonly encountered in everyday life, can eventually result in permanent hearing impairment. Because damage to the ear is usually painless and seldom visible, few people recognize the injury they are incurring until it is too late. The Occupational Safety and Health Administration (OSHA) has determined that exposure to daily noise levels averaging just 85 decibels (approximately the loudness of an electric shaver or a food processor) will result in irreversible hearing loss. For this reason, OSHA recommends hearing protection for workers whose 8-hour, time-weighted average noise exposure is at or above 85 decibels; for exposure to noise levels of 90 decibels and above, hearing protection is *required*.

The noise of city traffic, subways, power lawn mowers, motorcycles, certain household appliances, babies screaming, and even people shouting all exceed the decibel level considered "safe." Above 85 dB, progressively higher levels of noise exposure exert ever-increasing risk of damage—and the louder the noise, the shorter the exposure time required to wreak lasting harm. With each additional five decibels of loudness the time required to cause permanent injury is cut in half (Jaret, 1990). For revelers at a nightclub, where the intensity of sound may hit 120 dB, the damage is done in less than 30 minutes.

Mechanism of Hearing Loss

Noise results in hearing loss through its destructive effect on the delicate hair cells in the Organ of Corti within the cochlea of the inner ear. These hair cells convert fluid vibrations in the inner ear into impulses that are carried by the auditory nerve to the brain, resulting in the sensation of sound. The outer hair cells at the base of the cochlea, primarily associated with high-frequency sounds, are the first to be affected, but continued exposure to loud noise will eventually result in damage to hair cells in other areas of the cochlea. Over a period of time, prolonged exposure to excessive noise levels may result in the complete collapse of individual hair cells, thus affecting the transmission of nerve impulses. The average individual is born with approximately 16,000 sensory receptors within the Organ of Corti; while 30–50% of these hair cells can be destroyed before any measurable degree of hearing loss is detectable, losses above this level result inevitably in an impairment of hearing ability. Unfortunately, there is no method at present by which a doctor can diagnose the beginning stages of noise-induced hearing loss. The earliest warning signs—inability to hear high-frequency sounds—are unlikely to be noticed unless the affected individual has his or her hearing tested for some other reason. By the time enough hair cells have been lost to affect perception of lower-frequency sounds, a process that may require many years of excessive noise exposure, the damage has been done.

This type of hearing loss, categorized as **sensorineural**, is irreversible and cannot be restored by the use of a hearing aid since both the auditory nerve and cochlear structures have been affected. By contrast, hearing loss resulting from infections (e.g., "swimmer's ear," mumps, measles, etc.) or by trauma (e.g., a blow to the head that ruptures the eardrum or puncturing the eardrum with a cotton-tipped swab) is referred to as **conductive** hearing loss and can often be corrected by surgery or medication (Thurston and Roberts, 1991). To a limited extent the ear can protect itself against loud continuous noise by a tightening of the membrane at the entrance to the inner ear, thereby dampening sound. However, in situations where noise volume increases very rapidly or instantaneously, as when a military jet makes a low-altitude flyover or someone fires a rifle close to the ear, adaptation processes and reflex protective mechanisms don't have time to function effectively. In such cases, risk of damage to the inner ear is greater than it would be if the volume of noise were increasing more slowly (Ising et al., 1990).

Many people take it for granted that a gradual loss of hearing is one of the inevitable consequences of growing older, a belief bolstered by statistics which report that by the age of 65, one out of four Americans is experiencing hearing loss significant enough to interfere with communication; by the time they reach their 90s, nine out of ten seniors are so afflicted. Many researchers are convinced, however, that the extent of the problem is considerably greater than it need be. Some years ago, an audiologist traveled to a remote African village near the Sudan-Ethiopian border to test the hearing of tribe members who had never heard the blare of amplified music or the din of urban traffic. He found that 70-year-old Africans, unlike their American peers, could easily hear sounds as soft as a murmur from as far as 300 feet away (Jaret, 1990). While

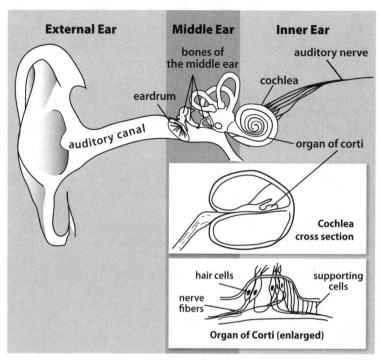

Sound waves enter the auditory canal, causing the eardrum to vibrate. The three small bones of the middle ear transmit these vibrations to the inner ear, through which they move as fluid-pressure waves. The Organ of Corti, running the length of the cochlea, converts these vibrations to nerve impulses, which are then carried to the brain by the auditory nerve.

Figure 14-1   How We Hear

some degree of age-related hearing loss (clinically described as **presbycusis**) may be inevitable, the Sudanese experience provides a meaningful lesson—one of the best ways to preserve lifelong sharpness of hearing is to limit as much as possible one's exposure to a noisy environment.

Effects of Hearing Loss

Hearing disability caused by noise can range in severity from difficulty in comprehending normal conversation to total deafness. In general, the ability to hear high-frequency sounds is the first thing to be affected by noise exposure; for this reason, tests for early detection of hearing loss should pay special attention to hearing ability in the 4,000 Hz range. People affected often have difficulty hearing such sounds as a clock ticking or telephone ringing and cannot distinguish certain consonants, particularly *s, sh, ch, p, m, t, f,* and *th*. Individuals suffering hearing loss not only have trouble with the volume of speech, but also with its clarity. They frequently accuse people with whom they are speaking of mumbling, particularly when talking on the telephone or when background noises interfere with conversation; listening to the radio or television may become impossible. The psychological impact of such difficulties—the fear of being laughed at for misunderstanding questions or comments, the frustration of not being able to follow a conversation, the feeling of isolation or alienation experienced as friends unconsciously avoid trying to converse—are frequently as severe as the physical disability. Individuals experiencing hearing loss tend to become suspicious, irritable, and depressed; their careers suffer and their social life becomes severely restricted, sometimes to the point of complete withdrawal (Perham, 1979). Some researchers even suspect that the confusion and unresponsiveness blamed on Alzheimer's disease may actually, in some cases, be due to hearing loss.

In addition to these problems, a person with partial hearing loss may suffer sharp pain in the ears when exposed to very loud noise and may experience repeated bouts of **tinnitus**—a ringing or buzzing sound in the head that can drive the victim to distraction, interfering with sleep, conversation, and normal daily activities. Probably the single most common side effect of noise-induced hearing loss, tinnitus can become a permanent condition, though it is usually only a temporary nuisance. To sufferers, the intensity of the noise in their heads can be maddening, likened by one victim to "holding a vacuum cleaner to your ear" (Murphy, 1989). The pitch of the ringing characterizing tinnitus can sound like a high scream, and volume levels as high as 70 dB have been measured. Among those afflicted with permanent tinnitus, certain medications, diet, or relaxation therapies may ease the symptoms, but the condition at this stage is essentially irreversible (Cohen, 1990).

OTHER EFFECTS OF NOISE

Hearing loss is the most obvious health threat posed by noise pollution, but it is by no means the only one. Noise can adversely affect our physical and psychological well-being in a host of other ways.

Stress and Related Health Effects

Exposure to unwanted noise involuntarily induces stress, and stress can lead to a variety of physical ailments including an increase in heart rate, high blood pressure, elevated levels of blood cholesterol, ulcers, headaches, and colitis.

Stressful reaction to loud or sudden noise undoubtedly represents an evolutionary adaptation to warnings signaling approaching danger. Bodily responses to the snarl of a predatory beast or the rumble of a boulder crashing down a mountainside cause a surge of adrenaline, an increase in heart and breathing rates, and the tensing of muscles—all physiological preparations for fight or flight that have important survival value. However, these same metabolic responses are today being triggered repeatedly by the innumerable noises of modern society. As a result, our bodies are subjected to a constant state of stress which, far from being advantageous, is literally making millions of people sick—even though they may not attribute their problems to noise. While many individuals insist that they have "gotten used to noise" and are no longer bothered by it, the truth is that no one can prevent the automatic biological changes that noise provokes.

Teratogenic Effects of Noise

The human uterus is not an inner sanctum of peace and quiet. Research has shown that fetal development proceeds amidst constant internal noise generated by the throbbing of maternal arteries and rumbling of bowels. Background noise levels within the pregnant uterus have been variously estimated as ranging anywhere from 56 to 95 dB (as compared with, for example, a typical office environment where decibel levels average about 50). Although the mother's body tissues to some extent attenuate penetration of external noise into the womb, both experimental and anecdotal evidence indicate that outside noise can provoke a physical response in the developing unborn child.

For over half a century, one method used by physicians for determining fetal viability has been to place a sound source near the mother's abdomen and expose the fetus to noise of 120 Hz frequency. Since a fetus' hearing ability is well developed by the 28th week of pregnancy, such noise exposure causes a noticeable increase in heart rate and kicking among third-trimester fetuses. Less scientific but equally persuasive testimony comes from pregnant women who have reported that they felt considerably more fetal movement while listening to music in a concert hall, the kicking reaching a peak when the audience began to applaud!

While the fact that noise exposure begins well before birth is undisputable, it is less clear whether such exposure presents any risk of hearing impairment to the unborn child. The question is of some concern because approximately 47% of the U.S. workforce is now female and many of these women will experience one or more pregnancies during their working years. Since occupational noise pollution control frequently is focused on providing ear protection to workers, the question of possible noise-induced hearing damage to the fetuses of pregnant employees is of more than academic interest. While a few epidemiologic studies have reported some degree of hearing impairment among children whose mothers received occupational noise exposures up to 100 dB during pregnancy, most of the limited research done to date indicates that hearing loss induced in a fetus by external noise is highly unlikely. The insulating effect of maternal

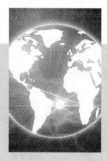

······· 14-2 ·······

The Noisy Seas

Humans aren't the only creatures forced to endure excessive levels of noise pollution. Throughout the world's oceans, whales, dolphins, sea lions, and other marine mammals are under increasing stress from human-generated sounds that threaten their hearing, health, and behavior—perhaps even their survival.

The oceans, of course, have never been serenely quiet. Marine life evolved in an environment permeated by underwater noises generated by wind-driven wave action, earthquakes, thunderstorms, cracking ice, and, in time, by the myriad sounds produced by sea animals themselves. Sea-dwelling mammals and fish rely heavily on sound to locate food, to navigate, and to communicate with other members of their species. All aquatic vertebrates have ears and auditory capabilities and they utilize sound as a critical means of learning about and surviving in their watery environment.

In recent years, awareness of the importance of sound to marine mammals has led to growing alarm among scientists and concerned citizens who fear that the steadily increasing underwater din produced by a wide range of human activities may be adversely affecting the lives of these creatures. Ocean noise levels that had remained more or less constant from primordial times until the mid-1800s began to escalate during the past century and a half as the Industrial Revolution accelerated and expanded across the globe. Commercial ship traffic early became, and still remains, the leading anthropogenic component of noise in the marine environment, as sailing ships gave way to mechanically powered vessels and as the number and size of ships steadily increased. In localized areas, high-speed yachts contribute significantly to underwater noise, as do outboard and inboard motorboats. In recent years the growing popularity of whale-watching has resulted in a documented change in the behavior of killer whales, as the animals increase the duration of their calls to compensate for the noise generated by numerous boatloads of tourists circling near their pods.

Over the past 65 years since the end of World War II, numerous other noise-generated activities have proliferated in or adjacent to the world's seas, raising fears of serious resultant harm to ocean mammals. Among these newer sources are activities related to offshore oil and gas exploration and production—seismic surveying utilizing air guns, drilling, emplacement and removal of drilling platforms, and provision of supplies to these platforms by noisy low-flying helicopters or power boats. Construction and other industrial activity along seacoasts further contribute to human-induced ocean sound levels. Dredging and pile-driving are both very noisy activities, as are power plant operations and certain types of industries; the increasing proliferation of near-shore power-generating windmills are a relatively recent addition to the long list of anthropogenic noise in the marine environment.

Attracting the most attention from environmentalists is the widespread use of sonar systems, employed for both civilian and military purposes, to characterize physical properties of the seabed and to locate underwater objects such as schools of fish, sunken ships, or enemy submarines. Proponents of sonar use correctly point out that, to date, sonar is the most powerful remote-sensing tool available for such tasks, a tool that has produced significant practical benefits and increased our general understanding of marine geology. Sonar also comprises an essential weapon for maintaining national security, providing a means to detect and track missile-carrying submarines, thus providing an early warning of potential danger to naval vessels in the general vicinity.

While the benefits of sonar and other types of underwater acoustical devices are undeniable, such technologies, nevertheless, raise legitimate concerns as to whether they affect the normal activities of marine mammals and their long-term ability to sustain healthy populations. As long ago as 1972, the Marine Mammal Protection Act mandated controls over noise sources that could negatively impact whales and other ocean mammals. However, there was limited public interest in the issue until 1992 when the Office of Naval Research (ONR) launched its Acoustic Thermometry of Ocean Climate project, utilizing high-intensity, low-frequency sound waves from a source deployed deep in the ocean and transmitted over thousands of kilometers to gather basic scientific information on the properties of ocean basins. The controversy generated by this project and the increasing levels of scrutiny it attracted from marine biologists, environmental groups, and other concerned parties have prompted ONR to require that all of its research programs utilizing underwater acoustic transmissions identify and mitigate against any possible harm to the marine environment and adhere strictly to all federal and relevant state environmental laws and regulations (National Research Council, 2003).

These safeguards have not silenced critics of such activities, however. In 2002 protests erupted when the U.S. Navy was given a permit to deploy its low-frequency active (LFA) sonar system, intended for submarine detection, across three-fourths of the world's oceans. Because the project calls for warships to tow a vertical line of up to 18 loudspeakers emitting an effective noise level of 235 dB through vast areas of the ocean, opponents alleged that whales or dolphins swimming nearby could be injured, deafened, or even killed by the excruciatingly loud noise. Even 300 miles from the source, they charged, noise levels would be high enough to interfere with the animals' normal activities. While research data pertaining to the effects of anthropogenic sound on marine life are scanty, there are valid reasons for such concerns. In 2001 in the Bahamas and 2002 in the Canary Islands, mass strandings of beaked whales (*Ziphius cavirostris*) occurred shortly after the navy engaged in military exercises testing high-energy, mid-frequency (1–10 kHz) sonar. A team of scientists from London's Institute of Zoology examined the whale carcasses soon after the strandings and concluded the animals died of decompression sickness, their livers and kidneys damaged by gas bubbles that formed in the whales' blood as they shot to the surface to escape the sonar. This study constituted the most direct evidence to date that sonar can be lethal to marine mammals (Jepson et al., 2003).

When news of the navy's LFA sonar permit was announced, environmental groups quickly rallied to block commencement of the research project. Leading the opposition, the Natural Resources Defense Council (NRDC) filed a lawsuit against the navy and the National Marine Fisheries Service (the agency issuing the permit), charging that deployment of the LFA system would violate the Marine Mammal Protection Act. In October 2002, just days before the navy intended to commence operations across 14 million square miles of the Pacific, NRDC won a preliminary injunction to block such action; in August 2003, a federal judge issued a final ruling barring the navy from pursuing its project as originally proposed, thereby protecting critical habitat of endangered whales and sparing countless marine mammals and fish from death and injury. However, the injunction permits the navy to test its sonar system in a limited area off the coast of northeastern Asia and allows use of the system in case of war.

Environmentalists were less pleased with the outcome of a more recent dispute with the navy regarding training exercises employing mid-frequency sonar off the coast of southern California. While admitting that these drills were likely to cause permanent injury to more than 450 whales and temporary hearing impairment to at least 8,000 more, the navy argued that such exercises were essential for antisubmarine warfare training. The Natural Resources Defense Council filed suit to curb the use of damaging sonar and in early 2008 a federal district judge and a federal appeals court both sided with the environmentalists, banning sonar use within 12 miles of the coast and requiring the navy to utilize safety measures to protect whales and dolphins during maneuvers. The navy appealed these rulings to the U.S. Supreme Court and in November 2008 the Court ruled that the navy's need to conduct realistic training exercises was more important than the health and welfare of marine mammals. The extent to which this situation adversely affects the well-being of sea creatures is as yet little understood and experts agree that far more broad-ranging research is needed to clarify and quantify the impact of human-generated noise on the health and behavior of these animals.

tissues, which limits the amount of outside sound penetrating the uterine environment, renders noise an unlikely teratogenic agent (Thurston and Roberts, 1991).

Much more research is needed to define the extent of the relationship, if any, between noise and birth defects, as well as to establish how high noise levels must be to cause developmental problems. Lacking definitive information, some doctors recommend that pregnant women try to avoid noise exposure to the greatest extent possible,

one such expert offering the tongue-in-cheek advice that "any expectant mother should get out of New York."

Effects of Noise on Learning Ability

It has long been recognized that noisy surroundings at school and in the home can adversely affect children's language development and their ability to read. A classic study in the early 1970s, comparing reading ability among children living on different floors of an apartment building located adjacent to a busy highway, revealed that youngsters living on the higher (i.e., quieter) floors had better reading scores than those living on lower (noisier) floors. It also showed that the longer a child had experienced excessive noise exposure, the poorer was his/her reading ability. Investigators concluded that a noisy home environment has more of an impact on reading skills than do such factors as parents' educational level, number of children in the family, or the child's grade level (Cohen, Glass, and Singer, 1973).

More recently, an important study conducted by a Cornell University researcher on first-and second-grade students whose school is located within the flight contour of a major New York metropolitan airport (overflights during school hours averaged one flight every 6.6 minutes) demonstrated convincingly that children constantly exposed to noise have poorer reading skills than children attending school in quiet areas. Investigators concluded

that the children's reading difficulties stem, at least in part, from noise-related impairment of their ability to recognize and understand spoken words. In order to cope with the constant noise to which they are subjected, children living and attending school near the airport unconsciously reduce their noise burden by "filtering out" certain sounds, including human speech (Evans and Maxwell, 1997). Given the large number of schools worldwide located near airports or busy highways, as well as the increase in residential area noise levels in developed and developing countries alike, the link between noise exposure and children's language development should be a serious concern to educators and parents.

Safety Aspects of Noise

Safety, as well as health, can be in jeopardy when noise levels are high. Both by interfering with shouts for help or by masking warning signals, high levels of back-

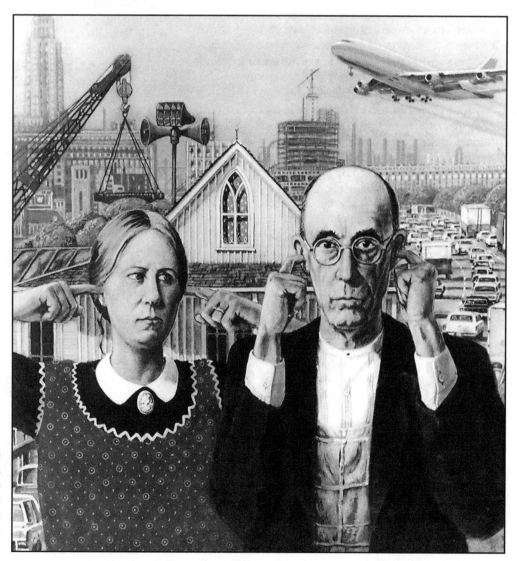

Contemporary American life is much noisier than in days gone by due in part to advanced technology, lifestyle changes, transportation habits, and population density. [*EPA Journal*]

ground noise pose a very real threat to public safety. A tragic case in point involved a Bloomington, Illinois, teenager who was killed when struck from behind by an Amtrak train while walking in the middle of the tracks en route to school. Investigators subsequently concluded that the young man failed to hear the approaching train because he was wearing large earphones while listening to a radio set at high volume. As a police officer at the scene remarked, "The engineer blew the horn, then laid on it to get this person off the tracks. It didn't work. We believe he never heard the train because he had his stereo on" (Simpson, 1997).

In the occupational environment as well, high noise levels can pose a safety hazard by preventing workers from hearing shouts of warning or cries for help. Many traffic accidents are thought to be caused by drivers' inability to hear emergency sirens. In a perhaps misguided effort to get around this problem, the New York Police Department unintentionally raised other noise concerns. In the fall of 2009, the NYPD installed "rumblers" on more than 150 of its patrol cars. Intended to catch the attention of drivers who have their windows rolled up and stereos on or pedestrians focused exclusively on their iPods, these new ground-shaking sound devices ensure that those who can't hear or see an approaching police car will be able to *feel* it up to 200 feet away. Anti-noise campaigners are aghast at the prospect of the "acoustic nightmare" New Yorkers will be forced to endure in the name of public safety—especially in light of a disclaimer by the rumbler's manufacturer, Federal Signal Corp., that users should wear hearing protection because the "audible equipment may cause hearing damage" (Feldman, 2009).

Table 14-2   Permissible Noise Exposures Established by OSHA

Duration per day (hours)	Sound level (dB)
8	90
6	92
4	95
3	97
2	100
1½	102
1	105
½	110
¼ or less	115

Source: OSHA, Occupational Safety and Health Standards, #1910.95.

Sleep Disruption

Sleep is a biological necessity. We need sleep to repair the wearing out of bodily tissues and to rejuvenate them; deprivation or disruption of sleep can thus directly threaten both physical health and mental well-being.

Noise can prevent people from going to sleep, can waken them prematurely, or can cause shifts from deeper to lighter stages of sleep. While individual response to noise in relation to its impact on sleep varies widely, in general adults are wakened by noise more easily than are children; the elderly are more sensitive than the middle-aged; sick people are more affected than healthy ones; and women are more easily disturbed than men (Bugliarello, 1976). In 1996 the World Health Organization cited noise as a significant health threat and the following year published guidelines that recommended lowering average nighttime noise levels suitable for undisturbed sleep from 35 to 30 decibels, with a peak nighttime maximum of 45 dB(A). Given such recommendations for healthful sleep, it is troubling to note that millions of people currently are subjected to noise levels well above the WHO guidelines. Indeed, a survey of traffic noise in western Europe estimates that 16% of Europeans are subjected to more than 40 decibels in their bedrooms every night (Bond, 1996). Given this situation, it shouldn't be surprising that results of a German study, discussed at a 2004 conference in Bonn on sleep and health, found that 80 million Europeans—20% of all EU residents—suffer from stress and sleep disorders serious enough to affect their health.

NOISE CONTROL EFFORTS

Historically, noise abatement efforts have consisted primarily of local ordinances directed at specific community nuisances. One of the earliest such laws was a London ordinance that went into effect in 1829, allowing stagecoach horses to be confiscated if they disrupted church services (Lipscomb, 1974). Over the years since then, cities have adopted a wide variety of local restrictions on noise sources. A brief sampling of such regulations include: requirements for mufflers on cars; bans on leaf blowers; prohibitions against construction activity, garbage collection, or lawn mowing during early morning or evening hours; bans on roosters or other noisy animals within city limits; restrictions on auto horn-blowing; bans on truck traffic through residential neighborhoods; and prohibitions on "boom cars" or other forms of amplified music outdoors.

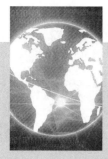

······· 14-3 ·······

Play Can Be Deafening!

The association between high noise levels and hearing loss in the occupational environment has been recognized—and regulated—for years. The Occupational Safety and Health Administration (OSHA) has set an eight-hour time-weighted average of 90 dB(A) as the maximum permissible noise exposure for the American worker. In recent years, however, it has become increasingly clear that dangerous levels of noise are found not only in factories but also in the home and in association with a wide range of recreational activities. The same individual whose hearing is protected by regulations while on the job may incur irreparable damage by engaging in noisy activities where sound levels are unregulated.

Perhaps most at risk of nonoccupational noise-induced hearing loss are millions of children and young adults whose ideas of fun are often inseparable from noise: listening to amplified music, playing electronic arcade games, participating in noisy sports events, playing in the school band. Researchers have been surprised to discover that noise-induced hearing loss can begin at 10–20 years of age, much earlier than they previously had thought possible. In 1990 a group of British researchers reported unexpected frustration in their efforts to study hearing damage among youths aged 15–23. Their project was stymied because they couldn't assemble a sufficient number of young people to serve as "controls"—virtually all the candidates had already been exposed to loud music (U.S. Congress, 1991).

Hearing impairment among rock musicians is legendary, as testimony by such notables as Pete Townshend, Ted Nugent, Joey Kramer, and others bears witness. Employees of nightclubs featuring loud music are also at risk. A survey of noise levels in a sampling of San Francisco dance clubs found that all violated the CAL-OSHA workplace noise regulations; club employees were resigned to hearing loss as an inescapable consequence of working in such a noisy environment. The impact on those whose exposure is limited to attending rock concerts or noisy nightclubs is probably less dramatic. Attendees are typically exposed to noise levels of 100 dB or higher (OSHA standards permit no more than two hours exposure to noise of this intensity in the workplace). They frequently experience temporary threshold shift (TTS) but generally recover within a few hours to a few days after exposure.

The roar of the crowd at athletic events may be endangering fans' hearing, particularly if the event in question happens to be a Minnesota Twins game at the Metrodome. Perhaps because its dome is smaller than average, with a roof configuration that returns noise to the field, the Metrodome may reverberate with noise levels exceeding 100 dB when the stands are full and the home team is winning. As in the situation with rock concerts, spectators who spend a limited amount of time in these raucous surroundings are at minor risk of long-term harm, but Twins players and the concessionaires who spend most of the season amidst the cheering throngs are at serious risk of permanent hearing impairment (Gauthier, 1988).

Many household appliances expose people of all ages to noise levels that frequently exceed the 85 dB "safe" level; fortunately the duration of exposure to such noises as the whir of a food processor or the drone of a vacuum cleaner is generally quite brief. On the other hand, certain power tools such as chain saws or leaf blowers could present a risk if used for prolonged periods without hearing protection. Similarly, farm equipment such as tractors can be a significant cause of hearing impairment for rural youngsters. A study conducted in Wisconsin revealed that more than half the children involved in farm work experienced some degree of noise-induced hearing loss, double the rate of children not working on farms.

Of all the dangerous forms of recreational noise exposure, however, the greatest toll is wrought by hunting and target shooting, activities regularly enjoyed by an estimated 13% of the U.S. population. With decibel levels frequently exceeding the threshold of pain, the crack of gunfire, or even cap pistols, can instantly destroy receptor cells in the inner ear and irreversibly damage hearing ability. Among a study group of 94 children or teenagers who were victims of noise-induced hearing loss, an analysis of the noise sources revealed that fully 46% suffered because of guns or fireworks; only 12% had been damaged by exposure to live or amplified music, 8% by power tools, and 4% by recreational vehicles (Clark, 1991).

Since noise-induced hearing loss is cumulative, growing slowly but steadily worse with continued exposure to a wide variety of high-decibel activities, people of all ages, but especially children, need to become more aware of the importance of wearing ear protection when engaged in noisy activities. Natural defenses unfortunately are insufficient; as an 18th century Englishman long ago commented, "I have often lamented that we cannot close our ears with as much ease as we can our eyes."

Overseas, governments are taking legislative action against nuisance noise as well. In Beijing, China, the municipal government regulates car alarms, requiring that they ring for no more than 35 seconds and then only when the engine catches fire; when a door, trunk, or hood is opened; or when the entire car is moved. These regulations were provoked by a flood of complaints about excessive noise from the city's 300,000 vehicles with anti-theft devices, some of which were so sensitive they began ringing when the car was merely touched or even when exposed to thunder, hail, or rain! New York City's new noise code targets barking dogs and Mr. Softee ice cream trucks as well as jackhammers, overly loud bars and nightclubs, and noisy air conditioning units—just to name a few. In Switzerland, public complaints about truck noise resulted in passage of a nationwide referendum requiring that heavy trucks transiting the country be put on trains when they cross the Swiss border to spare that small Alpine country the associated pollution, as well as the thundering noise that occasionally has been known to cause avalanches and landslides.

The federal government entered the noise control arena in 1972 with passage of the Noise Control Act—the first national law aimed at relieving overstimulated American ears by regulating certain commercial products considered to be major noise sources. The law called for noise emission limits to be set for products such as medium- and heavy-weight trucks, buses, motorcycles, power lawn mowers, jackhammers, and rock drills. In addition, the EPA was to draft noise labeling requirements for noisy products as well as conduct studies on the health impact of noise in order to provide an objective basis for the numerical noise standards yet to be promulgated.

In 1978 the Noise Control Act was amended by the Quiet Communities Act, which authorized EPA to work in partnership with state and local governments, helping them to develop antinoise programs appropriate to their own special needs and abilities. Federal funding provided aid in the form of grants, seminars, and training programs to assist lower levels of government. With the EPA serving as a coordinating agency and providing seed money for local initiatives, hundreds of community noise

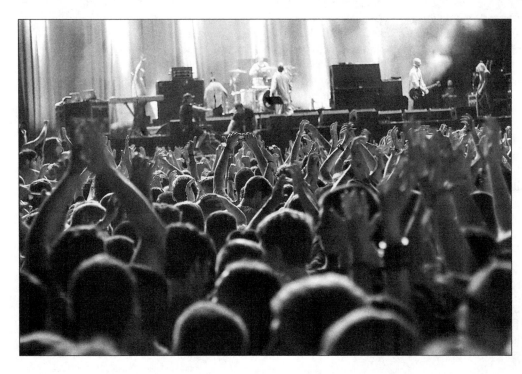

Loud rock concerts pose a risk of noise-induced hearing loss to those who attend as well as to the musicians themselves.

abatement programs were launched during the 1970s. Noise control efforts suffered a serious setback in the 1980s under President Reagan, who was committed to an antiregulatory agenda on environmental issues. In 1982, to the dismay of noise experts, EPA's Office of Noise Abatement and Control (ONAC) was disbanded and has yet to be restored. Without EPA leadership, technical assistance, or funding, research on the impact of noise on health and hearing has declined sharply since the early 1980s.

Most information on noise pollution appearing in current textbooks is still based on studies conducted during the 1970s. The promising proliferation of municipal noise abatement efforts that characterized the late 1970s has suffered a similar reversal. Although the Noise Control Act mandates are still theoretically in effect, they are not being enforced. Regulations that were about to be promulgated at the time ONAC closed were never completed and those that had been finalized have been ignored. Of the wide range of equipment targeted by the Noise Control Act, the only products for which noise emission standards have yet been promulgated are air compressors, motorcycles, trucks, and waste compactors. In 1991 hearing experts testified before a congressional committee, urging restoration of EPA leadership in national noise abatement efforts and calling for renewed noise emission information and warning labels on dangerously noisy equipment. Unfortunately, these initiatives were not followed by legislative action and noise pollution control remains an issue largely neglected by policy makers. Undoubtedly the most serious obstacle to implementing effective programs is the difficulty of convincing both policy makers and the public that noise pollution is really important. As one EPA official remarked, "Noise is something we grow up with, and it is very difficult to believe that such a common pollutant could be doing anything serious to our health or the environment." Until voters insist that excessive noise is a community health hazard that must be controlled, it is unlikely that elected officials will give noise abatement efforts the attention they deserve.

15

All the rivers run into the sea, yet the sea is not full;
to the place from whence the rivers come, thither they return again.
—Ecclesiastes 1:7

Water Resources

Although the ancient writer of Ecclesiastes expressed his scientific observations in poetic form, his statements relating to the cycling of water through the hydrosphere are basically correct, albeit overly simplified. Water moves in what is essentially a closed system, circulating from one part of the earth to another, changing in form from liquid to solid or gas and back to liquid again, yet remaining relatively constant in total amount. Water occurs as vapor in the atmosphere, as rain or snow falling on the earth or oceans, as ice locked in massive glaciers or ice caps, and as rivers, streams, lakes, seas, and subterranean groundwater. The manner by which water moves from place to place, changing from one form to another, is called the hydrologic cycle.

HYDROLOGIC CYCLE

The hydrologic cycle, like virtually all other processes on earth, is powered by energy from the sun that causes water to evaporate from the surface of the oceans, rivers, lakes, and from the soil. The movement of this water vapor in the atmosphere is an important factor in the redistribution of heat around the earth. Because heat is absorbed when water evaporates, the atmosphere becomes a reservoir of heat energy. This heat energy then drives the hydrologic cycle that gives rise to the atmospheric forces involved in weather and climate. The principal processes involved in the hydrologic cycle are:

1. Evaporation of water from surface waters and from the soil.
2. Transportation of water by plants; because both evaporation and transpiration produce the same result (i.e., the addition of water vapor to the atmosphere), the two processes are often collectively called evapotranspiration.
3. Transport of atmospheric water from one place to another as water vapor or as liquid water droplets and ice crystals in clouds.
4. Precipitation when atmospheric water vapor condenses and falls as rain, hail, sleet, or snow.
5. Runoff, whereby water that has fallen finds its way back to the oceans, flowing either on or under the surface of the continents.

The amount of time required for the completion of the cycle can vary widely from place to place and from one part of the cycle to another. On the average, a water molecule spends nine days in the atmosphere from the time it evaporates until it falls again as rain or snow (Ehrlich, Ehrlich, and Holdren, 1977). However, if it happens to fall as a snowflake on the Antarctic ice sheet, it may remain there for thousands of years before it breaks off as part of an iceberg and melts into the ocean; conversely, if it falls during a desert thunderstorm, it might evaporate in an hour or two.

Approximately 71% of the earth's surface is covered with water, a resource amounting to almost 1.5 billion km^3 in total volume. Of this amount, however, only a

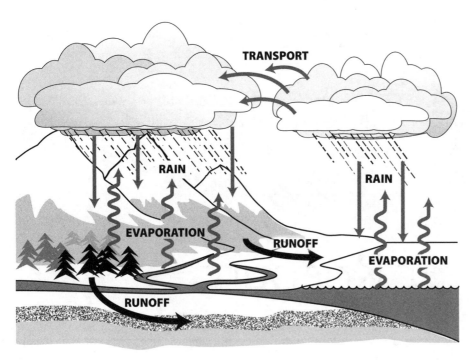

Figure 15-1   Hydrologic Cycle

very small percentage is readily available for human use. Most of the water on the planet, about 97.4%, is found in the world's seas and oceans—enormously abundant but too salty for drinking or agricultural use; 2% is freshwater locked up in glaciers and polar ice caps; the remainder, less than 1% of the total, consists of freshwater in rivers, lakes, groundwater, and water vapor in the atmosphere (World Resources Institute, 1992; Maurits la Riviere, 1989). Obviously, for humans this is the portion of greatest significance, since it constitutes the water we drink, bathe in, and use for irrigation and industrial purposes. Of this small percentage of water on which human life depends, only a minuscule portion is found in the rivers, streams, and lakes of the world. Likewise, at any given moment only a tiny amount of the world's water occurs as atmospheric water vapor. By far the greatest amount of all available freshwater, approximately 96.5% of the total, is found beneath the surface of the soil in the form of groundwater.

WATER QUANTITY AND HEALTH

The human body's absolute dependence on regular intake of water is second only to its need for oxygen. While an individual can, if necessary, survive for a number of weeks without food, deprivation of water will result in death within a few days at the most. Water makes up approximately 65% of the adult human's body, a somewhat higher percentage in children. Blood consists of 83% water, while bones contain 25%. Water is essential for the body's digestion of food, transport of nutrients and hormones, and removal of wastes. Depending on a person's size, weight, degree of activity, and the prevailing level of temperature and humidity, an individual requires approximately 1–3 liters of water daily just to maintain bodily functions.

To maintain good health and an adequate standard of living, however, 50 liters of water per day are considered the bare minimum essential for drinking, food preparation, cooking, dish washing, and bathing (Simon, 1998). The use of sewer systems for safe removal of human wastes—wastes that present serious problems when mismanaged—also requires considerable amounts of water. In typical urban residential areas, sewers will not transport wastes efficiently if per capita water use is less than 100 liters a day. In industrialized countries and among the more affluent segments of the urban population in developing nations, water quantity is generally more than ample to meet these basic human needs; average daily water consumption in such situations ranges between 200–400 liters per person per day.

In poor countries, however, the World Health Organization estimates that 1.1 billion people still lack access to safe drinking water and that 2.6 billion—40% of the world's population—don't have adequate water for basic hygiene. In many rural areas the problem is not the lack of water per se, but rather that the source of such water is far from the point of use. In some countries, women may spend several hours each day hauling water from a distant river, well, or standpipe to their homes, leaving little time for more economically productive tasks such as gardening or trading in the marketplace. Economists estimate that more than 10 million person-years of time and effort are spent each year in such water-hauling activities. If more conveniently located water supplies could enable these women to work just one additional hour per day at a minimum-wage job, the estimated cumulative income from such paid labor would be worth $63.5 billion annually (Hoffman, 2009). The sheer physical effort involved in carrying water long distances also exerts a toll on the health of rural women who, not infrequently, may be malnourished and overworked.

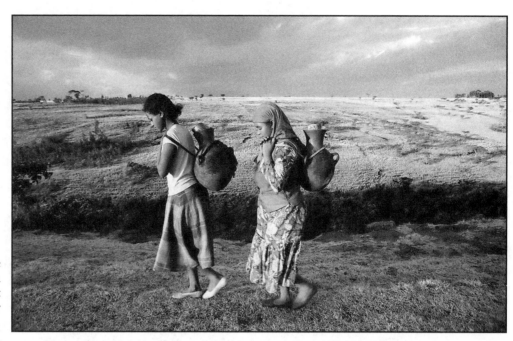

In developing countries like Ethiopia, women must often travel long distances on foot to obtain the daily water for their households.

In most urban areas of the developing world, water supply systems are in place, but frequently they are in poor condition or are unreliable, functioning perhaps only a few hours each day. While walking distances for the urban poor are less than for their country cousins, such people nevertheless spend hours waiting in long lines for their turn at the standpipe. Among many poor urban residents, water is obtained by purchasing it from vendors at a cost many times higher than the cost per unit of a piped-in municipal supply. The necessity of buying water imposes a heavy financial burden on family incomes; in Port-au-Prince, Haiti, 20% of a typical slum-dweller's household budget is spent on water.

In situations such as these, where safe water is in short supply, difficult or time-consuming to obtain, or exorbitantly expensive, important aspects of personal hygiene and basic sanitation such as washing hands and eating utensils are frequently neglected. In addition, there is a strong temptation to utilize polluted sources of water if higher-quality supplies are not easily accessible. A study published by the World Health Organization demonstrated that improved access to water reduced the incidence of diarrheal cases by 25%, while improvements in both water quality and access reduced such illnesses by fully 37%. Perhaps the most essential prerequisite for improving the health and living standards among the developing-world poor is an increase in readily available safe water (Briscoe, 1993).

WATER SUPPLY: OUR NEXT CRISIS?

Water scarcity may be the most underappreciated global environmental challenge of our time.
—WorldWatch Institute

While water is indeed a renewable resource, the rate at which it is renewed within the global hydrologic cycle is both fixed and slow. Water also is a finite resource—although human technologies can devise means for utilizing the existing supply more efficiently, science cannot create additional water nor alter the rate at which water is circulated through the biosphere. Faced with these realities, many water resource experts view current water use trends with alarm, warning that the approaching "water crisis" which they foresee could be the first resource constraint to impose serious limits on future world economic growth. Such fears are based on the fact that over the past 300 years worldwide, withdrawals from freshwater resources have increased more than 35-fold and continue to grow rapidly. Since the beginning of the 20th century, water consumption has risen more than twice as fast as the rate of population growth. A continuation of this trend in the years ahead appears likely, as water demand from growing cities, industry, and irrigated agriculture steadily increases.

Currently, according to a United Nations assessment of freshwater resources, about 40% of the world's people live in regions experiencing water "stress," defined as those with less than 1700 cubic meters of water per person annually—a state of affairs that could result in frequent water shortages. At levels below 1000 cubic meters

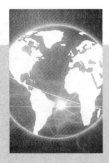

······· 15-1 ·······

Can Desalination Slake the World's Thirst?

Three years of drought may have been the deciding factor in the May 2009 decision by the San Diego County Water Authority to give final approval to Poseidon Resources' request to build a $320 million desalination plant in Carlsbad, California. First proposed in 1998, the highly controversial project took six years to go through the permitting process, with environmental groups arguing that the plant would be disastrous for marine life in the vicinity. Nevertheless, wider concerns about long-term water security in southern California ultimately proved decisive. As Carlsbad's mayor remarked to reporters, "Water is going to be very short until you have a new source—and the only new source is desalination." When it becomes operational in 2012, the Poseidon facility will be the largest desalination plant in the Western Hemisphere, taking in 100 million gallons of seawater and producing 50 million gallons of fresh drinking water daily. Expected to begin construction in 2010, the Carlsbad plant is but the first of more than 20 proposed large desalination plants along the California coast (about a dozen small facilities are currently operational), with major projects at Huntington Beach and Camp Pendleton also expected to break ground in 2010.

Desalination boosters in southern California can identify with inhabitants of arid coastal regions worldwide who have long dreamed of transforming seawater into a potable beverage. In recent years technological advances have turned that dream into reality for a growing number of water-short regions. Today some form of desalination is being used in approximately 130 countries, as well as in every U.S. state (Florida, California, Arizona, and Texas have most of the installed capacity). About 10,000 facilities larger than 100 cubic meters/day have been installed or contracted around the world, though not all are currently operational. Although these numbers may sound impressive, the total capacity of installed desalination plants represents just 3/1000ths of global daily freshwater use. Not surprisingly, fully half of world desalination capacity is in the oil-rich but water-poor countries of the Persian Gulf and North Africa. Saudi Arabia is the world's leading producer of desalted water, boasting 34 plants yielding over 800 million gallons a day. The United States ranks second in terms of desalination capacity (though several of the Gulf states, such as the United Arab Emirates, Kuwait, and Qatar get a significantly higher percentage of their daily freshwater supply from desalted seawater), with more than 2000 desalination plants, mostly small facilities, installed or contracted. However, unlike the situation elsewhere, most U.S. desalination plants treat only brackish waters or salt-laden river waters rather than seawater; in fact, in 2005 seawater represented less than 10% of U.S. desalination capacity. At present, prior to commencement of operations at the Carlsbad plant in 2012, the largest desalination facility in the United States, at 25 million gallons of freshwater per day, is the Tampa Bay Water plant in Florida, completed in 2003 but, thanks to financial and technical problems, not fully operational until 2007.

The technologies for desalting seawater are straightforward and relatively simple. The traditional fuel-intensive method, still used at most desalination plants in the oil-rich Middle East, employs a **multi-stage flash distillation (MSF)** process, in which water is heated under pressure and then injected into a low-pressure chamber where it instantly "flashes" into steam which is captured and condensed into pure water. The fact that pressurized hot water from a single source can be flashed into several chambers simultaneously makes it possible to produce large amounts of water quite dependably by this method. Elsewhere in the world, including the United States, a somewhat more energy-efficient approach known as **reverse osmosis (RO)** is the predominant technology, utilized at Tampa Bay, the plants in California, as well as by large facilities in Israel and Singapore. In this process, seawater is forced under high pressure through semi-permeable membranes that permit passage of water molecules but screen out the slightly larger ions of sodium and chloride.

The main problem with both methods—and the main factor limiting wider adoption of desalination—is the enormous amount of energy needed to power these processes, a requirement that translates into a high price per unit of water. In general, energy expenditures account for one-third to one-half the cost of desalted water. Although advances in RO technology have reduced desalination costs markedly in recent years, it is still considerably more expensive than obtaining the same amount from conventional freshwater sources. While the premium price associated with desalinated water may be acceptable to meet the escalating demand for drinking water in arid regions where other alternatives are scarce or nonexistent (or where abundance of domestic oil reserves render energy costs of trivial importance!), desalination is still far too expensive for the irrigation or industrial purposes that comprise the bulk of world water demand.

In addition to energy constraints, opponents of desalination plants point to several human health and environmental issues associated with such facilities. While desalted water is typically of high quality, concerns have been expressed that biological and chemical contaminants present in the source water could be hazardous to public health if desalted water doesn't undergo further treatment. Similarly, there are worries that desalination could introduce new contaminants into the finished product (e.g. brominated organic by-products of disinfection) or could remove essential minerals such as magnesium and calcium. Such problems can be mitigated by post-treatment of water, but emphasize the need for careful monitoring and regulation of desalination facilities.

The ecological impacts of desalination plants on the marine environment arouse even greater concerns and were responsible for much of the controversy surrounding the Carlsbad plant. Among the impacts wrought by desalination facilities is the impingement of adult fish, waterbirds, large invertebrates, and even marine mammals on intake screens when they get caught in the currents created by water intake pipes; smaller fish, eggs, larvae, and plankton that pass through the screens unharmed subsequently are killed as the saltwater is processed. All these organisms are eventually discarded back into the ocean, where their decomposition can deplete the oxygen content of surrounding waters.

Another serious environmental effect associated with desalination plants is ultimate disposal of the concentrated brine such plants produce. Typically these discharges are twice as salty as intake waters, as well as being more dense, and may contain toxic chemicals used during the desalination process to prevent fouling of membranes (e.g. chlorine and other biocides) as well as antiscaling agents (polyacrylic or sulfuric acid) that prevent salt formation on piping. Discharges also may contain coagulants (e.g. ferric chloride and polymers) used to bind together particles that are collected as the water passes through a filter. All these chemicals are discharged with the brine, though particulate matter, in some cases, is collected for landfill disposal. While coastal desalination plants theoretically could discharge brine to on-land evaporation ponds, contained aquifers, or saline rivers flowing into estuaries, these alternatives have their own problems and are more expensive than the most common expedient, ocean discharge. While desalination proponents argue that any adverse impacts of brine discharge will quickly be mitigated by dilution with much larger volumes of ocean water, problems associated with certain persistent toxic contaminants, especially heavy metals prone to bioaccumulation, are not so easily solved. Some of the heated debate surrounding siting of proposed desalination plants reflect the fact that certain marine environments—especially rocky habitats and kelp beds—are particularly sensitive to brine discharges, as are such benthic organisms as crabs, shrimp, and clams living close to discharge pipes. Unfortunately, to date there have been few comprehensive, long-term studies to collect reliable data on the impacts of desalination plant effluent on the marine environment; such information is sorely needed to assess the true nature of the problem and to find ways of minimizing damage to marine ecosystems by brine discharges.

One of the points most frequently raised in support of desalination projects is reliability of supply. At a time when climate change threatens increased likelihood of prolonged dry spells and a worsening of current water shortages, desalination offers a drought-proof solution to humanity's water supply needs. The fact that many of the regions currently most in need of water border oceans or seas is another reason proponents support aggressive pursuit of the desalination option. Unquestionably, populations in most of the Persian Gulf states, parts of North Africa, some islands in the Pacific, as well as several Caribbean nations even now are vitally dependent on desalted water for their municipal supplies—they have no other option and willingly pay the price. Nevertheless, in spite of notable advances in desalination technology in recent decades and the continued growth in world desalination capacity, it appears unlikely that desalination offers a "silver bullet" solution to the world's water woes. As water experts have pointed out, the freshwater produced by all the world's desalination plants in one year is equivalent in amount to that consumed globally in just a few hours. Certainly, desalination will continue to play an important role in meeting water needs in certain localities, but its high economic costs compared to alternatives—especially conservation of existing supplies—make it unlikely that desalination will be able to satisfy more than a small fraction of the world's water needs anytime in the foreseeable future (Gleick et al., 2006; Shankman, 2009).

per person, the situation is referred to as water "scarcity," while "acute scarcity" pertains to conditions where annual per person water availability is less than 500 cubic meters, insufficient for food production or, in some cases, even for adequate sanitation (Brown, 2008). The United Nations estimates that by 2025, 1.8 billion people will live in regions suffering from acute water scarcity, while fully two-thirds of the world's population could be experiencing water stress (Palaniappen and Gleick, 2009).

According to experts, recent water emergencies, precipitated by drought or water mismanagement, are harbingers of more difficult times to come, especially as climate change intensifies. In 1995, Ismail Serageldin, vice-president of the World Bank at that time, raised eyebrows when he predicted that *the wars of the next century will be about water.* Serageldin's concerns have subsequently been echoed by numerous observers citing the fact that, worldwide, more than 215 major rivers and 300 groundwater basins and aquifers are shared between two or more countries, with almost half the world's people living in such areas. Two-thirds of these basins have no treaty for sharing water and many downstream countries are dangerously dependent on upstream supplies, a fact that creates tensions and the potential for conflict over water rights. As a result, some, like the United Kingdom's former Defense Secretary, John Reed, warn that the global water crisis is becoming a global security issue (Barlow, 2007).

Certainly there are a large number of potential flash points, including the volatile Middle East, where all major rivers are shared and where several nations are overpumping groundwater from common aquifers; the Ganges basin in South Asia, where water diversions to boost Indian crop yields are depriving Bangladeshis of their traditional share of the river's flow; and the Nile River, indispensable to the life and economic survival of Egyptians who get 97% of their water from a river whose headwaters are in Ethiopia, a country that has recently expressed interest in greatly expanding its own irrigation canals by constructing hundreds of small dams across the upper reaches of the Nile. In 1979, Egyptian President Anwar Sadat remarked that "the only matter that could take Egypt to war again is water"—a comment aimed specifically at Ethiopia. Russia currently is upset over China's planned construction of a nearly 200-mile irrigation canal from Siberia's Irtysh River, shared by the two countries; the 450 million cubic feet of water the Chinese intend to divert to their own farmlands threaten to cut off water currently utilized by two million Russians. Similar concerns fuel the dismay expressed by both Syria and Iraq over upstream neighbor Turkey's Southern Anatolia Project, since dam construction on both the Tigris and Euphrates Rivers, intended to bolster development in arid southeastern Turkey, could significantly reduce the flow of these waterways into downstream Syria and Iraq.

In spite of these tensions—exacerbated by steadily increasing water demand, unequal distribution of water resources, and the prospect of dwindling supply resulting from climate change, many water experts are convinced that worries about "water wars" between nations are overblown and highly unlikely. They point out that an analysis of the history of water-related disputes over

Table 15-1   Observed Changes in North American Water Resources during the Past Century
(▲ = increase ▼ = decrease)

	Water Resource Change	Affected Region
	1-4 week earlier peak streamflow due to earlier warming-driven snowmelt	U.S. West and New England regions, Canada
▼	Proportion of precipitation falling as snow	Western Canada and prairies, U.S. West
▼	Duration and extent of snowcover	Most of North America
▲	Annual precipitation	Most of North America
▼	Mountain snow water equivalent	Western North America
▼	Annual precipitation	Central Rockies, southwestern U.S., Canadian prairies, eastern Arctic
▲	Frequency of heavy precipitation events	Most of U.S.
▼	Runoff and streamflow	Colorado and Columbia River basins
	Widespread thawing of permafrost	Most of northern Canada and Alaska
▲	Water temperature of lakes (0.1–1.5°C)	Most of North America
▲	Streamflow	Most of the eastern U.S.
	Glacial shrinkage	U.S. western mountains, Alaska and Canada
▼	Ice cover	Great Lakes, Gulf of St. Lawrence
	Salinization of coastal surface waters	Florida, Louisiana
▲	Periods of drought	Western U.S., southern Canada

Source: IPCC, *Climate Change and Water*, Technical Paper of the Intergovernmental Panel on Climate Change, Table 5.7. IPCC Secretariat, Geneva, Switzerland, June 2008.

many centuries reveals that very few resulted in armed conflict, with the vast majority of disagreements being resolved peacefully through cooperative agreements and they predict the same will hold true for current water-related disputes between nations (Grover, 2007). On the other hand, within countries the potential for conflict over water resources—between rival tribes, states, villages, or rural vs. urban interests—is likely to grow as a result of increasing water scarcity, inequitable access to existing supplies, pollution, and population growth. Such conflicts are likely to be related to disputes over economic development, water allocations, and equity—with a possible link to terrorism as well (Gleick, 2009c).

Whether or not water will be the defining crisis of the 21st century as some observers claim, ensuring adequate supplies to meet the basic health and sanitation needs of today's 6.9 billion people (and several billion more in the decades ahead), as well as for agriculture and industrial production, will be an enormous challenge. Even within regions where water supplies are usually adequate, periodic dry spells and increasing industrial and municipal demands may result in localized shortages. Compounding the problem of regional disparities in water supply is the fact that everywhere, both in water-rich and water-poor areas of the world, pollution is rendering much of the available supply unusable without extensive—and expensive—treatment.

Impact of Population Growth on Water Demand

To some extent, water demand within a society is determined by that society's level of affluence and technological development. On a per capita basis, today's largest water consumers are the rich nations of the industrialized world. Although data issued by the U.S. Geological Survey in 2004 revealed that per capita water consumption in the U.S. had dropped more than 25% since its peak in the late 1970s, thanks largely to water conservation initiatives, the average American still consumes, directly or indirectly, many times more water each year than the average developing-world resident.

However, in the years ahead the major factor accounting for increased water demand, especially in urban areas, will be the explosive growth of human populations. Within

any region, the amount of available water, determined primarily by precipitation, is finite. Thus, the amount available per capita is directly proportional to population size. While more efficient water management can help ensure more equitable distribution and prevent waste, unchecked population growth will inevitably result in chronic water shortages. The problem is particularly acute today for nations of the Middle East and North Africa, drought-prone regions with some of the world's highest population growth rates. Egypt and Morocco, with less than 1000 cubic meters of water per person per year, are nevertheless better endowed than neighboring Libya, Tunisia, and Algeria, whose populations must make do with less than 500 cubic meters per person, while Israel, Saudi Arabia, Kuwait, and Yemen cope with annual per capita water supplies of under 300 cubic meters (Brown, 2008). Most challenged of all are the 1.3 million residents of the Gaza Strip, each of whom has daily access to a mere 37 gallons of brackish groundwater (Pearce, 2006).

The impact of burgeoning population on water supplies promises to be most sorely felt in cities of the developing world. Even in countries where national averages indicate adequate water resources, runaway rates of urbanization and industrialization are seriously endangering both the quantity and quality of water supplies within many metropolitan areas. In China, over 400 of the country's 600 largest cities are experiencing water shortages, with 100 of these seriously affected. Periodic droughts, expected to become more frequent as climate change intensifies, are compounding problems caused by poor management, inadequate infrastructure, and increasing water demand fueled by urban population growth (Gleick, 2009a). To meet the growing water needs of its capital city, Beijing, China has been drilling deep wells

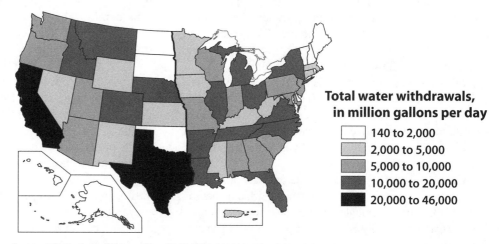

Total water withdrawals, in million gallons per day

☐	140 to 2,000
☐	2,000 to 5,000
☐	5,000 to 10,000
☐	10,000 to 20,000
☐	20,000 to 46,000

Source: U.S. Geological Survey, Fact Sheet 2009-3098, October 2009.

Figure 15-2   Estimated Water Demand in the U.S., 2005

more than half a mile down into nonrenewable groundwater reservoirs, causing the water table beneath some portions of the city to drop by more than 100 feet since the 1960s. By the mid-1990s, farmers in the surrounding rural areas were no longer permitted to draw irrigation water from nearby reservoirs because city dwellers' demands for existing water supplies took precedence over the needs of agriculture (Brown, 2008; Pearce, 2006).

Pollution of existing sources further reduces the usable water supply in many cities of the developing world. Bodily wastes generated by soaring numbers of urban poor lacking the most basic sanitation facilities have so polluted many urban water supplies with microbial pathogens that cities from Shanghai to Lima have been forced to divert millions of dollars from other urgently needed projects to finance increased levels of wastewater treatment. Such problems will become even more severe in the years ahead if current population growth trends persist.

GROUNDWATER

Mention "water resources" and most people immediately think of rivers, lakes, and constructed reservoirs—surface water sources that are visible, accessible, and useful not only for direct consumption but for transportation and recreation as well. However, as pointed out earlier, over 96% of all available freshwater supplies occur in the form of groundwater, a resource whose immense importance is often overlooked and little understood by the general public. More than 25% of the U.S. water supply consists of groundwater. Over half of all Americans and 1.5 billion people worldwide rely on underground sources for their drinking water (Glennon, 2002). In Asia, groundwater provides over half the drinking water in most countries, while in Europe the proportion of domestic supplies derived from groundwater is even higher—as much as 98% in Denmark, 96% in Austria, and 88% in Italy (Gleick, 1993). This vast, unseen reservoir flows very slowly toward the sea and is a major source of replenishment for most surface water supplies. Estimates indicate that most rivers receive as much of their flow from groundwater seepage as from surface runoff; such rivers may experience a drastic diminution of flow or dry up entirely if too much water is pumped from nearby wells.

Groundwater supplies constitute an invaluable natural resource—one that has long been regarded as having certain inherent advantages over surface water supplies. Groundwater is usually cleaner and purer than most surface water sources. This is true because the soil through which it percolates filters out most of the bacteria, suspended materials, and other contaminants that find easy access to rivers and lakes. In addition, because evaporation is virtually nil and seasonal fluctuations in supply are small, groundwater supplies are dependable year-round. In terms of cost, groundwater has advantages also. The expense of digging a well is generally less than that of piping surface water to its place of use, and because of its greater purity it is less expensive to treat prior to consumption.

Until recently, communities relying on groundwater for their municipal supplies tended to take this resource largely for granted. Today, however, a sense of alarm is spreading with the realization that the twin evils of pollution and overuse are threatening the integrity of groundwater supplies. To understand how this situation has come about, it is necessary to take a brief look at the physical characteristics of our groundwater resource.

Nature of Groundwater

When rain falls upon the earth, that which is not taken up by plant roots or lost as surface runoff percolates downward through the soil until it reaches the water table. Contrary to what some people think, the water table is not a vast underground lake or river, but the upper limit of what hydrologists call the **zone of saturation**—an area where the spaces between rock particles are completely filled with water. Such moisture-laden strata are called **aquifers** (Latin for "water carriers"). Above the zone of saturation lies the **zone of aeration**, where some soil moisture may be found as capillary water—useful for plants but incapable of being pumped out by humans. The zone of saturation extends downward until it is limited by an impermeable layer of rock. Sometimes there are successive layers of groundwater separated by impermeable rock layers. Aquifers may range from a few feet to several hundreds of feet in thickness and they may underlie a couple of acres or many square miles. They may occur just below the soil surface or thousands of feet below the earth, though seldom deeper than two miles.

The amount of water that any given aquifer can hold depends on its **porosity**—the ratio of the spaces between the rock particles to the total volume of rock. Sand and gravel aquifers are examples of rocks with high porosity. Additionally, if water is going to move through an aquifer, its pores must be interconnected. To qualify as a good aquifer, a rock layer must contain many pores, cracks, or both. The rate of water movement through an aquifer varies, not surprisingly, with the type of rock: through gravel it may travel tens or hundreds of feet per day; in fine sand only a few inches or less per day. When hydrologists measure the flow of surface streams, they do so in terms of feet per second; when measuring groundwater flow, figures in feet per year are the rule.

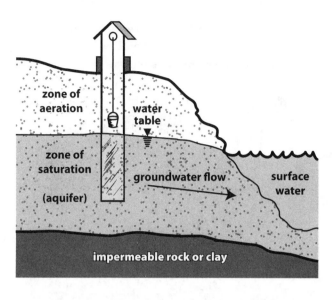

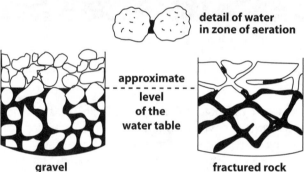

Source: U.S. Geological Survey, *A Primer on Groundwater.*

Figure 15-3   Nature of Groundwater

Groundwater Pollution

The inherent superiority of groundwater over surface water due to its supposed freedom from contamination can no longer be taken for granted. In recent decades, chemical, biological, and radiological contaminants from a wide variety of sources have been identified in groundwater deposits throughout the world. Although estimates by the National Research Council suggest the total geographic extent of groundwater pollution in the United States remains quite limited, such cases tend to occur in populated areas where the aquifer in question may be the principal or only source of local drinking water. Such findings have raised legitimate concerns regarding both acute and chronic health effects and have resulted in the closure of hundreds of wells, affecting the water supplies of millions of Americans. In numerous cases involving synthetic organic chemicals, levels of contamination have been many times higher than those found in the most heavily polluted surface waters.

Within affected communities, the discovery that wells are contaminated frequently has come as an unwelcome surprise since, contrary to the situation in lakes and rivers, groundwater pollution is in a sense hidden, out of sight and difficult to detect without sophisticated chemical analyses. Since many pollutants in groundwater are colorless, odorless, and tasteless, citizens may unknowingly consume health-threatening poisons for years. Because routine tests performed to ensure drinking water safety have only recently been expanded to include monitoring for toxic chemicals, well water pollution in the past was often detected only when noticeable numbers of people began to fall ill. Amendments to the Safe Drinking Water Act in 1986 significantly expanded the number of contaminants that public water systems must monitor in both surface and groundwaters. However, these regulations do not cover the millions of private wells, mostly in rural areas, which frequently are shallower and thus even more vulnerable to pollution than municipal wells (Sanford and Oosterhaut, 1991). Since well water traditionally has been regarded as pure enough to drink untreated, not all the public water systems in the U.S. that utilize groundwater sources disinfect the water prior to distribution. Likewise, very few of the noncommunity systems disinfect well water and a negligible number of private well owners chlorinate their supplies. Given this situation, it's not surprising that a large percentage of reported waterborne disease outbreaks in the United States are ultimately traced to the consumption of microbially contaminated well water.

Degradation of groundwater supplies by human-generated pollutants occurs largely due to faulty waste disposal practices or poor land management. The most significant sources of contamination include the following.

Waste Storage, Treatment, or Disposal Facilities

Unplanned seepage from open dumps, landfills, waste ponds, underground storage tanks, tailings piles—even graveyards!—constitutes a well-recognized and severe groundwater pollution threat if such facilities are improperly sited. In the U.S., petroleum products leaking from underground storage tanks constitute the leading source of groundwater pollution in most states, with landfill seepage close behind (EPA, 1998). Design requirements for the development of new landfills emphasize incorporation of barriers to prevent leachate migration, thereby protecting groundwater quality.

Septic Systems

On-site sewage disposal facilities constitute the third most commonly reported source of groundwater contamination in the United States. Such systems feature the deliberate discharge of wastewater effluent directly into the ground. If such facilities are properly sited, waste dis-

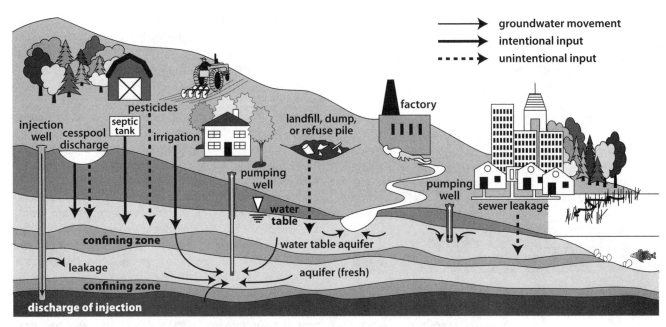

Source: EPA, "National Water Quality Inventory 1996 Report to Congress," EPA Office of Water, April 1998.

Figure 15-4   Groundwater Contamination

charges pose little hazard, but if located adjacent to or uphill from an aquifer or well, a potential for pollution exists. Contamination from septic systems, which serve approximately 25% of U.S. households, can be either microbial or chemical. A number of outbreaks of water-borne diarrheal diseases such as salmonellosis, hepatitis A, and typhoid fever have been traced to well water contaminated by sewage from septic systems.

Pipes, Materials Transport, Transfer Operations

Unintentional leakage from sewers or oil pipelines or accidental spills during transport or transfer of hazardous substances can be another source of groundwater pollution. Studies of well water contamination with agricultural chemicals conducted by the Illinois EPA revealed that the majority of problems—and all those involving high concentrations of pollutants—could be traced to locations where pesticidal formulations were routinely prepared (and routinely spilled on the ground!) prior to field application.

Nonpoint Sources of Pollution

Many instances of groundwater contamination can be traced to substances discharged as a result of other activities: irrigation practices, mine drainage, field application of farm chemicals or manures, de-icing of highways, and urban street runoff, among the most notable examples. Sources such as these are responsible for a host of water quality problems, among them the elevated nitrate levels found in numerous private wells in farming

areas and the high chloride content in wells in some northern states where large quantities of road salts are applied during the winter months.

The most disturbing aspect of groundwater pollution is the fact that by the time the problem is discovered, it is generally too late to do anything about it. Because of the very slow rate of groundwater flow, chemical pollutants will not be flushed out of an aquifer for many years after the source of contamination is cut off (conversely, and for the same reason, contamination of one part of an aquifer does not necessarily affect the use of other parts). Unlike the situation in surface waters, where naturally occurring microbes gradually break down organic pollutants, groundwater is largely devoid of the oxygen needed by the bacteria and other decomposer organisms that endow streams and lakes with their capacity for self-purification. Cleanup of a polluted aquifer, while theoretically possible, is so expensive and time consuming that it is usually not feasible. The process generally involves drilling numerous wells, pumping out enormous quantities of water, treating the water to remove the contaminants, and then reinjecting the water into the aquifer (Rail, 1989). For all practical purposes, a community that finds its groundwater seriously contaminated has little choice but to close the affected wells and seek a new water supply. Groundwater protection strategies, therefore, logically focus on preventing pollution in the first place rather than on efforts to clean up an aquifer after the damage is done.

Groundwater Depletion

With water demand and per capita water consumption increasing steadily in recent decades, many groundwater-dependent regions of the world have experienced an alarming decline in the water table, a direct result of overpumping. Periodic fluctuations in the level of the water table are normal, with levels rising during wet periods and falling during dry spells (generally the water table is highest in the late spring, sinks in summer, rises somewhat during the fall, and reaches its lowest point just before the spring thaw). However, when the water table lowers persistently it means that more water is being taken out of the groundwater reservoir than is being returned to it through precipitation or stream flow. Such a situation is akin to mining an aquifer, and if continued over an extended time period it can permanently deplete the groundwater supply or render it uneconomical to exploit due to excessive pumping costs.

Overextraction of groundwater has been accelerating in recent decades in response to the proliferation of well-drilling by farmers and municipal officials in many parts of the world where surface waters are no longer adequate to meet rising demand. As a result, in many regions the water table is declining at rates ranging from 3–10 feet (1–3 meters) per year. The countries most seriously impacted by groundwater depletion include some of the world's most populous: China, India, Pakistan, Mexico, and almost all of the nations in North Africa and the Middle East (Moench, 2004).

Instances of groundwater "mining" can occur even in well-watered areas when demand generated by rapid population growth, along with residential and commercial development, result in a sharp decline in groundwater reserves. In the United States, however, depletion is most acute in arid regions such as the Great Plains and Southwest, where the insatiable demand for irrigation water and the needs of homes and industries in the booming cities of the Sunbelt have resulted in serious groundwater overdrafts.

A classic case of groundwater depletion in the American West is exemplified by the exploitation of the Ogallala Aquifer, the world's largest underground water reserve. Underlying portions of eight states in the High Plains, the Ogallala supplies almost one-third of all the groundwater used for irrigation in the United States. This enormous sand and gravel formation was deposited millions of years ago as the eastern front of the Rocky Mountains eroded. The plentiful rains of Pleistocene times saturated the formation with water, but due to subsequent changes in the geology and climate of the region, replenishment of the aquifer by natural recharge ceased long ago. Consequently, the Ogallala in a very real sense represents "fossil" water—a nonrenewable resource much like coal or oil which, once gone, is gone forever.

Beginning in the early 1940s, heavy rates of groundwater withdrawal transformed 11 million acres of short-grass prairie into lush expanses of corn, cotton, and alfalfa. Such withdrawals also raised serious concerns about the region's long-term economic viability as the water table plummeted. Overpumping has been most pronounced in the Texas Panhandle where, by 1990, 24% of that state's portion of the aquifer had been depleted. Rates of extraction during the peak years of the early 1970s led some experts to project that the Ogallala's reserves would last only 40 more years and that production of corn, the crop with the highest water demand, would cease entirely within a few years. In fact, irrigated acreage in the High Plains of West Texas declined by

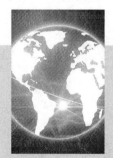

········ 15-2 ········

"A Fool's Paradise"—India's Groundwater Crisis

The years of bountiful harvests on India's most productive farmlands are coming to an end, threatening the livelihoods of millions of farmers who, according to Indian water expert Tushaar Shah, have been living in a fool's paradise of profligate water use. Unfortunately, what once seemed to be an endless supply of high-quality groundwater is now rapidly dwindling. Satellite remote sensing conducted since 2002 as a joint effort by NASA and the German Aerospace Center (Gravity Recovery and Climate Experiment) reveals that across a 2000-kilometer expanse of eastern Pakistan, northern India, and Bangladesh—the most intensely irrigated region on earth—groundwater supplies have been declining by 54 cubic kilometers a year (Kerr,

2009). States in western and southeastern India are also approaching a hydrologic crisis, with ominous implications for the food supply of hundreds of millions of Indians.

The current situation has its roots in the Green Revolution of the early 1970s, a period when agricultural production more than doubled, thanks to the introduction of improved, high-yielding varieties of wheat and rice. These new crops soon transformed chronically hungry India from a grain importer to a grain exporter, but these "miracle crops" came with a catch—they needed ample supplies of water to yield their full potential. During the early years of the Green Revolution the Indian government invested heavily in large surface irrigation projects, building dams and canals to store and carry water from the country's major river basins to fields of thirsty crops. However, these projects were often plagued by mismanagement and technical problems and by the mid-1980s only a quarter of the nearly 250 projects were operational. It was also becoming obvious that even if all the projects had been successfully completed, there simply was not enough surface water available to meet the competing water demands from farmers, industry, and rapidly growing urban populations.

As a result, Indian farmers by the millions turned to an alternative water source directly under their feet—deep aquifers only recently accessible, thanks to new tubewells and relatively inexpensive electric pumps. They quickly embarked upon an orgy of well-drilling that continues unabated today; it's estimated there are now 23 million private wells across India, up from just 2 million in the late 1970s, with another million going in every year. Regulation of these wells is nonexistent; government officials don't know where they are, who owns them, or how much water they extract—but judging from the rate at which water tables are falling, the amount is both huge and unsustainable. Tushaar Shah estimates that at least a quarter of Indian farmers are now engaged in "groundwater mining," removing water that will never be replenished through recharge. A World Bank study in 2005 ominously reported that 15% of India's food supply is now produced through groundwater mining.

Falling water tables first impact older, shallower hand-dug wells; half of these have already dried up in western Gujarat state, as have two-thirds in the southeastern state of Tamil Nadu. As shallower wells go dry, farmers scramble to drill wells still deeper, relying on pumps powered by artificially cheap, government-subsidized electricity to bring water to the surface. Fully half the electricity consumed in some states now goes for pumping water. As a result, widespread power outages have become increasingly common in these areas, as electric grids collapse under the strain. Overpumping is now leading to the failure of millions of deep tubewells also; when this happens, crops wither and economic disaster follows. In recent years the Indian press has been replete with tragic stories of thousands of farmers driven to suicide when crop failure rendered them unable to repay loans taken out to deepen wells that subsequently went dry.

Although groundwater now accounts for two-thirds of India's annual harvest, not all of the water being extracted is used for food production. In water-stressed Tamil Nadu, some former rice farmers are now pumping copious amounts of water from beneath their land, stockpiling it in reservoirs, and selling it to local factories who haul away numerous tanker truckloads on a daily basis. For the farmers who no longer need to worry about crop failure or do anything other than keep their reservoirs full and collect sales revenues, it's a win-win situation—at least until the water runs out. They admit that since they began selling water for industrial use the water table has been dropping by about 50 feet a year and will eventually be gone for good. Though most of the farmers realize that the good times won't last forever, no one is willing to change course. As one farmer's wife commented, "We are all trying to make as much money as we can before the water runs out."

Surprisingly, there seems to be little public indignation toward farmers who overexploit groundwater resources. It's a different story, however, when a foreign-owned company is the perceived culprit. In 2003 a village in the southwestern state of Kerala made headlines around the world when local farmers accused the local Coca-Cola bottling plant (the largest in Asia) of killing their coconut trees and rice fields by excessive groundwater pumping. Later that year a state court ordered Coca-Cola to halt local groundwater withdrawals and the plant shut down. Ironically, though the factory was taking 130,000 gallons daily via wells on its 40-acre site, collectively the area's farmers were using more water to irrigate their crops than Coca-Cola was extracting to fill its bottles—but a global corporation makes a better villain.

With each passing year, India's groundwater reserves shrink further and wells must be drilled deeper. The implications of this situation are aptly summed up by Tushaar Shah: "We are only just beginning to see the consequences. But I must say it looks like a one-way trip to disaster" (Pearce, 2006).

26% between 1979 and 1989. These cutbacks, along with more efficient irrigation techniques, have substantially reduced the rate of groundwater withdrawal in the region, but depletion is still estimated at 12 billion cubic meters annually (Postel, 1996). Over the past half-century, the Ogallala Aquifer has lost a volume of water equivalent to 18 years' worth of Colorado River flow—and that water is gone forever, never to be replenished. The region it serves now produces only half the crop yields harvested during the 1970s, but demand for the resource continues to grow (Barlow, 2007).

Elsewhere in the world, several governments are repeating the mistakes made on the American High Plains. Both Saudi Arabia and Libya have embarked on shortsighted efforts to irrigate desert fields with prodigious amounts of fossil groundwater reserves. Although food self-sufficiency is the stated objective of these undertakings, many experts question the economic wisdom of depleting a nonrenewable resource for agricultural commodities that could be purchased with petrodollars at a much lower price than they are currently spending to encourage domestic production.

The impact of groundwater overdrafts extends well beyond constraints on irrigated agriculture. Aquifer depletion can precipitate serious environmental problems, the most visible of which is the drying up of many surface lakes and streams (recall that many rivers, particularly in dry climates, receive the bulk of their flow from underground sources with which they are in hydrologic contact). In Arizona, approximately 90% of streams that used to flow year-round, including Tucson's Santa Cruz "River," have dried up completely or been seriously degraded due to overpumping of groundwater. While rivers in the arid West have suffered most, similar scenarios have played out in recent years in eastern states as well; Massachusetts' Ipswich River and the Flint River in Georgia have both experienced drastic declines in volume due to excessive groundwater withdrawals from the aquifers that supplement their flow (Glennon, 2002).

In coastal areas around the world, excessive pumping of groundwater to meet the demands of growing urban populations has resulted in migration of seawater into depleted aquifers, contaminating existing freshwater supplies. Saltwater intrusion is now a serious problem in such far-flung cities as Jacksonville, Florida; Dakar, Senegal; Jakarta, Indonesia; and Lima, Peru. Along Israel's Mediterranean shoreline, 20% of the important coastal aquifer is now polluted and officials fear that one out of five coastal wells may have to be abandoned within the next few years. In addition, as groundwater reserves are depleted, land subsidence is occurring, accompanied by the formation of fissures and faults that disrupt irrigation canals and highways, as well as endangering buildings. In Mexico City, where the pumping of groundwater to sup-

ply the needs of 18 million people greatly exceeds the rate of natural recharge, the 16th century Metropolitan Cathedral dominating the city's historic plaza is one of many structures now sagging precariously, and a main thoroughfare has assumed a roller-coaster configuration, both victims of land subsidence. Around Orlando and northern Tampa Bay, Florida, overexploitation of groundwater reserves has created huge sinkholes that virtually overnight swallow up chunks of roads, yards, and, occasionally, homes. Falling water tables are also resulting in the abandonment of hundreds of thousands of acres of irrigated lands, as energy costs render pumping too expensive to make such farming economically feasible.

Natural Recharge

Under natural conditions, aquifers are recharged by moisture filtering downward from the surface or by seepage from a lake or stream. The area of land that is the main source of the groundwater inflow is called the **recharge area** of the aquifer, and is characterized by permeable soils. This recharge zone may be many miles from the point at which the water is pumped out of the ground; and because groundwater flows so slowly, the natural refilling of an aquifer may be a very slow process, requiring many centuries in some cases.

In recent years it has become increasingly apparent that a major threat to both the quality and quantity of our groundwater supplies is the growth of industrial, commercial, and residential development within the critical recharge areas of an aquifer. When urban sprawl strips natural areas of most vegetation and covers what once was forest, farms, or pastureland with buildings and asphalt, the amount of precipitation that can penetrate the soil is greatly reduced. Even in rural areas, land degradation due to deforestation or overgrazing can have an adverse impact on groundwater recharge by reducing the absorptive capacity of soils and increasing the rate of surface runoff. Such factors assume heightened significance in regions where most of the annual precipitation falls during a distinct "rainy season." In some parts of India, for example, where 80% of the rainfall occurs during the summer monsoon, degraded soils can no longer capture as much of the deluge as in previous years and hence even high-rainfall areas now find themselves short of water during the nine dry months of the year.

Development within the recharge area can affect the quality as well as the quantity of groundwater. As human activities within such areas intensify, the potential for infiltration of contaminants from waste facilities, leaky sewage pipes, chemical spills, or street runoff increases. A growing realization of the importance of protecting groundwater resources has prompted many state governments to enact laws regulating the types of development and activities permitted within the critical recharge area of aquifers. In some areas, land-acquisition plans that are funded by either state or local governments have been instrumental in preserving sensitive recharge areas from potentially harmful development. Often, local citizens' groups have been extremely effective in generating the public support necessary for developing and implementing such programs.

WATER MANAGEMENT: INCREASING SUPPLY VERSUS REDUCING DEMAND

When the well's dry, we know the worth of water.
—Benjamin Franklin

In the past, as population increase and industrial development boosted urban water demand, cities typically sought to quench their growing thirst by searching for new sources to augment dwindling local supplies. Frequently their reach extended far beyond municipal borders to exploit previously untapped resources in the rural hinterlands. Doing so seemed an obvious solution for a number of reasons: the potential supply appeared limitless and, therefore, relatively cheap; such water generally was of high quality and required little expenditure for treatment; and legal rights to the watershed lands could usually be obtained easily, especially since rural residents seldom had the political savvy necessary to outmaneuver the urban interests that frequently dominated state legislatures. Thus today in places like southern California, where local sources supply only a third of the demand generated by a burgeoning population, the water that maintains lawns, fills swimming pools, and makes life pleasant in the Golden State is imported from the Colorado River, 170 miles to the east, and from sources in northern California as far as 400 miles distant. Similarly, when New Yorkers turn on the tap in Manhattan, the liquid that flows out could have originated from one of a thousand streams in the Catskills, Hudson, or Delaware River valleys. Hetch Hetchy Valley in Yosemite National Park provides much of the water supply for San Francisco; Denver taps the headwaters of the Colorado on the opposite side of the Rocky Mountains; and Oklahoma City pipes its supplies from reservoirs in the northeastern Oklahoma hill country more than 100 miles away (Ashworth, 1982).

In addition to pipelines for long-distance water transport, dams and reservoirs also have been key components of society's "hard path" to meeting water needs, the latter typified by reliance on centralized infrastructure and large, capital-intensive engineering projects. Although humans have been building small dams since ancient times to ensure adequate water for crop irrigation or for flood prevention, dam construction in the 20th century was also being promoted as a means of providing clean, cheap electrical power. Improvements in engineering technology and building skills ushered in a new era of megadam construction around the world. At the dawn of the 21st century, the World Commission on Dams counted 47,655 large dams (those 15 meters or more in height) in more than 140 countries. Although initially the United States was at the forefront of this trend—by 1945 the five largest dams on earth were all in the western U.S.—in recent decades the allure of megadams has been fading in this country and in Europe where few, if any, are expected to be built in the years ahead (the situation is quite different in the developing world, where large dams are still viewed as symbols of modernity and a highly visible source of national pride). In the United States, the prospects of future dam construction are dim, due to lack of suitable sites, high up-front costs, and mounting public opposition due to the serious environmental and social impacts associated with large dams.

As a result, since the 1970s water managers have tempered their once-automatic response of pursuing supply side solutions, opting instead to improve the overall productivity of water use. In fact, the era in which city planners attempted to solve water problems through a supply augmentation approach has basically been brought to a close due to:

- the scarcity of new untapped sources
- the sharply escalating costs of building dams and reduced federal funding for the same
- competition between urban and agricultural interests for existing supplies
- growing opposition to such projects on environmental grounds
- organized legal resistance by groups in areas targeted for water development

Today, in metropolitan areas as diverse as Los Angeles and Boston, the emphasis for ensuring adequate water resources has shifted decisively from increasing *supply* to managing *demand*. Demand management, more commonly referred to by environmentalists as **water conservation**, can include several components: reducing overall use, reducing waste, and recycling used water so it can be made available for other purposes.

Water Consumption

To understand how demand management strategies can help meet increased water needs, it is necessary to examine current water use patterns. Worldwide, irrigated agriculture accounts for the lion's share of water consumption—almost 70% of the total. In the United

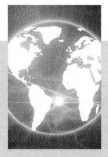

········ 15-3 ·······

Dams and Diversions: China's "Hard Path" to Water Security

Few countries today face more acute water supply challenges than does the People's Republic of China, a nation with 22% of the world's population but just 8% of its available freshwater supply (Hoffman, 2009). As national leaders emphasize the imperative of economic growth regardless of the consequences, demands for additional water by industry, urban residents, and farmers have been rising exponentially. Water use in China has quintupled since 1949 and shows no signs of tapering off, raising concerns about where additional supplies can be found. Compounding the problem is the reality of unequal distribution of water resources: four-fifths of the nation's water supply is in southern China, while more-populous northern China is relatively water-poor. Widespread contamination of existing water resources further reduces freshwater availability. Chinese government sources estimate that 40% of the nation's surface waters, even following treatment, are suitable only for agricultural or industrial use.

As surface water has become increasingly polluted, both farmers and municipalities have turned increasingly to groundwater reserves, particularly on the North China Plain. Since 1970, groundwater use has almost doubled and now accounts for 20% of China's total water use. As a result, water tables are falling precipitously, necessitating ever-deeper wells, while wetlands and natural streams are drying up. Overdrafts of surface water are resulting in a drop in the level of major rivers and, during periods of drought, some of these no longer reach the sea. Lake Baiyangdian, the largest natural lake in northern China, is gradually contracting and is badly polluted. Added to all this is the fear that current drought conditions in northern China are but an early manifestation of long-term increasing aridity in the region due to impending climate change. It appears unlikely that Nature herself will provide more water in the decades ahead (Yardley, 2007).

The response to these critical water supply challenges by Chinese leaders, several of whom are engineers by training, has been the classic supply side approach—constructing dams and diversions on a scale unequalled anywhere else on the planet. Approximately 22,000 large dams—close to half the world total— have been built in China since 1950. Of these, the iconic example is the mighty **Three Gorges Dam**, extending more than two kilometers across the Yangtze River in a spectacularly scenic area long famed for its steep canyons and towering limestone cliffs (hence its name, "Three Gorges"). Completed in 2008, 14 years after construction began in 1994, the Three Gorges Dam and its associated infrastructure constitute the largest water project in the history of the world. Nearly 200 meters high, the dam has a volume of 40 million cubic meters. The reservoir created behind the dam stretches for 600 kilometers (370 miles) upriver, with a total storage capacity close to 40 billion cubic meters. Electrical generating capacity at Three Gorges sets a world record as well—more than 22,000 megawatts.

From its inception, the Three Gorges project has been highly controversial, both in China and abroad, as experts continue to debate the benefits and risks of such a massive water management project. Supporters contend that the hydropower produced at Three Gorges helps to mitigate climate change, annually offsetting 100 million tons of carbon dioxide that would otherwise have been emitted by burning the 50 million tons of coal needed to produce an equivalent amount of electricity. Flood control along the Yangtze is another touted benefit, as is improved navigation along the upper stretch of the river, thanks to a significant increase in river depth.

Detractors, on the other hand, point to a dramatic degradation of the Yangtze River ecosystem, marked by a notable decline in local fisheries, endangerment of several rare aquatic species, and the likely extinction of the Chinese freshwater dolphin. They also worry that a drastic reduction in downstream sediment loads will result in coastal erosion and lowered biological productivity of the East China Sea. The potential for seismic activity has long been a worry, though government officials regularly downplay the risk. (As the reservoir is filled, it increases pressure on local faults.) A related problem that is already causing serious disruption, property damage, and occasional loss of life is the growing frequency of destructive landslides along the steep shores of the reservoir; in 2007 a Chinese official reported that the edge of the reservoir had collapsed in 91 locations and 36 km of shoreline had caved in.

The most bitter protests over the Three Gorges project center around the massive dislocation of an estimated 1.3–2 million Chinese villagers who were forced to move into resettlement areas after more than 100 towns, 14,000 hectares of farmland, and over 100 archeological sites were inundated as the massive reservoir filled with water. Although the Chinese government promised to give these people new homes and land equal to or better than those they were forced to evacuate, such lands simply don't exist in an already overpopulated country. Many of those displaced have been relocated to overcrowded marginal lands where living conditions are poor, job opportunities are scarce, and where tension and conflicts have been arising between the host population and relocated newcomers. Government funds for resettlement all-too-often find their way into the pockets of corrupt local officials and no channels for voicing grievances have been provided (Gleick, 2009b). Only time will tell whether the project's benefits are worth its costs; in the meantime, without waiting to learn whatever lessons the Three Gorges Dam may have to offer, Chinese water managers are moving forward on an even more ambitious undertaking intended to solve water deficiencies plaguing the rapidly growing urban areas of the North China Plain.

Whereas providing hydroelectric power was the main objective for constructing the Three Gorges Dam, alleviating northern China's chronic water shortages is the intent of China's latest water diversion scheme, the **South-to-North Water Transfer Project**. Officially launched in 2003 and not expected to be complete until 2050, the project's managers plan to divert 45 billion cubic meters of water each year from the Yangtze River basin in southern China through canals and tunnels to north China's Yellow River basin. Estimated to cost $62 billion, the project consists of three separate diversions, two of which are already underway while the third remains in the planning stage, with doubts as to whether it will ever materialize due to astronomical cost estimates and environmental concerns.

One of these diversions, the eastern route, takes water from near the Yangtze's mouth, transferring it northward through a 1,200-km-long canal to the major industrial city of Tianjin, suffering from water shortages since the 1990s. The middle route, also partially built, takes water from a reservoir on the Han River, a large tributary of the Yangtze, and sends it north across the North China Plain to Beijing. Both of these diversions are intended to relieve demand pressures on the Yellow River by using Yangtze waters. The primary beneficiaries of these diversions will be cities and industry—it's unlikely that the needs of farmers will outweigh the demands of metropolitan areas. The third planned diversion, the western route, aims to take water from the headwaters of the Yangtze high amidst Tibetan glaciers (assuming the glaciers haven't all melted by the time the project is complete!) and move it through tunnels and tributaries to discharge directly into the Yellow River to augment its flow—the only one of the three diversions to do this.

The Chinese government insists that up to 300 million people will benefit from these diversions, making the South-to-North Water Transfer Project worth its multibillion dollar cost. Many informed observers aren't convinced, however, pointing to numerous adverse environmental and social impacts as well as the escalating financial costs (estimates are that the western route alone will cost $36 billion). They question why the government doesn't focus instead on improving China's efficiency of water use, opting for managing demand rather than increasing supply. Chinese environmentalists point out that Chinese manufacturers use 3–10 times more water than their counterparts in developed countries, while Chinese farmers use twice as much. The fact that the government has for years heavily subsidized water prices, making the commodity artificially cheap and thereby encouraging wasteful use, has also prompted a new look at ways of managing water demand. Compared to other countries, China's water prices are quite low, one-tenth to one-fourth of those in Europe and less than half the cost paid by Americans. As a result, residential consumers in Beijing recently saw their water bills more than double, while prices for commercial uses such as car-washing increased even more dramatically. Elsewhere several local governments have imposed or are advocating higher prices to encourage water conservation and recycling or have imposed surcharges on householders for water use above a set limit. Separate quotas are being imposed on businesses, industry, and agricultural users, but far more could be done to employ rational pricing and economic policies to manage China's water demand (Gleick, 2009b).

In the meantime, China's leaders seem intent on moving forward with megaprojects to remedy the country's acute water supply problems, heedless of the potentially disastrous human and environmental consequences. Economic growth is the country's top priority, and as a senior engineer with a provincial water conservation bureau remarked, "We have a water shortage, but we have to develop—and development is going to be put first" (Yardley, 2007).

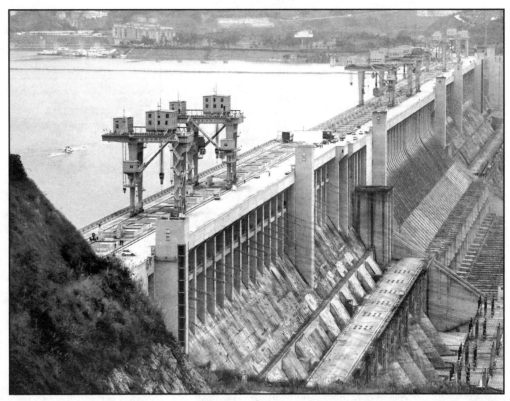

The world's largest hydro-electric project, China's Three Gorges Dam, is nearly 200 meters high and extends more than two kilometers across the Yangtze River. This massive water management project has generated considerable controversy due to the dislocation of some 1.3 to 2 million Chinese villagers as well as the dramatic degradation of the Yangtze River ecosystem. [*Imaginechina via AP Images*]

States, farmers account for about 40% of total freshwater withdrawals nationwide (but over 90% in some western states); in Europe, 30%, primarily in countries bordering the Mediterranean; and as much as 95% in many developing countries (Hoffman, 2009). Industries are the second largest consumers of water at 23% (more in heavily industrialized areas, less in others), while household use averages about 8% worldwide (obviously, in regions devoid of irrigated agriculture, the percentage of water use attributed to household and industrial use are considerably greater than world averages indicate). Focusing on these three major categories of water consumers, what opportunities do water managers have for reducing demand?

Agriculture

As the largest user—and the largest waster—of water, agriculture also offers the greatest potential for substantial reductions in water demand, in most cases without reducing crop yields. Because irrigation water is almost everywhere priced far below its true value, farmers are given the impression that the supply is plentiful and thus have little incentive to invest in more efficient irrigation technologies. As a result, in most parts of the world irrigators continue to channel or flood water across their fields in a manner that would have looked entirely familiar to their ancestors thousands of years ago. Such practices waste, on average, more than 60% of

the water applied, as evaporation or seepage from unlined channels robs thirsty plant roots of the moisture intended for them. More widespread use of advanced techniques such as the automated "drip irrigation" method developed by Israeli scientists can cut water loss to 5% and reduce energy expenses in the bargain.

Since the 1980s, farmers in West Texas have achieved dramatic savings by adopting techniques of "surge irrigation" or by installing low-energy precision application (LEPA) sprinklers that can achieve water-use efficiencies as high as 95%; buried droplines approach 100% efficiency. Experts estimate that if the world's farmers could reduce water losses due to inefficient irrigation practices by as little as 10%, the amount saved would be enough to double current domestic use (Postel, 1992). Unfortunately, even though the use of water-saving irrigation methods has grown impressively since the mid-1970s, it is still used on less than 1% of the world's irrigated croplands (WRI, 1998).

Industry

The huge amount of water needed by factories and power plants for processing, cooling, or generating steam accounts for a sizeable portion of total water use in Europe (55%), North America (47%), and other highly developed areas of the world (WRI, 1998). Since water used by industry is not "consumed" in the traditional sense (i.e., it may become heated or polluted but isn't

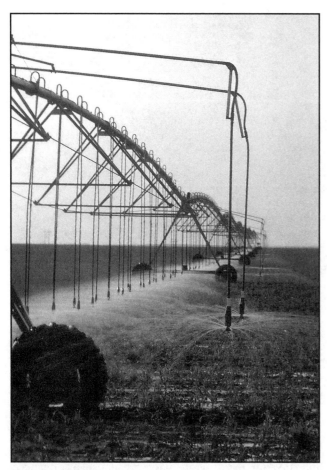

Irrigated agriculture consumes almost 70% of the world's water and therefore offers the greatest potential for water conservation through the application of new water-saving irrigation technology. The center pivot system shown here uses LESA (low-elevation spray application) sprinklers to reduce evaporation. [*Tim McCabe, Natural Resources Conservation Service*]

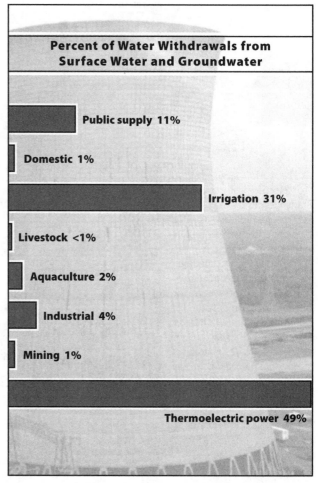

Source: U.S. Geological Survey, Fact Sheet 2009-3098, October 2009.

Figure 15-5   Estimated Water Use in the U.S. by Category, 2005

used up), industrial water use can be substantially reduced by recycling. Within the past decade or so, increasingly stringent federal mandates requiring treatment of industrial wastewater prior to discharge, coupled with the escalating costs of waste treatment and disposal, have given industry a strong incentive to embark on waste minimization strategies that entail recycling and reuse of process waters. Such efforts have resulted in sharp declines in water withdrawals in many industries. Further savings are likely in the years ahead as more and more industries recognize the advantages of climbing aboard the pollution prevention bandwagon.

Households

Although domestic water consumption averages far less than that used for agricultural and industrial purposes, societal norms and public health considerations require that such water be of very high quality, necessitat-

ing expensive treatment and distribution systems. In past years, municipal efforts in some areas to restrict residential water consumption were launched as a temporary reaction to drought conditions, largely abandoned when the rains returned or new supplies were tapped. Today urban planners are urging that water conservation become a way of life, even in areas of adequate rainfall, as a means of enhancing water availability and containing rising water costs. Contrary to popular belief, a call for water conservation is not a demand for citizens to change their lifestyle radically, nor does it necessarily imply deprivation. Rather, water conservation means making more efficient use of the resource available.

Water Conservation

Some of the major elements in an effective water conservation program include the following.

Rational Water Pricing

Pricing water to reflect its true cost is fundamental to the success of all other water conservation efforts. Ironically, in many cities current price structures reward profligate users through a system of declining block rates, whereby the cost of additional water units above a certain point is lower than the cost of the initial units. An opposite approach, now used in some major U.S. metropolitan areas, imposes higher unit costs on water use above a specified level, thereby encouraging conservation. Peak demand pricing (e.g., summer/winter price ratio of 3:1) can also help curtail water use for nonessential purposes. Studies conducted in the United States and elsewhere have shown that when water prices increase by 10%, household water consumption drops 3–7% (Bhatra and Falkenmark, 1992). Of course household water use can't be priced appropriately if it isn't metered. The failure of cities in many parts of the world to meter home water use actively discourages water conservation efforts, since consumers see no connection between the amount of water they use and the price they pay. Cities such as New York, Buffalo, Denver, and Sacramento witnessed declines in water use ranging from 10–30% after they installed residential water meters. Use of rational pricing as a tool for encouraging water conservation can be even more effective in the cost-conscious industrial sector. Faced with water prices substantially higher than those in the U.S., German industries use about half the amount of water consumed by their American counterparts (Ward, 2002).

Leak Detection/Correction Programs

Both at the household and municipal level, leaky plumbing can waste enormous volumes of water. In homes, leakage accounts for 5–10% of all residential water consumption. A faucet that loses 1 drop per second due to a worn out washer is wasting 7 gallons of water each day; that figure rises to 20 gallons per day with a steady drip. A leaky toilet tank can waste fully 200 gallons per day with-

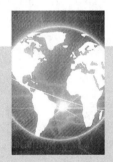

· · · · · · · 15-4 · · · · · · ·

A World Marketplace for Water?

The worldwide rush to open and integrate markets across national boundaries—a process known as "globalization"—has sparked one of today's most controversial water resource debates: should water continue to be regarded, as it has been for millennia, as a God-given "social good" available on an equal basis to all humankind or, with increasing scarcity, should it be viewed as a commodity for international trade, subject to the same marketplace rules as diamonds, steel, or toys? As mounting population pressures boost world water demand at the same time climate change, overexploitation, and pollution reduce supply, will countries experiencing water deficits look to the abundant, "unexploited" reserves of water-rich regions as something they should be free to purchase, regardless of whether the people living in those areas oppose such transactions?

Since the early 1990s, concerns among policy makers over the failure of massive international efforts to ensure that people everywhere have access to clean water have led many to conclude that such needs can never be met without a thorough reordering of water use policies and priorities, as well as improvements in the efficiency of water use. Such thinking led delegates to the 1992 International Conference on Water and Environment, held in Dublin, Ireland, to declare that "Water has an economic value in all its competing uses and should be recognized as an economic good." Such a statement has profound implications and immediately provoked a heated, ongoing debate. The idea that water should be regarded as a product, to be bought and sold like any other commodity, is especially alarming to public interest groups, worried that the world's poor could find themselves unable to afford one of life's most essential resources; some compare the idea of trading water for money with selling air and argue that governments are violating their citizens' human and civil rights if they don't provide everyone with water at the lowest possible cost. Environmentalists also fear that free trade in water would ignore ecosystem protection, failing to take into account the vital role played by freshwater in providing habitat for fish and other aquatic organisms, supporting vegetation and animal life along waterways, meeting the needs of water-based transportation and recreation, and contributing to society's aesthetic enjoyment in ways impossible to quantify in monetary terms.

On the other hand, the near-universal practice by which governments supply water at prices that bear little relationship to the true costs of acquiring and delivering that water all-too-frequently results in overuse and waste. While water subsidies vary widely from city to city, as a global average residents pay their municipal governments just 35% of what it costs to supply that water. All too often, financially strapped cities compensate for the shortfall by neglecting to maintain water storage and delivery systems or by failing to extend service to the poorest sections of the community. Water subsidies also encourage inefficient use, exemplified by the fact that irrigated agriculture consumes 80% of California's water supply yet represents but 10% of that state's economy. Industrial water in California is valued at 65 times that of agricultural water; regarding water as an "economic good" by taking competing uses into account and maximizing water's value to society would radically alter the current allocation of supplies in the Golden State and many other water-scarce areas where irrational water pricing currently prevails. Since subsidized water encourages wasteful use while a classic free market approach threatens to deprive the poor of sufficient water, the challenge facing decision makers is how to get the most value from available water while guaranteeing adequate supplies to those unable to pay and leaving enough water in place to avoid ecological damage.

One potential solution to water supply dilemmas, out-of-basin bulk water shipments, are not a new concept, but in the past they have been limited to transfers within the same country or to short-term emergency situations. Since 1955, St. Thomas and St. John in the U.S. Virgin Islands have received sporadic seaborne shipments of water from Puerto Rico; inhabitants of several of the smaller Fijian islands regularly receive water from their larger neighbors during periods of drought; Malaysia's offshore island of Penang gets a portion of its water via submarine pipelines from the mainland; and tiny Nauru, an island nation in the Pacific, receives up to a third of its water from Australia, New Zealand, and Fiji on ships returning to the island to pick up loads of phosphate, Nauru's primary export.

Visionary proposals for future international trade in water are more grandiose—and controversial—than these limited transfers, however. For years local boosters in the American Southwest have proposed schemes to divert vast quantities of water from Alaska and northwestern Canada to Arizona and southern California; Italians talk of building a pipeline under the Adriatic Sea to bring Albanian water to arid southern Italy; and Spain only recently dropped long-discussed plans to pipe water from France's Rhone River to Barcelona. As world water demand continues to mount, such proposals receive increasingly serious scrutiny.

Overshadowing all discussions about future transborder trade in bulk freshwater is confusion over the rules pertaining to international water trade. Uncertainty persists as to whether bulk water can be considered a "product" and hence subject to existing international trade requirements (the qualifier "bulk water" is important, since bottled water and other processed, value-added waters have been internationally traded for decades) and, if so, whether exceptions under the General Agreement on Tariffs and Trade (GATT) would apply to efforts by a government to block or limit water sales it deems objectionable. GATT currently allows a country to impose trade restrictions on a product if doing so is necessary to protect human, animal, or plant life or health and in situations where such restrictions are related to the conservation of natural resources. There is considerable debate among legal experts, however, as to whether these resource conservation principles could be invoked to halt bulk water sales, and few legal precedents exist to suggest how potential future disputes would be resolved. In 1999 the U.S.-Canadian International Joint Commission, an independent binational organization established to help resolve disputes relating to the use and quality of boundary waters, attempted to safeguard Great Lakes water from future export threats by declaring that the Great Lakes constitute a nonrenewable resource, inasmuch as the overwhelming bulk of water they contain was laid down in the distant geologic past. Whether such a statement ensures a GATT exception from the rules governing international trade remains to be seen.

In the near future, large-scale transborder commerce in bulk water is unlikely, due primarily to the high expense of moving water long distances. Reallocation of water among end users, improvements in water-use efficiency—even the construction of desalination plants—are usually less costly methods of increasing available supplies than shipping water from place to place by tanker. Nevertheless, over time the economics of water trading could change as demand escalates and new water transport technologies emerge. It is imperative that governments act now to formulate and institute national water policies to prevent the overexploitation and export of nonrenewable water resources and ensure that the water needed to safeguard human health and ecosystem stability is protected from the forces driving globalization (Gleick, 2002).

out making a sound. (To check for toilet tank leakage, simply pour a small amount of food coloring into the tank; if color appears in the toilet bowl before it is flushed, leakage is occurring, probably caused by a worn-out or defective flush ball.) Correcting these leaks is the easiest and cheapest way to reduce home water consumption.

Cities as well as households may suffer from leaky plumbing. The problem is particularly acute in many developing world cities. Plagued by chronic water scarcity, Amman, Jordan, loses 59% of the water flowing from its water purification plant to homes and institutions, thanks to leaky distribution pipes; in Manila, capital of the Philippines, the figure is 58%; in New Delhi, 50%; in Mexico City, about one-third (Simon, 1998).

Municipalities in the industrialized world are certainly not immune to such problems; until a few years ago London was losing 45 million gallons of water daily through leaks in the 10,000 miles of water distribution lines underneath the city. Of this amount, municipal authorities estimated that 25% was coming from residential pipes, so the city's water utility, Thames Water, took action. Customers were asked to attach a device, cleverly dubbed "Leakfrog," to their water meters to detect whether their pipes were indeed leaking. The program has been so successful that by 2008, just a few years after program initiation, water loss had dropped by 20%. In many older U.S. communities the pipes that carry water from a central treatment plant to thousands of homes, institutions, and businesses were installed during the 1800s or early 1900s and have for decades been in serious need of replacement. The current fiscal plight of many urban areas has resulted in shortsighted postponement of these urgently needed renovations. In those cities that have made the necessary investment, however, results have been striking. Prior to a major leak repair program, Boston was losing an estimated 20% of the water entering its distribution system each day; following completion of that program, officials credited leak repair with saving the city 35 million gallons daily.

Installation of Water-Saving Plumbing Devices

Technology now exists to cut household water use by close to one-half, with no loss of comfort or convenience. Since more water is used in the bathroom than any other room in the house, the focus of home water conservation efforts has been the installation of water-efficient toilets, showerheads, and faucet aerators. The prime candidate for replacement is the water-hogging conventional toilet which, at 5–7 gallons per flush (gpf), is the single largest water user in a typical American home. By the early 1980s, new low-flush (3.5 gpf) toilets became available, followed several years later by ultra-low flush (1.6 gpf) models offering significant water savings. Although early versions of the ultra-low flush toilets encountered cus-

tomer complaints of poor performance (mainly the need to double-flush), re-engineering of the bowl has largely eliminated this problem. Recent surveys indicate the vast majority of purchasers find ultra-low flush toilets as good as or better than the replaced models.

In 1992 Congress passed the federal **Energy Policy Act**, establishing mandatory nationwide water efficiency standards for all toilets, urinals, faucets, and showerheads installed in the United States after January 1994. These standards include the requirement that any new or replacement toilets sold or installed in the U.S. must be

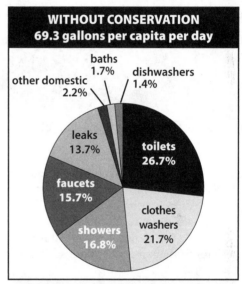

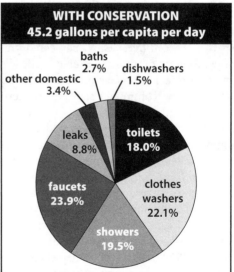

Source: Reprinted with permission from *Residential End Uses of Water.* Copyright © 1999, American Water Works Association (AWWA) and AWWA Research Foundation.

Figure 15-6   Water Use in U.S. Homes, With and Without Conservation (% of Daily Use)

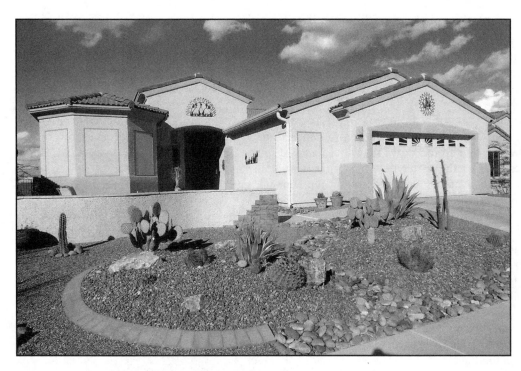

Residential landscaping that features rocks and drought-resistant horticultural varieties offers great water-saving potential without sacrificing beauty.

the ultra-low flush 1.6-gallon type. Since approximately 8 million new or replacement toilets are installed in the country each year, it is estimated that by 2025 water-conserving toilets will have replaced most of the pre-1994 stock currently in use. When complete, this transition is expected to result in nationwide water savings of 6.5 billion gallons per day.

Outdoor Water Conservation Measures

Americans' deeply held conviction that a broad, verdant expanse of weed-free, neatly manicured grass is an essential component of any respectable residence constitutes a major obstacle to meeting urban water conservation goals. In some communities in arid western states, watering lawns and gardens accounts for up to 70% or more of daily residential water consumption during summer months. Municipal programs aimed at reducing outdoor water waste by households can include outright prohibitions on landscape watering (usually imposed only during periods of severe drought); restrictions on the amount of yard space that can be devoted to turfgrass (a program in Las Vegas to replace turf in residential yards with more water-efficient plantings reduced water usage, on average, by 76%); rebates for homeowners to purchase and install censors to deactivate automatic sprinklers during precipitation events; requirements that owners of backyard swimming pools install pool cover to prevent excess evaporation when pools are not in use; and pro-

grams to encourage **xeriscaping**—the planting of drought-resistant horticultural varieties rather than those with a high water demand. The latter practice offers great water-saving potential without any sacrifice in landscape beauty. Studies in California's North Marin Water District found that xeriscaping could reduce household water use by up to 54%; a comparison of water use patterns of traditional vs. xeriscaped landscapes by the Southern Nevada Water District found that the latter consumed, on average, only 20–25% as much water as did traditional landscaping (Gleick et al., 2004).

Methods of managing water demand such as those just described, accompanied by intensive public information and conservation education programs, will play a major role in meeting future water needs. Encouraging results are already evident from recently launched programs in such disparate regions as southern California and metropolitan Boston, providing convincing evidence that water conservation not only will provide our largest single source of additional water within the next 20 years but will become an accepted way of life. Provided with appropriate technologies and a cost incentive, citizens, farmers, and industrialists alike will validate the assertion of water managers that the cheapest, quickest, most environmentally benign way to meet future water needs is to use existing supplies more efficiently.

Water, water everywhere
Nor any drop to drink . . .
—Samuel Taylor Coleridge
(*The Rime of the Ancient Mariner*)

Water Pollution

Back in the days when human settlements were relatively small and far apart, the issue of water contamination seldom occupied much attention on the part of the general public. Prevailing sentiment insisted that "the solution to pollution is dilution," and popular wisdom held that "a stream purifies itself every ten miles." While such statements have a certain amount of validity, they lost their relevance as villages mushroomed into crowded cities and as the expanse of countryside between towns steadily contracted under the impact of urban sprawl. The rapid growth of human population and of industrial output resulted in a corresponding decline in water quality, as both municipalities and industry regarded the nation's waterways as free, convenient dumping grounds for the waste products of civilized society. During the 19th century our careless waste-management practices turned most rivers into open sewers and many once-healthy lakes into algae-covered cesspools.

It is estimated today that most of the world's water drainage basins are polluted with such contaminants as toxic chemicals, human and animal excrement, heavy metals, pesticides, silt, and fertilizers. These contaminants are carried downstream where they are discharged into coastal estuaries and shoreline waters, effecting long-term changes in water quality. Such pollutants generate far more than unpleasant sights and odors. Waterborne disease outbreaks, fish kills, long-lasting changes in

aquatic ecosystems, and severe economic loss to sports and recreation-based industries are all directly related to degradation of water quality by human activities.

CONTROLLING WATER POLLUTION: THE CLEAN WATER ACT

Although water pollution had been recognized as a major environmental problem in the United States for many decades, it was not until 1972 that a tough, comprehensive federal program was enacted by Congress. Known originally as the Federal Water Pollution Control Act Amendments (Public Law 92–500), this landmark piece of legislation underwent some "mid-course corrections" in 1977, at which time its name was changed to the Clean Water Act. Prior to passage of this law, our nation's water pollution control strategy, such as it was, focused on attempts to clean up waterways to the point that they could be used for whatever purpose state governments had determined their function should be (e.g., drinking water, swimming, fishing, navigation, etc.). Thus each stream or portion of a stream might have a different water quality standard, and if that standard was not being met, it was up to the state water pollution control agency to determine which discharger was responsible for the violation and to seek enforcement action. This system was totally ineffective for a number of reasons:

1. designations of desired stream use were frequently modified to retain or attract industrial development

2. insufficient information was available on how pollutant discharges were affecting water quality

3. blame for violation was difficult, if not impossible, to assess when more than one source was discharging into a waterway

4. little attention was paid to the effects of pollution on the aquatic environment as a whole

5. only contaminants entering a waterway through pipe discharges were given much attention.

Undoubtedly the most serious drawback of the pre-1972 water pollution control strategy was the lack of enforcement power. State agencies had to negotiate with all the polluters along a given waterway, trying to persuade each individual source to reduce its discharges to the point at which water quality standards for the particular river or lake in question could be met. Not uncommonly, when industries disliked what they were being told, they would threaten to close down and move to a less demanding state. Also, due to the nature of river basins, many states discovered that in order to improve their own water quality, they had to persuade states upstream to pollute less.

Passage of the Clean Water Act radically altered this approach to water pollution control and took a new philosophical stance toward the problem, reflected in the 1972 senate committee's statement that "no one has the right to pollute . . . and that pollution continues because of technological limits, not because of any inherent right to use the Nation's waterways for the purpose of disposing of wastes." Stressing the need to "restore and maintain the chemical, physical, and biological integrity of the Nation's waters," Congress declared as national goals the attainment, wherever possible, of water quality "that provides for recreation in and on the water" (popularly referred to as the "fishable-swimmable waters" goal) by July 1, 1983, and the elimination of all pollutant discharges into the nation's waterways by 1985 ("zero discharge" goal). These goals were not the same as legal requirements—they could not be enforced and certainly were not attained by the dates indicated; nevertheless, they proved useful in providing objectives toward which to strive and against which progress could be measured.

Progress in moving toward congressional goals is difficult to assess on a comprehensive national basis because budgetary constraints, both at the federal and state levels, preclude the possibility of continuously monitoring the quality of all U.S. waterways. In addition, water quality at any one location changes from season to season and year to year. Even determining long-term trends for specific pollutants is somewhat problematic because of the lack of historical records and inconsistencies in the data. Also, since the various states and organizations that survey water quality utilize different monitoring strategies, it is often impossible to combine or compare survey results. Active efforts are currently underway to improve nationwide monitoring efforts and to establish an effective, uniform means of collecting, interpreting, and presenting water quality information.

In the meantime, policy makers must rely on the EPA's biennial *National Water Quality Inventory*—a compilation of data submitted to the EPA by individual states, territories, Indian tribes, Interstate Water Commissions, and the District of Columbia. Existing data, while incomplete, indicate commendable improvement in the nation's water quality during the years since passage of the Clean Water Act, when fully 95% of all U.S. watersheds were regarded as polluted. During several decades when both the economy and population size have grown substantially, the fact that overall surface water quality hasn't deteriorated gives evidence that the billions of dollars spent on water cleanup efforts have had a positive impact. Nevertheless, EPA's most recent water quality assessment reported that 44% of U.S. rivers, 64% of lakes, and 30% of coastal estuaries surveyed still suffer levels of pollution that impair their use for one or more designated purposes, indicating we have a long way to go before the goals of the Clean Water Act are fully met (it should be noted, however, that less than 30% of all U.S. waters were assessed for this report). While many of the conventional sources and types of water pollution are now being dealt with fairly adequately, more difficult-to-control problems such as farmland runoff and airborne fallout of mercury and PCBs have stymied pollution-abatement efforts (EPA, 2009b).

Elsewhere in the world, water quality issues rank high on the list of international environmental concerns. Not surprisingly, progress in controlling water pollution varies widely from one country to another. Most developed nations have imposed controls on industrial dischargers similar to those in the United States and the majority have financed the construction of sewage treatment plants. As a result, by the first decade of the 21st century the vast majority of North Americans and Europeans were served by wastewater treatment facilities. Similarly, in Japan and South Korea, notable progress has been made during the past few decades in expanding access to sewage treatment, particularly in urban areas.

Unfortunately, in many developing nations and most of the former Soviet republics the situation is bad and getting worse. Rapid industrial growth has given rise to numerous toxic "hot spots" of pollution, as industrial dischargers dump poisonous effluent into nearby waterways, unhindered by nonexistent or seldom-enforced water pollution laws. In China, for example, discharges from an estimated 20,000 chemical factories, half of them along the banks of the Yangtze River, are fouling waterways with both toxic and carcinogenic compounds. According to Chinese authorities, 40% of that nation's surface waters are suitable only for industrial or agricultural use, and even then may require preliminary treatment. In 2006 almost half of China's cities were using water that failed to meet national standards for drinking water quality, with the result that hundreds of millions of Chinese citizens have no choice but to consume water contaminated with heavy metals, agricultural chemicals, untreated wastewater from factories, and dissolved toxins leaching from municipal landfills (Gleick, 2009a). Though many people attempt to protect themselves by boiling water before using it for drinking or food preparation, doing so has no effect on most toxic contaminants. Throughout the developing world untreated sewage, as well as salt- and fertilizer-laden irrigation return flows, further contaminate lakes, rivers, and coastal waters.

To understand the worldwide impact of water pollution on the health of both ecosystems and their human inhabitants requires a look at the major sources and types of pollution and the problems posed by each. The remainder of this chapter will examine these issues and will describe the pollution control policies developed by the U.S. Congress and regulatory agencies as they strive to protect public health through improving water quality.

SOURCES OF WATER POLLUTION

Pollutants can enter waterways by a number of different routes. Strategies for preventing water contamination must take into consideration the nature of the pollutant source and must devise appropriate methods of control for each source category. Congress has coined two terms—**point source** and **nonpoint source**—to refer to the two general types of water pollution, and pollution control regulations adopted within recent years have by necessity been tailored according to source.

Point Sources

Pollutants that enter waterways at well-defined locations (e.g., through a pipe, ditch, or sewer outfall) are referred to as point source pollutants. Characterized by discharges that are relatively even and continuous, the approximately 100,000 traditional point sources of water pollution in the United States include factories, sewage treatment plants, and storm sewer outfalls. Point sources have been the most conspicuous violators of water quality standards, but because effluent from such sources is relatively easy to collect and treat, considerable progress has been made in reducing this type of pollutant discharge. The two major categories of point source pollution are

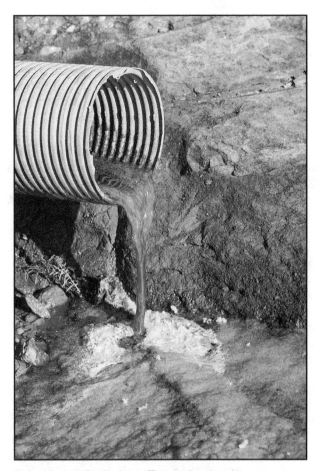

Point source of pollution: effluents that enter a waterway directly from a factory outfall, pipe, ditch, or sewage treatment plant are the most visible source of water pollution.

sewage treatment plants and industrial discharges. Each will be discussed in greater detail later in this chapter.

Nonpoint Sources

Until the 1980s, nonpoint source (NPS) pollutants—those which run off or seep into waterways from broad areas of land rather than entering the water through a discreet pipe or conduit—were largely overlooked as significant contributors to water contamination. However, when stringent effluent limitations on point sources failed to result in dramatic improvements in water quality, it became increasingly evident that in many waterways the largest pollutant contribution was coming from nonpoint sources. Today the majority of states identify pollutants coming from nonpoint sources as the main reason they have been unable to attain their water quality goals. Nonpoint source pollution (really just new terminology for old-fashioned runoff and sedimentation) results primarily from a variety of human land-use practices and includes the following.

Agriculture

In the United States as a whole, agriculture is the leading source of water pollution, adversely affecting the quality of 50–70% of the nation's surface waters. Among the various contaminants present in farmland runoff, the single most abundant is soil. While most people tend to think of erosion largely in terms of its adverse impact on agricultural productivity, soil entering streams or lakes can severely damage aquatic habitats as well. By increasing the turbidity of the water, sediment sharply reduces light penetration and thereby decreases photosynthetic rates of producer organisms; it buries bottom-dwelling animals, suffocating fish eggs and aquatic invertebrates. Storm-water runoff from fields and pastures carries more than just sediment into waterways, however. Manures from grazing lands or from large livestock management facilities located adjacent to streams or lakes can contribute five or six times as many nutrients to waterways as do point sources. Manure spread on fields can cause similar problems unless it is applied at rates moderate enough to permit complete uptake of nutrients by plants (i.e., at agronomic rates of uptake).

In the same way, chemical fertilizers and pesticides, when applied immediately prior to a storm or in amounts exceeding the assimilative capacity of the crop in question, can be carried by runoff water from fields into adjacent lakes or streams. Upon entering a waterway, farm chemicals can poison fish or promote algal growth; if runoff seeps through the soil into shallow aquifers, it can contaminate drinking water wells. Since these toxic pollutants generally enter waterways attached to soil particles, they can best be controlled by the same strategies used to prevent soil erosion—conservation tillage, terracing, contour plowing, and so on. Additional management strategies include: applying pesticides when there is little wind and the potential for heavy rain is low; using nonpersistent, low-toxicity pesticides; disposing of containers properly; applying fertilizers or manures only when they can be incorporated into the soil (i.e., not when the ground is frozen); and using chemicals in the proper amount and only when field checks indicate they are needed. Controlling runoff from pasturelands can be managed relatively easily by maintaining a buffer zone of vegetation along waterways and using fences to prevent livestock from walking into streams.

Construction Activities

Acre for acre, runoff from sites where homes, shopping centers, factories, or highways are under construction can contribute more sediment to waterways than any other activity—typically 10–20 times more than the amounts from agricultural lands. More than 500 tons of sediment per acre per year can wash off such sites into streams during the construction period, frequently carrying with them cement wash, asphalt, paint and cleaning solvents, oil and tar, and pesticides. These contaminants from construction sites have impaired an estimated 5% of U.S. surface waters. Fortunately the actual construction time during which land surfaces are unprotected is relatively short and the amount of land exposed is small in

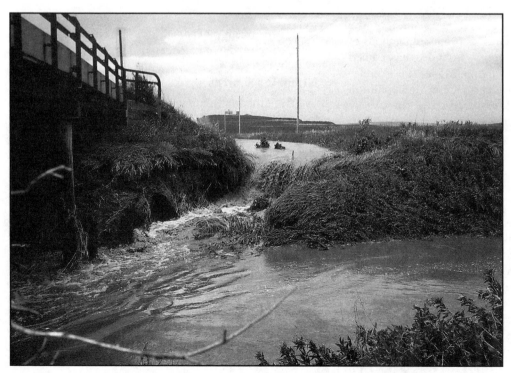

Nonpoint source of pollution: runoff from agricultural fields is the leading source of water pollution in the U.S., depositing large amounts of soil as well as manures, chemical fertilizers, and pesticides. [*Lynn Betts, Natural Resources Conservation Service*]

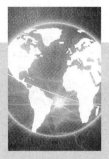

· · · · · · · 16~1 · · · · · · ·

Eutrophication, Pond Scum, and Coastal "Dead Zones"

Eutrophication, a term meaning "well-fed," is a process initiated when dissolved nutrients—primarily nitrates and phosphates—enter a body of water where they act as fertilizer to stimulate the growth and proliferation of algae. Anyone who has noticed the green scum that forms on shallow ponds or lakes during warm summer months is familiar with this phenomenon but may not realize that these algal "blooms" can cause serious problems for other aquatic organisms. Because some algal species produce powerful toxins, their sudden appearance may result in massive fish kills, so-called "red tides" that seem to be increasing in frequency in coastal waters worldwide. Even more important, as algal numbers increase exponentially, large numbers die and drift to the bottom where they constitute a feast for decomposer organisms, primarily bacteria. As bacterial populations explode in response to the increased food supply, their high rate of metabolic activity causes levels of dissolved oxygen in the water to plummet. The drop in oxygen content is particularly rapid in summer because high temperatures promote a speed-up in metabolism and because warm water holds less dissolved oxygen than does colder water. The ultimate effect of oxygen depletion is the loss of fish and other macro-organisms requiring high levels of dissolved oxygen and their replacement by species more tolerant of low-oxygen conditions.

Eutrophication of small lakes and ponds is a familiar and often seasonal phenomenon, regarded as a nuisance by those living nearby but largely ignored by everyone else. Since the 1960s, however, there has been growing alarm and discussion about eutrophication in many of the world's coastal waterways, where the formation of oxygen-deficient "dead zones" has caused most fish and other marine organisms in the vicinity to swim elsewhere or die. These **hypoxic zones**, as they are properly termed, are characterized by waters where the dissolved oxygen concentration is below 2 milliliters of oxygen per liter—the point at which most bottom-dwelling fauna begin to exhibit abnormal behavior patterns, reproductive impairment, and greater susceptibility to disease. Below 0.5 ml of O_2/liter, mass die-offs of benthic organisms can occur. Several major water bodies, including the Baltic Sea, Black Sea, and Chesapeake Bay, to name a few, have long experienced localized periodic bouts of hypoxia. However, during the past half-century the number of coastal dead zones has increased dramatically, doubling every decade since the 1960s, and their size has expanded as well. Today almost 450 hypoxic zones have been reported in the world's coastal oceans, collectively covering approximately 95,000 square miles (Diaz and Rosenberg, 2008).

Each summer one of the world's largest dead zones forms along the U.S. Gulf Coast, extending from the mouth of the Mississippi River westward to Texas. The Gulf hypoxic zone has attracted considerable attention and concern because of its rapid increase in size during the 1990s and due to its location in the midst of one of the United States' most important commercial and recreational fishing areas. Today's extensive Gulf dead zone—like the vast majority of dead zones around the globe—is unquestionably a human-caused phenomenon. The 2010 hypoxic zone was one of the largest measured since researchers began routine mapping in 1985. Extending 7722 square miles (20,000 square kilometers), it is roughly the size of New Jersey ("2010 Dead Zone," 2010).While a small hypoxic area probably always existed near the mouth of the Mississippi, there's general agreement that today's dead zone has been gradually created since the 1950s by increasing amounts of nutrients, primarily agricultural fertilizers, draining from the Mississippi watershed and discharged into the Gulf by the Mississippi and Atchafalaya rivers. Although these pollutants obviously come from a multitude of sources—sewage treatment plant effluent, urban storm-water runoff, atmospheric fallout from fossil fuel combustion and auto exhausts—the general consensus is that midwestern farmers bear most of the blame for the nitrates and phosphates flowing into the Gulf each year. As an economist at the University of Minnesota remarked, "The Gulf has become the end of the pipe for American agriculture."

Analyzing the cause of the problem is relatively straightforward, but reversing the situation is far more challenging. The key to solving the problem is a significant reduction in nitrogen loadings to the Mississippi watershed, a vast area draining over 40% of the land area of the continental United States. Phosphorus is usually the limiting nutrient whose overabundance causes eutrophication in freshwater bodies, but in marine environments like the Gulf, nitrogen concentrations are more critical. Since industrial and municipal point sources combined are estimated to contribute a mere 3–5% of all the nitrogen carried down the Mississippi, agriculture will bear the brunt of control measures, should they be imposed. Scientists are convinced that only a change in farming practices, such as not applying fertilizers in the fall, can reduce Gulf nitrogen loadings enough to ease hypoxic conditions in the dead zone. Another proposed approach is the restoration of major wetlands along river banks in the watershed to capture and contain farmland runoff—an undertaking that would provide flood control benefits as well. As policy makers debate how to resurrect the Gulf dead zone, biologists continue to research the diverse factors controlling algal blooms and hypoxia, seeking to better understand how well certain interventions, such as reducing fertilizer use, would actually impact the size of the dead zone (Berger, 2009).

Another major coastal estuary long beset by eutrophication and hypoxia is Chesapeake Bay, for over a quarter-century the focus of federal and state restoration and protection efforts. Stretching more than 190 miles inland from the Atlantic Ocean, Chesapeake Bay is the largest estuary in the U.S., with a watershed of 64,000 square miles extending over six states and the District of Columbia. Degradation of the Chesapeake Bay ecosystem first attracted attention in the 1950s, as nutrient enrichment of the bay provoked algal blooms, reduced water clarity, caused die-off of underwater grass beds, altered aquatic food chains, and precipitated a sharp decline in dissolved oxygen levels. By 1983 the need for government action to tackle a worsening problem resulted in signing of the Chesapeake Bay Agreement, a pledge by the governors of Maryland, Pennsylvania, and Virginia, along with the mayor of Washington, DC, and the Administrator of the EPA, to work cooperatively to restore the waterway. This group set a goal of reducing by 40% the amounts of nitrogen and phosphorus entering the bay, with 2000 set as the target year for achieving this objective.

Striving to reach this goal, states within the watershed agreed to limit pollutants at their source upstream in the bay's tributaries by upgrading sewage treatment, imposing more stringent regulations on large animal feeding operations, encouraging farmers to plant winter cover crops to reduce fertilizer runoff, and enacting stricter vehicle emission standards to reduce airborne fallout of pollutants. In 2000, New York and Delaware signed on as partners and in 2002 West Virginia became the last state in the Chesapeake Bay watershed to join the group. Despite the concerted efforts of all these parties and the expenditure of billions of dollars to reduce hypoxia, reports of record-size dead zones in Chesapeake Bay in 2003 and 2005 led to doubts as to whether the program was having any significant impact. Indeed, by 2008, only 21% of the established goals had been met and the quality of Chesapeake Bay water was still rated as "very poor."

In May 2009, President Obama issued an Executive Order announcing that the federal government would become more involved in the restoration effort. Federal agencies have since issued draft reports on approaches for reducing polluted runoff and for increasing accountability and public input. Among the initiatives outlined are new regulations to reduce runoff from urban and suburban areas, the fastest-growing source of pollution to Chesapeake Bay (agricultural runoff remains the single largest source). Agencies within the Department of the Interior are seeking to identify opportunities for establishing new wildlife refuges and parklands within the watershed, while federal agricultural officials are focusing on practices that can reduce runoff from large animal feedlots and croplands, while encouraging wider adoption of land conservation practices.

Long-time advocates of bay restoration are cautiously optimistic that the exercise of federal leadership may at last provide the impetus necessary for real progress. Unquestionably, the odds for success are sobering: to date, only 4% of the world's hypoxic zones have shown any signs of improvement—New York's Hudson and East Rivers and the Thames estuary in the U.K. are among the few examples of waterways where management of nutrients has largely eliminated dead zones. Similar efforts have not yet had a noticeable impact on dissolved oxygen levels in Chesapeake Bay (Diaz and Rosenberg, 2008). Nevertheless, federal officials are hopeful that this time things will be different. As EPA Administrator Lisa Jackson remarked to reporters in describing the administration's restoration strategy, "We need bold new leadership, collective accountability by all contributors to the bay's problems, and dramatic changes in policies using all the tools at hand if we are to fulfill President Obama's goal for clean water throughout the region" (ENS, 2009).

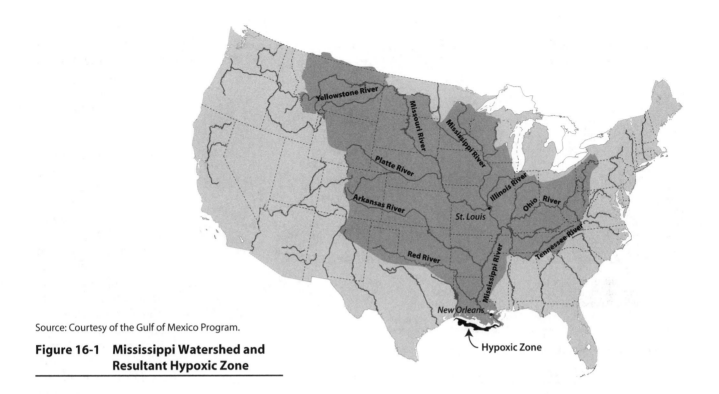

Source: Courtesy of the Gulf of Mexico Program.

Figure 16-1   Mississippi Watershed and Resultant Hypoxic Zone

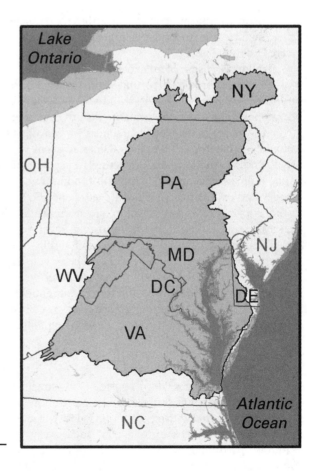

Source: Courtesy of the Chesapeake Bay Program.

Figure 16-2   Chesapeake Bay Watershed

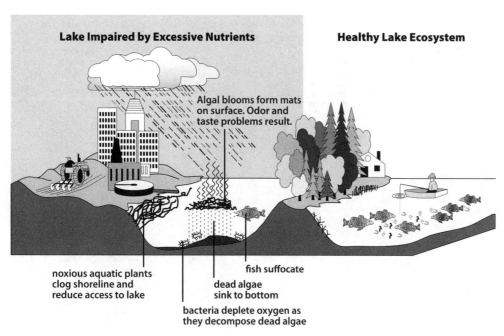

Source: EPA, *National Water Quality Inventory: 1996 Report to Congress,* April 1998.

Figure 16-3   How Excess Nutrients Degrade Water Quality

comparison with farm acreage. Nevertheless, damage to water quality due to construction site runoff can be severe and long-lasting.

To address this problem nationwide, a new EPA rule took effect in February 2010, and will be phased in over the next four years. The rule requires that owners and operators of construction sites that disturb one acre or larger use "best management practices" to ensure that soil and sediment aren't washed off into adjacent waterways. On construction sites impacting 10 acres or more at one time, owners and operators must monitor any discharges and ensure that they don't exceed specific limits in order to minimize construction site storm-water discharges. Using mulches and fast-growing cover vegetation, retaining as many existing trees and shrubs on the site as possible, roughening the soil surface or constructing berms to slow the velocity of runoff, and building retention basins to detain runoff water long enough to promote settling out of suspended sediment are all well-established management practices for reducing pollutant runoff from construction sites.

Urban Street Runoff

Although people seldom consider city streets and sidewalks as important sources of water pollution, studies have shown that during storm episodes, particularly storms that terminate a long dry spell, very large amounts of sediment and other pollutants are carried by runoff water into adjacent rivers, streams, or lakes. In many cities, the total pollutant load from urban runoff exceeds that from industrial discharges. Contaminants commonly found in urban runoff include sand, dirt, road salt, oil, grease, and heavy metal particles (lead, zinc, copper, chromium, etc.) from paved surfaces; pesticides and fertilizers from lawns; leaves, seeds, bark, and grass clippings; animal and bird droppings; and other substances too numerous to mention. The EPA has documented discharge of suspended solids from storm sewers in amounts far exceeding those entering waterways from sewage treatment plants. Urban runoff is the leading source of pollutants impairing U.S. bays and estuaries and the third-most important contributor to degradation of water quality in lakes. With over half of all Americans now living in coastal communities, polluted runoff from these densely populated urban areas is likely to be an even greater problem in the years ahead (Hoffman, 2009).

Reducing pollution from this source requires broad-based cooperation and effort on the part of both municipal officials and citizens: more frequent street-sweeping to prevent sediment accumulation on streets; proper disposal of pet wastes; careful and limited application of lawn and garden fertilizers and pesticides; litter control on both public and private property; judicious use of road salt and sand; application of organic mulches to reduce erosion on bare ground; incorporating more green space within urban areas and along waterways to allow runoff to filter into the ground; use of surface ponds, holding tanks, rooftop catchments, subsurface tunnels, or similar structures to hold, retain, and gradually release storm water.

Acid Mine Drainage

When the iron pyrite found in association with coal deposits is exposed to air and water during mining operations, a series of chemical reactions is initiated, culminating in the formation of a copper-colored precipitate (iron hydroxide) and sulfuric acid. The precipitate frequently covers the bottom of streams in mining regions, smothering bottom life and giving such streams a characteristic

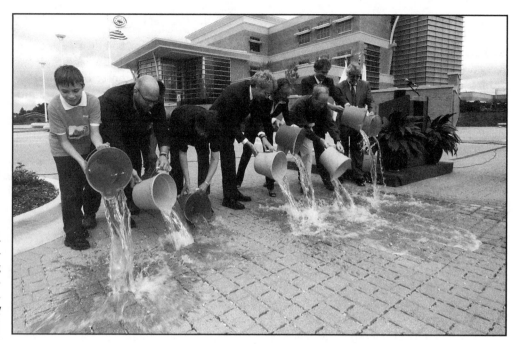

Local environmental and municipal officials demonstrate how permeable paving materials can reduce stormwater runoff from paved surfaces. [*Illinois Environmental Protection Agency*]

rusty appearance. The sulfuric acid lowers the pH of the water, eliminating many aquatic species that cannot survive or reproduce in the acidified water. Both operating and abandoned coal mines of either the underground or surface type are characterized by acid drainage, although only *abandoned* mines are termed nonpoint sources (*active* mines are classified as point source polluters). In West Virginia, the third largest coal-producing state in the United States and home to thousands of inactive mines, acid mine drainage constitutes the leading nonpoint pollution source—a problem shared by many other mining areas as well.

Acids, however, are not the only water quality problem posed by abandoned mines. Under the low pH conditions prevailing in such regions, metals such as iron, aluminum, copper, zinc, manganese, magnesium, and calcium are leached from soil and rock, contaminating streams. Large amounts of silt and sediment from slag heaps or refuse piles erode into waterways, clogging streams and burying bottom-dwellers under a thick layer of silt. Legislatively mandated regrading and revegetation of abandoned strip mines have been helpful in reducing runoff of sediment from abandoned mine sites, but have had minimal impact on acid drainage. Sealing openings to abandoned underground mines, thereby cutting off the supply of oxygen and water that permit acid formation, has been the chief means of combating acid mine drainage. Although this practice significantly reduces acid loadings, it doesn't eliminate them and efforts to find better ways of dealing with the problem continue. In recent years, the use of engineered wetlands to remove toxic chemicals from mine leachate has

yielded promising results. More advanced artificial wetlands have incorporated alkaline recharge zones designed to neutralize acids. These and other innovative approaches are undergoing active investigation and offer hope that a solution to acid mine drainage will eventually be found (Bennett, 1991).

Fallout of Airborne Pollutants

The situation represented by acid rainfall (see chapter 13) is but one example of pollution from the sky causing water quality problems. A great many of the particles released into the atmosphere through human activities eventually return to earth and enter rivers, lakes, or oceans either directly or in runoff. These airborne particles include many hazardous chemicals such as lead, asbestos, PCBs, mercury, fluorides, and various pesticides. The contribution to water pollution by synthetic chemical fallout is surprisingly large—the major portion of PCBs and other toxic chemicals in the Great Lakes, one-third of the nitrogen causing eutrophication in Chesapeake Bay, and a substantial amount of the hydrocarbons found in the oceans entered these waters through airborne deposition.

As point source pollutants decline in importance, thanks to improved pollution control technology and enforcement of effluent limitations, nonpoint sources such as those just described present the greatest single challenge to attaining our nation's clean water goals. The "top down" strategy, whereby federal and state governments promulgate regulations with which individual polluters must comply under threat of civil or criminal penalties, has served us well in reducing pollution from point sources but is entirely inappropriate for controlling poison runoff from broad land areas. Recognizing the near-impossibility of requiring discharge permits for every farm field or parking lot, regulators striving to control NPS pollution thus far have focused their efforts on altering harmful land-use practices. In 1987 Congress required states to conduct surveys and develop "assessment reports" describing the nature and extent of NPS pollution within their jurisdictions. Subsequently they were to implement management programs to combat the problems identified. Control strategies to deal with NPS pollution fall into one of two possible categories:

1. increasing the land's capacity to retain water, thereby reducing runoff (e.g., a wide variety of erosion control measures), or

2. minimizing the amount of pollutants available for runoff during storms (e.g., keeping manure piles away from streams, judicious application of farm chemicals, regular street sweeping, capturing potential air pollutants before they become airborne and subject to fallout).

Controlling nonpoint pollution unfortunately demands more than just a technological "fix"; it requires instead the cooperation of farmers, ranchers, municipal officials, developers, homeowners, and others in implementing better land management practices to prevent these diverse pollutants from running off the land and into the water.

Past regulatory efforts to deal with NPS pollution were not very successful. State runoff control programs varied widely in their focus, but few emphasized the watershed protection approach so critical to an effective program. Most even today continue to rely on voluntary compliance with recommended land management practices—a politically popular stance but not a particularly effective one. Insufficient monitoring data and a perennial lack of adequate funding to implement needed programs have further hindered progress to deal with NPS pollution in a meaningful way.

In an effort to rectify this situation and to improve national water quality management strategies, the federal government in 1998 launched a new initiative, the **Clean Water Action Plan**. Encompassing a wide range of water quality issues, the Action Plan addresses the problem of polluted runoff by encouraging states and tribes to adopt enforceable controls on nonpoint sources. It also has increased incentives and provided new funding to help farmers control polluted runoff from agricultural lands. Most significant for the long term, however, is that the Clean Water Action Plan finally emphasizes the importance of a watershed approach as the most effective means for further improving the quality of our rivers, lakes, and estuaries.

MUNICIPAL SEWAGE TREATMENT

In 1854 the city of London was reeling under a severe epidemic of Asiatic cholera, a disease characterized by the sudden onset of profuse watery diarrhea and vomiting, resulting in rapid dehydration and death of approximately half of those afflicted. Not all parts of the city were equally affected, however. Within a district called St. James Parish, the cholera death rate hit 200 per 10,000 population, while in neighboring Charing Cross and Hanover Square districts fatalities were considerably lower. Dr. John Snow, a member of the commission of inquiry appointed to investigate the outbreak, noted that the vast majority of individuals who had died of cholera obtained their drinking water from a well on Broad Street; in other respects there seemed to be no fundamental difference between conditions in St. James Parish and nearby districts where cholera rates were low. Although the cholera bacillus and its method of transmission had not yet been discovered, Snow recommended that the handle of the Broad Street pump be removed to prevent further consumption of water from the well. Shortly thereafter, the cholera epidemic subsided. Subsequent investigations disclosed that prior to the outbreak, residents of one house on Broad Street had been ill with an unidentified disease. Their fecal wastes had been dumped into an open cesspool near the well, a common method for disposing of human wastewater in those years. Unfortunately, the brick lining of the cesspool had deteriorated to the point that the liquid wastes could readily seep through the ground and contaminate the well water with still viable pathogenic organisms. The connection between poorly managed human wastes and serious human disease was clearly demonstrated (Cholera Inquiry Committee, 1855).

London's use of open cesspools as a method of sewage disposal was a well-established practice in many parts of the world until the late 19th and early 20th centuries. These pits in the ground simply collect wastes that are then stabilized by bacterial action. Seepage of liquids into the soil from such holes was common, and since no disinfection was used, contamination of wells and aquifers with human fecal pathogens frequently occurred. During the 19th century the growing popularity of flush toilets in urban areas resulted in greatly increased volumes of wastewater requiring disposal. This additional influx produced frequent overflowing of public cesspools and caused a further spread of filth and waterborne disease, particularly cholera and typhoid fever. Installation of sewer systems that carried wastes directly from homes into nearby rivers helped to alleviate problems of well contamination but caused severe degradation of surface water quality, eliminating many forms of aquatic life and enhancing the risk of waterborne disease in communities downstream that used surface water supplies for drinking.

By the end of the 19th century, rapid urban growth convinced city planners that sewage treatment facilities were needed to alleviate the health and aesthetic problems created by dumping raw sewage into waterways. Today in the United States, approximately 70% of the population live in areas where domestic wastes pass through a sewage treatment plant before being discharged. The remainder, for the most part, rely on on-site wastewater disposal systems—usually a septic tank and soil absorption field or sand filter. Provision of adequate methods of sewage treatment, along with the chlorination of drinking water, has done far more to reduce the incidence of epidemic disease and to upgrade standards of public health than has the more widely acclaimed introduction of modern medicines and vaccines.

The aim of sewage treatment is to improve the quality of wastewater to the point that it can be discharged into a waterway without seriously disrupting the aquatic environment or causing human health problems. Achieving these goals requires killing pathogenic organisms present in human wastes (within any human population there will always be some individuals suffering from various gastrointestinal diseases and releasing the causative bacteria, protozoans, etc., in their excreta; it is assumed, therefore, that domestic sewage entering the treatment facility is contaminated with pathogens capable of causing disease outbreaks) and, to the greatest possible extent, removing organic wastes or converting them to inorganic forms so that after discharge they will not deplete the oxygen content of the receiving waters as they

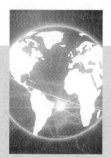

· · · · · · · **16-2** · · · · · · ·

For Want of a Toilet . . .

A clean, properly functioning toilet inside one's own home is an assumed fact of life among the vast majority of industrialized world citizens, living in relatively affluent societies where indoor plumbing and municipal sewers (or on-site septic systems) are near-universal. Not so among the poor in developing countries, where 48% of the population still lacks access to adequate sanitation (Bremner, 2010). The lack of toilet facilities in such areas is even more acute than the dearth of safe drinking water, and its impact on human health and well-being is equally profound. In Latin America as a whole, only 66% of the population lives in areas where toilets are connected to a sewer system; in parts of Asia and Africa that percentage is much lower, standing at 18% and 13%, respectively. Dismayed by such statistics, the United Nations in 2000 established what it referred to as Millennium Development Goals for reducing persistent poverty, one of which called for reducing by half the proportion of people lacking access to basic sanitation. Ten years later, it is clear that target will not be met; indeed, even the modest gains achieved in terms of absolute numbers of people with access to improved sanitation have largely been cancelled out by population growth.

The challenge is particularly acute in the squatter settlements that surround most cities in poor countries. Largely unplanned and overcrowded, these slum areas frequently lack even the most basic infrastructure. In Nairobi, Kenya, for example, 55% of the population in the mid-1990s lived in informal settlements where only a small minority of homes had toilets and a large percentage of residents had no access to showers or baths. Within the largest slum area, home to almost half a million people, traditional pit latrines provide the only method of excrement disposal. Frequently as many as 200 people are forced to use the same pit latrine; as a result, the pits fill up quickly, presenting a serious disposal problem because the narrow streets are difficult for removal vehicles to access. To make matters worse, little space exists for installing new pits. The situation is even worse in Tanzania's capital, Dar-es-Salaam, where 83% of households rely on pit latrines. Only 12% of the squatter camps in Karachi, Pakistan's largest city, are provided with sanitary facilities ("Water for People," 2003).

Although it may be unrealistic to expect the governments of low-income nations to provide all their citizens with indoor plumbing and a flush toilet anytime in the near future, international development agencies are urging them to ensure, at a minimum, "safe, convenient sanitation" as soon as possible. Doing so would require that human waste be disposed of in such a manner that it doesn't contaminate human hands, clothing, food, or water and that it not be accessible to disease-carrying houseflies. In this context, the current situation is discouraging. Reliance on public toilets or pit latrines is commonplace. Frequently such shared facilities are so filthy and poorly maintained that they constitute a genuine health hazard; because of this, they may be shunned and lapse into disuse. In addition, people living at a considerable distance from communal toilets may find them simply too inconvenient to access. Such facilities also are quite impractical for children, few of whom are able to walk the long distance to a public toilet or wait their turn in line once they decide they "have to go!" Reflecting such difficulties, a survey conducted in India found that only 1% of children under the age of 6 use public latrines; stools from an additional 5% are deposited in the latrines by their parents. Wastes from the remaining 94% ultimately end up in roadside ditches, streets, or open areas. Another deterrent to the use of public toilets by the urban poor is their cost. In one Ghanaian city, it costs 10–15% of the main breadwinner's daily wage for each member of the family to use the public latrine one time!

For a half-billion or so urban dwellers in developing nations, provision of sanitary facilities—even simple pit latrines—is so poor that people have no choice but to defecate outside on the ground or into a container such as waste paper or a plastic bag which they then throw away. In the Philippines the latter option is jokingly referred to as "wrap and throw"; in Ghana as "flying toilets"! Humor aside, the necessity of defecating in the open presents a humiliating dilemma for millions of women and girls who often feel that in order to avoid being seen and jeered at by men, they must wait until after dark to relieve themselves. In sub-Saharan Africa an estimated one-third of teenage girls drop out of school when they reach puberty due to lack of toilet facilities.

Unsanitary human waste disposal practices also have profoundly negative health consequences. Exposed feces attract flies that then carry human disease organisms to exposed foods. Excrement-saturated soil harbors parasites such as hookworms, the larvae of which burrow through the skin of bare feet, or several species of roundworms, whose eggs can be accidentally ingested with soil when children put dirty hands or objects in their mouths. Such helminthic infections afflict a billion or more people throughout the tropics and can be quite debilitating. Mosquito larvae thrive where sewage-polluted water pools due to inadequate drainage, facilitating transmission of malaria and filariasis. When human wastes contaminate wells or streams used for drinking water, outbreaks of microbial waterborne diseases such as dysentery, typhoid fever, and cholera may occur. Such problems are particularly common after periods of heavy rainfall in unsewered areas, when sewage-laden storm water fills streets, courtyards, and adjacent waterways.

Although the United Nations and numerous governmental and private organizations are actively striving to upgrade sanitation in developing world cities, some of the most successful projects have been carried out at the grassroots level by the residents most directly affected. In Pune, a city of nearly 3 million inhabitants in western India, 40% of the people live in shantytowns lacking plumbing and sewerage. The number of public toilets provided by the municipality is grossly inadequate and those that do exist are often poorly designed and constructed, provided with inadequate supplies of water for washing, and seldom cleaned. In 1999, a local nongovernmental organization allied with the slum dwellers signed an agreement with the municipality to construct and maintain new sanitary facilities. With capital costs provided by the city and local residents closely involved with management of the project, 114 toilet blocks were constructed, containing 2000 adult seats and 500 sized for children. In contrast to the older facilities, the new toilet blocks are well ventilated, bright, and feature better-quality construction. Large water storage tanks ensure that users have enough water to wash afterwards (toilet paper is an unknown commodity in most Indian households) and to clean the toilet after use. Additional improvements include separate sections of each toilet block for men and women, one block specially designed for children, and toilets designed for elderly or handicapped residents. Maintenance costs were reduced and the quality of service enhanced by including the construction of living quarters for caretakers and their families. Throughout the course of the project, ongoing communication between the government and residents, along with complete transparency in regards to costing and financing the project, established a high level of trust and cooperation between the parties involved. The end result was a major improvement in sanitation that both government and local users could afford ("Water for People," 2003).

Pune's example may not be widely transferable, however. In places where good governance is in short supply, it may take years before local residents can afford to invest in household toilets or communities install an adequate number of safe, accessible public facilities. Given the enormous health cost of improper management of human wastes, more effective action needs to be taken now to ensure that all the world's people are guaranteed access to the sanitary facilities most of us take for granted.

decompose. To accomplish these ends, several levels of sewage treatment are necessary.

Primary Treatment

The used water supply of a community, averaging about 100 gallons/person/day in cities having separate storm and sanitary sewers, flows from homes and institutions into the municipal sewer system, which carries the wastes to a treatment plant (in regulatory jargon a "POTW"—publicly owned treatment works). At this point sewage consists not only of human feces and urine, but also of wastes from laundry, bathing, garbage grinding, and dishwashing, as well as all the miscellaneous articles that find their way into the sewer system—sand, gravel, rubber balls, leaves, sticks, dead rats, and so on. Primary sewage treatment consists of several mechanical processes designed to remove the larger suspended solids through screening and sedimentation. Though there may be minor variations in the methods used by different treatment plants, in general the incoming flow first passes through one or more screens to remove large floating objects. After the waste-laden water has passed the screens, it enters a grit chamber where the reduced velocity of flow permits sand, gravel, and other inorganic material to settle out. Air is sometimes injected into the tank to maintain aerobic conditions and to remove trapped gases. Following several hours in an additional sedimentation tank (a primary clarifier), the wastewater enters the secondary treatment system or, in those POTWs having only a primary level of treatment, is chlorinated and discharged into the receiving waters. The solid material (sludge) that settles out in the sedimentation tank is regularly removed, dried, and disposed of by one of several methods.

While primary treatment is unquestionably better than no treatment at all, it does not result in an effluent of sufficiently high quality to prevent degradation of the receiving waters. During primary treatment approximately 50–65% of suspended solids are removed. In addition, the amount of pollutant organic material in the water, a measurement referred to as **biochemical oxygen demand**, or **BOD**, is reduced by about 25–40%. (When organic matter in wastewater discharged into streams or lakes is acted upon by bacteria, dissolved oxygen is rapidly depleted, resulting in fish kills and drastic alterations in the aquatic environment. Biochemical oxygen demand basically is an indication of how much putrescible organic material is present, with a low BOD indicating good water quality and a high BOD reflecting polluted conditions.) Because the pollution potential of wastewater following primary treatment is still quite high, the Environmental Protection Agency does not consider primary treatment by itself an adequate level of sewage treatment.

Secondary Treatment

Whereas primary treatment is based upon physical and mechanical methods of removing suspended solids from wastewater, secondary treatment depends on biological processes, similar to naturally occurring decomposition but greatly accelerated, to digest organic wastes.

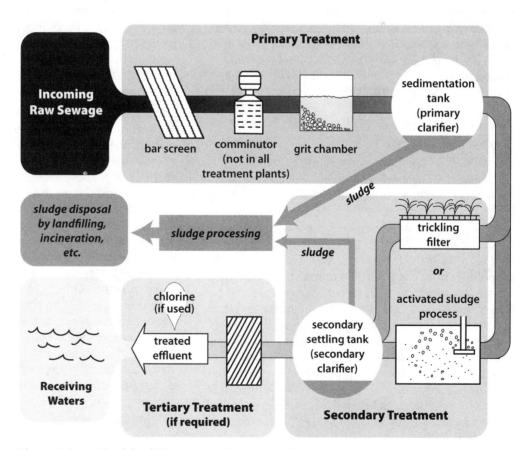

Figure 16-4   Municipal Wastewater Treatment Process

Microorganisms, predominantly aerobic bacteria, are utilized in the presence of an abundant oxygen supply to break down organic materials into inorganic carbon dioxide, water, and minerals. One method of accomplishing this is by use of **trickling filters**—beds of crushed stone whose surfaces are covered with a microbial slime consisting of bacteria, protozoans, nematodes, etc. that absorb the organic material as the wastewater is sprayed over the surface of the rocks. The more modern **activated sludge process** involves "seeding" a tank of sewage with bacteria-laden sludge, pumping compressed air into the mixture and agitating it for 4–10 hours. During this time the microbes adsorb most of the colloidal and suspended solids onto the surfaces of the sludge particles and oxidize the organic material. After the process is complete, the sludge is separated from the remaining liquid by settling (*secondary clarification*). Most of this sludge, consisting primarily of masses of bacteria, is removed, but some must be retained and fed back into the incoming sewage to perpetuate the process.

After wastewater has passed through both primary and secondary treatment, the level of suspended solids and of BOD has been reduced by about 90–95% (however, cold weather can reduce the efficiency of pollutant reduction because it slows the metabolic rate of the microorganisms on which secondary treatment depends). Secondary treatment is not effective in removing viruses, heavy metals, dissolved minerals, or nutrients (Koren, 1980). In the United States, a federally imposed mandate requiring that all POTWs provide at least secondary wastewater treatment took effect in July 1988.

Advanced Wastewater Treatment (Tertiary Treatment)

A third level of sewage treatment may be required in situations (1) where effluent from the secondary treatment process still contains substances that are causing water quality problems; (2) when the sheer volume of effluent is large enough that the remaining 10% of suspended solids and BOD are sufficient to initiate eutrophication; (3) or if the treated wastewater is to be used for purposes of drinking, irrigation, or recreation. Advanced wastewater treatment involves either one or a combination of several biological, chemical, or physical processes designed to remove such pollutants as phosphates, nitrates, ammonia, and organic chemicals. It also further reduces the concentration of remaining suspended solids and BOD to about 1% of that present in raw sewage. Recognition of a growing nitrogen pollution problem in many U.S. waterways and coastal estuaries has prompted requirements for many POTWs to install advanced technologies to remove nitrogen from their wastewater effluent—something that conventional secondary treatment

Table 16-1   Tertiary Treatment Processes

Tertiary Treatment Method	Pollutant Removed
Chemical coagulation, followed by filtration or sedimentation	phosphates, tertiary suspended solids, and BOD
Activated carbon adsorption	synthetic organic chemicals, tastes, odors
Nitrifying towers	ammonia
Air stripping	ammonia
Oxidation ponds and aerated lagoons	BOD, phosphates
Reverse osmosis	BOD, nitrates, phosphates, dissolved solids
Electrodialysis	dissolved minerals
Oxidation	organic material
Foam separation	organic chemicals
Land application	Phosphates, nitrates, BOD, suspended solids

fails to accomplish. The option most commonly chosen uses naturally occurring bacteria in a 3-step process called **biological nitrogen removal (BNR)**. BNR involves the microbial transformation of dissolved organic nitrogen through a series of steps to unreactive elemental nitrogen (N_2), which is released into the atmosphere and no longer poses any water quality threat. The technology to accomplish this is expensive, but treatment plants using BNR have substantially reduced their nitrogen loadings to receiving waterways (Driscoll et al., 2003).

Disinfection

Since the most common waterborne diseases are caused by pathogenic bacteria, viruses, or protozoans present in human excrement, one of the primary purposes of sewage treatment is to kill such organisms before they can infect new victims. Simple exposure to the hostile environment outside the human intestine is sufficient to reduce the number of bacteria appreciably as they pass through the treatment process. However, because a substantial number of live organisms still remain in the wastewater after primary and secondary treatment are complete, it was standard procedure for many years to disinfect treated effluent by adding chlorine prior to discharge in order to eliminate any remaining disease-causing organisms. More recently, the policy of chlorinating all sewage treatment plant discharges has met with increasing resistance and today more than half of all states no longer require that all sanitary wastewaters be disinfected. There are several reasons for this change in accepted practice.

1. Chlorine is effective in killing bacteria, but less so in relation to viruses and parasites (e.g., *Giardia, Cryptosporidium*), many of which survive this treatment.

2. Chlorine is very destructive of fish and other forms of aquatic life, many of which are eliminated for a considerable distance downstream from sewage treatment plants due to the presence of this chemical in the water. For this reason, many wastewater treatment plants that use chlorine as a disinfectant are now required to dechlorinate their wastewater prior to discharge in order to remove potentially harmful residual chlorine.

3. Chlorine treatment poses safety problems at the treatment plant in the eventuality of cylinder leaks or system disruption.

4. Chlorine disinfects only a fraction of the wastes in streams because bacteria-laden runoff from farmland and urban areas enters waterways untreated.

Proponents of chlorinating POTW discharges correctly point out, however, that this practice helps reduce outbreaks of disease that have been associated with swimming in sewage-polluted water or with consuming shellfish taken from contaminated waterways. Although disinfecting such effluent with chlorine does not sterilize the water, in the sense of killing every last microbe, it reduces their numbers significantly and thereby enhances the self-purifying capacity of natural waterways. As the controversy between wastewater chlorination opponents and proponents continues to rage, a compromise solution has been reached in some states where disinfection of discharge waters is required only during the summer bathing season, with the practice being discontinued during the winter when recreational contact with water is unlikely (Shertzer, 1986). In certain states, requirements for disinfecting POTW effluent have been dropped altogether, except in those situations where a drinking water intake point or a bathing beach is located a short distance downstream.

Unfortunately, as population density increases and the distance between POTW effluent discharge points and public drinking water intake pipes shrinks, fewer treatment plants may have the option of bypassing disinfection. This is especially relevant in states like Texas and California, where serious consideration is being given to proposals for discharging treated effluent directly into drinking water reservoirs as a means of augmenting water supplies. As a result, interest in nonchlorine methods of killing microbes is growing rapidly. While some POTWs now employ membrane filtration or ozonation as their method of disinfection, the most popular nontraditional disinfectant is ultraviolet (UV) light. UV kills microbes by disrupting their genetic material, preventing reproduction. Since the technology relies on radiation rather than chemicals, no harmful residual remains in the water posttreatment, eliminating any need to remove disinfectant from the effluent to protect aquatic life downstream. Industry surveys reveal that 25% of all U.S. and Canadian municipal wastewater treatment plants built or upgraded in 2000 opted to install UV systems as their primary disinfectant. UV disinfection technologies have been widely adopted in Europe as well, spurred by a European Union regulation that went into effect in 2005 requiring that all significant wastewater discharges must be pathogen-free. Since most European wastewater treatment plants, except for those in the U.K., weren't disinfecting their effluent at all, the new mandate prompted a large percentage to choose UV systems (Ultraguard Water Systems, 2004).

Biosolids Management

Ironically, the high degree of pollutant removal achieved at modern sewage treatment plants has created a new challenge for POTW operators—how to manage the steadily growing volumes of **sludge** (the term applied to untreated biosolids) that our increasingly efficient sewage treatment technologies are producing. The quantity of biosolids produced annually by U.S. municipal treatment plants has approximately doubled since passage of the Clean Water Act, thanks to continued population growth, further gains in the efficiency of wastewater treatment, and more widespread compliance with Clean Water Act requirements. Because sewage sludge itself can be a pollutant if improperly managed, its treatment, ultimate disposal, and potential use must be handled in ways that will not endanger public health or the environment.

Routinely removed at each step in the sewage treatment process, the watery sludge (before treatment, sludge consists of 93–99% water) generally is first thickened through the use of coagulant chemicals or dissolved air flotation. It is then stabilized through a two-step anaerobic digestion process in order to reduce problems associated with odors and the presence of pathogenic organisms—a process that takes approximately 60 days to complete. To reduce its volume for ease in handling, the sludge is then dewatered, either by mechanical processes or by drying on sand beds. At this point sludge has the appearance of rich black dirt and is largely odor free. A number of POTWs subsequently compost, heat-dry, or otherwise treat their sludge to kill remaining pathogens. Contrary to the negative public image of anything pertaining to sewage, the treated biosolids at this point represent a valuable resource rather than an objectionable waste. Indeed, the nitrates, phosphates, and organic matter present in sludge make it useful as a fertilizer and as a soil conditioner. Biosolids have a long history of use for improving marginal lands, increasing forest productivity (studies have shown that the rate of tree growth doubles on sludge-enriched soil), boosting home garden yields, and reclaiming lands devastated by strip-mining.

Since sewage treatment plants, particularly those in the larger metropolitan areas, generate enormous amounts of sludge during their normal course of operations, finding

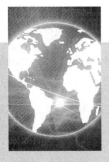

· · · · · · · · 16-3 · · · · · · · ·

**Watch Where You Swim—
Recreational Water Illnesses May Be Lurking**

A refreshing dip in the pool on a hot summer day, an afternoon at the beach, or a relaxing interlude in a hot tub are pleasures enjoyed by millions of people, totally oblivious to any disease hazard posed by such activities. In recent years, however, many are learning the hard way that microbes and parasites in both treated and natural recreational waters can make them sick. Since the CDC began compiling reports in 1978, the confirmed number of recreational water illnesses (RWI) has been steadily increasing and health authorities assume many more go unreported.

The most frequent outbreaks involve cases of gastroenteritis (diarrhea), acquired while bathing in pools or interactive fountains. Although such facilities are required to comply with state and local regulations regarding maintenance and disinfection, follow-up investigations have shown that the majority of pools implicated in waterborne disease outbreaks were poorly maintained and inadequately treated, characterized by disrupted chlorine disinfection. It should be noted that even when pool operators follow proper disinfection procedures, the protective chlorine residual can be depleted more rapidly than usual if the pool is overcrowded with swimmers, if organic material enters the water, or when the weather is particularly hot and sunny. Inadequate chlorine residual permits the survival of waterborne bacteria, which may then be ingested when swimmers accidentally swallow pool water (CDC, 2002c).

In most reported outbreaks involving pools, however, bacteria are not the culprits. The vast majority of illnesses are caused, instead, by the protozoan parasite, *Cryptosporidium parvum*, now recognized as the leading cause of diarrheal outbreaks associated with recreational water use. Sixty percent of all the disease outbreaks involving pools reported to CDC from 1995–2004 were caused by ingestion of this parasite. Cysts of *Cryptosporidium*, entering the water in fecal material, are highly resistant to chlorination and can remain viable in pools for several days, even when chlorine concentrations in the water meet the standards set by public health authorities. Victims of cryptosporidiosis experience profuse diarrhea that can persist for as long as three weeks. If they go back into the water during that time, they can recontaminate the pool and further spread the disease. Reducing recreational water outbreaks of cryptosporidiosis will likely require the use of ozone or ultraviolet light to inactivate this chlorine-resistant parasite, as well as enhanced filtration to improve *Cryptosporidium* removal. Equally important are public education efforts to inform swimmers how important it is to stay out of the water if they're experiencing diarrhea (Yoder and Beach, 2007).

While infections associated with swimming pools and interactive fountains most frequently involve gastrointestinal problems, those contracted in hot tubs are more likely to be a form of dermatitis called "hot tub rash." Caused by the bacterium *Pseudomonas aeruginosa*, this itchy skin condition often develops into a bumpy red rash, sensitive to the touch and sometimes featuring pus-filled blisters surrounding the hair follicles. The rash is often worse on areas of the skin covered by the victim's swimsuit, since wet fabric keeps contaminated water in contact with skin—a good reason for showering and changing into dry clothes as soon as possible after leaving the water. The causative pathogen, *P. aeruginosa*, is a common organism in soil and water but is effectively controlled through disinfection with chlorine or bromine and by maintaining proper pH levels in the water. To ensure water safety, chlorine/bromine and pH levels should be tested frequently because the warm temperatures typical of hot tub and spa water cause disinfectants to evaporate faster than is the case in swimming pools. Investigations of hot tub-related dermatitis outbreaks almost always identify treatment deficiencies as the causative factor.

Recreational water illnesses are certainly not restricted to treated pools or hot tubs. Swimming in fecally polluted lakes, marine waters, or untreated children's wading pools has led to a number of RWI outbreaks. The pathogen in most reported cases involving freshwater is *E. coli 0157:H7*, the culprit in many serious food-poisoning outbreaks as well. In some situations, just as in the pool incidents previously described, water contamination occurred as a result of infected children, usually toddlers, defecating in or near the water. In other cases, droppings of water birds or mammals introduce fecal bacteria into recreational waters. Point sources of pollution such as POTWs and storm sewers, if located near bathing beaches, may discharge pathogen-laden wastewaters that pose a health risk to swimmers. Malfunctioning septic systems, likewise, can be a source of water contamination. Nonpoint sources can degrade recreational waters when heavy rainfall washes animal wastes, soil, fertilizers, pesticides, and other pollutants off the land and into waterways. For this reason, beach water generally experiences much higher levels of pollution during and immediately after rainstorms, making swimming at such times inadvisable.

In addition to the risk of *E. coli 0157:H7* and other bacterial infections, swimming or playing in contaminated water may result in a parasitic infection properly termed cercarial dermatitis but more commonly known as "swimmer's itch." Caused by a species of flatworm related to the pathogen responsible for schistosomiasis in tropical regions, this temperate-zone pathogen alternates between a snail host and several species of warm-blooded animals, including ducks, geese, swans, gulls, beavers, and muskrats. The feces of infected animals contain worm eggs that hatch into free-swimming larvae when they come into contact with water. The larvae then parasitize snails, which subsequently release second-stage larvae called cercariae. These swim off in search of a host animal, one of those listed above, but sometimes encounter a human bather instead and burrow into the skin. Since humans are not the parasite's natural host, they soon die; before doing so, however, they provoke a tingling, burning, or itching sensation which may persist for as long as a week. Frequently, small reddish pimples appear, often developing into small blisters. Medical attention is seldom required, as the rash gradually fades away; however, since swimmer's itch is essentially an allergic reaction to the parasite, repeated exposures result in increasingly severe symptoms of discomfort. Because the cercariae are most likely to occur in shallow water near the shoreline where snails are common, small children tend to be the most frequent victims of swimmer's itch. Avoidance is the best approach for dealing with this recreational water illness: don't swim in areas where swimmer's itch is a known problem, shower or towel off immediately after leaving the water, and try to prevent the problem in the first place by not feeding (and thus attracting) waterfowl close to areas where people swim (CDC, 2002c).

Growing awareness of the health issues posed by RWIs has prompted greater scrutiny of beach conditions by federal, state, and local health and environmental agencies. Every year hundreds, even thousands, of beaches in the U.S. are posted with warnings or closed for a day or more due to known water contamination. EPA has established federal guidelines to assist states in setting standards for microbial water quality in lakes, ponds, and marine waters, but regulation remains the prerogative of state and local governments. As a result, these vary widely from one jurisdiction to another. Because many beaches are still not monitored at all, or monitored only sporadically, those who swim there have no way of knowing whether or not a hazard exists. To help rectify this problem, the EPA has instituted its BEACH Program (Beaches Environmental Assessment, Closure and Health Program), one feature of which is the agency's Beach Watch Web site (www.epa.gov/waterscience/beacon/) where those interested can access information regarding water quality and local protection programs at specific U.S. beaches.

Common-sense precautions and good personal hygiene on the part of bathers (particularly parents of toddlers and young children), combined with governmental public health efforts, can help ensure that fun in the water won't make you sick.

a place in which to dispose of this material poses major dilemmas for many such facilities. Incineration can present problems of air pollution, and in many communities where landfill space is at a premium, burying sludge is increasingly controversial—and increasingly expensive. In fact, biosolids management has become so expensive that, whatever the disposal option chosen, treatment and disposal of biosolids now account for over 50% of the operating costs of a typical POTW providing secondary sewage treatment.

Since the mid-1990s, EPA regulations have encouraged a marked trend toward "beneficial reuse" of biosolids; as a result, 55% of the estimated 8.2 million tons of biosolids produced annually by U.S. sewage treatment plants are being recycled, spread on the land as fertilizer; almost three-quarters of that amount is being used on farmlands, while the remainder is distributed to the public for a variety of uses, including landscaping and home gardening (NEBRA, 2007). The 1987 Clean Water Act amendments established a comprehensive program for reducing potential environmental risks posed by sludge through requirements that EPA (1) identify toxic substances that may be present in sludge at potentially dangerous levels, and (2) promulgate regulations that specify acceptable management practices and numerical limitations for sludge containing those pollutants. These regulations, referred to as the **Part 503** standards, were issued in February of 1993 and have now been implemented nationwide.

The main concern that has limited beneficial reuse of biosolids in the past is the fact that sewage sludge often contains toxic chemicals and pathogens as well as desirable nutrients such as phosphates and nitrates. In particular, sludge from POTWs receiving industrial wastewater discharges in addition to residential sewage may contain potentially dangerous concentrations of heavy metals and other toxics—cadmium and lead are of special concern, but copper, zinc, nickel, PCBs, and a number of other contaminants also may be present. EPA addressed this issue by setting maximum loading rates on soils for biosolids containing these contaminants, advising POTWs to police industrial discharges in their communities in an effort to eliminate toxic pollutants at the source. Regulatory standards for chemicals in biosolids were painstakingly developed through a risk assessment process that involved identifying those contaminants deemed likely to pose the greatest hazard, characterizing the most likely ways in which a person might be exposed, and then making science-based calculations on the maximum concentrations permissible in biosolids intended for land application and the amount of biosolids that could be applied to a given land area (i.e., loading rate).

EPA took a different approach to ensure that pathogen levels in biosolids wouldn't present a health risk. Rather than setting risk-based concentration limits for individual microbes, regulators established sludge treatment requirements, such as composting or heat drying, to reduce even further the already relatively low number of organisms present in digested sludge. Depending on the number of pathogens present following treatment, resulting biosolids are characterized as Class A or Class B. The former, characterized by pathogen densities below specified detection limits, can be applied to any lands, including home lawns and gardens, without restriction. Class B biosolids have a somewhat higher pathogen content and, to ensure public safety, Part 503 restricts their use to croplands, pastureland, and forests. Rules also specify the amount of time that must elapse between biosolids application and subsequent crop harvesting, animal grazing, or public access. During this interval it is assumed that environmental factors such as heat and sunlight will further reduce pathogen concentrations (though no on-site measurements are required to verify this assumption).

More than 30 years of research and practical experience have shown that food crops grown on lands fertilized with biosolids are safe for human consumption and the National Research Council (NRC) reports no documented scientific evidence to suggest that current biosolids regulations fail to protect public health. Nevertheless, some environmental groups cite anecdotal, though unsubstantiated, reports of people or animals sickened by exposure to land-applied biosolids, problems ranging from mild allergic reactions to severe and chronic health problems. Recognizing these concerns, the NRC has recommended that EPA reassess the existing Part 503 chemical standards using improved, up-to-date risk assessment practices and review whether additional chemicals should be added to the list of those currently regulated. They also suggest that although a direct link between biosolids exposure and human illness has never been scientifically proven, the EPA should conduct epidemiological studies focused on biosolids applicators, farmers using biosolids, and people living near land application sites in order to lay such fears to rest. Ensuring that existing rules pertaining to such management practices as loading rates and setback distances from waterways are rigorously enforced is another NRC recommendation to agency regulators, reflecting the fact that many complaints are related to excessive rates of biosolids application or to runoff contamination of streams when required setbacks were ignored (NRC, 2002). Responding to these recommendations, EPA is sponsoring scientific research and public health studies on the safety of biosolids use as a fertilizer. Perhaps as a reflection of public concerns, the rate of biosolids application to agricultural lands has not increased since the late 1990s, with biosolids continuing to be used on less than 1% of total U.S. farmland acreage (NEBRA, 2007).

Although agricultural lands are currently the destination for most of the biosolids being land applied, farmers are not the only ones interested in taking advantage of this "black gold." While some municipalities are giving biosolids away to anyone who will take it, the majority are selling the stuff to home gardeners, nurseries, or landscaping firms for use in commercial and residential areas. Milwaukee and Madison, Wisconsin, and Austin, Texas, have employed imaginative marketing skills in promoting their products, selling biosolids under such catchy trade names as *Milorganite*, *Metrogro*, or *Dillo Dirt*.

NEW APPROACHES TO WASTEWATER TREATMENT

Financing the improvements in municipal sewage treatment required by the 1972 Clean Water Act would have been impossible had Congress not included, in that same piece of legislation, the creation of a massive **Construction Grant Program**. This fund provided federal monetary assistance to communities that could not otherwise have afforded the multimillion-dollar expenditures necessary to construct new or upgraded POTWs capable of providing the mandatory secondary level of sewage treatment. Under the Construction Grant Program, the second-largest public works project in U.S. history (exceeded only by construction of the interstate highway system), the federal government agreed to provide fully 75% of the cost of such projects, an amount that was subsequently reduced to 55% by the Reagan administration in 1981. Over nearly two decades Washington contributed $57 billion for sewage treatment plant construction (state and local expenditures during the same period exceeded an additional $70 billion); as a result, by the late 1980s, 58% of the U.S. population was served by POTWs providing either secondary or secondary and advanced wastewater treatment. Since POTWs cumulatively serve about 70% of the American population, it is obvious that domestic wastewaters in the majority of sewered communities now receive a commendably high level of treatment prior to discharge.

Nevertheless, remaining sewage treatment needs are considerable. In the late 1980s, approximately one out of every ten Americans lived in communities providing less than secondary treatment—and some small towns still had no sewage treatment at all, discharging raw wastewaters directly into streams. In 1990, EPA estimated the total cost of bringing all municipal dischargers into compliance with CWA water quality requirements could exceed $110 billion—yet by 1990 the federal well had run dry (Adler et al., 1993). Amendments to the Clean Water Act passed by Congress in 1987 called for a phaseout of the federal Construction Grant Program by 1994, replacing it with a **State Revolving Fund** providing low-interest *loans* (no more free gifts from Uncle Sam!) to municipalities with unmet sewage treatment needs. Unfortunately, the demand for such loans exceeds the supply—but federal deadline dates for compliance with CWA requirements remain unchanged and potential penalties can be severe. Thus the fiscal and legal realities of the 1990s provided a major incentive to develop new, less costly, yet equally effective methods of treating sewage—alternatives to the highly engineered, energy-consuming, sludge-producing, exorbitantly expensive POTWs that offered a convenient "technological fix" during the era of free-flowing federal dollars but are an unrealistic option for communities of limited means.

In recent decades a variety of innovative approaches to solving wastewater problems have attracted considerable interest and a number are now in the pilot-project stage, undergoing extensive field studies; several are in full-scale use, having proven their ability to produce good quality effluent at a fraction of the cost of conventional sewage treatment. The majority of new systems are based on the concept that wastewater effluent, like biosolids, should be viewed as a nutrient-laden resource to be utilized rather than as a pollutant to be discarded.

One of the earliest and most widely adopted approaches to alternative treatment was land application of wastewater. This method involves spraying effluent from secondary treatment onto forest, pastures, or croplands. Land application not only helps prevent stream pollution by keeping nutrients out of the water, it also utilizes those same nutrients as fertilizer for the plants on which it is applied. A further advantage of this method is that the wastewater is largely purified as it percolates through the soil to recharge the groundwater supply. Early health concerns that dissolved metals or pathogens in the effluent might contaminate soils or vegetation have been dispelled by many years of problem-free experience with land application at Pennsylvania State University; in communities in Texas, Michigan, California, and New York; and in Germany, France, Israel, and Australia.

In the 1980s, emphasis shifted to the potential for artificial wetlands ("designer swamps"), duckweed systems (*Lemna spp.*), and water-purifying hydroponics-type systems inside greenhouses. In the United States, the Tennessee Valley Authority (TVA) has been at the forefront of research and development efforts focused on wetlands treatment. TVA views such systems as a viable wastewater treatment option for small communities that lack the expertise, as well as the financial resources, to operate highly sophisticated mechanical plants. Since the mid-1980s, TVA has designed and constructed engineered wetlands for a number of small towns in southern Appalachia, enabling such communities to comply with federal water quality standards at a fraction of the cost of conventional facilities. Although the sizeable land requirements for engineered wetlands have deterred many communities from giving such systems serious consideration, some larger cities such as Orlando, Florida, and Columbia, Missouri, have opted to utilize wetlands as one element in their treatment process.

Of the municipalities nationwide currently employing wetlands systems to treat sewage, the most renowned is Arcata, California, a community of 17,000 located on the north shore of Humboldt Bay. In the early 1980s, Arcata faced a serious fiscal dilemma: effluent from the town's POTW consistently violated discharge permit limitations and Arcata was being pressured by the state environmental agency to close the plant and join with neighboring municipalities in constructing a large regional facility. Wary of the exorbitant costs such an undertaking would entail, Arcata opted for a radically different solution. Assisted by faculty at Humboldt State University, the town proceeded to develop a series of ponds and marshes to remove the troublesome pollutants remaining in its effluent following primary treatment at the POTW. Today Arcata's wastewater receives secondary treatment in a 50-acre stabilization pond where suspended solids settle to the bottom, while dissolved organic materials are broken down through a symbiotic association between bacteria and algae. From here the effluent flows into a three-celled, five-acre "treatment marsh" where rooted aquatic plants such as cattails (*Typha latifolia*) and bulrushes (*Scirpus acutis*) flourish. The submerged stems of these plants harbor countless numbers of microorganisms that further metabolize dis-

solved organic nitrates and phosphates. Passage through the marsh also effectively breaks down pesticides, industrial solvents, and most of the heavy metals in wastewater. After passing through the treatment marsh, the effluent is pumped to a chlorine contact tank for disinfection and is subsequently discharged into an "enhancement marsh" for additional wetlands treatment. This enhancement marsh, open to the public, is interlaced with jogging and hiking trails, picnic areas, and a nature center; it also serves as a wildlife sanctuary, annually attracting more than 150,000 visitors and 160 species of birds and other wildlife—living proof that the impera-

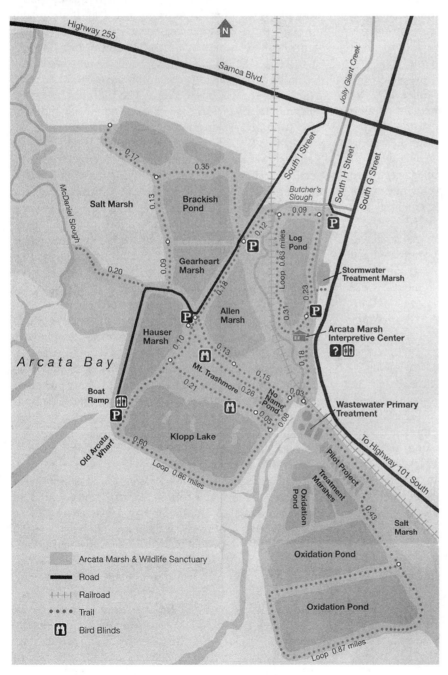

Figure 16-5

The Arcata Marsh & Wildlife Sanctuary is a municipal-wastewater-treatment success story. The series of ponds and marshes remove pollutants from the town's wastewater and produce an effluent that is cleaner than the seawater into which it is ultimately discharged. [*Leslie Scopes Anderson, Friends of the Arcata Marsh*]

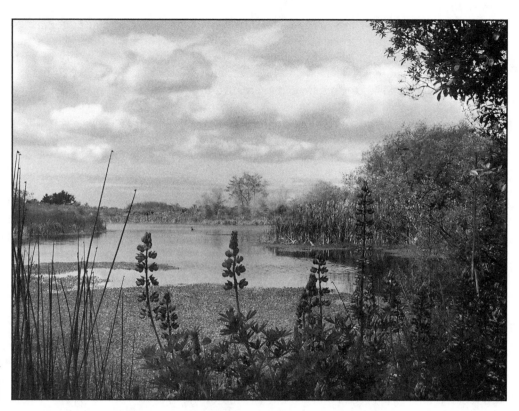

The log pond at Arcata Marsh. [*Leslie Scopes Anderson, Friends of the Arcata Marsh*]

tives of providing for society's urgent wastewater management needs and restoring valuable ecosystems are mutually compatible.

After treatment in the enhancement marsh, the effluent is chlorinated once again and finally discharged into Humboldt Bay (source of 60–70% of California's oyster crop), its levels of suspended solids and BOD by now well below the NPDES limits of 30 mg/L. Completed in 1986, Arcata's wetland system has been both an environmental and financial success. Once a polluter of Humboldt Bay, Arcata's wastewater treatment process produces an effluent that not only exceeds water quality standards but is even cleaner than the seawater into which it flows—and it does so at a cost far lower than that of a standard treatment facility. By the late 1990s, the obvious advantages of Arcata's natural approach to wastewater treatment had persuaded city officials in Davis and Pacifica, California, to construct their own wetlands treatment systems.

Why haven't more communities followed Arcata's example? The major limitation to such systems is the amount of land they require—about 20 acres for a town of 10,000 people. Unless a community already owns land on its outskirts, being able to afford, or even find, this much land may present serious difficulties. Perhaps the biggest obstacle is sheer ignorance and inertia. Only recently have adequate design guidelines become available for engineers and regulators; municipal officials fre-

quently are unaware of the advantages such systems offer; conventionally trained engineers are frequently reluctant to embark on new, little-tried technologies and often lack the understanding of environmental conditions needed to factor these into their designs. Despite these obstacles, the idea is gradually winning converts, and not only in small towns. In Phoenix, Arizona, the Tres Rios Ecosystem Restoration and Flood Control Project, underway since 2000, includes a constructed emergent wetland covering about 480 acres to treat effluent from its POTW. In addition to providing a more economical way of meeting effluent standards than upgrading its conventional treatment plant, the engineered wetland also provides wildlife habitat and a place where Phoenix residents can hike, picnic, and visit an environmental education center.

A more futuristic approach to meeting community wastewater treatment needs in an economical and environmentally benign manner is The Living Machine®, marketed by Worrell Water Technologies in Charlottesville, Virginia. Designed to treat both human wastewaters and high-strength industrial organic wastes, The Living Machine relies on a series of tanks and biofilters containing a wide spectrum of microorganisms, algae, snails, and plants, either inside a greenhouse-like structure or outdoors. After passing through this natural treatment system, the resulting effluent is clean enough to be discharged directly into a waterway or to be reused for toilet flushing, landscape irrigation, or, after reverse osmosis treatment, as potable water. By 2009, 23 Living Machines were in use or under construction in 14 states and three foreign countries (Ghana, the Netherlands, and Brazil), providing a low-cost, sustainable alternative to high-tech conventional wastewater treatment. As communities struggle to avoid stringent penalties for non-compliance with mandated effluent requirements in the absence of federal funding, it's likely that alternative natural systems will receive much wider and more serious attention in the years ahead.

Elsewhere in the world, a variant on wetlands treatment is the use of fishponds for treating sewage while simultaneously supporting aquaculture. In Lima, Peru, a portion of the city's sewage is directed to stabilization ponds where solids settle out and bacteria decompose the organic wastes. After three or four weeks the water is sufficiently cleansed of pollutants to use for irrigation and for fish culture. Similar systems are currently in operation in Hungary, Germany, Israel, and a number of countries in South and Southeast Asia. The largest of these can be found in Calcutta, India, where human wastewaters nourish algae in two large lakes. Herbivorous fish such as carp and tilapia feed upon these algae and are subsequently harvested to provide Calcutta markets with approximately 7,000 metric tons of fish each year. Obvious concerns about the potential for contamination of fish with human gastrointestinal pathogens can be allayed by retaining sewage in the stabilization lagoons for at least 20 days before allowing it to enter the fishponds or by transferring the fish to clean waters for a period of time prior to harvesting (World Resources Institute, 1992).

SEPTIC SYSTEMS

Approximately 30% of all Americans live in unsewered areas where they must utilize on-site septic systems for the disposal of wastewaters from bathrooms, kitchens, and laundries. Most on-site wastewater disposal systems consist of two basic parts: (1) a septic tank, buried in the ground at some distance from the house, to which it is connected by a pipe, and (2) a soil absorption field or sand filter.

The septic tank itself is a watertight container made of concrete or fiberglass with a minimum capacity of 750 gallons. Sewage entering the septic tank is partially decomposed by bacteria under anaerobic conditions. During this process, sludge settles to the bottom of the tank, while lighter solids and grease, as well as gases from the decomposing sludge, rise to the top to form a floating scum. The partially clarified liquid then passes through an outlet and the effluent is evenly dispersed

among several perforated pipes in a carefully designed absorption field, which must be of adequate size and proper soil porosity to ensure that the effluent seeping out of the perforated pipe moves quickly enough to prevent ponding, but not so rapidly as to infiltrate aquifers, wells, or surface water supplies before contaminants in the effluent have been filtered out or oxidized.

Since more than half of the solids in the wastewater settle out during the retention period in the septic tank, the accumulation of sludge at the bottom, as well as the scum layer at the top, must be removed periodically (usually every 3–5 years). If this is not done, the sludge build-up reaches the point that solids are discharged into the absorption field, resulting in clogging and ponding. This accumulation of particulates and scum in the pores of the soil prevents proper drainage of the effluent and eventually results in failure of the system. In addition to improper maintenance of the septic tank, other reasons for septic system failure may be: use of a septic tank that is too small for the householders' needs; excessive household water use (large parties in homes on septic systems can be disastrous); insufficient size of the absorption field; soil too impervious to receive effluent; or tree roots clogging the effluent distribution lines.

Although a well-located, carefully constructed, and properly maintained septic system can be a perfectly adequate method of sanitary wastewater disposal (and is the only feasible option in most rural areas), malfunctioning septic systems frequently give rise to serious NPS water pollution, as leachates containing pathogenic organisms and nutrients seep from absorption fields into water supplies. The rapid growth of rural subdivisions, many of which rely on septic systems installed on lots too small to provide adequate waste dispersal, ensures that pollution problems related to septic systems will continue to plague public health officials.

INDUSTRIAL DISCHARGES

Effluent discharges from industry comprise the second major category of point source water pollution and consist of a wide range of pollutants which, for regulatory purposes, have been subdivided into three major groups:

1. *Conventional pollutants.* These include organic wastes high in BOD, suspended solids, acids, oil and grease, etc. Such pollutants originate from food processing plants, pulp and paper mills, steel mills, oil tanker spills and cleaning operations, accidents involving offshore oil drilling, and so forth.

2. *Toxic pollutants.* A list of 129 priority toxic pollutants was developed by EPA in 1976 (three subsequently have been de-listed); substances listed include heavy metals such as cadmium, mercury, and lead, PCBs,

benzene, chloroform, cyanide, arsenic, 2,4-D, and a number of other pesticides. The electroplating and metal-processing industries, plastics manufacturers, and chemical companies are but a few of the industries discharging toxic effluents.

3. *Nonconventional Pollutants.* All the other pollutants not classified by EPA as either conventional or toxic are grouped into this third category—substances such as nitrogen and phosphorus, iron, tin, aluminum, chloride, and ammonia. As in the preceding categories, the sources of such pollutants can be traced to a wide variety of industrial processes.

The Clean Water Act requires EPA to develop technology-based national treatment standards for each category of industrial discharger (e.g., petroleum refiners, textile mills, iron and steel, leather tanning, etc.), directing that standards be reviewed periodically and made increasingly stringent as pollution control technologies advance. Industries discharging directly into the nation's waterways must obtain an NPDES permit, specifying the allowable amounts and constituents of pollutants in their effluent. Dischargers are required to monitor their effluent on a routine basis and violations of permit limitations can result in serious civil or criminal penalties.

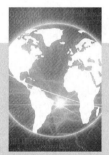

· · · · · · · 16-4 · · · · · · ·

Water and Terrorism: How Vulnerable is America's Drinking Water?

In 1984, Oregonians learned just how vulnerable municipal water supplies are to sabotage by groups intent on wreaking havoc. That year members of the Rajneeshee religious cult contaminated a city water supply tank in The Dalles with *Salmonella*, precipitating an outbreak that sickened over 750 people. At the time, most Americans regarded the incident as an outrageous but isolated event, but 17 years later after the tragedy of 9/11, the urgent focus on efforts to improve national security included a new realization of the need to safeguard U.S. water systems against potential terrorist threats.

Such threats are regarded as all too real; our water infrastructure provides attractive targets for those seeking to create chaos and calamity, since there is no substitute for water. Most water facilities are readily accessible and hence vulnerable either to physical attack, using explosives to destroy dams, pipelines, or treatment plants, or by introducing toxic chemicals or disease agents into the water supply. Fortunately, the public's most feared scenario of massive casualties caused by poisoning a municipal water supply is highly unlikely. Because of rapid dilution, it would take extremely large amounts of an introduced chemical contaminant to threaten large water supply reservoirs; also, routine water treatment processes would deactivate or remove most chemical contaminants. Similarly, many of the bacterial species and biotoxins considered likely biological warfare agents are rendered inactive by standard disinfection processes; others could be removed by such advanced treatment technologies as micro- and ultra-filtration and reverse osmosis filtration, although these technologies are not currently in place at most municipal water treatment plants (Gleick, 2006a). Until the terrorist attacks in 2001, the need to worry about such eventualities has seemed remote; over the past 100 years, medical records reveal only one death in the entire United States caused by intentionally contaminated water.

Unfortunately, the events of 9/11 and heightened awareness of an international terrorist threat have removed any sense of complacency regarding U.S. water security. Concerns increased in 2002 with the discovery of documents in Afghanistan indicating that al Qaeda operatives were considering various methods for massive disruption of American water supplies and water treatment plants. That same year, fearing more terrorist attacks within the U.S., Congress passed the 2002 Bioterrorism Act. The new law forced water utilities, whose existing emergency preparedness plans dealt solely with natural disasters or acts of vandalism, to focus instead on deliberate attempts by terrorists to disrupt or contaminate water supplies.

Such attacks, if successfully carried out, would have a devastating impact on public health, as well as on sanitation and fire-fighting capability, and could create widespread panic within affected communities. Under the Bioterrorism Act, EPA was required to prepare a baseline threat report, detailing likely threats that utilities should consider when assessing their vulnerability to terrorism. The utilities were then required to conduct vulnerability assessments, examining risks and identifying countermeasures for terrorist attacks against a wide range of water system components. After completing and submitting their vulnerability assessment to EPA, a process now accomplished, utilities must prepare an emergency response plan, based on the results of that assessment.

These new emergency response plans are fundamentally different from previous plans that focused primarily on major water main ruptures or potential tornado, hurricane, or earthquake damage. Although some types of terrorist attack, such as the use of explosives to inactivate a treatment plant or to blow up distribution lines, would be apparent within a matter of minutes, other equally devastating forms of sabotage might not be recognized for days. For example, if chemical or biological agents were somehow introduced into the post-treatment water distribution system (considered by experts a much more likely avenue of attack than dumping them into large reservoirs), it is unlikely this would be noticed until the utility started receiving customer complaints about the strange taste, odor, or color of water flowing from their taps—or until hospitals began to report a mysterious surge in emergency room visits. Even telling the public what to do in such a situation would be problematic. The standard "boil order" that typically accompanies a water main break might not be appropriate in a situation where the nature of the problem is still in question. Boiling water intended for drinking or cooking is generally effective in killing bacterial contaminants but does nothing to remove chemical pollutants—indeed, it simply increases their concentration. Similarly, as long as microbially contaminated water is used only for bathing it presents little danger, but the same may not be true for water containing chemical toxins. Until the identity of a presumed contaminant is definitive, the affected utility may have to advise the public not to use the water for any purpose. Currently, information on these and related water security topics is being exchanged among utilities nationwide via Water Information Sharing and Analysis Centers, which serve as an important link between service providers and government agencies dealing with homeland security, public and environmental health, intelligence, and law enforcement (Isenberg, 2002).

In addition to performing mandated vulnerability assessments and developing response plans, utilities have been altering many long-established policies and procedures to enhance the security of the water supply infrastructure. Examples of such changes include requirements that those delivering chemical supplies provide advance notification and undergo rigorous identity checks; strict procedures regarding access and parking for contractors and service providers; background checks on new employees; and coordination with local law enforcement agencies for increased surveillance and patrolling of utility grounds. Levels of vigilance have been particularly high in several cities thought to be at special risk. In Chicago, the local Coast Guard conducts regular patrols near that city's water intake site in Lake Michigan. New York City has increased the number of water samples it takes for testing each day and has blocked off some roads near its upstate reservoirs while stationing armed guards at some sites (AWWA, 2003).

Whether all the precautions will be sufficiently protective if terrorists are determined to attack water supply facilities is open to question. Some observers contend that water treatment plants are too large to protect against intrusion, given existing financial resources, and that water distribution pipelines, with hundreds of thousands of access points, are nearly impossible to protect everywhere. Pointing out that the nation's water infrastructure was never intended to withstand terrorism, such critics suggest decentralizing water treatment, perhaps establishing neighborhood package plants for drinking water treatment or even "point-of-use" treatment, utilizing under-the-faucet filters featuring advanced technologies that could reduce both biological and chemical hazards.

A final, and critical, element in protecting America's water supply is the active involvement of ordinary citizens. A number of utilities have already organized neighborhood watch programs, enlisting the help of residents living near pumping stations, storage tanks, or reservoirs to act as an extra set of eyes, contacting police or the utility if they notice any suspicious activity.

Although most experts regard a successful terrorist attack against America's water supply as unlikely, it is only prudent to establish proactive policies and procedures to ensure that this country continues to enjoy, as it has for many years, the safest drinking water in the world.

For the most part, industry has a better record of compliance with existing water pollution control regulations than do municipal dischargers (i.e., POTWs); EPA estimates that the use of best available pollution control technologies in 22 targeted industrial categories has reduced releases of certain toxic organic chemicals by 99% and heavy metals by 98% since passage of the Clean Water Act in 1972. Altogether, controls imposed on toxic industrial discharges have, according to EPA estimates, prevented the release of more than a billion pounds of toxics yearly into U.S. surface waters; even larger amounts of conventional pollutants have been controlled. Overall, stream monitoring data and self-reporting by industry both indicate a steady downward trend for industrial discharges in recent years—slow but encouraging progress toward the elusive goal of "zero discharge."

Direct Versus Indirect Discharges

Current water pollution laws distinguish two categories of industrial waste discharges: **direct discharges** that flow directly into a receiving stream or lake and **indirect discharges** that go into the sewer system, where they first pass through the municipal sewage treatment plant before entering a waterway along with sanitary wastewater effluent. When citizens think about industrial pollutant discharges, they generally envision the direct type— pipes from a factory leading straight to the water's edge, pouring a poisonous brew onto the back of some hapless fish. In point of fact, however, the majority of industrial discharges are of the indirect type, released by approxi-

mately 27,000 industrial users (IUs) who discharge huge volumes of industrial wastewaters into sewer systems every year. In cases where indirect industrial discharges consist primarily of biodegradable organic wastes, sending them to the sewage treatment plant is appropriate, since the same processes that decompose human excreta are effective on other organic materials as well. In situations involving toxic substances, however, indirect discharges via the sewer system have caused a number of very serious problems.

Structural Damage to Sewer System and Treatment Plant

Industrial discharges of strong acids or alkalis can corrode both sewer pipes and equipment at the POTW. Some chemicals react to produce toxic fumes that can present a serious health threat to workers at the treatment plant, and certain volatile substances can generate a build-up of gas in the sewers, occasionally resulting in explosions.

Interference with Biological Treatment Processes

When toxic chemicals like synthetic organic pesticides pass through a sewage treatment plant, they have the same effect on the microbes responsible for secondary treatment as they do on the target pests—they kill them, and in so doing render the sewage treatment plant ineffective.

Biosolids Contamination

Certain toxics such as cadmium, mercury, lead, and arsenic may pass through the sewage treatment plant without damaging equipment or interfering with biological treatment. Nevertheless, they pose major problems

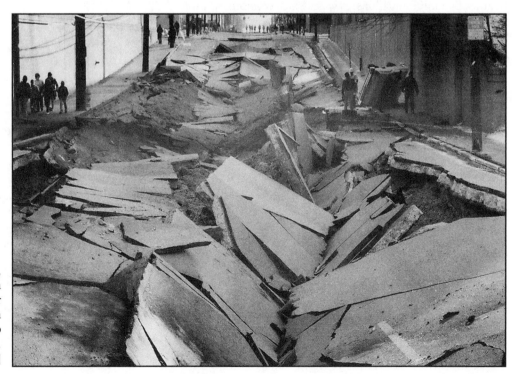

In Louisville, Kentucky, discharges of hexane from an industry into the city's sewer system caused an explosion in 1981 that destroyed two miles of city streets.
[© *The Courier-Journal*]

because they can be assimilated by the bacteria that provide secondary treatment and subsequently accumulate in the sludge, seriously limiting disposal options for biosolids. Sludge containing excessive concentrations of heavy metals cannot be land-applied due to concerns that toxics may be taken up by plants or leach into groundwater. Similarly, there are restrictions on incineration of metals-contaminated sludge (Banks and Dubrowski, 1982).

Violation of POTW Effluent Limitations

Because sewage treatment plants, like industries, must comply with the terms of their NPDES permit, toxic chemicals that pass through the treatment plant and pollute the receiving waters make it necessary for the POTW to install methods of advanced wastewater treatment to prevent such violations from occurring. This, of course, is a costly undertaking, the expense of which is borne by the tax-paying public.

Need for Pretreatment of Indirect Discharges

Problems such as those just described led Congress to legislate a national **pretreatment program** that requires industrial users to detoxify their effluent before discharging it into the sewer. EPA was charged with setting standards for specifically prohibited pollutant discharges as well as categorical pretreatment standards for groups of industries, comparable to the effluent limitations requiring best available technology for controlling pollution from direct dischargers. The work of developing, implementing, and enforcing the program has been assigned to approximately 1,600 local POTWs (those treating five million gallons of wastewater or more on a daily basis) that also have authority to set additional discharge requirements above and beyond the federal standards if such action is deemed necessary. Although originally mandated in 1972, the pretreatment program was extremely slow in getting started, in part because EPA did not formulate basic rules for the program until 1980. Implementation of the program by local sanitary districts moved into high gear by the mid-1980s and today most industries discharging wastewaters to municipal sewers have some form of pretreatment program in place. EPA reports that as a result of the national pretreatment program, industrial users have reduced the amount of pollutants they discharge to POTWs, a fact reflected most dramatically in the sharp reduction in metals present in sludge. Restrictions on industrial users can't solve every problem related to chemical discharges, however, since not all of the hazardous materials flowing into sewage treatment plants are of industrial origin. Of the regulated toxics entering POTWs, about 15% come from residences—all those bleaches, toilet bowl cleaners, paint thinners, outdated medications, etc., that we flush down the drain don't simply disappear but merge with the myriad of other substances moving through the sewers and eventually arrive at a sewage treatment plant. We all contribute to the problem.

Industrial Accidents, Spills, and Stormwater Runoff

In addition to direct and indirect effluent discharges, some industrial pollutants enter waterways due to transportation accidents, leaks in chemical containers, tanker spills or oil rig blowouts, or chemical runoff from industrial waste sites during storm episodes. Of these various events, the dramatic visual impact of oil spills at sea attracts the most public attention, the BP oil spill in the Gulf of Mexico in 2010 being but the most recent example. Fortunately, experience from numerous such events indicates their long-term ecological impact is frequently less serious than many fear. Studies of past marine spills show that while petroleum is toxic to many organisms, there is no strong evidence that oil spills have done any permanent damage to the world's ocean resources. Such spills, in fact, comprise a relatively small portion of the oil entering the seas each year. Routine tanker operations such as tank cleaning and ballasting contribute almost twice as many petro-pollutants to the ocean on an annual basis as do spills, even though they attract much less attention. While tanker accidents or offshore rig blowouts can have a catastrophic short-term impact on biotic communities, recovery begins within a matter of months and many such communities have returned to their pre-spill appearance within a year or two.

In 1987 mounting concerns about the adverse environmental impact of urban storm-water runoff prompted Congress to mandate a far-reaching new program to control storm-water discharges. Implementation of the first phase of the program began in 1995, with regulations imposed on more than 170 cities (those with populations of 100,000 or more), 47 counties, approximately 100,000 industrial facilities, and sites of construction activity disturbing five or more acres of land. Affected parties must identify the sources and types of pollutants that could be present in storm-water runoff from their premises and subsequently implement controls to prevent potential contaminants from washing into storm sewers. For municipalities, required preventive measures will include programs to detect and remove illegal connections, ending the improper dumping of used oil and other wastes into storm sewers, preventing and controlling spills, and adopting street de-icing methods less environmentally damaging than the use of road salt. Affected industries, which include those engaged in activities as diverse as manufacturing, airport operations, recycling, mining, wood treating, landfilling—virtually any facility where storm-water could come into contact with raw materials or wastes—must devise improved

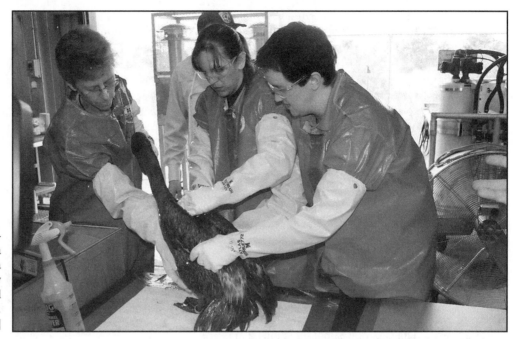

Workers at a wildlife rehabilitation center in Louisiana begin to remove oil from a brown pelican impacted by BP's Deepwater Horizon oil spill. [*Greg Thompson, U.S. Fish & Wildlife Service*]

methods for handling and storing materials and for preventing spills.

All potential contributors to storm-water contamination, municipalities and industries alike, are required to obtain discharge permits stipulating exactly how they intend to minimize polluted runoff. The second phase of the program, now underway, extends the requirement for storm-water discharge permits to small, municipal storm sewer systems located in urban areas with a total population of 50,000 or more, and to construction activities disturbing 1–5 acres of land. The number of urbanized areas that will be required to develop comprehensive storm-water management plans under phase II rules is estimated by EPA at 3,000–4,000, but due to the protracted schedule for filing permit applications and extended timetables for achieving compliance, it will likely be years before all sources of urban storm water are regulated. Nevertheless, after years of hand-wringing over urban water quality problems caused by storm-water runoff, meaningful steps to tackle this problem are finally underway (Hoffman, 2009).

WATER POLLUTION AND HEALTH

If a pollster were to conduct sidewalk interviews on what major concerns the average man or woman might have regarding water pollution, it's a safe bet that eutrophication of Chesapeake Bay, fish kills in the Mississippi, or New York City's sludge disposal headaches would rank far down on the list. Among the vast majority of respondents, the number one water quality priority undoubtedly

would be safe drinking water. Such public concerns stem from the recognition that human health is directly threatened by impure drinking water. There exists today a growing realization that the quality of drinking water is inextricably linked to the quality of our environment as a whole, inasmuch as air pollutants, agricultural chemicals, leachates from landfills, sewage, and industrial effluents all can invade public water supplies. While the nature of drinking water contamination problems differs somewhat in the developing nations versus more industrialized societies, the extent to which polluted water adversely affects health and well-being is a worldwide source of concern.

Microbial Waterborne Disease

Prior to the late 19th century, outbreaks of epidemic waterborne disease in every part of the world claimed a heavy toll in human lives and suffering. As late as the 1880s, typhoid killed 75–100 people per 100,000 population in the United States each year. A major outbreak of the disease in Chicago in 1885 claimed 90,000 victims and persuaded city officials to divert the flow of Chicago's sewage from Lake Michigan, also the source of municipal drinking water supplies, into the Sanitary and Ship Canal (completed in 1900) and ultimately to the Illinois River and the Mississippi—a policy decision that had the unintended side effect of seriously degrading the quality and attractiveness of the Illinois River. Cholera also was a feared disease in 19th-century America; a major outbreak in the Mississippi Valley during the 1870s claimed many lives and large numbers of westward-bound settlers died of cholera along the wagon trails.

In the developing world, contamination of waterways with a wide range of microbial pathogens found in human body wastes constitutes the most pressing environmental health problem. In October 2010 the first outbreak of epidemic cholera ever reported in Haiti (CDC, 2010b) made headlines worldwide. Over a period of several weeks, the deadly pathogen spread from densely settled rural areas to the capital city, Port-au-Prince, where survivors of the January 2010 earthquake were still living in squalid, overcrowded camps devoid of sanitary facilities and clean drinking water. As of early December, the Haitian Ministry of Public Health and Population reported over 91,000 cases of cholera and nearly 2,100 deaths. Epidemiologists fear that cholera will become endemic on the island and could afflict hundreds of thousands over the next several years. Elsewhere in the world, the WHO estimates that almost 5,500 people, most of them children, die every day due to fecally contaminated drinking water. The global toll due to infectious diarrhea among all age groups is estimated at one billion illnesses and between 2–5 million deaths annually. The gastrointestinal infections that occur when such pathogens are ingested are the leading cause of illness and death in most developing countries. Reducing the incidence of such disease requires not only the installation of water purification technologies, but also provision of sanitary wastewater disposal and public education regarding personal and household hygiene.

During the 1980s, designated by the UN as the "International Drinking Water Supply and Sanitation Decade," significant gains were made in expanding access to safe water supplies, particularly in rural areas where the number of people served increased by 240% worldwide (150% increase among city dwellers). Access to sanitation facilities improved as well, but these gains were largely offset by the continued rapid rate of population growth and urbanization in nations throughout the developing world. In spite of these Herculean efforts, 1.1 billion people today still lack safe drinking water and 2.6 billion remain without adequate sanitary facilities—a reflection of the inability of public works projects in developing nations to keep pace with the needs of rapidly growing populations, as well as the low priority given to such efforts by many developing world governments.

In 2000, the United Nations established its Millennium Development Goals (MDG) for tackling problems of persistent poverty in the developing world. Among the primary targets under this program are safe drinking water and basic sanitation, with a stated MDG goal of reducing by half the percentage of people without access to water and toilets by 2015, compared to baseline conditions in 1990. Although some progress has been made in the years since the goals were announced, especially in terms of improved access to safe drinking water, continued population growth in developing countries has left almost as many people in a water- and sanitation-deprived condition as was the case in 1990—even though the *proportion* so affected has declined. Even if the MDG is fully met by 2015, with a 50% reduction (from 1990) in the proportion of those lacking these basic amenities, the population increase from 1990–2015 will mean 800 million of the world's people lacking safe drinking water and 1.8 billion lack adequate sanitation. Almost all of them live in developing nations, but there is considerable variation in the statistics from one country to another.

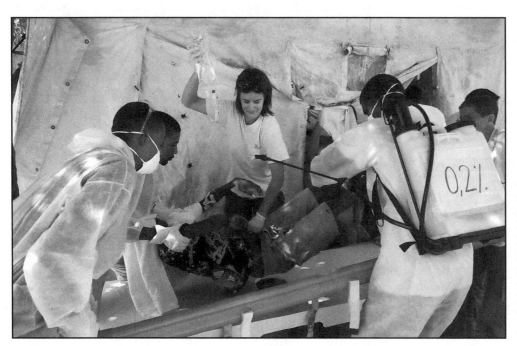

A patient suffering from cholera symptoms receives treatment at the Doctors Without Borders hospital in Port-au-Prince, Haiti, in November 2010. Epidemiologists fear that cholera will become endemic in Haiti, afflicting hundreds of thousands over the next several years. [*AP Photo/Ramon Espinosa*]

In general, the *percentage* of the population with access to safe drinking water is lowest in sub-Saharan Africa—just 44% in the region as a whole and only 22% in Ethiopia, the world's most-deprived country in terms of clean water. Regarding total *numbers*, however, China, heads the list of nations where people lack improved sources of drinking water, closely followed by several South Asian countries. Deficiencies in sanitation are most pronounced in South Asia and sub-Saharan Africa, where less than 40% of the population has access to a safe, clean, private place to go to the bathroom. Here again, Ethiopians are at the bottom of the heap, with only 13% enjoying improved sanitary facilities. Within developing countries, people in rural areas typically are worse off than those living in cities; by 2004, access to drinking water averaged 92% for urban residents, but only 70% for their country cousins. In terms of adequate sanitation, the urban/rural divide is even wider, at 73% for city dwellers versus 33% for rural residents (Palaniappan and Gleick, 2009).

In industrialized countries, disease caused by fecal pollution of waterways is much less common now than it was several generations ago. Nevertheless, outbreaks of gastroenteritis traced to microbial contamination of drinking water do occur from time to time, occasionally in headline-provoking magnitude. In the United States, despite the impression that waterborne disease is a thing of the past, periodic surveillance reports issued by the Centers for Disease Control and Prevention document numerous outbreaks, thousands of cases of illness, and occasional deaths caused by contaminated drinking water. Although most such occurrences in recent years have been associated with unregulated private wells (approximately 17 million Americans rely on private household wells for their water supply and more than 90,000 new wells are drilled each year) or small water systems where financial resources preclude the sophisticated equipment and highly trained personnel generally found in larger communities, a 1993 outbreak in Milwaukee, Wisconsin, sickened almost 400,000 people. These numbers, of course, represent only those illnesses that are reported to public health authorities. EPA estimates that for every case of waterborne disease identified, 25 more never appear in the statistics because of haphazard reporting.

Diarrheal illness may be caused by any of a large number of microbial species associated with sewage-tainted drinking water and fall roughly into one of the following groups.

Bacteria

Typhoid fever and cholera are the most notorious of the bacterial enteric diseases and over the centuries have been responsible for millions of human deaths and illnesses worldwide. Other bacterial waterborne ailments include dysentery (*Shigella*), paratyphoid, salmonellosis, *Campylobacter*, and some forms of *E. coli*—ailments which, like typhoid and cholera, can also be contracted by eating food harboring pathogens of fecal origin. Whereas typhoid and paratyphoid are characterized by headache, muscle pains, high fever, and constipation alternating with diarrhea (all symptoms being less severe in paratyphoid), cholera, dysentery, and salmonellosis are all typified by severe diarrhea (bloody in the case of dysentery) and vomiting.

Viruses

Noroviruses, hepatitis A, poliomyelitis, and rotavirus are among the most common of the several hundred species of enteric viruses associated with waterborne diarrheal illness. Many health authorities suspect that most waterborne ailments caused by unidentified pathogens are, in fact, viral diseases. Viruses are much more resistant to disinfection with chlorine than are bacteria, a fact which explains why outbreaks of hepatitis A have occasionally occurred in communities where drinking water was chlorinated and presumably was safe. While it was once thought that viral pathogens present a concern only in surface waters, it is now known that viruses also contaminate 20–30% of U.S. groundwaters, where they can survive for many months (NRC, 1999).

Protozoans

While more than 30 species of parasites may infect the human gut, only a few present a serious disease threat. Of these, the most common is giardiasis, caused by the flagellated protozoan *Giardia lamblia*, an inhabitant of the intestines of a wide variety of vertebrate animals. Over the past several decades *Giardia* has been blamed for numerous reported outbreaks in the United States, some of them in remote areas where the source of the problem was traced to infected beavers or deer that were polluting the water with feces containing protozoan cysts. Since *Giardia* is largely resistant to chlorination, filtration of drinking water supplies is important in forestalling outbreaks of giardiasis. Another chlorine-resistant protozoan parasite causing serious concern is *Cryptosporidium*, the culprit responsible for the massive disease outbreak in Milwaukee in April 1993. This parasite has now become the most frequently identified cause of diarrheal outbreaks associated with swimming pools and other recreational water venues. The CDC estimates that 300,000 cases of cryptosporidiosis occur in the United States each year, most of them affecting young children and their parents or caregivers (Yoder and Beach, 2007). Finally, amoebiasis (amoebic dysentery) is another widespread parasitic infection afflicting an estimated half billion people worldwide. Amoebic dysentery constitutes a major health problem in Mexico, eastern

South America, western and southern Africa, China, and throughout Southeast Asia.

Water Purification

At the beginning of the 20th century, a growing awareness of the link between waterborne pathogens and disease outbreaks prompted municipal officials in North America and Europe to institute various methods of drinking water treatment that largely succeeded in eliminating the serious water-related epidemic diseases of the past. The most important treatment method introduced at this time was chlorination, first used as a water disinfectant in Belgium in 1903. Introduced to the United States five years later, chlorine disinfection of municipal water supplies made its American debut on September 26, 1908, in Jersey City, New Jersey, and was swiftly adopted by larger communities nationwide (CDC, 2008a). Such advances in water treatment quickly effected a precipitous decline in deaths due to gastrointestinal waterborne disease and immeasurably improved public health. As a direct result, the number of typhoid deaths in the United States dropped from 25,000 in 1900 to less than 20 in 1960, with virtually none in recent decades; the incidence of other waterborne illnesses experienced a similar precipitous decline after chlorine disinfection became standard procedure at municipal water treatment plants (Hoffman, 2009). Nevertheless, the organisms that cause typhoid, cholera, dysentery, and other gastrointestinal ailments are still in our midst, ready to make their presence known whenever a breakdown in water treatment processes affords opportunity for such pathogens to penetrate our technological lines of defense.

Unlike sewage treatment, which is intended to reduce levels of wastewater contamination to the point where the effluent can be returned to a stream without provoking serious health or ecological damage, drinking water treatment theoretically should entirely remove all contaminants in the water, or at least reduce them to acceptable levels. All drinking water, regardless of its source, should be treated prior to consumption, since it can never be safely assumed that such water is totally free from contamination.

Although the precise details of drinking water treatment vary from plant to plant, depending largely on the quality of the local raw water supply (i.e., water from polluted surface sources will require more extensive treatment than does well water drawn from a high quality uncontaminated aquifer), the basic steps in the process can be described as follows:

1. *Sedimentation.* Incoming raw water is detained in a quiet pond or tank for at least 24 hours to allow heavy suspended material to settle out.

2. *Coagulation.* Alum (hydrated aluminum sulfate) is added to the water to cause smaller suspended solids to form flocs, which then precipitate to the bottom of the tank.

3. *Filtration.* Filtration through beds of sand, crushed anthracite coal, or diatomaceous earth further reduces the concentration of remaining suspended solids, including many bacterial cells and protozoans.

4. *Disinfection.* Most commonly accomplished with chlorine (ozone, bromine, iodine, or ultraviolet light also can be used for disinfection), disinfection is the most important method utilized for killing pathogens in water. An important advantage enjoyed by chlorine over other disinfectants is that it leaves a residual in the water that continues to provide germ-killing potential as the water travels through the distribution system to its point of use. Thus in the event of cross-contamination due to faulty plumbing or a break in water lines, some disinfectant is still present to kill intruding bacteria. However, disinfection in the absence of the preceding steps is not highly effective because organic materials and suspended solids in the water interfere with the germicidal action of the chlorine. In addition, occasional outbreaks of hepatitis, giardiasis, and cryptosporidiosis in cities where water has been disinfected indicate that chlorine is not as effective in killing viruses and protozoa as it is against other disease organisms.

In many water treatment plants, particularly those utilizing well water, preliminary treatment also includes aerating the water to remove iron and dissolved gases such as hydrogen sulfide, which impart objectionable tastes and odor to the water. In parts of the country where water contains excess amounts of dissolved calcium or magnesium (i.e., where the water is "hard"), lime and soda ash are added to precipitate these minerals out of solution, thereby "softening" the water. Ion exchange is an alternative method that can be used for this purpose. Finally, many treatment plants today add fluoride to the finished water to reduce the incidence of tooth decay (Koren, 1980).

To ensure that the water treatment process is working efficiently, laboratory tests of finished water samples are carried out on a regular basis. Historically, the presence of appreciable numbers of coliform bacteria in a water sample has been used as an indication that the water is unsafe to drink. In fact, coliforms themselves rarely cause disease; however, because they are common inhabitants of the intestines of warm-blooded animals, present in greater numbers than the pathogenic bacteria, and because they can survive for longer periods of time in water than do the latter, coliforms serve as indicators that the water is contaminated with fecal material and hence potentially hazardous. In other words, the presence of fecal coliform bacteria in a water sample warns health officials that less abundant, but more harmful organisms such as the dysentery bacillus or hepatitis virus might also be present, since all of these organisms live in the intestinal tract and are expelled with fecal material. The predictive value of the coliform test for establishing the safety of a given water supply is not absolute, however. As outbreaks of hepatitis A and cryptosporidiosis have demonstrated, disinfection that kills coliform bacteria may not always eliminate pathogenic viruses and protozoa.

Chemical Contaminants in Drinking Water

Standard water treatment processes, designed primarily to remove bacteria, hardness, and odors from water supplies, have been outstandingly successful in reducing the incidence of acute waterborne disease throughout the industrialized world. However, the public today is justifiably alarmed about the safety of water supplies due to recent revelations of toxic chemicals in drinking water. With purification processes aimed at preventing the microbial diseases of the past, few water treatment plants are equipped to remove—or even to detect—the 100,000 or more synthetic organic chemicals now in use, many of which are known to be present in drinking water supplies across the country. Although these substances may be present in concentrations measured in parts per million (ppm) or even parts per billion

(ppb), the fact that many of them are known to be mutagenic or carcinogenic raises unanswered questions concerning the long-term health effects of ingesting small amounts of poison on a daily basis. Indeed, the fact that some organic chemicals can be harmful to human health and to aquatic organisms at levels well below those currently detectable by standard analytical methods makes the issue particularly worrisome. A direct cause-and-effect relationship between toxic chemicals in drinking water and human health damage has not yet been conclusively demonstrated, but circumstantial evidence and the testimony of people who, unknowingly, consumed high levels of toxic chemicals with their water for a number of years are alarming.

Synthetic Organic Pollutants

The kinds of synthetic organic chemicals (SOCs, as they are now called) contaminating surface waters and aquifers worldwide consist of a vast array of pesticides, industrial solvents and cleaning fluids, polychlorinated biphenyls, and disinfection by-products. They originate from a wide range of activities such as chemical manufacturing, petroleum refining, iron and steel production, coal mining, wood pulp processing, textile manufacturing, and agriculture. They enter surface waters through direct and indirect discharges, by surface runoff, or by

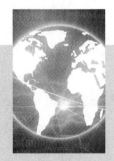

· · · · · · · · 16–5 · · · · · · · ·

Drugs Down the Drain

It seems we're always discovering something new to worry about. Over the past half-century drinking water treatment plants have done an increasingly good job of removing harmful microbes and chemicals from the water we drink. As water professionals' analytic methods improve, however, so does their ability to detect a wider range of pollutants, at lower levels of concentration, than were ever imagined a few decades ago. The latest water quality scare focuses on pharmaceuticals and personal care products—**PPCPs** in water industry jargon—which are now being detected almost everywhere researchers look; a nationwide survey of 139 U.S. streams conducted a few years ago found PPCP residues in 80% of the waterways sampled, albeit in very low concentrations.

PPCPs encompass a wide range of products, at least a few of which are used on a daily basis by almost everyone—shampoos, fragrances, painkillers, antibiotics, birth control hormones, blood pressure medications, antidepressants, sunscreen compounds, and many others. Deliberately or inadvertently we discharge them into the environment when we pour outdated or unused medications down the drain or flush unabsorbed pharmaceutical products in urine and feces down the toilet. Chemical residues on the skin are washed off while showering or bathing and household cleaning products flow into the sewer system as wastewater is discarded. Runoff from pasturelands and animal feedlots entering streams and groundwater frequently contains traces of excreted veterinary drugs, including hormones and antibiotics. While effluents from plants that manufacture pharmaceuticals and personal care products are closely monitored and regulated, discharges from individual homes via sewers and septic systems are not. At the municipal sewage treatment plants receiving home wastewater flows, PPCP residues are seldom measured, since POTWs have not been designed to deal with them.

There is no question that PPCPs are now ubiquitous in water supplies. Sampling conducted both in the U.S. and Europe has revealed trace amounts of these chemicals in surface water, drinking water, and POTW effluent. In the years ahead, PPCP concentrations are likely to increase further, both because of increasing per capita drug use and aging of the population. There are many questions, however, as to whether their presence is any cause for alarm. To date, there is no evidence that PPCPs in drinking water have had any adverse health impact on humans. Water professionals point out that the levels detected typically range from 1–10 parts per *trillion*, whereas drinking water standards for regulated contaminants are mostly set at parts per *billion*—a thousand times higher. They also remind a worried public that people regularly expose themselves to far higher concentrations of these substances via consumption of medicines, foods, and beverages or by liberally applying them to the skin than they ever encounter in public drinking water. An EPA scientist studying the issue contends that PPCP levels in drinking water are even lower than those in waterways because activated carbon filtration and chlorination—standard practices at most water purification plants—remove or break down many of the PPCPs in the treated water.

The major risk, if any, is to fish and other water-dwelling creatures living in a PPCP-tainted aquatic environment. Freshwater organisms chronically exposed to low levels of these compounds may be accumulating them so slowly that any adverse effects might not be noticeable until it's too late to do anything about it. Such fears were reinforced in 2006 when U.S. Geological Survey researchers found a number of "intersex fish"—male smallmouth and largemouth bass carrying immature eggs—in the Potomac River basin. Scientists couldn't explain the cause of this phenomenon or whether it was something new, but the discovery prompted speculation that hormone residues or "hormone mimics" might have a feminizing effect on some aquatic organisms (Dean, 2007).

Despite the lack of evidence that PPCPs in drinking water pose any real threat, environmental regulatory agencies and water professionals are paying close attention to this issue. The American Water Works Association, among others, is reviewing current water treatment techniques in an effort to determine how effective they are at reducing PPCPs. Among the technologies being investigated are those such as filtration, using membranes or granulated activated carbon (GAC), that physically remove compounds, as well as ozonation or ultraviolet radiation that break them down. On the regulatory side, the EPA maintains an active program, the Contaminant Candidate List, to identify drinking water contaminants the agency believes merit further study. In September 2009 EPA, for the first time, added 10 pharmaceutical compounds to the list, including one antibiotic (erythromycin) and nine hormones (Gerberding, 2009).

Beyond more research, however, policy makers remain unsure of how to proceed. Some argue that, given so many uncertainties, the "precautionary principle" should be applied, implementing actions to reduce risk even when the extent of that risk is unknown. Others insist that the benefits of costly actions, such as banning certain compounds or mandating widespread testing or treatment for others, should outweigh the costs—something that is questionable in this case. The challenge of estimating costs versus benefits is overwhelming, however, given the number of chemicals involved and the countless ways in which they could act in combination to augment—or diminish—their human health impact. As a professor at the Harvard Center for Risk Analysis commented, assessing the synergistic risk of such chemicals is a mathematical problem of impossible complexity (Dean, 2007).

In the meantime, the most direct and cost-effective approach to dealing with PPCPs in drinking water is to strive to keep source waters free from contamination in the first place. Consumers are urged never to flush unused medications down the sink or toilet. Some states and municipalities have established "take-back" centers at pharmacies or police stations while others include PPCPs in periodic hazardous waste collection events. If such options are not available, the local health department can be contacted for information about proper disposal of medications. Reducing pollution at the source is always the best management strategy; unfortunately, this approach, while certainly advisable, does nothing to curtail the other major source of the problem—the PPCPs passing through our bodies to enter the wastewater stream. Now if only someone could come up with a solution to address *that* issue!

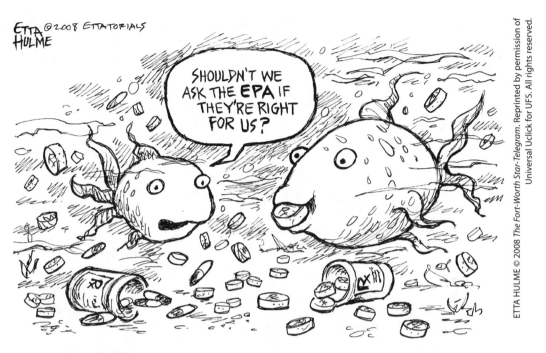

PRESCRIPTION DRUGS FOUND IN WATER SUPPLY

volatilization and subsequent fallout during precipitation episodes. Well waters can concentrate high levels of SOCs as a result of poor waste disposal practices or downward percolation of farm chemicals after heavy rains. The presence of SOCs in drinking water supplies has been a steadily growing source of public concern since the mid-1970s when several epidemiologic studies suggestively, though not conclusively, linked the presence of these chemicals with an elevated incidence of various types of cancer among exposed populations. Certain disinfection by-products called **trihalomethanes (THMs)** attracted the most attention and initiated a controversy over drinking water disinfection that persists in muted form even today. THMs, which include the carcinogen chloroform, are formed at the water treatment plant itself when chlorine is added to water containing the naturally occurring humic substances found in virtually any lake or river. The fact that traces of chloroform have been detected in almost every water system tested for this chemical led some people to call for the discontinuation of drinking water chlorination. However, since THMs usually are present only in minute amounts, many water experts argue that they pose a minimal health risk. More importantly, they contend that abandoning chlorination would result in a return of the microbial waterborne diseases that pose a much more immediate health threat than do THMs. Nevertheless, the controversy has prompted EPA to lower the maximum allowable level of THMs from 100 ppb to 80 ppb and the agency is considering lowering it even further. Concerns about THMs and the costs associated with their control have also caused a growing number of water treatment plant operators to switch from chlorine to UV radiation for drinking water disinfection.

While a number of the more than 100,000 SOCs currently in use (e.g., chloroform, benzene) are known or suspected carcinogens, establishing a direct causal relationship between polluted drinking water and cancer has been problematic. At present, the human health impact of exposure to organic chemicals in water supplies is thought to be relatively minor. Results of a U.S. Geological Survey study of 20 major U.S. river basins revealed that two or more pesticides were present in every stream sample taken and in half the well water samples. Fortunately, the amounts detected were almost always well below EPA's maximum contaminant levels for drinking water. However, over half the stream samples from both urban and agricultural areas contained at least one pesticide at concentrations that exceeded guidelines for the protection of aquatic life (some of the pesticides most frequently detected are suspected endocrine disruptors). Although public health does not appear to be seriously at risk from the low concentrations of pesticides detected, the survey raises some concerns. Health criteria and guidelines are still lacking for a number of the chemicals detected, nor do standards exist for their breakdown products—some of which are more toxic than the original pesticide. In addition, established guidelines fail to consider possible synergistic effects among the various chemicals present in the waterways sampled nor do they take seasonal pulses of higher-than-average concentrations into account. While not a cause for panic, the USGS report highlights some major challenges for improving protection of our nation's water resources (USGS, 1999).

Lead

That ingestion or inhalation of lead can cause human poisoning resulting in a wide range of health problems has been known for many years (see chapter 7). Government initiatives to lower the lead content of house paint and to phase out the use of leaded gasoline were prompted specifically by the desire to reduce human exposure to this toxic metal. However, in some areas of the country household drinking water may constitute a significant source of lead exposure. This situation does not mean that municipal water treatment plants are doing a poor job, for in almost all cases lead enters drinking water after it leaves the purification plant or private well. The problem arises either from lead service pipes leading from the water main to the house or from within the home plumbing system as a result of corrosion when water passes through lead pipes or through pipes soldered with lead, when brass fixtures are used, or in situations where the water itself is corrosive (i.e., low pH). This type of reaction is particularly likely with "soft" water; corrosion is also increased by the common practice of using water pipes for the grounding of electrical equipment, since electrical current traveling through the ground wire hastens the corrosion of lead in the pipes.

The age of a home's plumbing system is a major determinant of whether or not a lead problem exists. In older structures—those built prior to the 1930s—lead was commonly used for interior piping as well as for the service connections that joined the house to a public water supply. Obviously if a home has lead plumbing, a potential problem exists. After 1930, copper piping largely replaced lead for residential plumbing, but such pipes were typically joined with lead solder; it is this solder that many authorities consider the main contributor to drinking water contamination with lead. Over time, the amount of lead leaching into water from plumbing decreases because mineral deposits gradually form a deposit on the inside of the pipes, preventing water from coming into direct contact with the solder. For this reason, homes with the greatest likelihood of having high lead levels are those less than five years old (unless the plumbing is made of plastic, in which case there's no problem).

Although telltale signs of corrosion (rust-colored water, stained dishwasher or laundry, frequent leaks) or recognition that the house falls into one of the high-risk age categories mentioned above can alert residents to a potential problem, the only way to make a definite determination

of excess lead levels is to have the water tested at a certified laboratory (unfortunately, this is not a cheap procedure).

If lab analysis confirms high lead levels, abatement options short of total replacement of the plumbing system are somewhat limited. Reverse osmosis devices, cartridge filters, and distillation units can be installed at the faucet but are quite expensive and of variable effectiveness. Lead exposure can be minimized by two simple actions that should be taken by anyone who has, or suspects, a lead problem:

1. Don't drink water that has been in contact with pipes for more than six hours. The longer water has been standing, the greater the amount of lead likely to be present. Before using such water for drinking or cooking, flush out the pipes by allowing water to run for several minutes or until it is as cold as it will get (this water can be used for washing, watering plants, etc.).

2. Don't consume or cook with hot tap water, since lead dissolves more readily in hot water than in cold. If you need hot water, draw it cold from the tap and use the stove to heat it.

In response to this health hazard, Congress has prohibited the use of solder containing more than 0.2% lead (formerly, solder was 50% lead) and has banned any pipe or fittings containing more than 8% lead in new installations or for repair of public water systems. In addition, a number of states have now banned all use of lead materials in drinking water systems (EPA, 1987).

The realization that lead in drinking water presents a health hazard in many homes has prompted regulators to take a look at the school environment as well. In 1988, under the Lead Contamination Control Act, Congress urged both schools and day-care centers to test water from electric water coolers (some models of which were believed to have lead-lined tanks or other components made of lead) to ensure that children attending those facilities were not receiving excessive lead exposure. While the recommendations for testing and remediation were purely advisory and thus not legally enforceable, many schools complied with the government's request. Unfortunately, other potential sources of lead-contaminated water such as ice machines, non-cooled water fountains, and classroom and kitchen sinks were not mentioned in the advisory.

Continuing concerns about lead in drinking water have led to further EPA actions to reduce this hazard. In May 1991 the agency promulgated the Lead and Copper Rule, setting an "action level" (not the same as an enforceable standard) of 15 *ppb* lead at the water's point of use. Although EPA does not consider any level of lead in water as "safe," the agency believes that 15 ppb is the lowest level of control achievable by water systems, given current technology and financial resources. In cases where that level is exceeded, the rule calls for the water treatment plant to take steps to reduce the corrosivity of the water—an action designed to reduce the leachability of lead within the plumbing system (Gnaedinger, 1993).

New alarms were sounded in the spring of 1994 when EPA issued a warning to millions of private well owners, advising them to have their drinking water tested for possible high levels of lead contamination after research carried out by environmental groups at the University of North Carolina-Asheville revealed that the toxic metal was leaching into well water from lead-based brass and bronze alloys in submersible pumps, particularly from those recently installed (of the 11.8 million U.S. homes with private wells, approximately half feature submersible pumps, though not all such pumps have brass components). Environmental groups promptly urged pump manufacturers to recall all pumps containing lead components and replace them with safe, readily available lead-free models made of stainless steel.

Arsenic

Another toxic heavy metal, arsenic can contaminate groundwater supplies through dissolution of naturally occurring arsenic-containing minerals in the earth's crust or, in some cases, via agricultural and industrial effluents. Drinking arsenic-tainted water over a period of 10–20 years can lead to chronic arsenic poisoning, the earliest and most characteristic manifestation of which is a mottling of the skin, followed by the development of warts and open sores on the palms of the hands and soles of the feet. As arsenic body burdens gradually increase, affected persons often develop cancer of the skin, lungs, bladder, and/or kidneys. Since increased risk of such health problems has been observed in situations where arsenic drinking water concentrations were below 0.05 mg/liter, critics question why EPA's national drinking water standard for arsenic is still set at 0.05 mg/liter, rather than at the more protective provisional guideline of 0.01 mg/liter set by the World Health Organization (WHO), the standard adopted by many European countries.

Although arsenic contamination of groundwater is a worldwide problem, affecting the U.S., China, Mexico, and a number of other countries, nowhere is the problem more acute today than in the South Asian nation of Bangladesh, where an estimated 25 million people are at risk and two million are suffering from what the WHO has called "the worst mass poisoning in history." Ironically, the still-unfolding tragedy is the unintended result of a well-meaning development effort launched in the 1970s by the United Nations Children's Fund (UNICEF), working with the enthusiastic support of the government of Bangladesh. Attempting to reduce the burden of waterborne diarrheal diseases afflicting villagers dependent on hand-dug wells or polluted ponds, UNICEF initiated an ambitious effort to drill tubewells into deep underlying aquifers, intending to provide an abundant, pathogen-free supply of drinking water. Since it was assumed the aquifers were pollution-free, laboratory analysis of groundwater samples to test for possible contamination was considered unnecessary—until several decades later when thousands of villagers began exhibiting symptoms of chronic arsenicosis. Subsequent studies revealed that in many localities well water contains levels of naturally occurring arsenic that far exceeds WHO permissible limits. Unfortunately, millions of Bangladeshis, even when aware of the risk, continue to drink toxic water for lack of alternative supplies.

Nitrates

Contamination of drinking water supplies with inorganic nitrates from fertilizer or feedlot runoff, seepage from septic systems, or airborne fallout of nitrogen compounds emitted by industry or motor vehicles has been a concern since the 1940s. At that time a mysterious ailment called "blue baby disease" caused 39 deaths and several hundred illnesses among infants in rural areas. By 1945 the condition, more accurately known as **methemoglobinemia**, had been linked to the use of nitrate-polluted water from shallow farm wells to prepare infant formula. Bacteria in the babies' intestinal tract convert nitrates to toxic nitrites which bind to hemoglobin, displacing oxygen and producing a bluish discoloration of the skin; in extreme cases, death by asphyxiation can result. Although all members of a household typically drink from the same contaminated water supply, only infants under six months of age are at risk of developing methemoglobinemia because their stomach juices are less acid than those of older children and adults, and hence support a larger bacterial population.

Better understanding of the disease and regular monitoring of public drinking water supplies for nitrate content have greatly reduced the incidence of methemoglobinemia in recent decades. Nevertheless, risk of the disease still persists, particularly in agricultural areas of the Midwest where heavy use of nitrogen fertilizers is standard practice and where shallow aquifers supply much of the drinking water used by rural families (surface waters seldom contain concentrations of nitrates high enough to pose serious concerns). Monitoring of private wells for water quality is not a routine practice, but a 1994 national survey revealed that 22% of private farm wells contain nitrate levels in excess of the 10 mg/liter EPA standard for public water supplies (unpolluted water supplies contain an average of 2 mg/liter nitrogen). Because nitrates can persist in aquifers for many years, becoming increasingly concentrated as more nitrogen is applied to the land surface season after season, nitrates in drinking water will remain an ongoing health concern (EPA, 1995a).

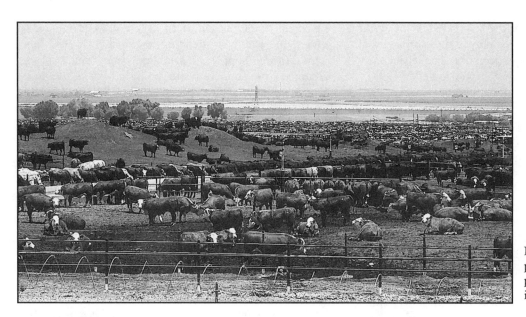

Nutrient runoff from manure piles in large cattle feedlots pose water challenges in California's Central Valley.

Safe Drinking Water Act

The federal program to protect drinking water quality in the United States is governed by the provisions of the Safe Drinking Water Act (SDWA), first passed by Congress in 1974 and subsequently amended in 1986 and again in 1996. Prior to 1974, regulation of drinking water supplies was the prerogative of the individual states, with federal involvement limited to developing advisory standards (which the states, for the most part, ignored) and to ensuring that interstate carriers such as railroads and airlines provided safe water to their passengers. Even the latter authority was limited to a focus on microbial pathogens only; not until passage of the SDWA were any enforceable provisions dealing with hazardous chemicals in drinking water incorporated into law.

Today the situation is quite different. The SDWA has established a federal-state partnership to ensure compliance with federal standards aimed at protecting U.S. residents from a wide range of contaminants potentially present in drinking water supplies. Under the act, by 2009 EPA had established **maximum contaminant levels (MCLs)** for 91 biological, chemical, and radioactive pollutants, the most recent added in 2000. These MCLs must be met by water supplied by every community water system (defined as one having at least 15 service connections used by year-round residents or regularly serving 25 or more people). Concerns about the hundreds of additional unregulated pollutants known to be present in various water supplies around the country prompted Congress to amend the SDWA in 1996. These most recent provisions require EPA to compile a list every five years of currently unregulated drinking water contaminants that may pose health risks. The agency

must then decide whether to develop standards for at least five of those contaminants, ensuring that the list of regulated drinking water pollutants will continue to expand in the decades ahead.

In addition to its requirements for setting MCLs, the Safe Drinking Water Act sets uniform guidelines for drinking water treatment and mandates that public water systems follow a prescribed schedule for monitoring and testing the quality of their treated water and report the results to the appropriate state agency. For regulation of some types of drinking water contaminants, specifically microbes, stipulating treatment techniques rather than focusing on maximum allowable concentrations has been the traditional basis for control. Demands that more be done to protect the public from such waterborne pathogens as *Giardia* and *Cryptosporidium* have resulted in amendments to the SDWA requiring water suppliers to employ filtration in addition to the standard practice of disinfection. Permission to forego the enormous expense of installing filtration technologies can be obtained only when suppliers can prove that effective watershed protection programs are in place to prevent pathogen-contaminated runoff from entering drinking water reservoirs (NRC, 1999). They also must be able to demonstrate that their disinfection controls are stringent enough to remove 99.9% of all viruses and *Giardia* cysts. These are difficult parameters to meet; EPA estimates that only 12% of the approximately 125,000 unfiltered public water systems serving populations over 10,000 will be able to meet these criteria.

The gradually evolving framework of state and federal drinking water legislation—beginning with simple disinfection requirements and culminating in the highly

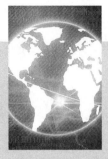

· · · · · · · 16~6 · · · · · · ·

The Case Against Bottled Water

Although public water supplies in the United States are among the highest-quality and safest in the world, more bottled water is consumed in this country than anywhere else on the planet. By 2008, according to the Beverage Marketing Corporation, sales of bottled water in the United States exceeded 8.6 billion gallons (33 billion liters), with the average American drinking close to 30 gallons of bottled water per year. Globally, the numbers are equally mind-boggling—over 200 billion liters sold in 2007, up from 163 billion just two years earlier (Gleick and Cooley, 2009). Although the United States, Mexico, and China (including Taiwan) are the three largest consumers in terms of total volumes purchased, on a per capita basis Europeans and Mexicans drink even more bottled water than Americans do, with Italians at the top of the list; growth in sales volume today is particularly rapid in Asia and South America. In the United States, far more people are now drinking bottled water than milk or beer; among beverages, only carbonated soft drinks are more popular—but per capita sales of the latter have begun to fall, while those of bottled water continue to rise.

Given the fact that, ounce-for-ounce, bottled water is 1000–4000 times more expensive than tap water, why do so many people opt for the former? To a large extent it's because many consumers perceived bottled water as safer than tap water, a perception that is quite valid in some high-use countries such as Mexico, Brazil, China, and Indonesia. In the United States, Canada, and Europe, by contrast, numerous analyses have shown virtually no difference in quality between water from public supplies and bottled water. The fact that tap water in most communities contains added fluoride while bottled water does not suggests that for consumers concerned about dental health, tap water is the better choice. In 1999 the Natural Resources Defense Council (NRDC), a prominent environmental advocacy group, published results from a four-year study that demonstrated industry claims of bottled water's superiority are simply untrue. NRDC found that nearly one-fourth of the 103 bottled water brands tested for the presence of chemical or biological contaminants had at least one sample that violated California's strict water quality regulations. Over the past decade there have been numerous enforcement reports or recalls of bottled water issue by the Food and Drug Administration (FDA) involving problems with such contaminants as benzene, coliform bacteria, algae, mold, glass chips, and crickets (Gleick, 2006b)! Bottled water unquestionably fills an important role as an alternative source of drinking water when emergency situations such as floods or pipeline ruptures render a public water supply subject to contamination, but such situations are exceptions to the rule. Unfortunately, most people are largely ignorant regarding the quality of their municipal water supply and hence tend to accept the bottling industry's deceptive advertising claims of superiority.

Aesthetic factors are another important determinant of bottled water's appeal, as evidenced by the fact that demand is highest in localities where the municipal supply is characterized by taste and odor problems caused by dissolved minerals or heavy chlorination. It is true that bottled water is free of the taint of chlorine detectable in some publicly supplied water, since most bottling companies disinfect their product with ozone, a chemical that leaves no residue. However, the widespread perception that bottled water tastes better is belied by the results of numerous blind taste tests that have shown few people can distinguish any difference in taste between bottled water versus tap water. From a taste standpoint, many municipal supplies are rated as good as or better than bottled water; New York City and Los Angeles municipal supplies, for example, consistently rank among the best-tasting waters in the nation (NRDC, 1999).

Convenience is another factor accounting for bottled water's popularity; available in almost every store and public venue, bottled water can be carried on the streets, to sporting events, class, or the office. Perhaps even more telling is the fact that skillful marketing, particularly of expensive imported brands such as Fiji Water and Evian, has made consumption of bottled water fashionable. With labels evoking such images as "natural alpine spring water," "glacier water," "pristine," or "prepared by Nature," pricey bottled water represents a fashion statement, even when that statement is decidedly misleading. A "truth in advertising" issue raised during the 1990s focused on the source of bottled water. Brand names and logos alike often suggest that water on supermarket shelves arrives direct from a wilderness mountain stream or Elysian spring. Many consumers are thus shocked to learn that at estimated 44% of the bottled water sold in the United States—including Coca Cola's Dasani and Pepsico's Aquafina—is obtained directly from municipal sources, sometimes given additional treatment, sometimes not. Bottling companies selling these brands simply fill their containers with public tap water, apply a fancy label, boost the price, and put them on the supermarket shelf.

While such water is perfectly safe, it's not the specialty product its purchasers were led to believe. Sources of the remaining 56% of bottled waters sold in the U.S. include springs, artesian wells, lakes, and rivers. In an effort to prevent misleading claims by bottlers, FDA—the federal agency in charge of regulating bottled water (public water supplies, by contrast, are regulated by EPA)—in 1995 issued rules specifying how bottled water should be labeled, according to source. Among the various categories, the two most common are "purified water"—basically tap water that has received some additional treatment such as distillation or deionization (without additional treatment, the product must be labeled "municipal water")—and "spring water," a term used to describe groundwater that flows naturally to a surface spring. According to FDA specifications, a product labeled as "spring water" can be collected either directly from a spring or from a well drilled into an aquifer that feeds a spring (Gleick and Cooley, 2009).

As the popularity of bottled water has soared in recent years, so has controversy regarding its use. The labeling issues that dominated much of the debate during the 1990s have now been eclipsed by concerns regarding the environmental and economic impacts of bottled water, with groups such as the Sierra Club, Natural Resources Defense Council, the World Wildlife Fund, and numerous religious organizations urging their members not to buy bottled water. Among their objections is the solid waste burden imposed by throwaway bottles; in spite of their inherent recyclability, according to the Container Recycling Institute, only 4% of discarded single-use bottles currently are being recycled to make new ones, while an estimated 30 million a year go to landfills. Environmental activists are also concerned about groundwater depletion that threatens ecosystems and local communities when large bottling companies extract huge amounts of water from aquifers shared with other users. Environmentalists' most often-cited objection to bottled water in an age of climate change awareness, however, is the amount of energy required for the production, packaging, chilling, and transport of bottled water—and the greenhouse gas emissions generated by such energy use.

Consider first the energy-intensive manufacture of the bottles. Most single-use plastic water bottles are made of polyethylene terephthalate (PET) and come in a variety of sizes, styles, and thickness. A detailed analysis of the energy required to produce PET and transform it into bottles, conducted at the Pacific Institute in California, concluded that approximately three million tons of PET were produced to make the 100 billion bottled water containers sold worldwide in 2007. Doing so required an estimated 300 billion megajoules of energy—the energy equivalent of about 50 million barrels of oil per year. And that's just for producing the containers. Additional energy, though far less, is used to treat the water before filling the bottles. The bottles are then rinsed, filled, capped, labeled, and packaged by power-consuming machines prior to being shipped to the marketplace.

Since water is heavy, moving it from one place to another consumes significant amounts of energy, particularly for spring waters that are usually packaged at one specific site and transported long distances to centers of demand. Fiji Spring Water, for example, is packaged on one small island in the South Pacific and shipped to spring water aficionados halfway around the world; a similar situation applies to Evian water, produced at one site in France but marketed globally. (Note that "purified water" generally doesn't need to travel as far, since the bottling plants that process and package what is essentially municipal water are usually located close to where they're sold). Overall, the Pacific Institute estimates that, in 2007, 0.34% of total U.S. primary energy use went to support the consumption of 33 billion liters of bottled water; satisfying the global demand required three times that amount (Gleick and Cooley, 2009).

Recognizing the absurdity of paying a premium price for a commodity that is qualitatively equivalent to tap water, a number of municipal governments, including those of San Francisco, Albuquerque, Minneapolis, and Seattle, now prohibit city purchase of single-serve bottled water, citing the unnecessary cost to taxpayers and the solid waste impact of disposable bottles. A number of churches, schools, and restaurants are following suit for similar reasons. With growing awareness of bottled water's environmental toll, minimal to nonexistent health and taste benefits, and its exorbitant price tag, consumers are beginning to realize that public water supplies provide Americans with a bargain product—inexpensive and, in most communities, of such good quality as to make bottled water a nonessential status symbol.

complex mandates embodied in the SDWA—has given Americans a high degree of assurance that the water they drink won't make them sick. Indeed, the provision of safe water supplies to the vast majority of the U.S. population was one of the great public health success stories of the 20th century. Nevertheless, continued sporadic outbreaks of waterborne disease remind us that vigilance can never be relaxed. Not surprisingly, conditions are most worrisome in impoverished rural areas where the USDA estimates that at least 2 million people are experiencing critical problems of drinking water quality and availability. Types of rural water-related difficulties include lack of running water, water contaminated by animal wastes running into streams, chemicals leaching into water supplies from waste disposal sites, inadequate sewage treatment, and water sources that are unprotected or inadequate to meet demand. EPA reports that the majority of violations involving drinking water quality in the U.S. since 2004 have occurred in communities with less than 20,000 residents. Because a number of states exempt operators of water purification plants serving fewer than 500 people from certification requirements, employees in these small treatment plants frequently have minimal training and qualifications. This fact, plus local financial constraints that limit the ability to upgrade facilities and equipment, may explain why a disproportionate share of U.S. waterborne disease outbreaks are associated with small public water systems (EPA, 2009b).

LOOKING AHEAD

As we enter the second decade of the 21st century, enormous water quality challenges confront societies worldwide. In the United States, despite significant improvement over the past 40 years, far too many of our rivers, lakes, and estuaries have yet to attain the "fishable, swimmable" goal set forth in the Clean Water Act. Policy makers increasingly acknowledge the need to do much more to reduce the contaminated runoff largely responsible for the degradation of American waterways. The need to address nutrient reduction more effectively is particularly urgent. A consensus is emerging among researchers, policy makers, and the general public that discharges of persistent toxics that bioaccumulate in aquatic organisms must be prohibited altogether; that more federal dollars must be allocated for State Revolving Funds; that enforcement actions be strengthened and applied more consistently at the state level; that technological innovation and market-based approaches to pollution control should be encouraged; and that our regulatory emphasis must shift from its past focus on "end-of-pipe" controls to a broad-based comprehensive watershed approach, using in-stream biological indicators as a yardstick for measuring progress in cleaning up the nation's surface waters.

In Europe, Japan, Canada, and most other industrialized regions of the world, water quality challenges parallel those in the United States. All have relied heavily in the past on expensive treatment technologies which deal with pollution problems after the fact and all need to refocus efforts on pollution prevention strategies and regional watershed management.

In the developing world the problems are far more daunting. Water quality is steadily deteriorating under the combined assault of human population increase, rapid urbanization, and growing volumes of toxic pollutant discharges. Simply quantifying water quality problems in these countries is difficult, since monitoring is virtually nonexistent and few data have been collected even on such basic concerns as sewage contamination and the frequency of microbial waterborne disease. Virtually nothing is known about the extent of toxic chemical pollution beyond anecdotal accounts of sickness and death wherever residents are forced to utilize waters tainted with industrial effluents. For the immediate future, data collection and interpretation will be high on the priority list. At the same time, however, existing knowledge must be used to protect as-yet undegraded waters since wide-scale construction of expensive treatment facilities to deal with pollution problems after damage has occurred is beyond the means of most less-developed nations.

Around the globe, in developed and developing countries alike, unrelenting human pressures on the environment have created unprecedented water quality challenges. Confronting these challenges will be expensive and will require some fundamental changes in our traditional approach to environmental protection. Nevertheless, the importance of clean water to human well-being—indeed, to our very survival—is so great that we have no choice but to make the effort. A generation ago the U.S. Senate's leading environmentalist, Senator Ed Muskie of Maine, urged his legislative colleagues to override then-President Nixon's veto of the Clean Water Act. His stirring appeal rings as prophetic today as it did in the autumn of 1972:

> Our planet is beset with a cancer which threatens our very existence and which will not respond to the kind of treatment that has been prescribed for it in the past. The cancer of water pollution was engendered by our abuse of our lakes, streams, rivers, and oceans; it has thrived on our half-hearted attempts to control it; and like any other disease, it can kill us.

Everyone wants you to pick up the garbage
and no one wants you to put it down!
—William Ruckleshaus (1990)

Solid and Hazardous Wastes

Throughout the modern world, the "waste not, want not" ethic of past generations has long since been replaced by the consumerist lifestyle of a "throwaway society." The inevitable result of our proclivity to "use once and throw away" has been an ever-increasing volume of refuse which, for both sanitary and aesthetic reasons, must be regularly collected and disposed of in a manner that will not degrade the environment or threaten public health. As pointed out by former EPA Administrator William Ruckleshaus in the statement quoted above, doing so presents major challenges to waste managers because of public opposition to the siting of waste management facilities. The sometimes explosive "politics of garbage" will only be resolved through a deeper public understanding of the issues involved in waste management, and by a societal shift in attitudes and behavior regarding the materials we use and discard.

WASTE DISPOSAL—A BRIEF HISTORY

Human generation of wastes is, of course, as old as humanity itself. Anthropologists and archaeologists have gleaned illuminating information about the everyday lives of our primitive ancestors by excavating the rubbish heaps outside early cave dwellings and other ancient set-

tlements. Among rural or nomadic peoples, however, discarded wastes seldom accumulated to an extent great enough to threaten human well-being. The advent of the first cities after the Agricultural Revolution of approximately 10,000 years ago presented humankind with its first serious problems of refuse disposal. The poor sanitary conditions and frequent epidemics that characterized city life from ancient times until the late 19th century derived primarily from the perpetuation of country habits in a crowded urban environment. Human body wastes, garbage, and discarded material items were typically left on the floors of homes or thrown into the streets. A rudimentary awareness of the link between refuse and disease led to the establishment in Athens, Greece, of what was perhaps the first "city dump" in the Western world around 500 BC; this innovation was accompanied by what is believed to be the world's first ban against throwing garbage into the streets, as well as by a regulation requiring scavengers to dump wastes no closer than a mile from the city walls. The Athenian example regarding waste management was not widely emulated, however. Throughout the Roman period and the Middle Ages in Europe, open dumping of wastes in streets or ditches remained the prevailing method of urban waste disposal. An ancient Roman signpost warning citizens to "take your refuse elsewhere or you will be fined" suggests that governmental anti-littering efforts in those days had a very limited focus!

Attempts by municipal authorities to cope with their citizens' slovenly habits were limited and sporadic. In 1388 the English Parliament prohibited dumping of wastes in public waterways; after the 13th century Parisians were no longer permitted to throw garbage out their windows (they obviously pitched it elsewhere, however, for by AD 1400 the mounds of garbage outside the city gates of Paris were so high that they obstructed efforts by the military to defend the city). As medieval towns gradually developed into modern cities, and particularly after the onset of the Industrial Revolution in Europe at the end of the 18th century, the solid waste problem became even more acute. Urban areas became grossly overcrowded, polluted, noisy, and dirtier than ever. Rising levels of affluence among some segments of society, as well as sheer growth in population size, resulted in the generation of increasing amounts of waste. It gradually became apparent to civic leaders that the accumulation of filth and refuse in urban centers was directly related to disease outbreaks. Thus by the late 19th century, city-sponsored efforts at improving urban sanitation were launched both in Europe and North America. Refuse, previously regarded simply as a nuisance, was finally perceived as a serious threat to human health—a problem so massive that it could be effectively tackled only by municipal governments, not simply by private individuals acting on their own initiative (Melosi, 1981).

Throughout the 20th century and into the 21st, the "garbage problem" has continued to mount at a rate several times higher than the rate of population growth. In contrast to the situation in centuries past, the major forces determining waste output since the 1950s have been an affluent lifestyle and changes in marketing techniques (e.g., multiple packaging), which result in more waste materials. While tossing garbage into the streets is no longer considered socially acceptable, modern methods of waste disposal, for the most part, are not a great deal more advanced than they were at the end of the 19th century. Today the enormous volume of refuse generated by homes, businesses, and industry, coupled with the realization that many of these wastes are of a toxic or otherwise hazardous nature, has prompted a concerted effort on the part of both government and the private sector to develop safer, more effective methods for managing the unwanted by-products of modern society.

MUNICIPAL SOLID WASTES (MSW)

Every sector of the national economy—farms, mines, and factories as well as businesses, institutions, and households—contributes to the mounting mass of unwanted materials requiring disposal. Nevertheless, municipal wastes, although proportionally far smaller in amount than agricultural and mining wastes, arguably represent our greatest waste management challenge (with the possible exception of industrial hazardous wastes). This is because urban wastes are generated where people live and must be quickly removed and properly disposed of in order to prevent serious environmental health problems. Municipal wastes are also much more heterogeneous than are the wastes produced by agriculture, mining, or specific industries. Paper and paper products constitute the single largest portion of household rejects, but an examination of a typical garbage container would also reveal glass, metal, and plastic containers; rubber, leather, and cloth items; food wastes; discarded furniture and electronic equipment; and numerous other items.

The quantity of these discards steadily increased from 1960 until the peak year of 1994, after which volumes declined slightly. Waste generation dropped noticeably in 2009–2010 due to the global economic recession and as a result of changes in materials usage. Perhaps most notable has been the steady decline in the amount of newsprint in the waste stream, a function of falling newspaper circulation and size as increasing numbers of readers turn to online sources of information (Miller, 2010). EPA reported that in 2008 the United States generated almost 250 million tons of wastes from households, businesses, and institutions, technically referred to as **municipal solid waste (MSW)**. This amount is equivalent to 4.5 pounds of daily refuse tossed away by every man, woman, and child in the country. Reported MSW tonnages include organic wastes and tires, but do not take into account industrial, agricultural, or construction and demolition wastes, all of which contribute significantly to the nation's nonhazardous solid waste stream (EPA, 2009a).

Since the late 19th century, Americans have regarded the collection and disposal of urban wastes as a primary responsibility of municipal governments. Today many cities rely on private haulers to collect wastes, and the majority of disposal facilities are privately owned and operated. Nevertheless, municipal officials bear the ultimate responsibility for seeing that waste management services are provided to the satisfaction of their constituents and in compliance with increasingly stringent state and federal environmental regulations.

Municipal Waste Collection and Disposal

The piles of refuse and unsightly, unsanitary conditions that quickly accumulate during a garbage workers' strike provide a dramatic illustration of the importance of regular, frequent urban refuse collection. Any breakdown in this essential service, particularly during the warmer months of the year, can result in odor and litter problems or in the rapid growth of fly and rat populations. To prevent such problems, the Public Health Service recommends that refuse be collected twice weekly in residential areas and daily from restaurants, hotels, and large apartment complexes. This is particularly important during the peak of the summer fly-breeding season when eggs may hatch in less than a day and larval stages can be completed in three to four days. Historically, because the public has been far more concerned that refuse be regularly removed than with what happens to it once the garbage truck rounds the nearest corner, municipal solid waste budgets traditionally allocated a significantly greater proportion of their resources to refuse collection than to disposal.

From a public health and environmental quality standpoint, proper disposal of urban refuse is just as important as regular collection. Until the 1970s this aspect of solid waste management was given scant attention, resulting in cities utilizing the cheapest method available, with little or no consideration given to the often severe pollution problems thereby created. A new ecological awareness on the part of both the public and policy makers gradually led to the legal prohibition of many long-established practices, such as feeding municipal refuse to hogs or dumping it into waterways. Recognition that garbage-fed hogs frequently were infected with the parasite that causes trichinosis in people who consume undercooked pork diminished the popularity of this waste disposal option. Outbreaks of such diseases as hog cholera among herds of swine fed on raw garbage also provoked second thoughts. By the late 1950s, the U.S. Public Health Service and a number of state health departments passed regulations prohibiting the feeding of uncooked garbage to hogs. Since cooking the wastes made the practice uneconomical, this method of urban refuse disposal has now virtually disappeared.

Dumping of municipal wastes into the nearest body of water—a disposal method relied upon for many years by cities such as New York, Chi-

cago, and New Orleans—was halted many decades ago. In 1934 the U.S. Supreme Court banned the dumping of municipal wastes at sea, though certain industrial and commercial wastes were exempted from this ruling. The

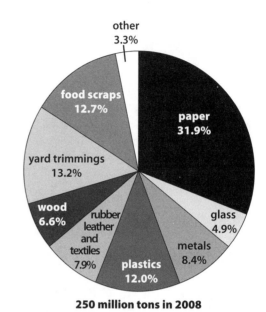

250 million tons in 2008

Source: EPA, *Municipal Solid Waste Generation, Recycling, and Disposal in the United States: Facts & Figures, 2008.* EPA 530-F-009-021, November 2009.

Figure 17-1   What's in Our Trash?

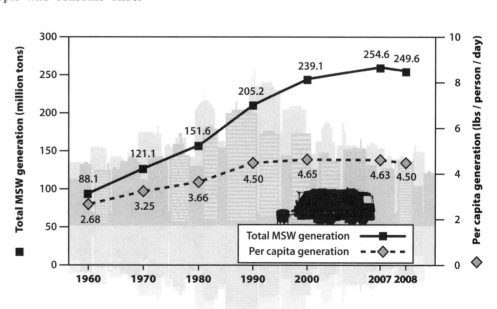

Source: EPA, *Municipal Solid Waste Generation, Recycling, and Disposal in the United States: Facts & Figures, 2008.* EPA 530-F-009-021, November 2009.

Figure 17-2   Municipal Solid Waste Generation Rates, 1960 to 2008

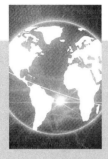

······· 17-1 ·······

The Great Pacific Garbage Patch

Careless waste disposal practices have far-reaching and unintended consequences—and the ecological damage wrought by humanity's proclivity to litter may sometimes be impossible to remediate. One of the best examples of this fact is a vast marine area officially known as the North Pacific Subtropical Gyre, but more commonly referred to as "the Great Pacific Garbage Patch."

This immense expanse of floating trash was first reported in 1997 by Charles Moore, an American oceanographer who accidentally came upon the waterborne debris while taking a shortcut back to California after a sailing race in Hawaii. The "garbage patch" has subsequently attracted the attention of environmentalists and marine research groups who are now conducting scientific studies in the area while using it as a showcase for why we, as a society, need to transform our throw-away lifestyle.

Covering an area variously described as "about the size of Quebec," "twice the size of Texas," or "twice the size of the continental United States," the floating mass of detritus constitutes what some observers call "the largest landfill in the world," located in an area of the ocean where strong currents and little wind keep millions of pounds of refuse from all over the world circling in a giant whirlpool. The Great Pacific Garbage Patch is actually made up of a western and an eastern mass—the former extending from an area east of Japan to west of Hawaii, the latter between Hawaii and California—linked together by a narrow 6,000 mile long current called the Subtropical Convergence Zone.

Researchers sampling the oceanic debris report that approximately 80–90% of the total consists of plastic items—discarded fishing lines and nets, buoys, food and beverage containers, condoms, beach toys, and plastic bags, among other detritus. This trash represents far more than just an aesthetic affront because it persists for years, breaking down very slowly, if at all, and poses a serious threat to marine wildlife. While plastics don't *bio*degrade, they may be broken into smaller pieces by wave action or may *photo*degrade through exposure to sunlight, fragmenting into tiny bits of plastic called "nurdles" that act as nuclei, attracting toxic chemicals that may be widely diffused in the surrounding seawater and concentrating these on their surface. When nurdles are ingested by filter-feeding organisms, the poisons they contain become ever more concentrated as they move up the marine food chain.

Sources of the debris swirling in the "garbage patch" include materials dumped overboard, either deliberately or by accident, by ocean-going vessels and fishing boats. Most, however, originate on land; it's estimated that approximately 80% of ocean trash is washed out to sea via land-based storm-water discharges, combined sewer overflows, beach littering by tourists, runoff from landfills located in low-lying coastal areas, and spillage during loading or unloading at port facilities.

Sea creatures feel the impact of such carelessness in a number of ways. Entanglement in discarded fishing lines or nets, as well as in six-pack rings, can result in strangulation, suffocation, drowning, or injury. Seals and sea lions have been particularly affected, but whales, porpoises, turtles, and seabirds have also suffered considerable mortality due to entanglement in marine debris. Discarded fishing gear is responsible for a phenomenon known as "ghost fishing," resulting in the capture and death of large numbers of fish, lobsters, crabs, and other sea creatures. Birds and turtles are impacted when they ingest plastic debris, presumably mistaking it for prey. Plastic bags, plastic pellets, or fragments of larger plastic items can get stuck in their throats, block their digestive tracts, or fill up their stomachs with indigestible material, resulting in malnutrition and slow starvation. The UN Environment Programme estimates that, worldwide, plastic debris in the oceans kills more than a million seabirds and 100,000 marine mammals each year, reporting that autopsies of dead birds revealed such unnatural items as cigarette lighters, syringes, and toothbrushes in their stomachs.

The extent to which oceanic garbage is imperiling marine wildlife populations, and especially the impacts of nurdles in the marine food chain, are now the focus of serious scientific investigation by the Algalita Marine Research Foundation, a nonprofit group created by Mr. Moore in 1999 expressly to study the situation he had discovered in the Pacific gyre just two years earlier. Having developed a standard methodology for sampling the ocean surface for floating micro-plastics, as well as methods for processing these samples, Algalita researchers aboard the research ship *Alguita* are striving to determine their long-term effects, both on the ocean ecosystem and on human health—effects which are potentially wide-ranging but as yet poorly understood.

Cleaning up the existing mess is widely acknowledged as impossible, both because of the magnitude of the problem and because the areas most severely affected are beyond the territorial waters of any nation; even if the task were technically feasible, governments simply aren't willing to invest massive sums of money to clean up areas that aren't "theirs" and that don't directly harm their economies. To forestall further worsening of the situation, however, 122 countries have ratified the International Convention of the Prevention of Pollution, which bans the dumping of most garbage and all plastic wastes at sea. Nevertheless, since the majority of plastic wastes in the sea originate on land, improving waste management practices on shore, accompanied by public education efforts, would have a greater impact. Unfortunately, the only lasting solution would be to abandon the use of plastic, replacing this now-omnipresent, nondegradable material with an innovative, acceptable alternative. Until that happens, "garbage patches" are likely to continue proliferating throughout the world's oceans. As the first mate of the *Alguita* remarked, today's growing mass of marine rubbish is "just a reminder that there's nowhere that isn't affected by humanity" (Hoshaw, 2009; Allsopp et al., 2006).

Marine Protection, Research, and Sanctuaries Act, passed in 1972 and subsequently strengthened by a series of amendments, gradually imposed increasingly strict limitations and now prohibits ocean dumping of industrial waste, sewage sludge, radioactive wastes, and all radiological, chemical, and biological warfare agents.

Until the 1970s, the most common method of urban refuse disposal was **open dumping**, a practice that simply involved hauling collected garbage to a location at the edge of town (usually on "the wrong side of the tracks") and dumping it on the ground. Regarded today as environmentally unacceptable, open dumping epitomizes the problems that can arise when solid wastes are mismanaged. Employed primarily because they are cheap and convenient, open dumps support large populations of rats, flies, and cockroaches that frequently invade nearby dwellings. They contaminate adjacent surface or groundwater supplies when **leachates** (liquids resulting from the interaction of water with wastes) containing dissolved pollutants run off or seep downward through the soil from the dump site. If burned over to prevent litter from blowing about or to reduce the volume of wastes, open dumps can pose air quality problems. They are odorous, unsightly, and have a negative impact on property values of adjacent lands. Open dumping as a method for disposing of municipal refuse was outlawed by the federal government in 1976 (earlier by some state governments), and there has been a concerted effort, largely successful, to phase out all open dumping in the United States. In many less-developed areas of the world, however, open dumping remains the most prevalent form of urban waste disposal.

CURRENT WASTE DISPOSAL ALTERNATIVES

Sanitary Landfilling

In recent decades, most municipalities seeking an economically feasible yet environmentally acceptable alternative to open dumping have opted for sanitary landfills. A sanitary landfill differs from an open dump in that collected refuse is spread in thin layers and compacted by bulldozers. When the compacted layers are 8–10 feet deep, they are covered with about 6 inches of dirt, which is again compacted. At the end of each working day another thin layer of soil is placed over the fill to prevent litter from blowing about, to keep away insect and rodent pests, and to minimize odor problems. When the landfill has reached its ultimate capacity, a final earth cover two feet deep is placed over the entire area and the land can then be used for a park, golf course, or other kinds of recreational facilities.

When properly sited, well designed, and efficiently operated, a sanitary landfill can be a perfectly adequate means of urban refuse disposal, free from offensive odors, vermin, or pollution problems. Unfortunately, in the past most so-called "sanitary" landfills were not well sited, properly designed, or well run. As a result, many landfills caused environmental contamination problems little different from those of open dumps and made sanitary landfills unwelcome neighbors wherever they were located. In the mid-1970s it was reported that of 17,000 land disposal sites surveyed, 94% failed to meet the minimum requirements of a sanitary landfill—requirements that in the 1970s were far less stringent than those prevailing today.

Nevertheless, landfills became the overwhelming waste disposal method of choice nationwide, largely because they were (and still are in most places) the most economical of the legal options. In 2006 the average cost for landfilling one ton of MSW (the **"tipping fee"**) ranged from a low of $15 in Oklahoma to a high of $96 in Vermont, with the majority of states featuring tipping fees of $42 per ton (Arsova et al., 2008). In northeastern states such as Vermont, Massachusetts, New Jersey, New Hampshire, and Connecticut, significantly higher-than-average landfill tipping fees make other alternatives economically attractive. Landfills also appealed to municipal officials because they were capable of receiving any type of waste and could, after completion, be used for facilities popular with the public such as parks, ski slopes, or golf courses.

Landfills, of course, are not trouble-free: uneven settling of the land may occur, making them unsuitable as sites for constructing buildings after operations have ceased; anaerobic decomposition of landfilled materials may result in the accumulation of dangerous amounts of methane, which can cause explosions or fires if the gas migrates into nearby structures; perhaps the most serious environmental impact associated with landfills is their potential for polluting nearby surface streams or underlying aquifers with leachates. This problem can be minimized by careful site selection, choosing locations underlaid by impervious clay formations and far removed from any bodies of surface water. In the past such considerations were frequently neglected, with siting decisions typically based on the price of the land. Unfortunately, in many communities wetland areas, once considered "worthless" because of the cost of developing them for residential or commercial purposes, have been utilized as cheap landfill sites. Aside from the fact that wetlands have intrinsic value for their biologic productivity and flood control attributes, the fact that they are usually in hydrologic contact with groundwater makes wetland areas the *least* appropriate siting choice for a sanitary landfill.

Although landfills have been regarded with increasing public disfavor in recent years, largely due to the long-term environmental liability they represent (approximately 20% of the federal Superfund sites slated for multimillion dollar cleanup efforts are former municipal landfills), sanitary landfilling remains the most prevalent method of MSW disposal in the United States. In 2008, according to EPA's Office of Resource Conservation and Recovery (formerly known as the Office of Solid Waste), 54% (135 million tons) of MSW generated in the United States was landfilled, down from 89% in 1980.

In the mid-1980s, anxious talk about a so-called national "garbage crisis" dominated discussion of MSW issues in the United States. The tragi-comic voyage of the Islip, New York, "garbage barge" during the spring and summer of 1987 focused media attention on the problem of where to deposit society's refuse. Loaded with over 3,000 tons of commercial trash banned from a local landfill reserved for residential refuse, the barge *Mobro* cruised the Atlantic and Gulf coasts for five months, searching in vain for a disposal facility that would accept its increasingly odorous cargo. Eventually the *Mobro* returned to New York, festooned with an enormous Greenpeace banner advising, "Next Time Try Recycling," and its cargo was ultimately burned in a Brooklyn incinerator. Commentators at the time cited worrisome statistics indicating a rapidly dwindling number of landfills in many states and sharply escalating tipping fees at those facilities still in operation. Pointing to rising rates of waste generation, they warned that half of all American cities would soon have no place to send their garbage. Compounding the problem—indeed, the essence of the dilemma in a country where open spaces still abound—

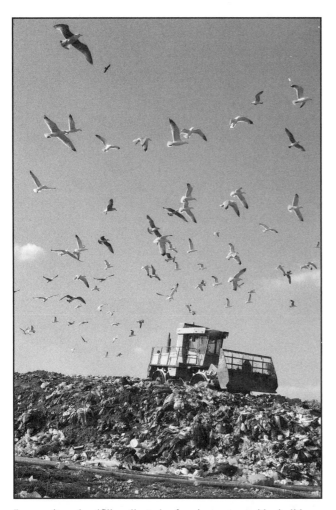

In a sanitary landfill, collected refuse is compacted by bulldozers to a depth of about 8-10 feet. Each compacted layer is then covered by 6 inches of dirt.

was the political reality of intense public opposition to landfill siting, a situation which time and again has stymied efforts by local government officials or private waste management firms to develop needed replacement facilities.

The new public focus on MSW concerns sparked intensive efforts by local and state officials to develop new, more sustainable waste management strategies for the decades ahead—and to insist that new and existing landfills be better designed and operated than earlier facili-

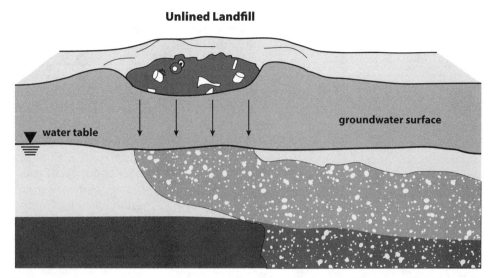

Unlined Landfill

water table

groundwater surface

Figure 17-3   Groundwater Contamination as a Result of Unlined Landfill Disposal

ties. A major step toward the latter objective was EPA's promulgation of its new **RCRA Subtitle D** landfill requirements, now in effect nationwide. Mandating that all landfills install groundwater monitoring wells and methane detection systems, Subtitle D has sharply increased the cost of landfill operations but has also ensured that leachates or potentially explosive gases migrating from the fill don't go unnoticed and neglected. Requirements that new cells within a landfill be constructed with double liners and a leachate collection system to remove standing water means that new MSW landfills will be virtually indistinguishable in design from land disposal facilities licensed to accept hazardous wastes. The design features of such landfills render them essentially "dry tombs" where, in the near-absence of moisture and sufficient oxygen, organic wastes degrade very slowly, if at all.

A relatively new concept in landfill design—**bioreactors**—is attracting attention and a number of pilot experiments and demonstration projects are underway in several states across the country, as well as at a site in Quebec, in order to assess their performance. Bioreactors differ from conventional landfills in that the leachate removed from the bottom layer is not discarded but recirculated into the landfill to promote microbial activity. In aerobic bioreactors (an anaerobic version is currently being tested as well), air is injected into the waste mass via wells. This greatly accelerates the decomposition and biological stabilization of landfilled wastes compared to that occurring in conventional landfills. Bioreactors also are expected to generate greater volumes of methane, which can be recovered and sold; leachate disposal costs and post-closure care should be less than for conventional landfills, another economic advantage. Since waste decomposition in a bioreactor decreases its volume, the

resulting increase in airspace may permit landfill operators to extend the useful lifespan of the facility. Because bioreactors will be more expensive to build and operate than conventional landfills, it remains to be seen whether the aforementioned cost savings outweigh the increased capital expense of such facilities. The EPA has been collecting information from studies carried out at existing bioreactor landfills in order to assess their advantages and disadvantages and has been gathering additional data in order to identify specific bioreactor standards and to recommend operating parameters.

Compliance with Subtitle D requirements, of course, is expensive and owners of many smaller landfills opted to go out of business rather than invest the sums necessary to continue operations under the new regulations. As a result, after the federal rules went into effect in October 1993, the number of operating U.S. landfills dropped from 5,386 to just 1,831 in 2006 (compared to approximately 8,000 in 1988). The sharp decline is much less of a problem than the statistics might suggest, however, for while the *number* of landfills has fallen, remaining landfill capacity has not taken a similar nosedive. Although remaining landfill space varies widely across the U.S., many states (Texas, California, Pennsylvania, Illinois, Virginia, etc.) now have adequate capacity to accommodate their needs for the foreseeable future; Wyoming reports its landfills won't be full for at least 100 years! Overall, landfill capacity in the United States is now at its highest level in two decades, with over 40 states reporting that they are currently in the process of expanding existing landfill space. It appears earlier apocalyptic predictions of garbage piling up in the streets have now largely been discredited. Current trends indicate that for the foreseeable future, MSW will be transported longer distances to fewer, large regional facilities designed and operated in a manner that provides a considerably higher level of environmental protection than the leaky landfills of the past (Arsova et al., 2008).

In the meantime, waste planners are broadening their perspective, searching for more environmentally friendly MSW management approaches and striving to bring about a paradigm shift in societal attitudes toward the materials we use and throw away. Rather than focusing on one "technological fix" to solve every community's problems, most waste management experts view the solution as a combination of approaches, tailored to the specific needs and realities of individual municipalities. The EPA has formulated a recommended three-tiered hierarchy of methods for managing wastes, ranking **waste reduction and reuse** as the most desirable option, **recycling and composting** second, and **waste combustion** and **landfilling** as methods of last resort, to be replaced to the greatest extent possible by the first two alternatives.

Source Reduction

The best—and cheapest—way of managing wastes is not to produce them in the first place. Accordingly, policies of reducing wastes at their source are top-ranked in every priority listing of waste management options. First raised as a possible approach at a 1975 EPA-sponsored Conference on Waste Reduction, the goal of conserving materials and energy through waste prevention or by reducing the volume or toxicity of wastes generated was given little more than lip service until the so-called "garbage crisis" of the mid-1980s. The sense of urgency to relieve pressures on existing disposal facilities prompted a more serious look at the potential for source reduction strategies, which most advocates estimated could cut urban waste streams by about 5%. Approaches to source reduction variously target consumers, manufacturers, or government and can include either voluntary or mandatory components.

Appealing to consumers to use their considerable purchasing power in a more environmentally aware manner has been a key component of source reduction efforts for years. By shopping selectively—buying only the amount of a product that will be used, choosing items without excessive amounts of packaging, buying products that have fewer toxic ingredients than comparable items, avoiding single-serve disposable packages, or participating in waste exchanges (garage sales might be regarded as an effective source reduction strategy!) are all ways of reducing the garbage we throw away. Another approach involves substituting reusable consumer items for single-use throwaway products—cloth napkins and terry towels instead of paper ones; china or plastic dishes instead of paper plates; handkerchiefs instead of Kleenex; reusable cloth grocery bags. Backyard composting of kitchen scraps and garden debris, as well as "grasscycling"—allowing grass clippings to fall and decompose on the lawn or using them for mulch—are other examples of waste reduction that can easily be practiced by individuals.

Opportunities for source reduction of wastes in business or institutional settings are similarly plentiful. Simply asking employees to use their own coffee mugs rather than the ubiquitous Styrofoam cup can noticeably reduce daily waste volume. Copy-machines designed to print on both sides of a sheet of paper can save thousands of dollars in business expenditures on paper supplies—as well as on reduced waste disposal fees. Using e-mail rather than paper for interoffice memos, or simply circulating one document rather than making multiple copies, are practices being adopted by thousands of waste-conscious firms.

Manufacturers must play a pivotal role in any national source reduction effort, since their decisions regarding product composition, design, packaging, and durability have such far-reaching implications. Already industry's efforts to reduce packaging and transportation costs through "lightweighting" have had a positive impact on waste reduction trends. When General Mills reduced the thickness of the plastic liners in its cereal boxes, it simultaneously cut the amount of plastic used—and thrown away—each year by half a million pounds. Similarly, since the early 1970s, lightweighting has reduced the weight of a steel can by 43% and decreased that of a one-gallon plastic milk container from 95 grams to under 60 grams today. Aluminum beverage containers are now half the thickness of those manufactured in 1959 when they were first introduced by Coors; lightweighting of aluminum cans has resulted in considerable savings in metal, transportation costs due to lighter loads, and even in refrigeration costs, since thinner cans chill more rapidly (*The Economist*, 2009). Many observers feel that manufacturers could do much more, however, by substituting less hazardous components for toxic ones (e.g., Apple Computer several years ago began using brown cardboard packaging containers to replace chlorine-bleached white boxes) and by designing products for easier repair and increased durability, thereby moving away from a corporate policy of "planned obsolescence."

Finally, there are a number of options government could pursue to advance source reduction goals. Aside from efforts at public education—providing citizens with the information they need to make wise purchasing decisions—governments could employ a mix of economic incentives and disincentives, fees, taxes, subsidies, or outright bans to influence consumer choice or manufacturers' behavior. For example, thousands of U.S. municipalities have adopted unit-based pricing (commonly known as "pay-as-you-throw") rather than the traditional flat fee for residential garbage pickup. Essentially a user fee based on the amount of waste discarded, this approach to funding waste management services provides a financial incentive to householders to reduce waste generation and simultaneously encourages recycling and composting. EPA reports an average 14–27% drop in the amounts of MSW discarded in communities that have adopted pay-as-you-throw programs, as well as a 32–59% increase in recycling. Although most unit-based pricing schemes are volume-based (i.e., per-container fees), a few communities have adopted weight-based systems. While a number of municipalities have hesitated to opt for unit-based pricing for fear it would encourage illicit dumping, experience in the communities that have chosen this approach indicates minimal or short-lived problems in this regard.

Another option involves taxes at the time of purchase on certain hard-to-dispose-of items. While this may not deter their purchase, it can at least provide funds to help offset recycling or disposal costs. Thirty-six states now impose such a tax on tires; motor oil, automobiles, lead-acid batteries, antifreeze, and major appliances are additional products upon which certain states levy taxes that reflect their environmental impact. Outright bans on certain troublesome items have been more difficult to impose due to possible conflict of such mandates with laws governing regional or interstate commerce. Nevertheless, a few have been successfully implemented, most notably the nationwide prohibition against flip-top openers on beverage containers and a ban on plastic bags in ahead-of-the-curve San Francisco.

The ultimate success of source reduction efforts hinges upon a fundamental shift in society's basic approach to waste management—a refocusing of attention toward ways to prevent wastes from being generated in the first place rather than trying to deal with them after the fact. Source reduction, if wholeheartedly pursued, would also necessitate a different national lifestyle, though not necessarily a less satisfying one. While the concept has yet to capture the hearts and minds of most Americans and has encountered resistance from certain industries that would be directly affected by such policies, the benefits of source reduction programs in reducing waste management costs, saving natural resources, and easing humanity's impact on the environment guarantee a growing commitment in the years ahead to the *practice*, not just the *promise*, of source reduction (League of Women Voters, 1993).

Recycling

More broadly referred to as **resource recovery**—any productive use of what would otherwise be a waste material requiring disposal—recycling and composting are ranked second, after source reduction and reuse, on the EPA's list of most environmentally desirable strategies for

municipal solid waste management. Perceived by many as "the right thing to do" and by local officials as a way of extending the remaining lifespan of existing land disposal facilities (thereby postponing politically prickly decisions regarding the siting of new landfills or incinerators), recycling of MSW has made impressive gains since the late 1980s. According to EPA, of the 250 million tons of MSW generated across the nation in 2008, 83 million tons—33.2% of the total—were either recycled or composted. In some states the recycling rate is considerably higher than the national average, with Minnesota, Oregon, California, Illinois, and Maryland among the leaders in national resource recovery efforts.

Recycling, of course, is not a new phenomenon. An earlier generation of Americans diligently recycled during World War II, when saving valuable resources to aid in the war effort was widely regarded as a patriotic duty. However, interest in resource conservation waned during the prosperous 1950s and 1960s and only revived with the emergence of the ecology movement and the energy "crisis" of the 1970s. At that time increased emphasis on recycling was promoted for its very real ecological benefits in conserving natural resources, saving energy, and reducing the pollutant emissions inherent in manufacturing products from virgin materials (e.g., producing aluminum from recycled materials cuts both energy use and pollutant emissions by 95%). More recently, recycling's role in diverting wastes from landfills, thereby extending the lifespan of those facilities, and in reducing greenhouse gas emissions has given added impetus to municipal recycling efforts.

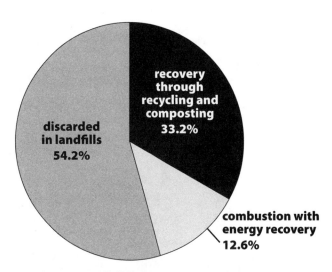

Source: EPA, *Municipal Solid Waste Generation, Recycling, and Disposal in the United States: Facts & Figures, 2008.* EPA 530-F-009-021, November 2009.

Figure 17-4   Management of MSW in the United States, 2008

To encourage more aggressive development and implementation of municipal recycling programs, 46 states, plus the District of Columbia, have set recycling goals that local governments within those states are required to meet, specifying deadline dates for achievement (so-called **"rates and dates"**). Many have also enacted legislation requiring that local governments develop long-range comprehensive waste management plans, detailing how they intend to comply with state-mandated recycling goals. These planning requirements have forced local officials and citizen advisory groups to look much more closely at waste management problems and solutions in their own communities, leading to a number of innovative approaches for reducing the amount of refuse destined for landfill burial or incineration. While states and municipalities retain primary responsibility for solid waste management within their jurisdictions and have taken the lead in recycling legislation, the federal government is seeking to emulate these state initiatives. In 2002 EPA launched its **Resource Conservation Challenge (RCC)**, one goal of which was to boost the national recycling rate to 35%.

To attain these admittedly ambitious goals, waste managers must devise innovative strategies for eliciting greater participation in recycling efforts by householders, businesses, and institutions. One of the most successful approaches has been the introduction of curbside collection programs that make household recycling as easy as setting out the weekly garbage. From just 1,000 programs nationwide in 1988, curbside collection was provided by approximately 8,660 U.S. municipalities in 2008. Requirements regarding co-mingling or separation of recyclables into one or several containers vary from program to program, as does the range of materials accepted for curbside pickup, with newspapers, glass, and aluminum cans among the items most commonly included. A number of cities that provide curbside collection have mandates penalizing those who don't remove recyclables from their waste stream. In 2009 San Francisco imposed one of the most stringent recycling laws in the country, requiring every residence and business in that city to have three color-coded waste bins: black for nonrecyclable trash, green for compostable material, and blue for recyclables. If garbage collectors find food scraps, paper, beverage containers, or other recyclable materials in the black bin, they are required to leave a warning tag reminding the perpetrator of the violation; several warnings may result in a fine. City officials hope that this mandate will enable San Francisco to divert fully 75% of its wastes from landfills by 2010—with an ultimate goal of zero waste by 2020!

Once materials are collected through **source separation** programs (which can include curbside collection, neighborhood recycling centers, community drop-boxes, or periodic recycling drives), they must be sorted and baled prior to being shipped to buyers for reprocessing. These tasks are carried out by **materials recovery facilities (MRFs**—referred to in recycling jargon as "murfs") where mixed recyclables are prepared for marketing.

In some regions of the country, municipal leaders have opted for an alternative approach to source separation. Since even curbside programs, convenient though they are, almost never achieve 100% public participation, some cities don't even make an attempt to involve citizens in recycling efforts. Instead, they simply collect the

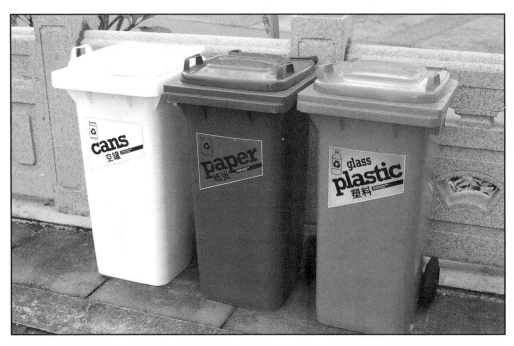

Source separation programs can include curbside collection, neighborhood recycling centers, community drop-boxes, and periodic recycling drives.

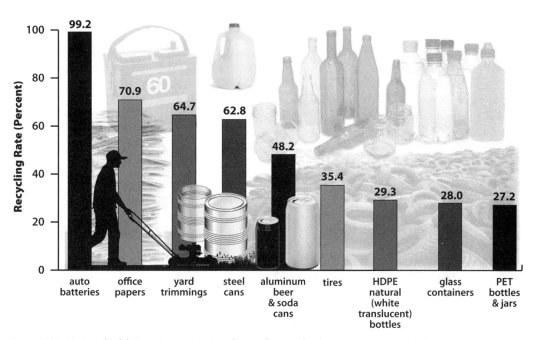

Source: EPA, *Municipal Solid Waste Generation, Recycling, and Disposal in the United States: Facts & Figures, 2008*. EPA 530-F-009-021, November 2009. Note: Does not include combustion (with energy recovery).

Figure 17-5   Recycling Rates of Selected Products, 2008

mixed residential wastes jumbled together in the garbage can—food scraps, old newspapers, dirty diapers, junk mail, empty milk cartons, and so on—and truck them off to a mixed waste processing facility (not-so-affectionately known in recycling circles as a **"dirty MRF"**). There the recyclable components are pulled out of the waste stream and diverted for processing, while the remainder is either landfilled or made into pellets for burning in an incinerator. Proponents of "dirty MRFs" admit that the facilities are expensive to construct and operate, but point out that, in comparison with source separation programs (i.e., separation by the person who generates the waste), mixed waste recovery facilities are theoretically capable of diverting a much higher percentage of recyclables from the waste stream. Some local officials favor such facilities because they don't require any public education efforts to persuade or coerce residents into altering long-established waste-generating behavior. Conversely, opponents contend that, aside from their high cost, "dirty MRFs" are environmentally unsound because the quality of potentially recyclable materials pulled from the mixed waste stream is so poor as to have little or no value to a secondary materials industry that demands as clean and homogeneous a waste stream as possible (i.e., who would want to buy paper for recycling once it's smeared with tomato sauce from discarded pizza?). As a case in point, Chicago's "Blue Bag" program, launched with much fanfare in 1995, achieved the abysmally low recy-

cling rate of just 6%, largely due to the fact that the blue bags containing source-separated recyclables were intermixed in the garbage trucks with nonrecyclable refuse (Pellow, 2002). As a result, Chicago officials in 2008 decided to phase out the Blue Bag program over a three-year period, replacing it with city-wide "Blue Cart" curbside recycling by the end of 2011. These realities have sharply limited the appeal of "dirty MRFs," which comprise less than 15% of all recycling processing facilities nationwide (Berenyi, 1999).

In an effort to promote recycling, governments at the federal, state, and local levels are pursuing a number of options to boost the supply of high-quality recyclables or to stimulate market demand. Among the legislative approaches to increase the amounts of material diverted through source separation efforts are the setting of "rates and dates" as previously described, as well as the passage of **"Bottle Bills,"** laws currently in effect in 11 states (Oregon, Vermont, Maine, Michigan, Iowa, Connecticut, Massachusetts, Delaware, California, New York, and Hawaii) which require consumers to pay a refundable deposit on beer and soft drink containers (California and Maine recently added noncarbonated beverage containers to their deposit laws and other states are considering similar action). Similar mandates are in effect throughout Canada, where most provinces require refundable deposits on a variety of beverage containers; Manitoba is the sole exception, imposing a deposit on beer containers only. First adopted by the province of British Columbia in 1970 and the state of Oregon in 1972, bottle bills were originally intended to combat littering. Surveys performed a few years after bottle bills took effect documented a 75–86% drop in the number of beverage containers discarded along roadsides (although some slovenly individuals persist in tossing cans and bottles away even in bottle bill states, there is now financial motivation for others to retrieve them). Bottle bills have subsequently proven themselves equally effective at boosting recycling rates for aluminum, glass, and PET plastic. Data from bottle bill states indicate that, on average, over 70% of the beverage containers sold in these states are ultimately recycled (95% in Michigan where the deposit is 10¢, as opposed to 5¢ or less in the other ten states). By contrast, in nondeposit states the aggregate rate of beverage container recycling is just 27.9% (Gitlitz, 2004).

Another popular legislative move in recent years has been prohibiting landfill disposal of such materials as yard wastes, lead-acid batteries, whole tires, white goods (large appliances), electronics, and used motor oil. While the main purpose of these bans has been to conserve landfill space or to prevent the formation of toxic leachates, their enactment has greatly enhanced the amount of these materials diverted to recycling centers or composting facilities since there's now nowhere else for them to go.

Minimum recycled content mandates have become an increasingly popular way of creating market demand for old newspaper, glass, and plastic—even telephone directories! Such laws require that targeted products contain a certain percentage of recycled material. For exam-

ple, 27 states have enacted voluntary or mandatory requirements that newspapers sold in those states contain specified percentages of recycled fiber (Miller, 2010).

Government procurement policies that require government agencies, state universities, and public schools to purchase supplies that are recyclable or contain recycled material have long been advocated as a way to promote market demand for recyclables. Since the purchases of goods and services by federal, state, and local governments in the United States cumulatively amount to 20% of the GNP, use of government purchasing power in favor of secondary materials could provide an important boost to the recycling industry.

Take-back programs in which manufacturers are required to take back and recycle their products and packaging are becoming an increasingly important component of MSW management. The economic slowdown that began in late 2008 has had a significantly adverse impact on recycling; as prices for recyclables plunged, a number of commercial recycling facilities went bankrupt, leaving many municipalities scrambling for a place to send collected materials. Moreover, it has become obvious that municipal governments are incapable of managing certain waste streams effectively, since the design of many products—appliances, furniture, and electronic equipment being notable examples—render resource recovery of their various components difficult or impossible. This realization has led to a growing conviction that the *manufacturers* of these products—not local taxpayers, government officials, or waste reprocessors—should bear most of the responsibility for their end-of-life management.

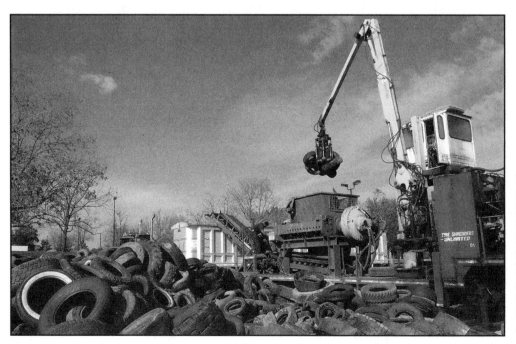

Most states have banned landfill disposal of whole tires and have instead instituted collection and recycling programs. Shredded tire material can be used for such things as road base, running tracks, playgrounds, horse arenas, and as a component in tire-derived fuel. [*Illinois Environmental Protection Agency*]

Such thinking has given rise to a concept known as **Extended Producer Responsibility (EPR)**. EPR policies, in essence, force manufacturers to consider the environmental impact of products throughout their life cycle, a process which, ideally, will result in the elimination of unnecessary parts and excessive packaging, as well as promote product design that facilitates repair, recycling, or reuse. In Europe, where the EPR concept was first introduced with Germany's 1991 "Ordinance on the Avoidance of Packaging Waste" and complimentary "Green Dot" (Grüne Punkt) system, many countries now have legislation requiring producers to take back and recycle packaging waste free of charge—a mandate credited with dramatic reductions in manufacturers' use of unnecessary packaging materials. EPR laws in a number of European nations have expanded their initial focus on packaging to include producer **take-back requirements** for discarded electric and electronic equipment, batteries, and automobiles. In most cases, European EPR legislation prohibits the landfilling or incineration of products targeted under the take-back laws and establishes minimum recycling and reuse requirements. The EU now requires auto manufacturers not only to take back vehicles their owners no longer want, but also mandates that 80% of their components by weight be recycled or reused; by 2015 that proportion will rise to 85% (*The Economist*, 2009). As intended, mandatory EPR requirements have motivated European manufacturers to

develop materials or products that can easily be reused or which break down readily once discarded. Examples include a new, infinitely recyclable nylon-6 fiber, produced by the German chemical firm BASF, and a Swiss-manufactured upholstery fabric that naturally decomposes at the end of its useful life (Renner, 2004).

In the U.S., proposed federal EPR legislation has made little headway due to strong opposition by manufacturing interests. Nevertheless, the threat of regulation has prompted several voluntary programs by producers, involving product redesign or limited take-backs of certain products (Canada, like the U.S., has a number of voluntary initiatives at the national level, but all ten provinces have various mandatory EPR programs in operation). Except for the 11 state bottle bills and state mandates regarding take-back of discarded electronic products, laws enacted by a number of U.S. states assign waste management responsibility for specified products not to the producers of those items, as in Europe, but to government, consumers, or retailers. Examples include used motor oil recycling programs financed by consumer fees or state money, government-managed scrap tire collections funded by fees collected from customers by tire dealers, and retailer take-back programs for used lead-acid batteries, now in effect in 37 states. Thanks to effective lobbying, producer trade organizations have successfully avoided any significant take-back responsibility. An industry-wide voluntary take-back program for recovery

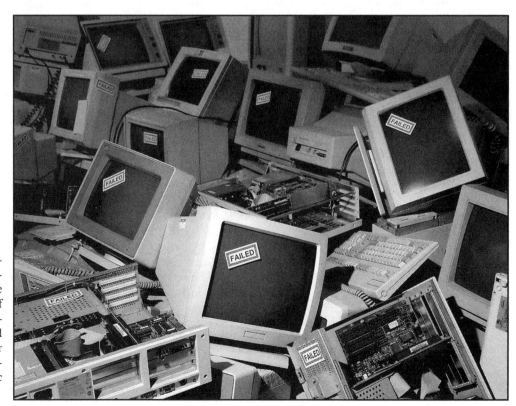

Extended producer responsibility policies force manufacturers to consider the environmental impacts of their products and packaging. This philosophy has led to take-back requirements for a number of product categories, including electronic equipment.

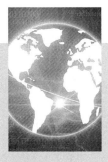

········ 17-2 ········

E-Waste Recycling—Not Always "Green"

Electronic wastes—or "e-wastes"—today represent one of the world's most urgent waste management challenges. The sheer volume of such materials, including personal computers, printers, mobile phones, TVs, and household appliances, discarded each year is staggering. The United Nations estimates current annual e-waste generation at roughly 40–50 million tons worldwide (the GAO reports that in 2006 alone, Americans threw away more than 300 million electronic devices). Over the next decade the situation will only get worse, as developing nations such as India and China bridge the "digital divide" and as large regions in Africa and Latin America also experience a sharp rise in the sale of electronic products. The UN projects that within the next ten years, e-wastes from discarded computers will increase by as much as 200 to 400% over 2007 levels in China and by 500% in India; during that same period, e-waste from old mobile phones will increase seven-fold in China and eighteen-fold in India!

At the same time their domestic e-waste generation is soaring, many developing countries—especially China and other Asian nations—are serving as the final destination for massive quantities of discarded electronic goods from the United States and other developed nations where increasingly-tight restrictions on their disposal make export the cheapest management option (Schluep et al., 2009).

The impact that their unwanted TVs, PCs, and cell phones are having on the environment and human health in the far-away communities receiving such discards remains largely unrecognized by most Americans. As e-waste volumes began to mount in this country, there was a growing awareness that dumping such materials in municipal landfills represented a colossal waste of resources as well as a serious environmental hazard. On average, computer monitors and older TV picture tubes contain four pounds of lead, as well as other toxic substances, necessitating responsible e-waste management. In response to the domestic e-waste challenge, many states now have laws banning the landfilling of e-wastes and require that they be recycled. Other programs have established **reuse and donation** as the primary e-waste goal, reasoning that if outdated equipment remains in working order, donating it to those who couldn't otherwise afford it benefits society and protects the environment by diverting such materials from the waste stream. Several hundred nonprofit organizations in the U.S. and Canada accept donations of unwanted computers which they then refurbish and send to schools, low-income residents, or organizations in developing countries. Federal legislation such as the 21st Century Classrooms Act has made such donations increasingly attractive to large corporations by granting tax incentives for donations of computer equipment to schools. For nonworking, nonrepairable items, e-waste recycling opportunities have expanded rapidly and in recent years the processing of electronic scrap has become the fastest-growing segment of the North American recycling industry.

Unfortunately, while many e-waste recyclers strive to conduct their business in an ethical, environmentally sound manner, many others have yielded to market pressures and are exporting e-wastes, either directly or through brokers, to buyers in Asia. It has been estimated by industry insiders that of all the e-wastes collected in the western U.S. for domestic recycling, between 50–80% is loaded onto container ships headed for China (about 90% of total e-waste exports) or other low-wage Asian countries. Once there, recycling technologies are anything but "green" and have resulted in shocking levels of air, water, and soil pollution—and are believed to be seriously harming human health. Surveys conducted by the UN Environmental Programme found that so-called "recycling" operations typically involve skimming off the most valuable components for resale, with the remaining items being dismantled under hazardous conditions by low-paid workers unaware of the dangers to which they are being exposed. Such practices include open-air burning of wire and other plastic-coated computer parts to recover copper, steel, and other metals; de-soldering and removing computer chips from printed circuit boards; and chemical stripping of computer chips and other gold-plated components in open acid baths. Laborers engaged in such activities typically work bare-handed, wear no protective gear, are not provided with ventilation fans, and hence incur such occupational hazards as dermal and inhalation exposure to heavy metals (lead, cadmium, mercury, etc.), dioxins, and carcinogenic polycyclic aromatic hydrocarbons. Residual toxic wastes from such operations are simply dumped onto the ground where they seep into the soil or are washed into nearby waterways, endangering not only the workers themselves, but entire communities.

Unlike the situation in Asian countries where most foreign e-wastes are shipped for recycling, those exported to Africa are, for the most part, intended for reuse. However, it has been standard procedure among U.S. exporters to include a large number of broken, unusable computers and other electronic equipment along with those still in working condition. Sometimes as much as 40% of the total shipment may consist of junk units that are simply dumped in the countryside and burned without any attempt made to prevent the release of toxic components (GAO, 2008).

For years environmental groups have been urging both the U.S. government and the scrap recycling industry to tighten export controls on potentially hazardous used electronics. The United States remains the only advanced industrial nation not to have ratified the Basel Convention, an international treaty banning the export of all hazardous wastes to developing countries for any reason, including recycling. Under the Resource Conservation and Recovery Act (RCRA), e-wastes are specifically exempted from regulations requiring that importing countries receive prior notification of hazardous waste shipments (Schluep et al., 2009). With the exception of cathode-ray tubes (CRTs), used electronics can be legally exported without restriction from the U.S.—and EPA does little to enforce the CRT export ban. EPA officials in 2008 stated they had neither plans nor a timetable to develop an enforcement program. This is unfortunate, because that same year federal investigators found that 43 U.S. recycling firms were violating the CRT export regulations— while simultaneously bragging about their "green" credentials on their company Web sites (GAO, 2008)!

In the absence of federal action on the issue, a number of states in recent years have been enacting their own laws for dealing with e-wastes. With the exception of California's Electronic Waste Recycling Act which requires consumers to pay an Advanced Recovery Fee to retailers at the point of purchase, with fees being used to reimburse e-waste collectors and recyclers, most of the state mandates are "extended producer responsibility" (EPR) laws—sometimes referred to as "producer take-back" requirements. Under EPR, electronics *manufacturers*, as opposed to consumers or governments, must take responsibility for the environmentally safe management of their products after they are discarded. Similar mandates have been in effect in a number of European countries since the early 1990s and have proven very effective in motivating manufacturers to design more durable products that last longer and are easier to recycle.

Some companies aren't waiting for government to tell them what to do but are voluntarily taking responsibility for e-wastes they manufactured. A prime example of such corporate good citizenship is Dell, whose 2009 announcement of a policy prohibiting the export of hazardous electronic waste to any developing country has been praised by environmentalists and consumer groups as the highest standard in the industry. A company spokesman urged his fellow manufacturers to follow Dell's example, proclaiming that "as one of the world's leading providers of technology, we recognize our responsibility to ensure that technology is disposed of properly at the end of its usable life" (BAN, 2009).

To provide assurance to those, like Dell, who seek to manage their e-waste in an environmentally sound manner, an independent accreditation and certification program—the **e-Stewards Standard for Responsible Recycling and Reuse of Electronic Equipment**®—has been created by the Basel Action Network (BAN) and was launched in early 2010. The e-Stewards program has been hailed as the "gold standard" of the electronics recycling industry, regarded as a certification program customers can rely on to differentiate the truly conscientious recyclers from those less scrupulous, whose quest for profits without regard for workers or the environment have given rise to the steadily worsening e-waste export crisis.

In the meantime, as advocates for reform continue to press for tougher e-waste regulations and greater corporate responsibility in the United States, developing countries need to act to improve their own e-waste recycling practices. With millions of newly affluent consumers of iPhones, laptops, and TVs in China, India, and elsewhere, domestic e-wastes could become an even bigger problem than imports in the years ahead.

and recycling of nickel-cadmium rechargeable batteries, launched with considerable fanfare in the mid-1990s by the Rechargeable Battery Recycling Corporation (RBRC) has been a dismal failure, with a recovery rate hovering around 10%, as opposed to RBRC's 70% stated goal.

The unimpressive results of voluntary initiatives by American industry and the unlikelihood of mandatory federal requirements in the foreseeable future have prompted legislative activity in a number of states. In 2001 Maine became the first to enact a manufacturer take-back law for mercury-containing waste products and to require that car manufacturers pay a bounty to auto salvagers who recover mercury-containing switches. By March 2010, 22 states had passed, and many more were considering, laws either banning mercury in consumer products or requiring that such products bear warning labels. Types of products targeted by these mandates include fever thermometers containing mercury, mercury-added thermostats, certain instruments and measuring devices, and some pharmaceutical and cosmetic products. In 2004 Maine again set a national precedent, becoming the first state to require that industry take back and recycle discarded television sets and computer monitors. Since then, a number of other states have chosen to emulate Maine's example; by early 2010, 20 states, as well as New York City, had passed laws mandating statewide electronics waste recycling and several others had similar legislation pending.

These producer responsibility mandates have been welcomed by some electronics manufacturers. Hewlett Packard (HP) insists that it has consistently aimed at "cradle-to-cradle" product design to facilitate recycling at the end of an item's useful lifespan. As a result, according to a company spokesman, 90% of HP laptops manufactured in 2008 were recyclable, as were at least 70% of HP printers. In that year Hewlett Packard recycled more than 450,000 tons of discarded equipment and aimed to double that figure by 2010. Eventually the company hopes to design computers so they can easily be upgraded instead of replaced, further reducing the volume of electronic waste (*The Economist*, 2009).

Composting

Since the late 1980s, proliferation of state mandates prohibiting the landfilling of yard wastes has led to an explosive increase in municipal composting facilities in the United States. By 2010, 23 states had enacted such bans and more than 3,200 yard-waste composting facilities were operating in the United States (bans on the landfilling of yard wastes have also contributed to booming sales of mulching mowers; results from a four-year demonstration project conducted by the Rodale Institute concluded that use of mulching mowers produces health-

ier lawns with fewer weeds and no thatch buildup). While a number of European countries have long recognized that composting of organic household waste can reduce the amount of refuse requiring disposal, consideration of composting as a viable waste management alternative in the United States is a much more recent phenomenon. Even though readily decomposable food and yard wastes make up almost 26% of the U.S. urban waste stream (considerably more during the warmer months of the year, less during the winter), perceived lack of demand for the finished product, plus the ease and low cost of landfilling, led city officials to dismiss composting as an impractical venture. That attitude has now been transformed by the realization that it makes little sense to devote valuable landfill space to grass clippings and autumn leaves when such materials could be converted into a useful and environmentally beneficial product. Nor are yard wastes the only potentially compostable materials in MSW. In 2008, 13 mixed-waste composting plants located in 11 states were processing the entire organic portion of residential and commercial wastes—food scraps, soiled paper, etc.—removing only noncompostable (but still recyclable) glass, metal, and plastics, as well as any hazardous materials (Spencer and Yepsen, 2008). Though questions have been raised about the quality of mixed-waste compost, efforts to educate citizens on the importance of source separation have helped to prevent contamination of the final product and to avoid the loss of potentially compostable materials.

A form of resource recovery, composting utilizes natural biochemical decay processes to convert organic wastes into a humus-like material, suitable for use as a soil conditioner. Although its nutrient content is too low to consider it a fertilizer, compost greatly improves soil structure and porosity, aids in water infiltration and retention, increases soil aeration, and slows erosion. Co-composting of yard wastes with municipal sewage sludge (another increasingly difficult-to-dispose-of waste product), now being practiced in a number of communities, enhances the nitrogen content of the finished product and makes it more valuable for agricultural uses.

A variety of methods for converting wastes to compost are currently in use, ranging from the low-tech, relatively inexpensive **windrow** technique, where long rows of wastes are piled outdoors and mechanically turned periodically to aerate the mass, to highly sophisticated, expensive **in-vessel** operations or processes in which pumps mechanically aerate windrows (**aerated static pile**), hastening decay and eliminating the need for frequent turning. Choice of the most appropriate composting method depends on the needs and resources of the community in question: if land is abundant and funding scarce, the windrow method may be the best option—though it often requires two or three years for complete

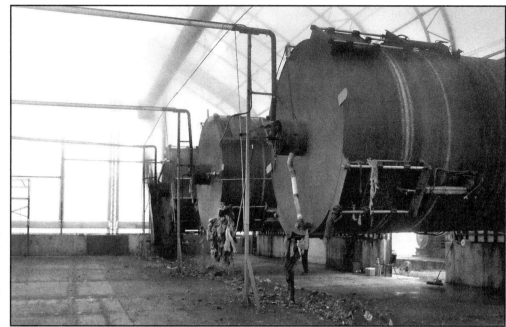

Composting utilizes natural biochemical decay processes to convert decomposable food and yard wastes into a finished product suitable for use as a soil conditioner. In more sophisticated operations like that shown here, rotary drums mechanically aerate the wastes, hastening decay. [*Robert Spencer, www.BioCycle.net*]

breakdown of wastes to occur if the piles are turned only once or twice annually. If available space is at a premium and rapid turnover of wastes desirable, a community might be wise to choose a more high-tech method, provided it can afford the considerably higher price tag associated with such facilities. Whatever the technology, the composting process consists of four basic steps:

1. *Preparation.* Incoming wastes are shredded to a relatively uniform size; in most composting operations, nonbiodegradable materials such as glass, metal, plastics, tires, and so on are separated from the compostable wastes. In some composting operations, sewage sludge or animal manures are added to the refuse at this point.

2. *Digestion.* Microbes naturally present in the waste materials or special bacterial inoculants sprayed on the refuse are utilized to break down organic waste materials. While digestion may be either aerobic or anaerobic, aerobic systems are generally preferred due to shorter time periods required and fewer odor problems. In aerobic decomposition, heat given off by microbial respiration raises the temperature in the windrows well above the 140°F necessary to kill fly eggs, weed seeds, or pathogenic organisms.

3. *Curing.* After digestion of simpler carbonaceous materials is complete, additional curing time is allowed to permit microbes to break down cellulose and lignin in the waste.

4. *Finishing.* To produce an acceptable finished product, compost may be put through screens and grinders to remove nondigested materials and create a uniform

appearance. Some composting facilities bag or package the finished product to facilitate marketing or distribution.

While the public rightly regards composting as an environmentally desirable method of organic waste management, composting facilities do not always make good neighbors. Some have been forced to close due to problems with objectionable odors—problems that are gradually being solved as operators compare notes and learn techniques for managing trouble-free facilities. Another public health issue related to composting operations is their potential to emit **bioaerosols**, tiny airborne particles of microorganisms whose inhalation has been blamed for ailments ranging from a runny nose and watery eyes to flu-like symptoms. Bioaerosols, such as spores of the ubiquitous fungus *Aspergillus fumigatus*, were first cited as a potential environmental health concern in 1992 when a New Jersey epidemiologist testified before Congress about potential health risks to people living within a two-mile radius of composting sites. Since that time bioaerosols have attracted intensive scrutiny and have prompted organized community opposition to siting of compost facilities in several localities. Representatives of the composting industry argue that any fears are vastly exaggerated, stating that public exposure to Aspergillus emissions from composting are negligible when the process is performed correctly. A report jointly sponsored by the EPA, USDA, NIOSH, and the Composting Council tends to support industry's contention. Conceding that exposure to bioaerosols could be life-threatening if inhaled by individuals with suppressed immune systems, the report nevertheless points out that the level of such

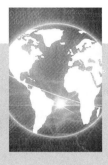

· · · · · · · 17-3 · · · · · · ·

Waste-Eating Worms

While many components of the municipal solid waste stream are now effectively targeted by recycling programs, management of the enormous quantities of food waste discarded daily by households and the food service industry continues to rely heavily on landfill disposal or discharge to municipal sewer systems via home garbage grinders. Recently, however, a somewhat unconventional method of food waste management has been winning enthusiastic converts—a practice known as **vermicomposting**. Derived from the Latin word vermis (worm), the term describes a method by which certain species of redworms, most commonly *Eisenia foetida*, feed on organic wastes, converting them into worm castings that are now widely regarded as the best soil amendment available.

Redworms are amazingly voracious little creatures, eating over half their body weight in organic matter daily and creating high-quality compost in the process. Not surprisingly, home gardeners, horticulturists, and organic growers have been leading the vermicomposting bandwagon, but soil scientists and agricultural researchers now support the practice, citing studies that demonstrate a significant increase in seed germination, plant growth, and crop yields when vermicompost is added to growth media or soils. Why worm castings produce such beneficial results is now the subject of scientific investigation at a number of universities; researchers hypothesize that plant growth enhancement by vermicompost is due to a worm-stimulated increase in the populations of hormone-producing fungi and bacteria. The water-soluble hormones present in vermicompost stimulate plant growth much more effectively than do the mineral nutrients present in conventional finished compost. Preliminary experiments indicate that vermicompost also markedly suppresses certain soil-based plant diseases and pests such as nematodes, mites, and several species of insects. As a result, use of vermicompost by commercial growers is expanding rapidly—a trend that is giving a major boost to organic waste recycling efforts by the food service industry, feedlot managers, wood pulp producers, and large-scale agricultural operations. For such waste generators, utilizing worms to eat their garbage is a win-win situation, converting wastes into a saleable product (Edwards and Aracon, 2004).

Fortunately, vermiculture offers the same rewards at the household level as it does on an industrial scale, giving individuals and families an opportunity to turn kitchen scraps into "brown gold" to nourish houseplants and gardens (it can also provide a fun classroom project for school children and an ecologically beneficial way to dispose of lunch box leftovers!). Unlike the standard outdoor compost pile where decomposition slows to a halt during winter, worm bins for vermicomposting are best kept indoors and hence function year-round—a definite advantage since kitchen waste generation proceeds regardless of the weather.

For those wishing to launch a home vermicomposting project, only a few basic ingredients are needed.

1. **A worm bin**, either purchased or homemade. Numerous types of containers suitable for home vermicomposting are available on the Internet, but bins also can be constructed at home using large plastic or wooden containers (detailed instructions for building a simple worm bin are available online or in numerous publications such as *Worms Eat My Garbage* by Mary Appelhof). In general, containers should be relatively shallow (about 8–12" deep) with holes in the bottom for aeration and drainage; they also need a lid to maintain high humidity and exclude light from the bin. Bricks or wooden blocks should be placed underneath to permit air circulation and drainage. If kept indoors, a tray placed beneath the bin is useful to collect any liquids leaking from the container; these can then be used to fertilize plants.

2. **Bedding** composed of shredded corrugated cardboard or shredded paper (ink poses no problems). To prepare it for use, the dry bedding should be thoroughly soaked with water (it may take several hours to become well saturated), then drained and as much of the excess water as possible squeezed out. The moist bedding should then be fluffed up and placed in the bin to 2/3 its depth.

3. **Redworms**, favored for their rapid reproduction rate and tolerance of high population densities, are available on the Internet, in garden catalogs, or bait shops. Don't try to economize by using night crawlers or other garden worms—they won't survive in the confines of a worm bin. The amount needed depends on how much food waste is generated daily; for a typical family, one pound of worms is usually sufficient. When starting a new worm bin, simply scatter the worms on top of the bedding; they quickly move down into the shredded material to avoid light. Redworms prefer temperatures in the 55–77°F (13–25°C) range; they are likely to die if temperatures fall below freezing or exceed 84°F (29°C).

4. **Kitchen scraps**, including vegetable and fruit peelings, coffee grounds, tea leaves, and nongreasy table scraps. Avoid fat, meat, and bones; citrus peels also may be problematic, since they contain a chemical toxic to redworms. A small amount of gritty material such as cornmeal, coffee grounds, or finely crushed eggshells should be added occasionally to help the worms digest the food. These food scraps can either be spread in a thin layer on top of the bedding or the bedding can be pulled back at one location, the food scraps dumped in, and the bedding pulled back over them (if the latter method is used, vary the location each time more food is added). If odors develop, reduce the amount of food being added or cut it up into smaller pieces.

Assuming that proper environmental conditions have been maintained, the redworms go to work rapidly. Within 3–4 months nearly all of the food scraps and bedding material will be converted to a dark brown material the consistency of coffee grounds. At this point the vermicompost should be harvested, before it becomes odorous and sludge-like. Harvesting essentially means separating the compost from the worms, a process than can be accomplished in one of several ways. One method involves dumping the contents of the bin onto a tarp in bright light, causing the worms to wriggle downward toward the bottom of the pile; the castings at the top can then be scraped away, a process repeated several times until all that is left is a pile of worms which can then be placed in a newly prepared bin. Alternatively, new bedding can be placed on one side of the existing bin, the other side being left undisturbed. Over a period of several weeks, most of the worms will move into the new bedding, allowing the castings on the other side to be removed.

To use the finished compost for container plants, either add it directly to potting mix prior to planting or, for already established plants, spread it thinly on the surface of the soil. When setting out seedlings in the garden, a small amount of vermicompost can be placed in each hole at the time of planting; more can subsequently be worked into the soil around the base of individual plants and watered in. Whatever the application method, the result is beneficial, since worm compost contains 5 times more nitrogen, 7 times more phosphorus, and 11 times more potassium than average soil. Giving a boost to home gardening while also diverting food waste from landfills, vermicomposting is an idea whose time has come (Cochran, 2003).

---

particles is no higher in the vicinity of composting operations than in the general environment. A person is just as likely to inhale *A. fumigatus* spores while mowing the lawn, raking leaves, or cleaning the attic as by living near a composting facility. Experts report that *Aspergillus* at composting sites originates primarily from the storage of bulking agents such as wood chips, with airborne spores being released at the time of initial mixing (the steam rising off the top of windrows does not appear to be a major source). Operational considerations such as moisture and dust control and minimization of handling can significantly mitigate bioaerosol emissions. While authorities agree that more research is needed, the general consensus at present is that bioaerosols do not present concerns serious enough to warrant a reconsideration of municipal composting operations (Greczyn, 1994).

In the past, the difficulty of finding outlets for municipal compost was a major stumbling block in convincing local officials to consider composting as a waste management strategy. Poor quality of the finished product from some mixed-waste composting facilities restricts its use to landfill cover material, filter berms, construction projects, and erosion control. Better-quality municipal compost, however, is being sold or given away free to farmers, landscapers, and home gardeners for use as a soil conditioner, mulch, turf blend, potting mix, or for landscaping purposes (Spencer and Yepsen, 2008).

Waste Combustion

Prior to passage of the 1970 Clean Air Act, many communities chose to burn urban refuse at large municipal incinerators because the high cost of land, unavailability of suitable sites, or neighborhood opposition to siting made landfilling unfeasible. By the 1960s, almost 300 municipal incinerators were operating in the United States. As the decade of the 1970s ushered in an era of strict air quality control regulations, however, most of these incinerators closed down, unable to comply with the new emission standards. Studies indicated that in some large cities, close to 20% of all particulate pollutants were coming from municipal incinerators (Melosi, 1981).

By 2008, according to EPA data, incineration was the management option for only 12.6% of U.S. municipal solid wastes, a figure considerably lower than that predicted two decades earlier. During the 1980s, as the nation's garbage woes mounted, interest in burning as an attractive waste management option was revived by the advent of a new generation of incinerators: **waste-to-energy (WTE)** plants. These facilities not only burn refuse, thereby reducing its volume by 80–90%, but also capture the heat of combustion in the form of salable electricity or process steam. Many communities, particularly in the northeastern U.S. where landfill tipping fees were skyrocketing, committed themselves to this new technology as the most feasible alternative to disappearing landfill space. By the mid-1990s, however, increasing landfill capacity and a drop in tipping fees shifted the economics in favor of landfilling. As a result, some municipalities that had been considering construction of combustion incinerators decided to forego that option; elsewhere small, economically marginal incinerators were shut down. By 2006, just 103 municipal solid waste incinerators were operating nationwide, most of them in New England, the Middle Atlantic states, and Florida. Among states, Connecticut is the most reliant on incineration for MSW disposal, burning 64% of wastes generated (Arsova et al. 2008).

From an environmental standpoint, the enthusiasm that welcomed WTE incinerators as the ideal solution to our disposal dilemmas is now giving way to a more cautious appraisal, as concerns are raised about possible toxic air emissions, especially dioxins, furans, and heavy metals (e.g., lead, cadmium, and mercury). Proponents of the technology insist such problems can be minimized through good emission controls and proper plant operation. In 1991 tighter emissions limitations required by Clean Air Act Amendments for municipal incinerators were approved by EPA, requiring that facilities install state-of-the-art equipment to control acid gases, metal particulates, and organic products of incomplete combustion, such as dioxin. Smokestacks are now being fitted with acid gas scrubbers, baghouse filters for trapping metal particulates, and activated carbon injection systems for capturing mercury vapors. By utilizing advanced combustion controls, plant operators can maintain furnace temperatures high enough to prevent dioxin formation and to ensure a more complete burn.

Disposal of the considerable volumes of incinerator ash generated by large WTE facilities has been another contentious issue. Incineration is not a complete waste management method; in general, for every three tons of refuse burned, a ton of ash remains, requiring disposal. Until recently the most prevalent method for managing incinerator ash was to bury it in ordinary sanitary landfills or in "monofills"—facilities that accepted only incinerator ash for disposal. However, concerns that this material frequently contains dangerous levels of heavy metals (particularly the fly ash captured by pollution control equipment), have led to demands that incinerator ash be classified as "hazardous waste," thereby necessitating its disposal at a hazardous waste landfill—at an anticipated 10-fold rise in tipping fees. In May 1994, the U.S. Supreme Court settled the dispute by ruling that ash from municipal incinerators must be tested, using specified laboratory procedures, and if results indicate that the waste is indeed toxic, it must be managed as hazardous waste. This ruling, while greeted initially with dismay by municipalities reliant on incinerators, gave a major boost to resource recovery programs aimed at removing toxics-containing components of the MSW stream—items such as batteries, paint cans, and electrical equipment. Also, by halting the standard practice of combining the often-toxic fly ash with the far more voluminous but much less dangerous bottom ash, incinerator operators could greatly reduce the amount of ash requiring disposal as "hazardous" (Greenhouse, 1994).

Nevertheless, opponents remain wary, fearing that cities opting for incineration are going to find they've simply traded one set of environmental problems for another. Perhaps the major question regarding the future of WTE incineration, however, is financing their construction and operation. To remain economically viable, incinerators need a steady supply of trash and a dependable market for the energy they produce—but recent developments make both difficult to guarantee. Competing demands from recycling programs for high-BTU trash and recent court invalidation of local "flow-control" ordinances (which communities have imposed to ensure incinerators a predictable daily volume of waste) have resulted in a number of municipal incinerators operating considerably below their design capacity—a money-losing proposition. WTE incinerators are exorbitantly expensive to construct and operate (as a rough rule-of-thumb, WTE projects average $100,000–125,000 per ton of daily waste capacity; a city contemplating construction of a typical 1,000 ton-per-day facility can thus count on investing well over $100 million). Costs are recovered (hopefully!) through tipping fees (which a *Bio-Cycle* survey of nine states found averaged $64.88 per ton in 2006) paid by haulers bringing wastes to the facility and through sales of electricity or process steam produced by the plant. Since prevailing regional rates for electricity determine what this amount will be, low power demand reflected in falling prices has caused some communities to cancel plans for incinerator construction, since anticipated revenues from energy sales turned out to be less than originally projected.

The future role of WTE incineration in a comprehensive waste management strategy thus depends on a number of economic and political considerations, including trends in landfill tipping fees (increases make incineration more cost-competitive and vice-versa); demand for energy (high demand equals brighter future for WTE combustion); congressional initiatives (will Congress impose a legislative moratorium on incinerator construction?); and EPA decisions (will the agency further tighten emissions requirements or mandate that communities achieve specified recycling goals before building new incinerators?). WTE combustion remains the most important MSW management method in Japan, accounting for over 50% of that country's municipal waste disposal, and is popular in many European countries as well. Worldwide, approximately 700 WTE plants are simultaneously generating power while significantly reducing the flow of MSW to land disposal sites (*The Economist*, 2009). However, given the current abundance of landfill capacity in the U.S. and the large discrepancy between per unit disposal charges at landfills versus incinerators, it is unlikely that the percentage of MSW managed by combustion will increase significantly in the years immediately ahead.

HAZARDOUS WASTES

Late in the summer of 1978 the name of a small residential subdivision in the city of Niagara Falls, New York, entered the American vocabulary and became a household word almost overnight, symbolizing the dangers of our chemical age. The tragic sequence of events that unfolded at Love Canal epitomizes the dangers facing millions of citizens in thousands of communities across the nation as a result of our indiscriminate use and careless disposal of hazardous chemicals.

The Love Canal Story

The origin of the chemical dump site that became the focus of worldwide attention in the late 1970s can be traced to the mid-1890s, when William T. Love began construction of a canal intended to serve as a navigable power channel, connecting the Upper Niagara to the Niagara Escarpment about seven miles downstream, thereby bypassing the Falls. At the point where Mr. Love's canal was intended to reenter the river, the intention was to construct a model industrial city that would

be provided with cheap, abundant hydroelectric power. Unfortunately for Mr. Love, his development company went bankrupt shortly after construction of the canal had begun; the project was abandoned, leaving a waterway approximately 3,000 feet long, 10 feet deep, and 60 feet wide. For many years, residents of this area on the outskirts of town used the canal for recreational fishing and swimming; in 1927 the land was annexed by the city. In 1942 Hooker Chemical Company (now a subsidiary of Occidental Petroleum), one of several major chemical industries located in Niagara Falls, received permission to dump chemical wastes into the canal, which it proceeded to do from that time until 1952 (in 1947 Hooker purchased the canal, along with two 70-feet-wide strips of land adjacent to the canal on each side). During this time more than 21,000 tons of chemical wastes—acids, alkalis, solvents, chlorinated hydrocarbons, etc.—were disposed of at this site. Only a few homes were present in the area at that time, but old-time residents recall the offensive odors, noxious vapors, and frequent fires that accompanied the dumping.

By 1953 the canal was full and so was topped with soil and eventually acquired a covering of grass and weeds. Hooker then offered to sell the land to the Niagara Falls School Board for the token fee of $1. At the same time, company officials pointedly advised school and city administrators that although the site was suitable for a school, parking lot, or playground, any construction activities involving excavation of the area should be avoided to prevent rupturing the dump site's clay lining, thereby allowing escape of the impounded chemicals. In 1955 an elementary school and playground were constructed on the site; in 1957 the city began laying storm sewers, roads, and utility lines through the area, disregarding the warnings received a few years earlier. In the years that followed, several hundred modest homes were built in the neighborhood parallel to the banks of the now-invisible canal. Most of the newer residents had no knowledge of the site's past history and, in spite of occasional chemical odors (not considered unusual in a city where chemical manufacturing was a leading industry), few outward signs of trouble were apparent.

Unusually heavy precipitation in the mid-1970s, however, was accompanied by some alarming phenomena. Strange-looking, viscous chemicals began oozing through basement walls, floors, and sump holes. Vegetation in yards withered and appeared scorched. Large puddles became permanent backyard features. Holes began to open up in the field that had once been a dump site and the tops of corroded 55-gallon drums leaking chemicals could be seen in places protruding from the soil surface. Complaints and fears expressed by citizens were generally downplayed by local authorities who assured them there was nothing to worry about.

By early 1978, pressure from a local congressman and regular critical coverage of events in the *Niagara Gazette* prompted the U.S. Environmental Protection Agency to undertake a program of air sampling in the basements of Love Canal homes. New York State authorities also began conducting soil analyses and taking samples of residues in sump pumps and storm sewers. The results of these studies indicated that the area was extremely contaminated with more than 200 different chemicals, including 12 known or suspected carcinogens. Benzene, known to be a potent human cancer-causing agent, was readily detected in the air inside many of the houses sampled. Dioxin was subsequently found in high concentrations in some of the soil samples analyzed. State officials in New York estimated that as many as 10% of the chemicals buried at Love Canal were mutagens, teratogens, or carcinogens. On August 2, 1978, the Health Commissioner of New York publicly proclaimed "the existence of a great and imminent peril to the health of the general public" at Love Canal and advised all pregnant women and families with children under the age of two to leave the area if they could do so. Five days later, President Carter officially declared Love Canal a national emergency.

The months that followed witnessed mass relocation at public expense of residents living closest to the dump site, as well as openly expressed fears by those left behind on adjacent streets that their health was similarly endangered. A number of health studies, whose methodology and conclusions remain highly controversial, suggested that Love Canal residents had experienced statistically significant elevated rates of miscarriage, birth defects, and chromosomal abnormalities. Ultimately 1,004 families were evacuated from Love Canal, their homes purchased by the state. Over 300 of the residences closest to the canal were demolished and the area covered with a protective layer of clay and a synthetic liner to exclude rainwater. Most of the remaining homes were boarded up, awaiting a pending EPA assessment of whether they could ever again be inhabited. Trenches were dug around the old canal site to capture contaminated groundwater, which was then pumped to a treatment center for detoxification. Nearby creeks where high levels of dioxin seepage were detected were fenced off to protect children and animals. Combined federal and state expenditures for relocating residents, investigating environmental damage, and halting chemical seepage from the site total $150 million, and an additional $32 million has been spent to clean up contaminated creeks and sewers and to determine the future habitability of the neighborhood. The Congressional Office of Technology Assessment estimated that if Hooker had employed current disposal standards and practices, its wastes could have been safely managed for about $2 million in 1979 dollars (Levine, 1982).

Occidental Chemical, which acquired Hooker in a 1968 buy-out, has paid $20 million in out-of-court settlements to affected residents; a federal district court ruling in 1988 held Occidental liable for the cost of previous, ongoing, and future cleanup of the Love Canal site—a figure approximating $250 million. Two years later, the State of New York sued Occidental for an additional $250 million in punitive damages, claiming that its subsidiary Hooker had "displayed reckless disregard for the safety of others." In the spring of 1994, a federal judge ruled against the plaintiff, saying the evidence in the state's case was insufficient; this decision, however, did not alter Occidental's liability for cleanup costs.

In the fall of 1988, after reviewing a five-year habitability study of the affected area, New York State Health Commissioner David Axelrod declared that most of the Love Canal neighborhood could be safely resettled by former residents. While the decision was controversial, with some environmentalists warning that "Love Canal is a ticking time bomb," by the summer of 1990 over 200 people had expressed interest in renovated homes selling for 20% less than the prevailing market price. Reassured by government claims that the area no longer presented any threat, new residents began reoccupying homes in the Love Canal neighborhood, renamed "Black Creek Village." Eventually more than 200 abandoned homes were renovated and sold to new owners and 10 new apartment buildings constructed in the area. In 1995 Occidental Chemical agreed to pay the federal government $129 million to cover costs for the pollution cleanup at Love Canal. Hailing the final agreement concluded by the U.S. Department of Justice, EPA Administrator Carol Browner remarked that it represented "this administration's firm commitment to ensuring that polluters, not the American people, pick up the tab for cleaning up toxic waste dumps." The final chapter in this saga concluded in September 2004 when the EPA officially removed the Love Canal site from the Superfund National Priority List, declaring that all work at the site had been completed and cleanup goals achieved.

The events that transpired at Love Canal cannot be shrugged off as a unique tragedy that unfortunately victimized a few thousand people in western New York State. Health authorities and environmental agency officials regard Love Canal as but the "tip of the iceberg" in alerting society to the widespread nature of the hazardous waste problem. EPA has released a report projecting that as many as 350,000 sites across the nation may require cleanup over the next 30 years due to contamination with hazardous wastes or petroleum products. If current remediation standards are maintained, the total cleanup costs could be as high as $250 billion. Little wonder that public opinion polls show citizens ranking hazardous waste management issues among their top environmental quality concerns.

What Is "Hazardous" Waste?

In the 1976 Resource Conservation and Recovery Act (RCRA), Congress legally defined hazardous waste as "any discarded material that may pose a substantial threat or potential danger to human health or the environment when improperly handled." EPA has established a two-tier system for determining whether a specific waste is subject to regulation under current hazardous waste management laws:

1. If the substance in question is among the more than 500 wastes or waste streams itemized in Parts 261.31–33 of the Code of Federal Regulations, it will automatically be subject to regulation as a hazardous waste. Wastes may be placed on the list because of their ability to induce cancer, mutations, or birth defects; because of their toxicity to plants; or because even low doses are fatal to humans. However, the Administrator of EPA can exercise a wide measure of discretion in deciding whether to list a particular waste, so a number of potential carcinogens, mutagens, and teratogens are not yet listed as officially "hazardous."

2. In addition to the wastes listed in the federal code, any waste that exhibits one or more of the following characteristics is defined as hazardous and subject to regulation:

   Toxic—wastes such as arsenic, heavy metals, or certain synthetic pesticides are capable of causing either acute or chronic health problems.

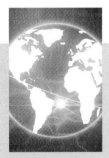

⋯⋯⋯ 17-4 ⋯⋯⋯
Plants vs. Pollution

Several years ago the Army Corps of Engineers launched an innovative pilot project to clean up wastes contaminating approximately 600 acres of residential and university property near American University in northwestern Washington, DC. The area, used during World War I for testing chemical weapons, is tainted with traces of arsenic from those long-ago experiments and a hazardous waste cleanup operation had been ordered. However, the Corps' conventional remediation project had stalled because residents resisted seeing the lovely old trees in their neighborhood removed or damaged during soil removal operations. Responding to such concerns, the Corps opted to deal with problems remaining on more than 100 private properties by utilizing a relatively new waste treatment method known as **phytoremediation**, planting 2,800 arsenic-absorbing brake ferns (*Pteris vittata*) at three different locations within the affected area. The ferns will pull arsenic out of the soil and accumulate the toxic metal in their stems and fronds, concentrating it to more than 50 times soil levels—and do so without any harm to the surrounding trees. Corps personnel subsequently harvest the ferns, analyze them for arsenic, and then safely dispose of the plants at a hazardous waste facility if arsenic levels are extremely high.

The ability of brake ferns, a common southeastern species, to accumulate arsenic was discovered in 1998 when researchers from the University of Florida tried growing 14 different plant species in arsenic-contaminated soil at a lumberyard in central Florida (arsenic compounds from wood preservatives are often found in soils where treated lumber has been stored). While few plants even survive in arsenic-tainted soil (arsenic is an effective ingredient in some weed-killers), the brake ferns thrived in this environment and the Florida researchers proudly announced their discovery of the first plant species able to accumulate arsenic in high concentrations. They subsequently patented their discovery and the so-called "edenferns" are now sold by Edenspace, a Virginia-based bioremediation company. Edenferns are currently being used to remove arsenic from soil and drinking water at various locations across the United States, proving themselves a cost-effective alternative to conventional remediation technologies that typically involve excavation, acid-washing, and landfill disposal of contaminated soils (Ruder, 2004).

Edenferns are by no means the only plants to prove their worth in cleaning up chemically contaminated sites. At present, over 440 plant species have been identified as possessing the natural ability to take up quantities of metals such as lead, zinc, cadmium, and uranium from soils and to accumulate them in quantities that would kill most other species. Referred to as **hyperaccumulators**, such plants can store as much as 2.5% of their dry weight in heavy metals in leaves without suffering any reduction in yields. Researchers have now identified the gene that produces phytochelatins, the substance that allows plants to detoxify heavy metals, and hope to use this information to enhance further the natural ability of hyperaccumulator plants to take up toxic metals. Field studies are currently underway in a number of countries to identify which plants are best suited for phytoextraction purposes.

Among those so identified is Indian mustard (*Brassica juncea*), a hyperaccumulator of lead. At a contaminated DaimlerChrysler site in Detroit, a mixed planting of Indian mustard and sunflowers, another lead-absorbing species, reduced existing soil lead concentrations 43%, bringing contaminant levels below legal limits; the cost of the remediation project was $1 million less than conventional soil excavation would have been, and waste from the project consisted merely of a few cubic yards of lead-laden plant material. Indian mustard has also been used to remove selenium from contaminated soils in California's San Joaquin Valley, where toxic selenium in agricultural drainage water severely disrupted the ecosystem at Kesterson Reservoir. The state has set a high priority on remediating high-selenium soils and on minimizing movement of the chemical from soil to irrigation effluent. Since most of the conventional methods investigated were either very costly or only marginally effective, phytoremediation attracted considerable interest as an economical, environmentally friendly alternative. Long-term field studies have shown that the top 24 inches of soil experienced nearly a 40% reduction in selenium content when planted with Indian mustard. Most of the selenium taken up was incorporated into plant tissue, while some was biologically volatilized into the air, primarily via the roots. Mustard plants with elevated concentrations of selenium have the potential to become a high-value crop for farmers, as well as a cheap method of soil improvement. Because selenium is an essential trace element for mammals, selenium-containing mustard could be blended with alfalfa and feed to produce nutritious livestock forage—a win-win situation (Banuelos et al., 1997).

For cleanup of soils contaminated with zinc or cadmium, the humble Alpine pennycress (*Thlaspi caerulescens*) appears to be one of the most promising candidates. The plant has long been recognized in Europe as a good biological indicator of metal ore deposits. Studies have shown that pennycress takes up 35 times more zinc than other plant species growing in the same vicinity, concentrating the metal in its shoots.

Sunflowers have proven effective in remediating water tainted with low-level uranium, a situation where other methods either don't work or are prohibitively expensive. An experiment conducted in 1995 on a small radioactively contaminated pond near Chernobyl utilized sunflowers grown on Styrofoam rafts to extract strontium-90 and cesium-137 from the water. With their dense roots dangling in the water, the sunflowers quickly took up radioisotope concentrations several thousand times higher than those in the pond. The uranium taken up by the plants remains localized in the roots, simplifying waste disposal since only the roots need to be managed as low-level wastes, generally by incineration and land disposal of the residual ash.

Another plant successfully employed in wetlands systems to treat wastewaters contaminated by heavy metals is water hyacinth (*Eichhornia crassipes*). Water hyacinth multiplies rapidly, absorbing dissolved metals and accumulating them in plant tissues, especially the roots. Since *E. crassipes* floats on the water's surface, the plant can easily be harvested and, following incineration, its toxic metal component either recovered for reuse or land disposed. Water hyacinth is regarded as having good potential for in-situ remediation of hexavalent chromium, as well as a number of other toxic metals contaminating industrial wastewaters or sediments.

Poplar and willow trees are now employed at numerous locations to pump and treat solvent-contaminated groundwater. During the peak of the growing season, each poplar tree takes up more than 15 gallons of water daily, pulling organic contaminants into the root zone where they are biodegraded by soil microbes or by the plants themselves. Poplars planted near landfills or other potential sites of leachate migration can also be effective in capturing migrating pollutants, pulling them out of the ground before they infiltrate aquifers or surface waters (Revkin, 2001).

At a time when the estimated cost of remediating the nation's hazardous waste legacy using conventional technologies exceeds $700 billion, phytoremediation has the potential to revolutionize our approach to cleanups, especially in situations where levels of contamination are low, dispersed, but nevertheless in violation of standards. Phytoremediation's chief drawback is time; reducing concentrations of toxic metals to safe levels may require several years, depending on initial levels of contamination. Researchers hope that in the not-too-distant-future genetically engineered hyperaccumulators capable of accomplishing the cleanup task more expeditiously will be developed. Nevertheless, for nonemergency situations where toxins are not immediately threatening human health, phytoremediation holds great promise as an affordable, effective, nonintrusive way to restore contaminated sites.

Ignitable—organic solvents, oils, plasticizers, and paint wastes are examples of wastes that are hazardous because they have a flash point less than 60°C (140°F) or because they tend to undergo spontaneous combustion. The resultant fires are dangerous not only because of heat and smoke, but also because they can disseminate toxic particles over a wide area.

Corrosive—substances with a pH of 2 or less or 12.5 and above can eat away at standard container materials or living tissues through chemical action and are termed corrosive. Such wastes, which include acids, alkaline cleaning agents, and battery manufacturing residues, present a special threat to waste haulers who come into bodily contact with leaking containers.

Reactive—obsolete munitions, wastes from the manufacturing of dynamite or firecrackers, and certain chemical wastes such as picric acid are hazardous because of their tendency to react vigorously with air or water or to explode and generate toxic fumes.

Two other categories of wastes that might logically be considered hazardous—radioactive wastes and potentially infectious medical wastes from hospitals and clinics—are not presently regulated under the same laws as the groups listed above. Radioactive wastes are managed according to regulations adopted by the Nuclear Regulatory Commission under the Atomic Energy Act, while biomedical waste disposal laws vary from state to state. In 1988, public outrage over incidents of used syringes and other medical wastes washing up on East Coast beaches led to passage of the Medical Waste Tracking Act, which set up a two-year pilot project to attempt regulation of biomedical wastes through a procedure similar in nature to the manifest system currently required for off-site shipments of hazardous wastes. With the expiration of that program, individual states have, for the most part, adopted medical waste management programs of their own involving the manifesting of such wastes shipped off-site and, in several states, requiring that infectious wastes be "rendered innocuous" in specially licensed high-temperature incinerators—a form of disposal considerably more expensive than sanitary landfilling. Many authorities deplore what they regard as exaggerated public fears about the threats posed by medical wastes. Pointing out that wastes generated by hospitals are no more dangerous than many of the items tossed into the trash by householders (e.g., used syringes from home insulin injections, bloody bandages, outdated medications, etc.) and that not a single case of human illness has been traced to contact with infectious medical waste, they question the public health benefit of strict new regulations that significantly increase national costs for health care. Ironically, the highly sensationalized beach littering incidents that provoked the federal legislation, initially attributed to illegal ocean dumping by waste haulers, were subsequently traced to sewer discharges of discarded medical devices from private residences.

Generation of Hazardous Wastes

By the first decade of the 21st century, more than 20,000 U.S. manufacturers were sending approximately 7 million tons of hazardous wastes and wastewaters to commercial hazwaste landfills, incinerators, treatment, or recycling facilities each year (Perket, 2004), a figure that does not take into account wastes managed by the generators on-site. Production of these wastes is not evenly distributed among industries, however. More than 85% of all hazardous wastes are produced by just three major categories of generators: chemicals and allied products, metal-related industries, and petroleum and coal products. Geographic location of these industries, as well as population density, are major determinants of which states are the leading hazardous waste generators.

At the time when new federal waste management regulations went into effect in November 1980, EPA estimated that fully 90% of all hazardous wastes were being disposed of by methods that would not meet government standards. Thanks to what is widely regarded as the most stringent hazardous waste management program in the world, that situation has now markedly improved.

Threats Posed by Careless Disposal

Mismanagement of hazardous wastes can adversely affect human health and environmental quality in a number of ways.

Direct Contact

Direct contact with wastes can result in skin irritation, the initiation of serious chronic illness, or acute poisoning—as in the case of two 9-year-old Tampa boys who were killed in June 1992, while playing inside a municipal waste bin. Subsequent investigations revealed that the bin, located behind an industrial firm, contained toluene- and acetone-contaminated waste, leading officials to conclude the boys had died due to inhalation of toxic chemical fumes.

Fire and/or Explosions

In April 1980, a spectacular blaze destroyed a riverside warehouse complex in Elizabeth, New Jersey, where 50,000 chemical-containing drums had been sitting for almost 10 years. Such accidents are a constant threat when hazardous wastes are in transit, carelessly stored, or roughly handled. Explosions are a particular threat to workers at landfills accepting hazardous wastes. In Edison, New Jersey, a bulldozer operator who inadvertently crushed a container of flammable phosphorus was burned so quickly that his corpse was discovered with his hand still on the gearshift.

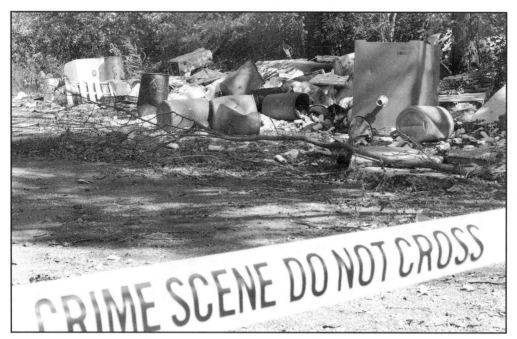

Containers of unknown chemicals leak their contents into the ground at an illegal dump site in Illinois. Such careless disposal of hazardous wastes can result in ground-water or surface water contamination, pose a poisoning threat to humans and wildlife, and constitute a fire/explosion hazard. [*Illinois Environmental Protection Agency*]

Poison via the Food Chain

Biomagnification of toxic wastes discharged into the environment can result in the poisoning of animals or humans who consume the toxin indirectly. The tragic outbreak of methyl mercury poisoning at Minamata, Japan, typifies this sort of situation.

Air Pollution

When toxic wastes are burned at temperatures insufficiently high to completely destroy them, serious air pollution problems can result. Only specialized types of equipment are licensed for the incineration of hazardous wastes, and even these must be carefully monitored while operating to ensure a complete burn.

Surface Water Contamination

Accidental spills or deliberate dumping of hazardous wastes can easily pollute waterways. The extent and duration of environmental damage to surface waters varies widely, depending on the size of the water body in question and the rate of flow, but short-term damage to aquatic ecosystems can be severe. In Butte, Montana, location of the largest Superfund complex in the nation, several hundred snow geese died in 1995 soon after landing on a lake of toxic wastewater that had formed at an open-pit mine. Post-mortem analyses of the birds revealed acid-burned esophagi, indicating they died from drinking the highly polluted water. Public drinking water supplies also can be endangered by hazardous waste discharges; municipal water intake points occasionally must be closed until the plume of pollution from an accidental spill flows past.

Groundwater Contamination

The most common problem associated with poor hazardous waste management is the pollution of aquifers with toxic leachates percolating downward through the soil from landfills or surface impoundments. This type of pollution is particularly insidious because it is seldom discovered until it is too late to do anything about it. Citizens in numerous communities around the nation have discovered to their horror that they had unknowingly been consuming well water contaminated with a variety of toxic chemicals that entered the groundwater supply via seepage from disposal sites.

Methods of Hazardous Waste Disposal

Historically, the largest percentage of hazardous wastes has been disposed of on land, primarily because land disposal, particularly prior to government regulation of hazardous waste management, was by far the cheapest option. During the mid-1970s, for example, almost half of all hazardous wastes, the majority of which were in the form of liquids or sludges, were simply dumped into unlined surface impoundments, technically referred to as "pits, ponds, or lagoons," located on the generators' property. These wastes eventually evaporated or percolated into the soil, often resulting in groundwater contamination. Other wastes, about 30% of the total, were buried in sanitary landfills, easily subject to leaching, and another 10% were burned in an uncontrolled manner. None of these methods would be in compliance with current regulations.

Although many citizens are convinced that no methods exist for the safe disposal of hazardous wastes, a number of new technologies have been developed which avoid most of the shortcomings inherent in past hazardous waste management practices. All such methods, not surprisingly, are considerably more expensive than simply dumping wastes in a pit or a municipal landfill, and thus were not widely utilized until strict regulatory action was taken by Congress. A listing of legal hazardous waste disposal options would include the following.

Secure Chemical Landfill

Generally, the cheapest method of hazardous waste disposal is the so-called "secure" chemical landfill, a specially designed earthen excavation constructed in such a way as to contain dangerous chemicals and to prevent them from escaping into the environment through leaching or vaporization. In the past, secure landfills frequently differed from sanitary landfills only in that they were topped with a layer of clay to keep water out of the trenches in which chemical drums had been placed. This of course did not prevent chemical seepage from contaminating water supplies. Under current RCRA standards, a secure chemical landfill must be located above the 100-year floodplain and away from fault zones; it must contain double liners of clay or synthetic materials to keep leaching to a minimum; a network of pipes must be laid to collect and control polluted rainwater and leachate accumulating in the landfill; and monitoring wells must be installed to check the quality of any groundwater deposits in the area (surface water supplies must also be monitored by the landfill operator). In spite of these precautions, most experts agree that there is no way to guarantee that sometime in the future contaminants will not migrate from the landfill site. Liners eventually crack; soil can shift or settle. Since many chemical wastes remain hazardous more or less indefinitely, serious pollution problems can occur many years after a secure chemical landfill has been closed and forgotten. Many authorities feel that although chemical landfills are legal, they are the least acceptable method of managing hazardous wastes.

Since 1984 when more stringent requirements for groundwater monitoring, minimum technology standards, and financial guarantees for post-closure activities took

effect, the number of operating facilities has dropped substantially. By 2010 there were just 21 commercial hazardous waste landfills operating in the United States and five in Canada, compared to more than 1,000 during the 1970s. Over the past two decades, the list of wastes for which disposal in landfills is prohibited has been steadily growing; federal legislation enacted in 1984 and fully implemented by 1990 imposed a ban on the landfilling of virtually all hazardous wastes, unless such materials undergo prior treatment to minimize their toxicity and ability to migrate. The explicit intent of such legislation is to reduce reliance on land disposal and to encourage the use of alternative technologies to the greatest extent possible.

Deep Well Injection

The use of deep wells for waste disposal dates back to the late 19th century when the petroleum industry employed this method to get rid of salt brine, but its use for liquid hazardous waste disposal began only during the 1940s. A number of industries, most notably petroleum refineries and petrochemical plants, now utilize this disposal method. Commercial deep well injection currently is practiced only in the Midwest and in Texas and neighboring states, although many other injection wells operated by private firms solely for the disposal of their own wastes are widely scattered across the United States. The process involves pumping liquid wastes through lined wells into porous rock formations deep underground, well below any drinking water aquifers. Some critics point out that cracks in the well casing or undetected faults in the earth that intersect the disposal zone could result in outward migration of wastes. EPA contends that deep wells

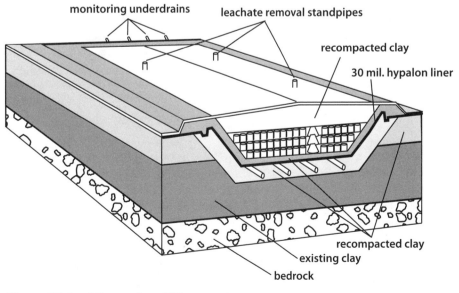

Figure 17-6 A Secure Landfill

are safe, provided that they are constructed, operated, and maintained in accordance with agency regulations.

Various Chemical, Physical, or Biological Treatment Processes

Processes that render wastes nonhazardous or significantly reduce their volume or toxicity have assumed major importance in recent years, particularly as more and more "land bans" have been implemented, prohibiting the landfilling of untreated wastes. With economic motivation spurring invention, a number of promising new technologies are now in the pilot project phase or fully operational, promising safer, more effective ways of cleaning up past mistakes and ensuring that wastes currently being generated are properly managed.

Physical methods include **evaporation** to concentrate corrosive brines, **sedimentation** to separate solids from liquid wastes, **carbon adsorption** to remove certain soluble organic wastes, and **air-stripping** to remove volatile organic compounds from groundwater.

Chemical techniques involve processes such as **neutralization** to render wastes harmless, sulfide **precipitation** to extract certain toxic metals, **oxidation-reduction** processes to convert some metals from a hazardous to a nonhazardous state, and **stabilization/solidification**, in which the waste material is detoxified and then combined with a cement-like material, encapsulated in plastic, blended with organic polymers, or combined with silica to form a solid, inert substance that can be disposed of safely in a landfill or incorporated into road beds. Another innovative technology is **in-situ vitrification (ISV)**, a process that relies on large amounts of electricity (about 750 kilowatt-hours per ton of soil) delivered by giant electrodes fixed at several locations in the soil surrounding the area undergoing cleanup. Suitable for detoxifying soils contaminated with toxic organics (e.g., chlorinated pesticides), heavy metals, or radioactive wastes, ISV actually melts the soil as the electricity flows through it, fusing the toxics into a solid block of glassified material, similar to natural obsidian. The solidified

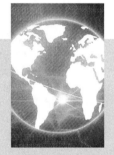

· · · · · · · 17-5 · · · · · · ·
Pollution Prevention

Just as municipal waste management strategies emphasize the value of waste prevention as opposed to cleanup, so does national policy for hazardous waste management stress the importance of reducing the amount and toxicity of waste generated—an approach referred to among waste managers as **P2 (pollution prevention)**. P2 is a concept that has gradually been winning adherents since 1984, when Congress passed the Hazardous and Solid Waste Amendments to RCRA and decreed that "the generation of hazardous waste is to be reduced or eliminated as expeditiously as possible." EPA was told to issue waste minimization regulations designed to increase awareness among industrial managers of waste reduction possibilities and to encourage voluntary initiatives aimed at lowering the amounts of waste generated. In 1990, pollution prevention became an official environmental policy of the United States when Congress enacted the **Pollution Prevention Act**. Subsequently, under its Waste Minimization Program, EPA has made reduced generation of wastes containing any of 30 "priority chemicals" its top goal, urging manufacturers to employ production methods that minimize, substitute, or completely eliminate such chemicals wherever possible.

Although the corporate world's initial response was tentative, P2 has now become a buzzword among savvy managerial types who recognize that implementing effective pollution prevention programs is a key to economic competitiveness. Not simply a public-relations ploy to appease the "green faction," corporate policies to reduce waste at the source constitute economically sound business decisions, since in today's highly regulated world it is far cheaper and more efficient to avoid the generation of waste rather than try to clean it up after the fact. Not only can effective P2 strategies save money on pollution abatement costs but by using raw materials more efficiently they also contribute to lower production costs. Fears of potential liability under the federal Superfund program have also been a strong motivating force for the adoption of pollution prevention programs—the fewer wastes shipped off-site for disposal, the less a company needs to fret about being cited as a "potentially responsible party" when a land disposal facility springs a leak!

The opportunities for significantly reducing the industrial waste stream are numerous—and often require minimal capital investment. Methods that can be employed with significant results include:

1. *Changing manufacturing processes.* By switching from an acid spray to a mechanical scrubber using pumice and rotating brushes to clean copper sheeting at its electronics plant in Columbia, Missouri, the 3M Corporation reduced its generation of liquid hazardous wastes by 40,000 pounds annually. Similarly, the need to reduce generation of lead waste during cab-salvaging operations led Springfield, Ohio-based International Truck and Engine Corporation to replace their use of lead solder with a portable device that pulls dents out of metal, eliminating the need for solder to fill in defects; by doing so, the company not only eliminated a workplace health hazard but also reduced the time required for repairs from two hours to five minutes per cab.

2. *Reformulating the product.* In a plastics factory in New Jersey, Monsanto changed the formula for an industrial adhesive it was producing; in doing so, it eliminated the need for filtering the product and thus no longer had any hazardous filtrate or filters requiring disposal.

3. *Substituting a nonhazardous chemical for a hazardous one in the manufacturing process.* In Pennsylvania, American Video Glass Company (AV) instituted a number of innovative strategies to minimize releases of lead while manufacturing TV picture tubes. By replacing lead oxide with zirconium oxide as shielding in the glass panel, AV reduced its lead consumption by 1,800 tons/year and its generation of lead-containing wastes by 125 tons annually. Performance of the new zirconium oxide shielding compares favorably with that of lead shielding; the substitution of zirconium oxide shielding allowed AV to increase the size of its glass panels, enhancing the company's competitive position and thereby benefiting both the environment and AV's bottom line.

4. *Changing equipment.* Simply by adding a condenser to an existing piece of equipment, a USS Chemicals plant in Ohio was able to capture escaping emissions of cumene, returning them to the phenol process unit. By so doing, the company solved an air quality problem and recaptured a major raw material.

5. *Altering the way hazardous wastes are handled in-plant.* Basically housekeeping changes, efforts at minimizing spills and using chemicals more conservatively can make a considerable difference in the amount of hazardous wastes generated. Segregating wastes to reduce contamination can also have a major impact. In Fremont, California, the Borden Chemical Company reduced the phenol content of its wastewater by 93% simply by separately collecting and reusing rinsewaters used to clean resin-contaminated filters. Formerly the company had allowed this rinsewater to flow into floor drains where it contaminated all the wastewater that flowed from the factory to a sewage treatment plant. American Video prevented accidental release of toxics-contaminated wastewater into city sewers simply by eliminating floor drains.

Not only do the approaches just described reduce the amounts of hazardous waste requiring disposal, they also save the companies that utilize them a great deal of money. The catch phrase "Pollution Prevention Pays," coined by the 3M Corporation, rings true in case after case. In one year after changing its process for cleaning copper sheeting, 3M saved $15,000 in raw materials, waste disposal, and labor costs; International Truck and Engine estimates that its $1,700 investment in the LP-1000 Lenco dent puller saves the company approximately $125,000 annually in labor and materials costs; by recovering 400,000 pounds of cumene after installation of a $5,000 condenser, USS Chemicals saved $100,000 in raw materials.

Until recently, many companies failed to take a comprehensive view of their waste streams—pinpointing precisely where wastes were generated and the exact management cost of each waste. By lumping all waste treatment, disposal, and oversight expenses together, corporate accountants denied themselves the opportunity of identifying specific process control points where considerable savings could be achieved. More recently, assisted and encouraged by state and federal voluntary programs such as EPA's National Partnership for Environmental Priorities, as well as by enlightened self-interest, a growing number of firms are conducting intensive waste audits, instituting cost-accounting procedures, and involving employees at all levels to identify opportunities for pollution prevention. While wholehearted endorsement of P2 principles within conservative corporate boardrooms is not yet universal, the transition is now well underway (EPA Office of Solid Waste, 2004).

material can simply be left in place, no longer posing any environmental threat.

Bioremediation, based on the ability of microbes, fungi, or plants to break down or absorb organic pollutants or toxic metals, is increasingly used for cleanup of oil spills and remediation of contaminated soil and groundwater. The largest number of projects utilizes various species of naturally occurring bacteria. By far the most widely used method of bioremediation is **biostimulation**, in which oxygen and/or nutrients are added to contaminated material to promote more rapid growth of indigenous microbes, resulting in faster, more efficient metabolism of wastes than would have occurred without human intervention. In situations where resident bacteria are too few in number, even with biostimulation, to degrade wastes effectively or when the microbes naturally present are genetically incapable of breaking down a particular waste, it may be necessary to utilize **bioaugmentation**. In such situations, nonindigenous species are added to "lend a hand," working in concert with the local microbes to accomplish pollutant removal more rapidly and completely. In a quest to create new bacterial strains better able to degrade chemicals under specific environmental conditions, scientists have been working to develop genetically engineered microbes (GEMs) to destroy pollutants that have proven resistant to breakdown by naturally occurring species. In order to avoid any possible risk to human health or the environment, the use of GEMs is strictly regulated under the Toxic Substances Control Act, which requires that they undergo a rigorous safety review prior to approval for field use.

Controlled Incineration

Because burning at very high temperatures actually destroys hazardous wastes (as opposed to storing them out of sight underground as is essentially the case with various land disposal methods), many hazardous waste management experts regard controlled incineration as the best and, in some cases, the only environmentally acceptable means of disposal. In spite of its relatively high cost compared to other hazwaste management options, controlled incineration is assuming increased importance as land disposal regulations grow more restrictive. Waste generators, fearful of legal liability if their wastes migrate from a land disposal site, are increasingly likely to consider a management method that ensures total waste destruction. A controlled incinerator burns at temperatures ranging from 750–3000°F, with wastes, air, and fuel being thoroughly mixed to ensure complete combustion. Afterburners, which are part of the incineration system, destroy any gaseous hydrocarbons that may have survived the initial incineration process, while scrubbers and electrostatic precipitators remove pollutant emissions from the stack gases.

In 1999, EPA further tightened nationwide standards for air emissions from hazwaste combustors. The new regulations required all commercial hazardous waste incinerators (22 operating in the U.S. in 2010), cement kilns, and other facilities that burn hazwastes to achieve a 70% reduction in dioxins and furans as well as reductions in mercury and lead emissions up to 86%. The technologies employed to lower concentrations of these pollutants also reduce emissions of particulates, carbon monoxide, hydrocarbons, hydrochloric acid, and other toxic metals. The stringent requirements were justified as necessary to protect the health and environment of the 37 million U.S. residents living in the vicinity of hazardous waste combustors.

Waste Exchanges

The ideal way to manage hazardous materials would be to recycle them, thus preventing their entry into the waste stream and eliminating the disposal problem. This is the idea that prompted the establishment of waste exchanges, which act as helpful third parties in establishing contact between waste generators and potential waste users. For example, a paint manufacturer, faced with the problem of how to dispose of hazardous sludges from a mixing operation, contacts a waste exchange and is referred to another company which willingly purchases the sludge to use as a filler coat on cement blocks. Thus, the paint manufacturer avoids the high cost of disposal in a secure chemical landfill or controlled incinerator and also makes a modest profit on the sale of the waste. The buyer, too, is pleased with the arrangement because a needed raw material is obtained for a lower price than unused filler would have cost; and society is well served because a potentially hazardous substance has been prevented from entering the environment.

The first waste exchange program began in the Netherlands in 1972. The Midwest Industrial Waste Exchange, started in 1975 in St. Louis, was the first U.S. program, the forerunner of approximately 160 waste and materials exchanges throughout the U.S. and Canada, some coordinated by state or local governments, others run by private, for-profit businesses. Although waste exchanges were originally developed exclusively for industrial hazardous waste trading, the concept has now expanded to include many exchanges dealing in nonhazardous waste materials (technically these are referred to as *materials exchanges*, while those dealing in hazardous wastes are termed *waste exchanges*). While some exchanges exist as actual waste warehouses that utilize printed catalogs to advertise their available commodities, many others are strictly Web sites that serve basically as information clearinghouses, connecting buyers and sellers. Subscribers are allowed to post notices regarding materials wanted for purchase of sale and those interested in the posted commodities then contact each other directly. The success of business-oriented materials exchanges has inspired individuals to get involved as well. In recent years The Freecycle Network™, a grassroots, nonprofit movement of nearly 5,000 local groups has spread worldwide, involving over 7 million people who give—or receive—unwanted items for free, keeping them in use and out of disposal facilities (to join a local Freecycle group, go to www.freecycle.org, find your community by entering it into the Search box, and sign up; membership is free). As waste disposal costs increase and familiarity with Internet-based trading expands, utilization of the services provided by materials and waste exchanges will continue to grow.

Siting Problems: From "NIMBY" to "BANANA"

Everyone wants hazardous wastes to be managed in ways that present the least possible threat to health or the environment, but no one wants to live near the site chosen for such storage, treatment, or disposal. Get rid of such wastes in the next county, a neighboring state, out in the desert, anyplace else—but "Not In My Back Yard!" (referred to as the "NIMBY" problem). This, in essence, is the siting dilemma which represents one of the most difficult obstacles faced by those trying to deal with municipal or hazardous wastes (not to mention *radioactive* refuse!) in a safe and responsible manner. Certainly waste disposal horror stories from Love Canal and countless other places across the nation have made citizens understandably nervous at the prospect of seeing hazardous waste management facilities locate in their communities. Nevertheless, if society desires to continue using products whose manufacture entails the production of hazardous wastes, improved waste-handling facilities are urgently needed. Inevitably, the best location for some of those facilities will be in someone's "back yard." Responsible decision making demands that citizens carefully evaluate the pros and cons of a site under consideration before automatically rejecting it. Laws governing the siting of hazardous waste facilities provide for public information and public participation programs during the siting process, though the scope for public input into the decision-making process varies widely from state to state. Before opposing or supporting a proposed facility, citizens should gather information on the following points:

- characteristics of the wastes involved
- nature of the proposed waste management process
- the design and manner of operation of the proposed facility
- the topographical, hydrogeological, and climatic characteristics of the site
- transportation routes to the site

Table 17-1   The ABCs of Waste Disposal

(Wall poster seen at the Environmental Protection Agency)

NIMBY	Not In My Back Yard
NIMFYE	Not In My Front Yard Either
PIITBY	Put It In Their Back Yard
NIMEY	Not In My Election Year
NIMTOO	Not In My Term Of Office
LULU	Locally Unwanted Land Use
NOPE	Not On Planet Earth

Source: *A Dictionary of Environmental Quotations*, Barbara K. Rodes and Rice Odell, eds., Simon & Schuster, 1992.

- safeguards to be employed at the facility
- potential for human or ecological exposure to hazardous chemicals released into the air, water, or soil
- location of the site in reference to population centers, farmland, or valuable natural areas (e.g., wetlands, endangered species' habitat, etc.)
- possible uses of site after closure

Public opposition has stymied acquisition of new hazardous waste management sites in recent years, with objectors mobilizing from far beyond the locality directly affected. Indeed, the sentiment prevailing among many activist groups has moved well beyond the familiar NIMBY to BANANA (Build Absolutely Nothing Anywhere Near Anything!). Unless society is willing to adopt a lifestyle in which no wastes whatsoever are generated (assuming this is even possible), a more reasonable, middle-ground approach to waste management decisions must be adopted. Protection of public health requires a new willingness on the part of citizens to sanction the siting of new facilities when a thorough review of site and operational considerations indicate that such facilities will not present serious environmental health problems.

HAZARDOUS WASTE MANAGEMENT LEGISLATION: RCRA

An evaluation of the types of hazardous waste incidents that have occurred indicate that we are basically dealing with two different categories of hazardous waste problems: how to manage the new volumes of chemical wastes being generated daily by American industry and what to do about wastes improperly disposed of years ago.

In order to tackle the first of these issues, the problem of newly created wastes, Congress in 1976 enacted the **Resource Conservation and Recovery Act (RCRA—** pronounced "rickra" in bureaucratese) which mandates that EPA:

- define which wastes are hazardous

- institute a "manifest system" to track the movement of hazardous wastes from the place they were generated to any off-site storage, treatment, or disposal facility

- set performance standards to be met by owners and operators of hazardous waste facilities

- issue permits for operation of such facilities only after technical standards have been met (operating licenses specify which types of wastes may be managed at that facility; thus most hazardous waste disposal sites are authorized to accept only certain classes of wastes)

- help states to develop hazardous waste management programs of their own which may be more stringent than the federal program, but which cannot be less so

RCRA took effect in 1980 when EPA finally issued its generator and transporter regulations (i.e., manifest requirements) and marked an important step forward in responsible hazardous waste management. However, it soon became apparent that the 1976 law featured some glaring loopholes that needed to be plugged. There was also mounting sentiment in Congress and elsewhere that land disposal of hazardous wastes is the least desirable method of managing these substances and that legislation should encourage reliance on alternatives. Accordingly, when RCRA came before Congress for reauthorization in 1984, the original legislation was substantially strengthened with the enactment of the **Hazardous and Solid Waste Amendments (HSWA)**. Among the key provisions of this law are mandates that (1) significantly reduce the types of hazardous wastes which can be buried in landfills; (2) strengthen requirements for landfill design and operation; (3) bring into the regulatory framework hundreds of thousands of previously exempt "small quantity generators"—those who produce 100 kg (220 lbs.) per month or more of hazardous wastes (under the original law, only those generators producing 1,000 kg or more per month were subject to regulation); and (4) create a whole new program for detecting and controlling leakage of hazardous liquids (mainly petroleum products) from underground storage tanks. Implementation of these new requirements, while making hazardous waste management considerably more expensive than it had been previously, gave new impetus to safer, more environmentally responsible waste management strategies.

While confronting the issue of newly generated wastes with an array of regulatory approaches, RCRA does nothing to deal with the serious problem posed by leaking abandoned dump sites. Even in the relatively few cases where the owners can be found, they often lack the financial resources to clean up the site, making litigation a futile exercise. Since EPA estimates there may be as many as 350,000 abandoned hazardous waste sites in the United States, the potential for future problems is obviously significant.

"Superfund"

Spurred by public demands that something be done to alleviate problems caused by old, leaking dump sites, Congress in December of 1980 enacted the **Comprehensive Environmental Response, Compensation, and Liability Act (CERCLA**, dubbed the "Superfund"), authorizing the expenditure of $1.6 billion over a five-year period for emergency cleanup activities and for the more long-term containment of hazardous waste dump sites (the legislation, however, did not include funds to compensate victims for health damage incurred by exposure to such sites—an issue which was the focus of considerable debate). EPA, in cooperation with the states, was charged with compiling a **National Priority List (NPL)** of sites considered to be sufficiently threatening to public health or environmental quality to make them eligible for Superfund cleanup dollars. These funds can be used either to remove hazardous substances from the site (a process which may also include temporary relocation of people in the area and provision of alternative water supplies) or for remedial measures such as storage and confinement of wastes, incineration, dredging, or permanent relocation of residents. In the years following passage of CERCLA, many states enacted their own "mini-Superfund" laws, aimed at forcing similar cleanups on sites where contamination wasn't bad enough to qualify for placement on the NPL but sufficiently threatening to warrant remediation.

Table 17-2   2007 CERCLA Priority List of Hazardous Substances

1 Arsenic
2 Lead
3 Mercury
4 Vinyl chloride
5 Polychlorinated biphenyls
6 Benzene
7 Cadmium
8 Polycyclic aromatic hydrocarbons
9 Benzo(A)pyrene
10 Benzo(B)fluoranthene
11 Chloroform
12 DDT, P, P'-
13 Aroclor 1254
14 Aroclor 1260
15 Dibenzo(A,H)anthracene
16 Trichloroethylene
17 Dieldrin
18 Chromium, hexavalent
19 Phosphorus, white
20 Chlordane

Source: Agency for Toxic Substances and Disease Registry. Accessed November 2010 from http://www.atsdr.cec.gov/cercla/07list.html

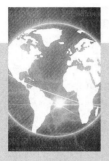

$\cdots\cdots$ 17-6 $\cdots\cdots$

Underground Storage Tanks

In the early 1980s, as citizens became increasingly alarmed by the widespread scope of hazardous waste problems, people assumed that the threat was largely confined to industrial sites, leaky landfills, or out-of-the-way illegal dumps. It came as a shock, therefore, to discover that virtually every community in America, no matter how small, harbored invisible sources of potential contamination in the form of **underground storage tanks (USTs)** containing petroleum or other hazardous liquids. By 1984 the extent of the problem was regarded as so serious that when Congress enacted the Hazardous and Solid Waste Amendments (HSWA) to the Resource Conservation and Recovery Act, it created a whole new federal program to deal with the situation. "Subtitle I," the Underground Storage Tank Program, required EPA to develop comprehensive regulations to protect public health and the environment from leaking underground storage tank systems. Groundwater pollution was the primary concern, since even small amounts of pollution can render groundwater supplies unusable without expensive treatment.

At the time the new regulations were issued in 1988, EPA estimated the U.S. had over 2 million underground storage tank systems (i.e., underground tanks with their associated piping) at approximately 700,000 locations nationwide. Of those, between 25–30% were believed to be leaking their contents into the surrounding soil and aquifers; an additional 50% posed a significant threat of leakage and environmental harm. This sorry state of affairs stemmed from the fact that, until the mid-1980s, most tanks were made of bare steel without any form of corrosion protection and hence were subject to gradual deterioration. Subtitle I banned the installation of any new unprotected tanks as of 1985, but the older tanks remained an overwhelming problem.

Today that situation is well on its way to being resolved. Final UST regulations adopted in September of 1988 required that existing tank systems be replaced, upgraded, or closed (i.e., removed from the ground or filled with sand) by 1998. Owners failing to meet this deadline were advised they would face stiff fines for not complying with the law. The regulations further stipulated that all new tanks must conform with minimum standards that require corrosion protection as well as spill and overflow prevention equipment for the great majority of USTs that contain petroleum. In addition, secondary containment (i.e., essentially a double lining) and interstitial monitoring to detect potential leaks are mandated for the estimated 25,000 USTs that contain hazardous substances (Nordi, 1995).

Most tank owners lacked the financial resources to comply with these requirements, since upgrading a tank can cost more than $12,000 while a new one is about $30,000. Simply closing a tank carries a tab of $5,000–11,000. Accordingly, in 1986 Congress created the Leaking Underground Storage Tank Trust Fund, providing funds for cleanups at sites where the owner of a tank is deceased or can't be located, is financially incapable of responding, or in cases requiring emergency action. Many state governments similarly have created special funds to expedite tank removals. By the time the federal deadline expired in December 1998, the majority of tank owners had complied with EPA regulations. During the preceding ten-year period, a million USTs had been closed or replaced, while an additional 600,000 were upgraded to prevent leakage. Four years later, in December 2002, 81% of the remaining 698,000 federally regulated USTs were in compliance with rules pertaining to spill and overflow prevention and corrosion protection; 74% met the requirements for leak detection. These figures mark a vast improvement over the situation a decade earlier, but indicate that problems still remain; accordingly, EPA is focusing on improving compliance with UST regulations. In addition, since a number of releases have been reported from USTs that were in full compliance with existing regulations, the agency is now conducting field investigations and working in partnership with industry and academic researchers to analyze the components and processes of UST systems in order to determine what improvements might be needed (EPA, 2003b).

Tank removal, replacement, and performance evaluation are only partial solutions to USTs' past legacy of pollution, however. Expensive cleanup efforts at thousands of sites where corroding tanks silently leaked their contents into soil and groundwater for years have been underway since the 1990s, and by mid-2009 almost 381,000 government-financed cleanups had been completed; nevertheless, another 100,000 UST-contaminated sites were still awaiting remediation. Addressing these remaining problems will be facilitated by the $200 million included in the 2009 American Recovery and Reinvestment Act—stimulus dollars that EPA estimates will pay for at least 1,600 UST cleanup projects. The task remaining is immense and will likely continue for several decades; nevertheless, notable progress has been made in the decades since attention first focused on the "ticking time bombs" buried in every community across the land.

The original federal Superfund bill expired in September 1985, and in spite of public demands for speedy reauthorization so that cleanup work could proceed without interruption, the law was not renewed until late the following year. Extreme congressional dissatisfaction with the excruciatingly slow rate of progress during Superfund's first years led to several significant changes in the 1986 **Superfund Amendments and Reauthorization Act (SARA)**. Realizing that 1980 funding levels were inadequate, Congress in 1986 increased Superfund allocations to $8.5 billion to be spent over the next five years and in 1990 allocated an additional $5.1 billion for the program. EPA was given mandatory deadlines for initiating site-specific cleanup plans and remediation activities. Concerned that previous cleanup actions represented little more than moving contaminated wastes from one site to another site, which would itself then become eligible for Superfund status, Congress specified a preference for cleanup actions which "permanently and significantly" reduce the volume, toxicity, or mobility of hazardous substances. This mandate has given a major impetus to development of treatment or disposal technologies (e.g., mobile incinerators that can be moved from one Superfund site to another) which permit hazardous wastes to be destroyed or detoxified on site, thereby avoiding the risks of transporting such wastes to another facility where they might cause future problems.

Several contentious policy issues have provoked heated debate among Superfund supporters and critics since the program's inception. One involves the extent of remediation necessary—how clean is clean enough? While many citizens demand that remediation restore a contaminated site to its original condition, critics complain that it makes no sense to spend millions of dollars to remove every last trace of contamination on a site destined to be paved over for a parking lot. Carol Browner, EPA Administrator during the Clinton administration, acknowledged the validity of such criticism and predicted ". . . there will be different levels of clean." Undoubtedly, the most controversial feature of the Superfund program has been its liability provisions that can hold the owner of a contaminated site (i.e., the **potentially responsible party**) responsible for multimillion dollar cleanup costs, even if that person or company was not directly responsible for the contamination (e.g., a small businessman who unknowingly purchased a property where a former owner, now deceased, dumped hazardous liquids that subsequently contaminated soil and groundwater can himself be held responsible for remediating the site). While business interests demand changes in what they regard as an inherently unfair provision, environmental

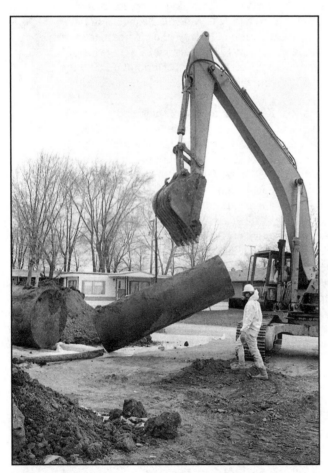

Workers with the Illinois EPA oversee the removal of a leaking underground storage tank. [*Illinois Environmental Protection Agency*]

advocates strongly support the status quo, insisting that concerns about **Superfund liability** alone have caused generators to be much more conscientious about managing their wastes in a responsible manner and have given major impetus to serious pollution prevention efforts.

Since passage of Superfund legislation in 1980, the number of listed NPL sites has grown from an original 400 to 1,281 as of October 2010, with an additional 62 proposed for listing. By early 2010 construction had been completed at 1,082 of these sites and cleanup finished at 341. Although most Americans enthusiastically support

the concept of cleaning up the nation's hazardous waste mistakes of the past, congressional support of the program has waned in recent years. Until the mid-1990s, the lion's share of funding to pay for cleanup of abandoned sites came from a tax on the petroleum and chemical industries—a "superfund" whose creation reflected the prevailing "polluter pays" principle. For obvious reasons, this tax had always been unpopular with the targeted industries and in 1995 federal legislators yielded to corporate pressure and refused to reauthorize the tax. For the next few years EPA continued to finance cleanups

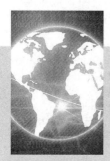

· · · · · · · 17-7 · · · · · · ·

Revitalizing Communities through "Brownfields" Redevelopment

In cities across America, particularly in the industrial Northeast and Midwest, aging cities are pockmarked by boarded-up gas stations, abandoned factories, and rubble-strewn lots. Although located in close proximity to transportation services, utilities, and a willing workforce, these properties have been bypassed by developers and constitute a visual and economic blight on urban neighborhoods. Known as **brownfields**, these underused, idled, or abandoned sites are shunned because of actual or suspected environmental contamination. Fearing legal liability for cleanup costs, prospective buyers have chosen to avoid any potential headaches, opting instead for construction on "greenfields" in the suburbs. In doing so, they have thwarted inner-city residents' dreams of economic development, put still-clean lands at risk of future contamination, and exacerbated concerns about urban sprawl. Far from being irrational or discriminatory, developers' decisions have been based on the reality that, under CERCLA's "strict, joint and several" liability provisions, property owners could find themselves responsible for multimillion dollar cleanups, even though the contamination problems were caused by a previous owner many decades earlier. In addition, a developer's likelihood of being able to obtain financing for construction on a brownfield property was virtually negligible, as lending institutions have been extremely reluctant to finance development for fear that they, too, could incur unlimited liability under Superfund if the property owner were to default or disappear.

This seemingly intractable dilemma was confronted head-on in January 1995, when EPA launched its **Brownfields Action Agenda**. A visionary and aggressive program for restoring blighted properties to productive use while promoting job development and community participation in decision-making, the brownfields initiative has brought entrepreneurial activity and a new sense of hope to urban areas long mired in depression and decay.

The potential scope of brownfields reclamation efforts is immense. Estimates of the number of contaminated sites nationwide range from 350,000 to as many as a million. On most of these properties levels of contamination are low to moderate; Superfund-type sites that present a serious environmental health risk are not included in the brownfields program. A sizeable portion of brownfields are sites contaminated by gasoline leaking from underground storage tanks. Others may be old dry-cleaning establishments where solvents were dumped on a back lot or abandoned factories with heavy metals contamination. Although most designated sites are urban, brownfields can be found in suburban and rural areas as well.

The Brownfields Action Agenda includes four major initiatives.

1. Grants for brownfields projects comprise the foundation of EPA's program by providing funds for site assessment, remediation, and job training. Federal dollars invested in brownfields projects have had a multiplier effect, leveraging over $6.5 billion from private, state, and local sources for cleanups and redevelopment.

2. Clarification of liability and cleanup issues. Since uncertainty regarding future liability for cleanup at polluted sites has been the main deterrent to restoration of brownfields, several important actions have been taken under this initiative. A major step was EPA's removal of approximately 25,000 locations from the list of potential Superfund sites. The sites deleted were ones already designated by the agency as "no further response action planned," meaning they were not sufficiently contaminated ever to make the NPL. Nevertheless, the fact that they had been retained in the Superfund archives was a deterrent to potential developers, making their deletion from the list a symbolically reassuring action. Equally important was congressional enactment in 2002 of the Small Business Liability Relief and Brownfields Revitalization Act, which limited the potential liability of brownfields purchasers to cleanup costs known at the time of purchase, thereby removing one of the major deterrents to brownfields cleanup. Although a number of states had already enacted similar legislation, passage of the federal law freed developers from any worry that unpleasant surprises discovered later on could entail large, unanticipated expenses for remediation. For those whose property lies above an aquifer contaminated by groundwater flow from an adjacent polluted site, the law guarantees freedom from liability for groundwater cleanup so long as they did not cause or contribute to the pollution.

One of the most critical issues addressed by the brownfields initiative was the "How clean is clean enough?" question. Insistence on the near-pristine standards required for remediated Superfund sites would doom the brownfields program by making such ventures cost-prohibitive. Accordingly, EPA and many state environmental agencies have introduced the concept of **risk-based corrective action (RBCA**—referred to in agency jargon as "Rebecca"). Originally applied to the remediation of petroleum-contaminated UST sites, RBCA is a decision-making process in which the required level of cleanup is based on real-life exposure risks, rather than on the assumption that the entire population of an area will be exposed to the maximum level of contamination present. Thus the degree of cleanup is based on the intended future use of a site. For example, a piece of land where trace amounts of lead remain in the soil could be covered with asphalt and used as a shopping mall parking lot without endangering anyone. If the same property were intended for use as a children's playground, higher cleanup standards would be in order.

3. Partnerships and outreach. Every brownfields project aims to establish a cooperative working relationship among federal agencies, states, cities, and community groups. Issues of environmental justice and the empowerment of brownfields area residents, encouraging their participation in decision-making, are key elements in this initiative.

4. Job development and training. A report issued by the Northeast-Midwest Institute categorically stated that "Brownfields and employment problems go together." EPA emphasizes the importance of ensuring that brownfields redevelopment benefits area residents by providing both short- and long-term employment opportunities. To guarantee the availability of a locally based, well-trained labor pool, the Brownfields Action Agenda is establishing partnerships with local educational institutions, striving to develop long-term programs for worker training.

Since the Brownfields program was created in 1995, estimates of the number of eligible sites across the nation have been estimated as exceeding 450,000 and hundreds of projects have gotten underway. Geographically, these projects span the nation and include a computer-controlled greenhouse for tomato production in Buffalo, New York; a greenway featuring a bike path linking a series of linear parks in Providence, Rhode Island; an upscale shopping and restaurant district in Charlotte, North Carolina; and a community day care facility for more than 200 children on Chicago's West Side. All were built on abandoned, contaminated sites long viewed as worthless.

Recently the EPA has launched a new program—Re-Powering America's Land (RE-PAL)—aimed at recovering brownfields and other potentially contaminated land and mine sites for renewable energy generation. Since brownfields often have roads, water, and electric transmission lines already on site and are usually appropriately zoned for such uses, developing them for wind, solar, or biomass projects offers both economic and environmental benefits. A case in point is Steel Winds Wind Farm in Lackawanna, New York, where eight wind turbines have been installed on an old slag pile at the Bethlehem Steel site, producing enough electricity to power 7,000 homes.

Brownfields initiatives throughout the country are revitalizing American communities. By restoring degraded sites to new uses, increasing property values, and stimulating tax revenues, brownfields developments are improving the quality of life in hundreds of low-income neighborhoods.

Table 17-3   States with the Most Listed NPL Sites (2010)

New Jersey	111
Pennsylvania	95
California	94
New York	86
Michigan	67
Florida	54
Washington	48
Texas	48
Illinois	44
Wisconsin	38
North Carolina	35
Ohio	34
Indiana	32
Massachusetts	31
Virginia	31
South Carolina	26
Minnesota	25
Total, October 2010:	1,281

Source: EPA, 2010.

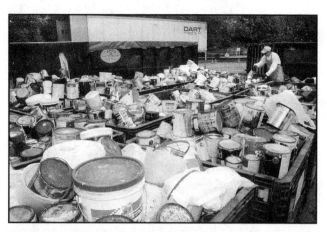

Household hazardous wastes are separated at a state-wide collection event in Illinois. [*Illinois Environmental Protection Agency*]

with the dollars remaining in the rapidly dwindling Superfund account. Once that source of funding was exhausted, however, the agency became wholly dependent on general tax revenues annually appropriated by Congress. Remediation activities at many of the nation's most contaminated sites proceeded at a crawl or halted altogether for several years until passage of the 2009 American Recovery and Reinvestment Act (ARRA) allocated $600 million specifically to facilitate further cleanup at Superfund sites. Hopes are high that in the years immediately ahead many more NPL sites will undergo the removal of immediate threats and long-term protection through site remediation.

Household Hazardous Wastes

Comforting references to "Home Sweet Home" are slightly less reassuring today than in years past. The invisible hazards posed by radon and other indoor air pollutants make us wonder if we'd be safer inhaling deeply at a busy intersection than in our paneled family room. More recently, the righteous indignation directed at corporate polluters who disregard public well-being by careless disposal of their toxic by-products is being tempered somewhat by the realization that all of us—whatever our occupations—contribute to the nation's hazardous waste woes through our use, misuse, and thoughtless disposal of hundreds of potentially dangerous household chemicals.

It is estimated that the average American generates about 20 pounds of household hazardous waste each year. Typical examples of such discarded materials include pesticides, paints and varnishes, brush cleaners,

ammonia, toilet bowl cleaners, bleaches and disinfectants, oven cleaners, furniture polish, swimming pool chemicals, batteries, motor oil, outdated medicines, and many others. Although these substances may be every bit as toxic, corrosive, flammable, or explosive as the industrial wastes regulated under RCRA, federal and state hazardous waste laws do not apply to the comparatively minor household sources. Nevertheless, the cumulative environmental impact of even small amounts of these materials being carelessly discarded by millions of individuals can be significant.

Household hazardous waste disposal presents a variety of concerns:

1. Stored inside the home, hazardous chemicals pose poisoning risks, particularly for children; some, such as paints and solvents, pose problems of indoor air pollution; others, ammonia and chlorine bleach, for example, can result in highly toxic emissions when inadvertently mixed; still others pose serious fire hazards.

2. The welfare of public employees can be threatened by hazardous household products. Home fires involving hazardous chemicals can result in explosions or the generation of toxic fumes that can kill or seriously injure firefighters. Refuse collectors frequently suffer injury when they throw garbage bags into compactor trucks, unaware that they contain corrosive or flammable materials. In November 1996, a refuse collector in New York was killed when doused with acid from a discarded battery mixed with the trash he tossed into the compacter of his garbage truck; one worker was killed and another critically injured in a fire at a recycling plant caused by aerosol cans fed into a baler (Pellow, 2002).

3. The environment itself can be seriously degraded when householders pour hazardous liquids into drains and flush them down toilets or into septic systems.

People who pour waste motor oil into storm sewers or dump paint cans in the woods can cause long-lasting damage to ground and surface water supplies. Throwing such hazardous materials in the trash may ultimately result in the threat of contaminated incinerator ash and air pollution or, alternatively, in the formation of toxic leachates at municipal landfills.

In an effort to raise public awareness about these problems and to provide concerned citizens with a safe and responsible way of getting rid of hazardous household wastes, an increasing number of communities, state environmental agencies, and public interest groups have been sponsoring household hazardous waste collection programs in recent years. These events have attracted large numbers of householders who are happy to take advantage of the opportunity to clean out the basement or garage and safely get rid of those old bottles of pesti- cides, paints—even ammunition—that may have been sitting on a shelf gathering dust for 20 years or more. Once wastes are brought to a collection center, they must be separated by type, packaged, and manifested as RCRA hazardous wastes by trained personnel (usually licensed hazardous waste transporters). They are then taken to a licensed facility for treatment, disposal, or recycling. The cost of running such programs, as well as concerns about legal liability, has limited their more widespread adoption. Nevertheless, these widely publicized efforts have had an impact far beyond the city limits of their sponsoring communities, enhancing public awareness of the fact that each one of us is a part of America's solid waste problem and pointing the way toward safer, more responsible ways of managing the hazardous by-products of our national lifestyle.

Appendix
· · · · · · · · A · · · · · · · ·

Environmental Agencies of the Federal Government

National policy-making regarding environmental health issues has been delegated among several different federal agencies and cabinet-level departments. Among the more important groups dealing with issues discussed in this book are:

Environmental Protection Agency (EPA)
www.epa.gov

Created by President Nixon in December 1970, the EPA is an independent agency formed to coordinate the administration of a wide range of environmental programs which, prior to that time, had been scattered among a number of governmental agencies and departments, several of which frequently worked at cross-purposes. EPA has been charged with setting and enforcing standards pertaining to air and water pollution, solid and hazardous waste management, noise, public water supplies, pesticides, and radiation (excluding that associated with nuclear power plants). All EPA actions are published in the *Federal Register* as proposed regulations, with time being allowed for public comment prior to their adoption as legally enforceable final regulations.

The Administrator of the EPA is appointed by the President of the United States and confirmed by the U.S. Senate. Although EPA headquarters are in the nation's capital, the agency has ten regional offices, each with its own regional administrator, responsible for the states within its region.

Council on Environmental Quality (CEQ)
www.whitehouse.gov/CEQ

Established by the National Environmental Policy Act signed by President Nixon on January 1, 1970, the CEQ operates within the Executive Office of the President. The CEQ coordinates federal environmental efforts and works closely with agencies and other White House offices in the development of environmental policies and initiatives. The council's chairperson is appointed by the president and serves as principal environmental policy advisor to the president.

Nuclear Regulatory Commission (NRC)
www.nrc.gov

A five-member civilian board that began operations on January 19, 1975, the NRC was created by the Energy Reorganization Act of 1974, which broke up the old Atomic Energy Commission (AEC) into the research-oriented Energy Research and Development Administration (subsequently absorbed by the Department of Energy) and the NRC. The Nuclear Regulatory Commission has jurisdiction over the licensing and regulation of nuclear reactors and also over the processing, transportation, and security of nuclear materials.

Office of Science and Technology Policy (OSTP)
www.ostp.gov

Established in 1976 within the Executive Office of the President, this agency advises the president on scientific and technological considerations involved in a wide range of national concerns, including health and the environment.

Consumer Product Safety Commission (CPSC)
www.cpsc.gov

This independent regulatory agency seeks to reduce unreasonable risks of injury associated with consumer products by encouraging the development of voluntary standards related to consumer product safety, requiring the reporting of hazardous consumer products and, if justified, recalling for corrective action hazardous products already on the market. The commission conducts research on consumer product hazards, can establish mandatory standards, and, if necessary, has the authority to ban hazardous consumer products.

Public Health Service (PHS)
www.usphs.gov

An office within the Department of Health and Human Services, the U.S. Public Health Service helps states and communities develop local health resources, conducts and supports medical research, and oversees other public health functions. Among the various subdivisions within the Public Health Service, a few are of particular environmental health interest:

Centers for Disease Control and Prevention (CDC)
www.cdc.gov

This agency is charged with protecting public health by providing leadership and direction in the prevention and control of disease. It administers programs related to communicable and vectorborne diseases, urban rat control, control of childhood lead-based paint poisoning, and a range of other environmental health problems. CDC also participates in a national program of research, information, and education regarding smoking and health. The nine major offices of the CDC are those dealing with epidemiology, international health, laboratory improvement, prevention services, environmental health, occupational safety and health, health promotion and education, professional development and training, and infectious diseases.

Food and Drug Administration (FDA)
www.fda.gov

The FDA's activities are aimed at protecting public health against impure and unsafe foods, drugs, cosmetics, and other possible hazards such as radiation. In carrying out its responsibilities, the FDA conducts research and develops standards for food, drugs, medical devices, veterinary medicines, and biologic products. Through its National Center for Toxicological Research, the FDA studies the biologic effects of potentially toxic chemicals in the environment.

Agency for Toxic Substances and Disease Registry (ATSDR)
www.atsdr.cdc.gov

This agency, based in Atlanta, Georgia, is a federal public health agency within the U.S. Department of Health and Human Services. The agency focuses on minimizing human health risks associated with exposure to hazardous substances. Although ATSDR is an independent operating division within the Department of Health and Human Services, the Centers for Disease Control and Prevention (CDC) perform many of its administrative functions. The CDC director also serves as the ATSDR administrator, and ATSDR has a joint Office of the Director with the National Center for Environmental Health (NCEH).

Unlike the Environmental Protection Agency (EPA), ATSDR is an advisory, non-regulatory agency. It conducts research on the health impacts of hazardous waste sites and provides information and recommendations to federal and state agencies, community members, and other interested parties. However, ATSDR is not involved in cleanup of those sites, nor can it provide or fund medical treatment for people who have been exposed to hazardous substances. Its functions include public health assessments of waste sites, health consultations concerning specific hazardous substances, health surveillance and registries, response to emergency releases of hazardous substances, applied research in support of public health assessments, information development and dissemination, and education and training concerning hazardous substances.

National Institute of Environmental Health Sciences (NIEHS)
www.niehs.nih.gov

One of 27 institutes of the National Institutes of Health (NIH), the mission of the NIEHS is to reduce the burden of human illness and disability by understanding how the environment influences the development and progression of human disease. NIEHS focuses on basic science, disease-oriented research, global environmental health, and multidisciplinary training for researchers. The institute funds centers for environmental health studies at universities across the United States.

National Toxicology Program (NTP)
www.ntp.niehs.nih.gov

This program was established in 1978 to coordinate toxicological testing programs within the Department of Health and Human Services. NTP develops and validates improved testing methods, generates data to strengthen scientific knowledge about potentially hazardous substances, and communicates with stakeholders. NTP is at the forefront in providing scientific information that improves our nation's ability to evaluate potential human health effects from chemical and physical exposures. NTP maintains a number of complex, interrelated research and testing programs that provide unique and critical information needed by health regulatory and research agencies to protect public health.

Occupational Safety and Health Administration (OSHA)
www.osha.gov

Operating within the Department of Labor, OSHA develops and promulgates safety and health standards and regulations for the American workforce. It conducts investigations and inspections of workplaces to ensure compliance with those regulations and can issue citations and propose penalties for employers who violate such standards.

Fish and Wildlife Service (FWS)

www.fws.gov

A bureau within the Department of the Interior, the Fish and Wildlife Service has jurisdiction over matters regarding endangered species, certain marine mammals, wild birds, inland sports fisheries, and wildlife research. The bureau carries out biological monitoring for effects of pesticides, heavy metals, and thermal pollution; it maintains wildlife refuges, enforces game laws, and carries out programs to control livestock predators and pest species. The bureau maintains a number of fish hatcheries, conducts environmental education and public information programs, and provides both national and international leadership regarding endangered fish and wildlife species.

Office of Surface Mining Reclamation and Enforcement (OSM)

www.osmre.gov

Another agency within the Interior Department, this office is charged with assisting states in developing a nationwide program to protect society and the environment during coal mining and reclamation and to reclaim mines abandoned before 1977.

Bureau of Land Management (BLM)

www.blm.gov

The BLM is responsible for managing the nation's 341 million acres of public lands, most of which are located in the West. In doing so, the bureau manages the timber, minerals, rangeland vegetation, wild and scenic rivers, wilderness areas, endangered species, and energy resources of these lands. A division of the Interior Department, BLM also is involved in watershed protection, development of recreational opportunities, and programs to protect and manage wild horses and burros. The bureau provides for the protection, orderly development, and use of public lands and resources under principles of multiple use and sustained yield. Criticism in recent years has focused on the bureau's overemphasis on permitting exploitation of public resources for private gain and insufficient protection and conservation of these resources.

Natural Resources Conservation Service (NRCS)

www.nrcs.usda.gov

An agency of the Department of Agriculture, the NRCS develops and carries out soil and water conservation programs in cooperation with landowners and operators, land developers, and community planning agencies. NRCS also is active in programs to control agricultural pollution and to bring about environmental improvement.

Emergency and Environmental Health Services (EEHS)

www.cdc.gov/nceh/eehs

CDC's National Center for Environmental Health/ Division of Emergency and Environmental Health Services (EEHS) provides national leadership in the development of environmental and emergency public health policy and prevention programs. EEHS provides consultation and technical and resource assistance to state and local health departments and to other agencies at the federal, state, local, and international levels. It also responds to national and international emergency and recovery assistance situations, especially after natural or technologic disasters, and provides technical support for public health activities during emergencies such as famines, disasters, and civil strife.

The division's major activities are chemical weapons elimination, environmental health services, healthy community design, lead poisoning prevention/healthy homes, and cruise ship sanitation.

National Response Center (NRC)

www.nrc.gov

Operated by the Coast Guard, the NRC is the U.S. government's sole point of contact for reporting all oil, chemical, radiological, biological, and etiological discharges into the environment anywhere in the U.S. and its territories. In addition to gathering and distributing spill data and serving as the communications and operations center for the National Response Team, the NRC maintains agreements with a variety of federal entities to make additional notifications regarding incidents meeting established trigger criteria.

U.S. Global Change Research Program (USGCRP)

www.globalchange.gov

The USGCRP coordinates and integrates federal research on changes in the global environment and their implications for society. It began as a presidential initiative in 1989 and was mandated by Congress in the Global Change Research Act of 1990, which called for a program which would help the U.S. and the world understand, assess, predict, and respond to human-induced and natural processes of global change.

National Oceanic and Atmospheric Administration (NOAA)

www.noaa.gov

The NOAA, part of the Department of Commerce, dates back to 1807, when the nation's first scientific agency, the Survey of the Coast, was established. Since then, NOAA has emerged as an international leader on scientific and environmental matters. Its mission is to understand and predict changes in Earth's environment and conserve and manage coastal and marine resources to meet our nation's economic, social, and environmental needs.

Office of Environmental Management (EM)

www.oem.gov

The Office of Environmental Management, within the Department of Energy, is charged with the safe cleanup of the environmental damage brought about by five decades of nuclear weapons development and government-sponsored nuclear energy research. The program is one of the largest, most diverse, and technically complex environmental cleanup programs in the world and includes responsibility for the remediation of 108 contaminated nuclear weapons manufacturing and testing sites across the U.S.

U.S. Geological Survey (USGS)
www.usgs.gov

The USGS is a scientific agency that provides information on the health of our ecosystems and environment. USGS scientists collect, monitor, and analyze information relating to atmosphere and climate, the impacts of land-use and climate change, environmental issues, natural hazards, water resources, and numerous other topics. Moreover, it is the nation's largest civilian mapping agency.

Appendix
...... B ......

Environmental Organizations

American Lung Association
www.lungusa.org

American Society of Professional Wetland Engineers
www.aspwe.org

Atlantic Coast Watch
www.atlanticcoastwatch.org

Basel Action Network
www.ban.org

Center for Health, Environment, and Justice
www.essential.org/cchw/

Center for Science in the Public Interest
www.cspinet.org

Clearwater
www.clearwater.org

Climate Action Network
www.climatenetwork.org

Cool Climate Jobs
www.coolclimatejobs.com

Cool the Earth
www.cooltheearth.org

Defenders of Wildlife
www.defenders.org

Ducks Unlimited, Inc.
www.ducks.org

Earth Policy Institute
www.earth-policy.org

Earthworks
www.earthworksaction.org

Energy Action Coalition
www.energyactioncoalition.org

Environmental Defense Fund
www.edf.org

Friends of the Earth
www.foe.org

Greenpeace USA, Inc.
www.greenpeace.org

International Union for Conservation of Nature (IUCN)
www.iucn.org

League of Conservation Voters
www.lcv.org

League of Women Voters
www.lwv.org

The Marine Mammal Center
www.marinemammalcenter.org

National Audubon Society
www.audubon.org

National Environmental Health Association
www.neha.org

National Geographic Society
www.nationalgeographic.com

National Religious Partnership for the Environment
www.nrpe.org

National Wildlife Federation
www.nwf.org

The Nature Conservancy
www.tnc.org

Natural Resources Defense Council
www.nrdc.org

Oil Change International
www.priceofoil.org

Pesticide Action Network North America
www.panna.org

Planned Parenthood Federation of America
www.plannedparenthood.org

Population Action International
www.populationaction.org

Population Connection
(formerly Zero Population Growth)
www.populationconnection.org

Population Reference Bureau
www.prb.org

Rainforest Action Network
www.ran.org

Rainforest Alliance
www.rainforestalliance.org

Sierra Club
www.sierraclub.org

Silicon Valley Toxics Coalition
www.svtc.org

Union of Concerned Scientists
www.ucsusa.org

The Wilderness Society
www.wilderness.org

Worldwatch Institute
www.worldwatch.org

World Resources Institute
www.wri.org

World Wildlife Fund
www.worldwildlife.org

References

Abramovitz, Janet N. 1998. "Taking a Stand: Cultivating a New Relationship with the World's Forests." *Worldwatch Paper* 140 (April).

Acid Rain: What It Is. 1982. National Wildlife Federation.

Action on Smoking and Health (ASH). 2004. "International Tobacco Treaty Has Strong Provisions . . . But We Must First Get It Ratified." *ASH Smoking and Health Review* 34, no. 1 (Jan/Feb): 4–5.

Adler, Robert W., Jessica Landman, and Diane Cameron. 1993. *The Clean Water Act: 20 Years Later.* Natural Resources Defense Council.

Adler, Tina. 2010. "Better Burning, Better Breathing: Improving Health with Cleaner Cookstoves." *Environmental Health Perspectives* 118, no. 3 (March): a124–a129.

Agency for Toxic Substances and Disease Registry (ATSDR). 1999. *Toxicological Profile for Mercury.* U.S. Dept. of Health and Human Services, Public Health Service.

———. 2000. *Public Health Statement for Polychlorinated Biphenyls (PCBs).* Accessed March 24, 2004, from http://atsdr1.atsdr.cdc.gov/ToxProfiles/phs8821.html

Agricultural Research Service (ARS). 2004. *Technologies in the Marketplace: Better Traps, Fewer Bugs.* Accessed March 16, 2009, from http://www.ars.usda.gov/business/docs.htm?docid=769

Air Pollution Primer. 1969. National Tuberculosis and Respiratory Disease Association.

Akre, Roger D., and Elizabeth A. Myhre. 1994. "The Great Spider Whodunit." *Pest Control Technology* 22, no. 4 (April).

Aldy, J. E., and R. N. Stavins. 2008. "Climate Policy Architectures for the Post-Kyoto World." *Environment* 50, no. 3 (May/June): 7–17.

Allison, Graham. 2004. *Nuclear Terrorism: The Ultimate Preventable Catastrophe.* New York: Time Books, Henry Holt and Company.

Allsop, Michelle, Adam Walters, David Santillo, and Paul Johnston. 2006. *Plastic Debris in the World's Oceans.* Amsterdam: Greenpeace.

Alston, Julian M., Jason M. Beddow, and Philip G. Pardy. 2009. "Agricultural Research, Productivity, and Food Prices in the Long Run." *Science* 325 (Sept. 4): 1209–1210.

Altman, Lawrence K. 1993. "Big Health Gains Found in Developing Countries," *New York Times*, July 7.

American Cancer Society. 2010. *Cancer Facts and Figures—2010.* Atlanta: American Cancer Society, Inc.

American Chemical Society. 1998. *Understanding Risk Analysis.*

American Council for an Energy Efficient Economy. 2007. *2007 Federal Energy Legislation: Estimates of Energy and Carbon Savings from Energy Bill Passed in Senate, Dec. 14.* Accessed from http://www.aceee.org/energy/national/07nrgleg.htm

American Council on Science and Health (ACSH). 2003. "Irradiated Foods." Accessed from http://www.acsh.org/publications/pub ID.198/pub_detail.asp

American Water Works Association (AWWA). 2003. *Protecting the Water: Drinking Water Security in America after 9/11.*

American Wind Energy Association (AWEA). 2008. *Wind Power—Clean AND Reliable.* Factsheet. Accessed June 2009 from www.awea.org

———. 2009. *Offshore Wind Energy.* Factsheet. Accessed June 2009 from www.awea.org

Anderson, Sarah. 2009a. "States Cool to Hosting DOE Long-Term Mercury Storage Site." *RadWaste Monitor* 2, nos. 16 & 17 (Double Edition): 12–14.

———. 2009b. "WCS Receives Final Disposal License From State Regulators." *RadWaste Monitor* 2, no. 20 (Sept. 21): 8–9.

Applied Foodservice Sanitation. 1985. John Wiley & Sons in cooperation with the Educational Foundation of the National Restaurant Association.

Armstrong, G. L., et al. 1999. "Trends in Infectious Disease Mortality in the United States During the 20th Century." *Journal of the American Medical Association* 281, no. 1 (Jan. 6): 61–66.

Arnet, E. B., M. Schirmacher, M. M. P. Huso, and J. P. Hayes. 2009. *Effectiveness of Changing Wind Turbine Cut-In Speed to Reduce Bat Fatalities at Wind Facilities.* Annual report submitted to the Bats and Wind Energy Cooperative, Bat Conservation International, Austin, Texas.

Arnold, S. F., D. M. Klotz, B. M. Collins, P. M. Vonier, L. J. Guillette, Jr., and J. A. McLachlan. 1996. "Synergistic Activation of Estrogen Receptor with Combinations of Environmental Chemicals." *Science* 272 (June 7): 1489–1492.

Arsova, Lyupka, Rob van Haaren, Nora Goldstein, Scott M. Kaufman, and Nickolas J. Themelis. 2008. "The State of

Garbage in America: 16th Nationwide Survey of MSW Management in the U.S." *Biocycle* 49, no. 12 (Dec): 22–29.

Ashford, Lori S. 1995. "New Perspectives on Population: Lessons from Cairo." *Population Bulletin* 50, no. 1 (March).

———. 2002. *Hidden Suffering: Disabilities from Pregnancy and Childbirth in Less Developed Countries.* Population Reference Bureau, MEASURE Communication (Aug).

Ashworth, William. 1982. *Nor Any Drop to Drink.* New York: Summit Books.

———. 1986. *The Late Great Lakes: An Environmental History.* New York: Alfred A. Knopf.

Ayres, Ed. 2004. "The Hidden Shame of the Global Industrial Economy." *World Watch* 17, no. 1 (Jan/Feb).

Baird, P. A., A. D. Sadovnick, and I. M. L. Yee. 1991. "Maternal Age and Birth Defects: A Population Study." *Lancet* 337: 527.

Bakir, R., et al. 1973. "Methylmercury Poisoning in Iraq." *Science* 181: 230–241.

Baliles, Gerald L. 2001. "Aircraft Noise: Addressing a Potential Barrier to Global Growth." *Virginia Lawyer* (June/July).

Bamber, J. L., R. E. M. Riva, B. L. A. Vermeersen, and A. M. LeBrocq. 2009. "Reassessment of the Potential Sea-Level Rise from a Collapse of the West Antarctic Ice Sheet." *Science* 324 (May 15): 901–903.

Band, Pierre R., Nhu D. Le, Raymond Fang, and Michele Deschamps. 2002. "Carcinogenic and Endocrine Disrupting Effects of Cigarette Smoke and Risk of Breast Cancer." *The Lancet* 360, no. 9339 (Oct. 5): 1044–1049.

Banks, James T., and Frances Dubrowski. 1982. "Pretreat or Retreat"? *The Amicus Journal* (Spring). Natural Resources Defense Council.

Banuelos, G.S. et al., 1997. "Phytoremediation of Selenium-Laden Soils: A New Technology." *Journal of Soil and Water Conservation* 52, no. 6 (Nov/Dec): 426–431.

Barboza, David. 2007a. "2nd Ingredient Is Suspected in Pet Food Contamination," *New York Times,* May 9, C3.

———. 2007b. "China's Seafood Industry: Dirty Water, Dangerous Fish," *New York Times,* Dec. 15, A1, 10.

Barlow, Maude. 2007. *Blue Covenant: The Global Water Crisis and the Coming Battle for the Right to Water.* New York: The New Press.

Barringer, Felicity. 2009. "Environmentalists in a Clash of Goals," *New York Times*, March 24, A17.

———. 2010. "Solar Power Plants to Rise on U.S. Land," *New York Times*, Oct. 5.

Basel Action Network (BAN). 2009. "Environmentalists and Consumer Groups Applaud Dell's Policy on E-Waste Export." *Toxic Trade News*, BAN/ETBG Media Release (May 12).

Baskin, Yvonne. 2002. *A Plague of Rats and Rubbervines: The Growing Threat of Species Invasions.* Washington, DC: Island Press/Shearwater Books.

Battisti, David, and Rosamund L. Naylor. 2009. "Historical Warnings of Future Food Insecurity with Unprecedented Seasonal Heat." *Science* 323 (Jan. 9): 240–244.

Beek, Jim. 1994. "Man-Made Minerals Could Be Key to SBS." *Indoor Air Review* 3, no. 11 (Jan).

Beeson, W. Lawrence, David E. Abbey, and S. F. Knutson. 1998. "Long-Term Concentrations of Ambient Air Pollutants and Incident Lung Cancer in California Adults: Results from the AHSMOG Study." *Environmental Health Perspectives* 106, no. 12 (Dec): 813–828.

Behar, Michael. 2009. "Selling the Sun: A Man, A Plan, and the Dawn of America's Solar Future." *On Earth* 31, no. 1 (Spring): 26–37.

Bell, Michelle L., Aidan McDermott, Scott Zeger, Jonathan M. Samet, and Francesca Dominici. 2004. "Ozone and Short-Term Mortality in 95 U.S. Urban Communities, 1987–2000." *The Journal of the American Medical Association* 292, no. 19 (Nov. 17).

Benbrook, Charles M. 1996. *Pest Management at the Crossroads.* Yonkers, NY: Consumers Union.

Bender, W., and M. Smith. 1997. "Population, Food, and Nutrition." *Population Bulletin* 51, no. 4 (Feb).

Bennett, B. G. 1997. "Exposure to Natural Radiation Sources Worldwide." In *Proceedings of 4th International Conference on High Levels of Natural Radiation: Radiation Doses and Health Effects*, edited by L. Wei, T. Sugahara, and Z. Tao. Beijing, China, Oct. 1996.

Bennett, Lyle. 1991. "Abandoned Mines: Report from West Virginia." *EPA Journal* 17, no. 5 (Nov/Dec).

Beral, Valerie, Carol Hermon, Clifford Kay, Philip Hannaford, Sarah Darby, and Gillian Reeves. 1999. "Mortality Associated with Oral Contraceptive Use: 25-Year Follow up of Cohort of 46,000 Women from Royal College of General Practitioners' Oral Contraceptive Study." *British Medical Journal* 318, no. 7176 (Jan. 9): 96–100.

Berenyi, Eileen Brettler. 1999. "Whither MRF-based Recycling?" *Resource Recycling* 18, no. 4 (April): 12–17.

Berger, Eric. 2009. "Ocean Dead Zones Hard to Predict," *Houston Chronicle,* Nov. 6.

Bernstein, Mark, and David Whitman. 2005. "Smog Alert: The Challenges of Battling Ozone Pollution." *Environment* 47, no.8 (Oct): 28–41.

Bever, Wayne et al. 1975. *Illinois Pesticide Applicator Study Guide.* Cooperative Extension Service, University of Illinois College of Agriculture, Special Publication 39.

Bhatra, Ramesh, and Malin Falkenmark. 1992. "Water Resource Policies and the Urban Poor: Innovative Approaches and Policy Imperatives." *International Conference on Water and the Environment: Development Issues for the 21st Century.* Dublin, Ireland, Jan. 26–31.

Birnbaum, Linda S. 1994. "The Mechanism of Dioxin Toxicity: Relationship to Risk Assessment." *Environmental Health Perspectives* 102 (Nov) (Suppl. 9): 157–167.

Black, Edwin. 2008. *The Plan: How to Rescue Society the Day the Oil Stops—or the Day Before.* Washington, DC: Dialog Press.

Blackmore, Carina. 2009. "Compendium of Measures to Prevent Disease Associated with Animals in Public Settings." *Morbidity & Mortality Weekly Report.* Recommendations and Reports (May 1) 58(RR05): 1–15.

Blair, Aaron et al. 1987. "Cancer and Pesticides Among Farmers." *Pesticides and Groundwater: A Health Concern for the Midwest.* The Freshwater Foundation.

Blancher, Peter. 2002. "Importance of Canada's Boreal Forest to Land Birds Final Report." *Bird Studies Canada* (Dec).

Block, Ben. 2008. "DNA Forensics May Prevent Elephant Poaching." Accessed August 20 from http://www.worldchanging.com/archives/008392.html

Bond, Michael. 1996. "Plagued by Noise." *New Scientist* 152, no. 2056 (Nov. 16): 14–15.

Bowker, Michael. 2003. *Fatal Deception: The Untold Story of Asbestos—Why It Is Still Legal and Still Killing Us.* New York: Rodale.

Boyle, Robert, and R. Alexander Boyle. 1983. *Acid Rain.* New York: Schocken Books/Nick Lyons Books.

Bradley, Don J. 1997. *Behind the Nuclear Curtain: Radioactive Waste Management in the Former Soviet Union.* Columbus, OH: Battelle Press.

Bradley, Rob. 2009. Director, International Climate Policy Initiative, World Resources Institute. Testimony to the U.S. House of Representatives Select Committee on Energy Independence and Global Warming (Feb. 4).

Bremner, Jason. 2010. "Improved Sanitation." *Population Bulletin* 65, no. 2. Population Reference Bureau, www.prb.org

Bremner, Jason, Carl Haub, Marlene Lee, Mark Mather, and Eric Zuehlke. 2009. "World Population Highlights: Key Findings from PRB's 2009 World Population Data Sheet." *Population Bulletin* 64, no. 3 (Sept.).

Bright, Chris. 1998. *Life Out of Bounds: Bioinvasion in a Borderless World.* New York: W.W. Norton.

Briscoe, John. 1993. "When the Cup Is Half Full: Improving Water and Sanitation Services in the Developing World." *Environment* 35, no. 4 (May).

Brockerhoff, Martin, and Ellen Brennan. 1998. "The Poverty of Cities in Developing Regions." *Population and Development Review* 24, no. 1 (March): 75–114.

Broder, John M. 2009. "Bush to Protect Vast New Pacific Tracts," *New York Times,* Jan. 6.

———. 2010. "Climate Talks Reach Final Day With No Deal," *New York Times,* December 10.

Bronner, Eric C., et al. 1994. "Mutation in the DNA Mismatch Repair Gene Homologue hMLH1 Is Associated with Hereditary Non-polyposis Colon Cancer." *Nature* 368 (March 17).

Brown, Lester. 2003. *Plan B: Rescuing a Planet under Stress and a Civilization in Trouble.* Earth Policy Institute. New York: W.W. Norton.

———. 2008. *Plan B 3.0: Mobilizing to Save Civilization.* Earth Policy Institute. New York: W.W. Norton.

———. 2009. *Plan B 4.0: Mobilizing to Save Civilization.* Earth Policy Institute. New York: W.W. Norton.

Brown, Lester R., Christopher Flavin, and Hilary F. French. 1999. *State of the World 1999.* New York: Worldwatch Institute/W.W. Norton.

Brunekreef, B., and S. T. Holgate. 2002. "Air Pollution and Health." *The Lancet* 360: 1233–1242.

Bryner, Gary C. 1993. *Blue Skies, Green Politics: The Clean Air Act of 1990.* Washington, DC: CQ Press.

Budyko, M. I. 1986. *The Evolution of the Biosphere.* Dordrecht, the Netherlands: D. Reidel Publishing.

Bugliarello, George, Ariel Alexandre, John Barnes, and Charles Wakstein. 1976. *The Impact of Noise Pollution.* Pergamon Press.

Bush, Mark. 2000. *Ecology of a Changing Planet.* 2nd ed. Upper Saddle River, NJ: Prentice Hall.

Bushmeat Crisis Task Force (BCTF). 2003. *Bushmeat: A Wildlife Crisis in West and Central Africa and Around the World.* Silver Spring, MD: BCTF. Accessed January 2004 from www.bushmeat.org

"Buying Farmland Abroad: Outsourcing's Third Wave." *The Economist* 391, no. 8632 (May 23).

Caldeira, Ken. 2009. "Geoengineering to Shade Earth." In *2009 State of the World: Into a Warming World.* The Worldwatch Institute. New York: W.W. Norton.

California Energy Commission. 2006. *Choices for the Home: Geothermal or Ground Source Heat Pumps.* Accessed from http://www.consumerenergycenter.org/home/heating_cooling/geothermal

Calvert, G.M. et al. 2008. "Acute Pesticide Poisoning among Agricultural Workers in the United States, 1998–2005." *American Journal of Industrial Medicine* 51, no. 12 (Dec): 883–898.

Campbell, Kurt M., ed. 2008. *Climatic Cataclysm: The Foreign Policy and National Security Implications of Climate Change.* Washington, DC: Brookings Institution Press.

Canadell, J. G. et al. 2007. "Contributions to Accelerating Atmospheric CO_2 Growth from Economic Activity, Carbon Intensity, and Efficiency of Natural Sinks." *Proceedings of the National Academy of Sciences,* 104 (47): 18866–18870.

Cappiello, Disia. 2010. "White House Solar Panels to Provide Obamas' Green Power," *Christian Science Monitor,* Oct. 5.

Carpenter, Kent E., et al. 2008. "One-Third of Reef-Building Corals Face Elevated Extinction Risk from Climate Change and Local Impacts." *Science* 321 (July 25): 560–563.

Carson, Rachel. 1962. *Silent Spring.* Boston: Houghton Mifflin.

Carter, L. J. 1977. "More Burning of Coal Offsets Gains in Air Pollution Control." *Science* 198.

Cascio, Jamais. 2009. "It's Time to Cool the Planet," *The Wall Street Journal,* June 15, R1.

Casselman, Ben. 2009. "U.S. Gas Fields Go From Bust to Boom," *The Wall Street Journal,* April 30.

Centers for Disease Control and Prevention (CDC). 1992. "Elevated Blood Lead Levels Associated with Illicitly Distilled Alcohol—Alabama, 1990–1991." *Morbidity & Mortality Weekly Report* 41, no. 17 (May 1).

———. 1993a. "Lead Poisoning in Bridge Demolition Workers—Georgia, 1992." *Morbidity & Mortality Weekly Report* 42, no. 20 (May 28).

———. 1993b. "*Vibrio vulnificus* Infections Associated with Raw Oyster Consumption—Florida, 1981–1992." *Morbidity & Mortality Weekly Report* 42, no. 21 (June 4).

———. 1994a. "Human Plague—United States, 1993–1994." *Morbidity & Mortality Weekly Report* 43, no. 13 (April 8).

———. 1994b. "Water Hemlock Poisoning—Maine, 1992." *Morbidity & Mortality Weekly Report* 43, no. 13 (April 8).

———. 2001. "Fatal Pediatric Lead Poisoning—New Hampshire, 2000." *Morbidity & Mortality Weekly Report* 50, no. 22 (June 8): 457–459.

———. 2002a. "Outbreak of *Salmonella* Serotype Kottbus Infections Associated with Eating Alfalfa Sprouts—Arizona, California, Colorado, and New Mexico, Feb.–April, 2001." *Morbidity & Mortality Weekly Report* 51, no. 1 (Jan. 11).

———. 2002b. "Outbreaks of Gastroenteritis Associated with Noroviruses on Cruise Ships—United States, 2002." *Morbidity & Mortality Weekly Report* 51, no. 49 (Dec. 13).

———. 2002c. "Surveillance for Waterborne Disease Outbreaks—United States, 1999–2000." *Morbidity & Mortality*

Weekly Report, Surveillance Summaries vol. 51, no. SS-8 (Nov. 22): 1–28.

———. 2003a. "Hepatitis A Outbreak Associated with Green Onions at a Restaurant—Monaca, Pennsylvania, 2003." *Morbidity & Mortality Weekly Report*. Dispatch 52 (Nov. 21).

———. 2003b. "Prevalence of Current Cigarette Smoking Among Adults and Changes in Prevalence of Current and Some Day Smoking—United States, 1996–2001." *Morbidity & Mortality Weekly Report* 52, no. 14 (April 11): 303–307.

———. 2003c. "Surveillance for Elevated Blood Lead Levels Among Children—United States, 1997–2001." *Morbidity & Mortality Weekly Report*, Surveillance Summaries, Sept. 12, 2003/52 (SS10): 1–21.

———. 2005. "Information on *Aedes albopictus*." Accessed from http://www.cdc.gov/ncidod/dvbid/arbor/albopic_new.htm

———. 2006a. "Botulism Associated with Commercial Carrot Juice—Georgia and Florida, September 2006," *Morbidity & Mortality Weekly Report*. Dispatch 55 (Oct. 6): 1–2.

———. 2006b. "Human Plague—Four States, 2006." *Morbidity & Mortality Weekly Report*. Dispatch 55 (Aug. 25): 1–3.

———. 2007. "Surveillance for Foodborne Disease Outbreaks—United States, 2007." *Morbidity & Mortality Weekly Report* 59, no. 31: 973–979.

———. 2008a. *A Drop of News*. (Nov): 2.

———. 2008b. "Asbestosis-Related Years of Potential Life Lost Before Age 65 Years—United States, 1968–2005," *Morbidity & Mortality Weekly Report* 57, vol. 49 (Dec. 12): 1321–1325.

———. 2008c. "Cigarette Use among High School Students—United States, 1991–2007." *Morbidity & Mortality Weekly Report* 57, no. 5 (June 27): 686–688.

———. 2008d. "Surveillance for Lyme Disease—United States, 1992–2006." *Morbidity & Mortality Weekly Report*, Surveillance Summaries vol. 57, no. SS-10: 1–9 (Oct. 3).

———. 2008e. "Update on Overall Prevalence of Major Birth Defects—Atlanta, Georgia, 1978–2005." *Morbidity & Mortality Weekly Report* 57, no. 1 (Jan. 11): 1–5.

———. 2009a. "Anaplasmosis and Ehrlichiosis—Maine, 2008." *Morbidity & Mortality Weekly Report* 58, no. 37 (Sept. 25): 1033–36.

———. 2009b. "Children with Elevated Blood Lead Levels Related to Home Renovation, Repair, and Painting Activities—New York State, 2006–2007." *Morbidity & Mortality Weekly Report* 58, vol. 3 (Jan. 30): 55–58.

———. 2009c. "Cigarette Smoking Among Adults and Trends in Smoking Cessation—United States, 2008." *Morbidity & Mortality Weekly Report* 58, no. 44 (Nov. 13): 1227–1232.

———. 2009d. "Malaria Surveillance—United States, 2007." *Morbidity and Mortality Weekly Report*, Surveillance Summaries, vol. 58, no. SS-2 (April 17).

———. 2009e. "Multistate Outbreaks of *Salmonella* Infections Associated with Live Poultry—United States, 2007." *Morbidity & Mortality Weekly Report* 58, no. 2 (Jan. 23): 25–29.

———. 2009f. "State-Specific Prevalence and Trends in Adult Cigarette Smoking—United States, 1998–2007." *Morbidity & Mortality Weekly Report* 58, no. 9 (March 13): 221–226.

———. 2009g. *Tobacco Use and Pregnancy*. Accessed from www.cdc.gov/reproductivehealth/tobaccousepregnancy/index.htm

———. 2010a. *Fetal Alcohol Spectrum Disorders (FASDs)*. Fact-sheet. Accessed September 2010 from http://www.cdc.gov/ncbddd/fasd/data.html

———. 2010b. "Update: Outbreak of Cholera—Haiti, 2010." *Morbidity & Mortality Weekly Report*, 59, no. 48 (Dec. 10): 1586–1590.

Chao, Jason, M.D., and George D. Kikano, M.D. 1993. "Lead Poisoning in Children." *American Family Physician* (Jan).

Charles, Daniel. 2003. *Lords of the Harvest: Biotech, Big Money, and the Future of Food*. Cambridge, MA: Perseus.

The Chernobyl Forum. 2005. *Chernobyl's Legacy: Health, Environmental and Socio-Economic Impacts*. Austria: International Atomic Energy Agency.

Chivian, Eric, M.D., et al., eds. 1993. *Critical Condition: Human Health and the Environment. Physicians for Social Responsibility*. Cambridge, MA: The MIT Press.

Cholera Inquiry Committee. 1855. *Report on the Cholera Outbreak in the Parish of St. James, Westminster, During the Autumn of 1854*. London: J. Churchill.

Chu, Junhong. 2001. "Prenatal Sex Determination and Sex-Selective Abortion in Rural Central China." *Population and Development Review* 27, no. 2 (June): 259–281.

"Chu Presents 'Blue Ribbon' Panel to Study Yucca Mountain Alternatives." 2010. *Nuclear Waste News* 30, no. 3 (Feb. 11): 1, 7.

Chung-En Liu, John, and Anthony A. Leiserowitz. 2009. "From Red to Green? Environmental Attitudes and Behavior in Urban China." *Environment* 51, no. 4 (July/Aug): 32–45.

Clare, Dennis. 2009. "Reducing Black Carbon." In *2009 State of the World: Into a Warming World*. The Worldwatch Institute. New York: W.W. Norton.

Clark, Claudia. 1997. *Radium Girls: Women and Industrial Health Reform, 1910–1935*. Chapel Hill: Univ. of North Carolina Press.

Clark, William W. 1991. "Noise Exposure from Leisure Activities: A Review." *Journal of the Acoustic Society of America* 90, no. 1 (July).

Cochran, Soni. 2003. *Vermicomposting—Composting with Worms!* Educational Resource Guide #107, University of Nebraska, Lincoln.

Coffin, Tristam, ed. 1993. "The Damage Done by Cattle-Raising." *The Washington Spectator* 19, no. 2 (Jan. 15).

Cohen, C. J., L. C. Grothaus, and S. C. Perrigan. 1982. "Effects of Simulated Sulfuric and Sulfuric-Nitric Acid Rain on Crop Plants: Results of 1980 Crop Survey." *Special Report* 670, Agricultural Experiment Station, Oregon State University, Corvallis.

Cohen, Peter. 1990. "Drumming: How Risky Is It to Your Hearing?" *Modern Drummer* (Oct).

Cohen, S., D. C. Glass, and J. E. Singer. 1973. "Apartment Noise Auditory Discrimination and Reading Ability in Children." *Journal of Experimental Social Psychology* 9: 407–422.

Colborn, Theo, Dianne Dumanoski, and John P. Myers. 1996. *Our Stolen Future*. New York: Dutton.

Colchester, Marcus. 1994. "The New Sultans." *The Ecologist* 24, no. 2 (March/April).

Cole, Philip, and Brad Rodu. 1996. "Declining Cancer Mortality in the United States." *Cancer* 78, no. 10 (Nov): 2045–2048.

Coleman, David. 2006. "Immigration and Ethnic Change in Low-Fertility Countries: A Third Demographic Transition." *Population and Development Review* 32, no. 3 (Sept.): 401–446.

Collier, Paul. 2008. "The Politics of Hunger: How Illusion and Greed Fan the Food Crisis." *Foreign Affairs* 87, no. 6 (Nov/Dec).

Connolly, Scott, Katie Elmore, and William Ryerson. 2008. "Entertainment-Education for Social Change." *World-Watch* 21, no. 5 (Sept/Oct): 28–29.

Cooper, George, Jr. 1973. "The Development of Radiation Science." In *Medical Radiation Biology*, edited by Glenn V. Dalrymple, M. E. Gaulden, G. M. Kollmorgen, and H. H. Vogel, Jr. Philadelphia: W. B. Saunders.

Costello et al. 2009. "Managing the Health Effects of Climate Change." *The Lancet* 373 (May 16): 1693–1733.

"Creatures of the Night." 2009. *Science* 323 (Jan. 23): 443.

Crooks, Ed, and James Blitz. 2009. "Split on the Atom," *Financial Times*, Sept. 9, 7.

Curtis, Jennifer, Tim Profeta, and Laurie Mott. 1993. *After Silent Spring: The Unresolved Problems of Pesticide Use in the United States.* New York: Natural Resources Defense Council.

Dahl, T. E. 2006. *Status and Trends of Wetlands in the Conterminous U.S., 1984–2004.* U.S. Dept. of the Interior, Fish and Wildlife Service.

Dahlquist, G., and L. Hustonen. 1994. "Analysis of a Fifteen-Year Prospective Incidence Study of Childhood Diabetes Onset: Time, Trends, and Climatological Factors." *International Journal of Epidemiology* 23: 1234–1241.

Dalrymple, Glenn V. 1973. "Microwaves." In *Medical Radiation Biology*, edited by Glenn V. Dalrymple et al. Philadelphia: W. B. Saunders.

Dasgupta, Partha S. 1995. "Population, Poverty, and the Local Environment." *Scientific American* 272, no. 2 (Feb): 40–45.

Davis, Debra Lee. 1990. "Natural Anticarcinogens: Can Diet Protect Against Cancer?" *Health & Environment Digest* 4, no. 1 (Feb).

Davis, Lucas W. 2008. "Driving Restrictions and Air Quality in Mexico City." *Resources* 170 (Fall): 6.

Dean, Cornelia. 2007. "Drugs Are in the Water. Does It Matter?" *New York Times*, April 3.

———. 2009. "The Beaver Came Back and It Won't Go Away," *New York Times,* June 9, D1.

Derr, Mark. 1993. "Redeeming the Everglades." *Audubon* (Sept/Oct).

Dessler, A. E., and S. C. Sherwood. 2009. "A Matter of Humidity." *Science* 323, no. 5917 (Feb. 20): 1020–1021.

DeWeerdt, Sarah. 2009. "Is Local Food Better?" *WorldWatch* 22, no. 3 (May/June): 6–10.

Diaz, Robert J., and Rutger Rosenberg. 2008. "Spreading Dead Zones and Consequences for Marine Ecosystems." *Science* 321 (Aug. 15): 926–929.

Dickson, L. C., and S. C. Buzik. 1993. "Health Risks of Dioxins: A Review of Environmental and Toxicological Considerations." *Veterinary and Human Toxicology* 35, no. 1 (Feb).

Dieben, Tom, F. J. Roumen, and D. Apter. 2002. "Efficacy Cycle Control and User Acceptability of a Novel Combined Contraceptive Vaginal Ring." *Obstetrics and Gynecology* 100(3): 585–593.

Dockery, Douglas W. et al. 1993. "An Association Between Air Pollution and Mortality in Six U.S. Cities." *The New England Journal of Medicine* 329, no. 24 (Dec. 9).

Dodman, David, Jessica Ayers, and Saleemul Huq. 2009. "Building Resilience." In *2009 State of the World: Into a Warming World.* The Worldwatch Institute. New York: W.W. Norton.

Doll, Richard. 1996. "Nature and Nurture: Possibilities for Cancer Control." *Carcinogenesis* 17, no. 2 (Feb): 177–184.

Drews, Carolyn D., Catherine C. Murphy, Marshalyn Yeargin-Allsopp, and Pierre Decouflé. 1996. "The Relationship between Idiopathic Mental Retardation and Maternal Smoking during Pregnancy." *Pediatrics* 97, no. 4 (April): 547–553.

Driscoll, Charles, David Whitall, John Aber, Elizabeth Boyer, Mark Castro, Christopher Cronan, et al. 2003. "Nitrogen Pollution: Sources and Consequences in the U.S. Northeast." *Environment* 45, no. 7 (Sept).

Dubrova, Yuri E., Rakhmet I. Bersimbaev, Leila B. Djansugurova, Maira K. Tankimanova, Zaure Zh. Mamyrbaeva, Ritta Mustonen, et al. 2002. "Nuclear Weapons Tests and Human Germline Mutation Rate." *Science* 295, no. 5557 (Feb. 8).

Dulitzki, M., D. Soriano, E. Schiff, A. Chetrit, S. Mashiach, and D. S. Seidman. 1998. "Effect of Very Advanced Maternal Age on Pregnancy Outcome and Rate of Cesarean Delivery." *Obstetrics and Gynecology* 92, no. 6 (Dec): 935–939.

"Easy Guide to the Air Toxics Law." 1993. *The Environmental Manager's Compliance Advisor*, no. 344 (Feb. 1).

Eckholm, Erik, and Kathleen Newland. 1977. "Health: The Family Planning Factor." *Worldwatch Paper* 10, Worldwatch Institute.

"Economics Focus: Does Population Matter?" 2002. *The Economist*, Dec. 7.

The Economist. 2009. "A Special Report on Waste." (Feb. 28).

Economy, Elizabeth C. 2004. *The River Runs Black: The Environmental Challenge to China's Future.* A Council on Foreign Relations Book. Ithaca & London: Cornell University Press.

Edwards, Clive A., and Norman Q. Arancon. 2004. "Vermicomposts Suppress Plant Pest and Disease Attacks." *Biocycle* 45, no. 3 (March).

Ehrlich, Paul R., and Anne H. Ehrlich. 2008. *The Dominant Animal: Human Evolution and the Environment.* Washington, DC: Island Press/Shearwater Books.

Ehrlich, Paul R., Anne H. Ehrlich, and Gretchen C. Daily. 1993. "Food Security, Population, and Environment." *Population and Development Review* 19, no. 1 (March).

Ehrlich, Paul R., Anne H. Ehrlich, and John P. Holdren. 1977. *Ecoscience.* New York: W. H. Freeman.

Eisenbud, M. 1973. *Environmental Radioactivity.* San Diego: Academic Press.

Enserink, Martin. 2008. "Malaria: Signs of Drug Resistance Rattle Experts, Trigger Bold Plan." *Science* 322 (Dec. 19): 1776.

Environmental Law Handbook. 12th ed. 1993. Government Institutes, Inc.

Environmental News Service (ENS). 2009. *Obama Administration Releases Chesapeake Bay Restoration Plans* (Sept. 10).

Environmental Protection Agency (EPA). 1987. *Lead and Your Drinking Water.* EPA-87–006 (April).

————. 1994. "Deposition of Air Pollutants to the Great Waters." EPA-453A/R-93–055 (May).

————. 1995a. *National Water Quality Inventory: 1994 Report to Congress.* EPA 841-R-95-005. Washington, DC: Office of Water.

————. 1995b. "Report on the National Survey of Lead-Based Paint in Housing: Base Report." EPA A747–R95–003.

————. 1998. *National Water Quality Inventory: 1996 Report to Congress.* EPA 841-R-97-008 (April).

————. 2003a. *America's Children and the Environment: Measures of Contaminants, Body Burdens, and Illnesses.* 2nd ed. EPA 240–R-03–001, Office of Children's Health Protection (Feb).

————. 2003b. *Introduction to the Underground Storage Tank Regulations and Policy* (March).

————. 2009a. *Municipal Solid Waste Generation, Recycling, and Disposal in the United States: Facts and Figures for 2008.* EPA-530-F-009-021 (Nov). Accessed from http://www.epa.gov/wastes

————. 2009b. *National Water Quality Inventory: Report to Congress for the 2004 Reporting Cycle.* EPA-841-R-08-001 (Jan.). Washington, DC: Office of Water.

————. 2010. *Air Quality Trends.* Accessed from http://www.epa.gov/airtrends/aqtrends.html

Environmental Working Group (EWG). 1998. "Same As It Ever Was." Press Release, May 21.

"EPA Study Links Pesticide Use with Ground Water Contamination." 1992. *Environmental Health Letter,* Jan. 28.

Epstein, John H. 1998. "Sunscreens and Skin Cancer." *Southern Medical Journal* 91, no. 6 (June).

Erickson, Wallace P., Gregory D. Johnson, and David P. Young, Jr. 2005. *A Summary and Comparison of Bird Mortality from Anthropogenic Causes with an Emphasis on Collisions.* USDA Forest Service General Technical Report PSW-GTR-191.

Estes, James A., Martin T. Tinker, Terrie M. Williams, and Daniel F. Doak. 1998. "Killer Whale Predation on Sea Otters Linking Oceanic and Nearshore Ecosystems." *Science* 282: 390 (Oct. 16).

Eustace, Larry W., Duck-Hee Kang, and David Coombs. 2003. "Fetal Alcohol Syndrome: A Growing Concern for Health Care Professionals." *Journal of Obstetric, Gynecologic, and Neonatal Nursing* 32, no. 2 (March/April): 215–221.

Evans, Gary W., Monika Bullinger, and Steffan Hygge. 1998. "Chronic Noise Exposure and Physiological Response: A Prospective Study of Children Living Under Environmental Stress." *Psychological Science* 9, no. 1 (Jan): 75–77.

Evans, Gary W., and Lorraine Maxwell. 1997. "Chronic Noise Exposure and Reading Deficits: The Mediating Effects of Language Acquisition." *Environment and Behavior* 29, no. 5 (Sept): 638.

Evelyn, John. 1661. *Fumifugium.* London National Society for Clean Air, reprinted 1969.

Ewing, Rodney C., and Frank N. von Hippel. 2009. "Nuclear Waste Management in the United States—Starting Over." *Science* 325, no. 5937 (July 10): 151–152.

Eyles, John, and Nicole Consitt. 2004. "What's At Risk? Environmental Influences on Human Health." *Environment* 46, no. 8 (Oct).

Ezzati, Majid, and Alan D. Lopez. 2003. "Estimates of Global Mortality Attributable to Smoking in 2000." *The Lancet* 362, no. 9387 (Sept. 13): 847–852.

Fachelmann, Kathleen. 1998. "Do Sunscreens Protect Against Cancer?" *Consumers' Research* 81, no. 8 (Aug): 23–26.

Farb, Peter. 1963. *Ecology, Life Nature Library.* New York: Time Inc.

Fargione, Joseph, Jason Hill, David Tilman, Stephan Polasky, and Peter Hawthorne. 2008. "Land Clearing and the Biofuel Carbon Debt." *Science* 319, no. 5867 (Feb. 29): 1235–1238.

Faris, Stephan. 2009. "The Last Straw." *Foreign Policy* (July/Aug): 92–93.

Fawcett, Howard H. 1988. *Hazardous and Toxic Materials: Safe Handling and Disposal.* New York: John Wiley & Sons.

Feldman, Emily. 2009. "NYPD to Shake Up Streets With Siren-Sound Device." NBC New York (Oct. 26). Accessed from http://www.nbcnewyork.com/news/local-beat/NYPD-To-Shake-Up-Streets-With-Siren-Sound-Device-65983997.html

Feshbach, Murray. 1995. *Ecological Disaster: Cleaning Up the Hidden Legacy of the Soviet Regime.* New York: The Twentieth Century Fund Press.

Fingerhut, Marilyn A., et al. 1991. "Cancer Mortality in Workers Exposed to 2,3,7,8–Tetrachlorodibenzo-p-Dioxin." *The New England Journal of Medicine* 324, no. 4 (Jan. 24).

Finkleman, R.B. et al., 1999. "Health Impacts of Domestic Coal Use in China." *Proceedings of the National Academy of Sciences* 96 (March): 3427–3431.

Fishel, Richard, et al. 1993. "The Human Mutator Gene Homolog MSH2 and Its Association with Hereditary Nonpolyposis Colon Cancer." *Cell* 75 (Dec. 3).

Flannery, Tim. 2005. *The Weather Makers: How Man Is Changing the Climate and What It Means for Life on Earth.* New York: Atlantic Monthly Press.

Flavin, Christopher, and Robert Engelman. 2009. "The Perfect Storm." In *2009 State of the World: Into a Warming World.* The Worldwatch Institute. New York: W.W. Norton.

Flint, M. L., and R. VandenBosch. 1981. *Introduction to Integrated Pest Management.* New York: Plenum Press.

Florini, Karen L. 1990. *Legacy of Lead: America's Continuing Epidemic of Childhood Lead Poisoning.* Environmental Defense Fund.

Floyd, R. L., and J. S. Sidhu. 2004. "Monitoring Prenatal Alcohol Exposure." *American Journal of Medical Genetics* 127 C (May 15): 3–9.

Foden, W., et al. 2008. "Species Susceptibility to Climate Change Impacts." In J.-C. Vié, C. Hilton-Taylor, and S. N. Stuart (eds.), *2008 Review of the IUCN Red List of Threatened Species.* Gland, Switzerland: IUCN.

Food and Agriculture Organization of the United Nations (FAO). 1998. "Expert Committee: No Danger to Humans from Milk and Meat from BST-Treated Cows." *News & Highlights* (March 5).

————. 2001. *State of the World's Forests 2001.* Rome: FAO.

————. 2002. *The State of Food Insecurity in the World 2002.* Rome: FAO.

————. 2009a. *The State of Food Insecurity in the World 2009.* Rome: FAO.

————. 2009b. *The State of the World's Fisheries and Aquaculture 2008.* Rome: FAO.

————. 2010. *Global Forest Resources Assessment 2010: Main Report.* FAO Forestry Paper 163. Rome: FAO.

Food and Drug Administration (FDA). 1998. "Once-Feared Drug Provides Relief for Leprosy Symptoms." *FDA Consumer* 32, no. 6 (Nov): 2.

Foulke, Judith E. 1993. "A Fresh Look at Food Preservatives." *FDA Consumer* (Oct).

Fradin, Mark S., and John F. Day. 2002. "Comparative Efficacy of Insect Repellents against Mosquito Bites." *The New England Journal of Medicine* 347, no. 1 (July 4): 13–18.

Franklin, Deborah. 1991. "Lead: Still Poison After All These Years." *Health* 5, no. 5 (Sept/Oct).

Frenzen, P., A. Majchrowicz, B. Buzby, M. Imhoff, and the FoodNet Working Group. 2000. "Consumer Acceptance of Irradiated Meat and Poultry Products." *Agriculture Information Bulletin* 757: 1–8.

Friedman, Thomas L. 2008. *Hot, Flat, and Crowded: Why We Need a Green Revolution—and How It Can Renew America.* New York: Farrar, Straus, and Giroux.

Fuhrmans, Vanessa. 2009. "German Nuclear Plants Get a New Lease," *The Wall Street Journal,* Oct. 17–18, A8.

Gardner, Gary, and Brian Halweil. 2000. "Underfed and Overfed: The Global Epidemic of Malnutrition." *Worldwatch Paper* 150 (March). Worldwatch Institute.

Gardner, Gerald T., and Paul C. Stern. 2008. "The Short List: The Most Effective Actions U.S. Households Can Take to Curb Climate Change." *Environment* 50, no. 5 (Sept/Oct): 12–24.

Garland, Cedric F., et al. 1992. "Could Sunscreens Increase Melanoma Risk?" *American Journal of Public Health* 82, no. 4 (April).

Garrett, Laurie. 1994. *The Coming Plague.* New York: Farrar, Straus, and Giroux.

Gauthier, Michele M. 1988. "Clamorous Metrodome Hard on Ears and Foes." *The Physician and Sports Medicine* 16, no. 3 (March).

Gelband, Hellen. 2008. "Malaria: It's Not Neglected Any More (But It's Not Gone, Either)." *Resources,* no. 168 (Spring).

General Accounting Office (GAO). 2001. *Management Improvements Needed to Further Promote Integrated Pest Management.* GAO-01-815, Agricultural Pesticides (Sept. 28). Washington, DC: U.S. GPO.

Gerberding, Dr. Julie. 2009. *Pharmaceutical and Personal Care Products (PPCPs) in Drinking Water.* American Water Works Association. Accessed from http://www.drinktap.org

Giovanucci, E., A. Ascherio, E. G. Rimm, M. J. Stampfer, G. A. Colditz, and W. Willett. 1995. "Intake of Carotenoids and Retinol in Relation to Risk of Prostate Cancer." *Journal of the National Cancer Institute* 87, no. 23 (Dec. 6): 1767–1776.

Gitlitz, Jenny. 2004. "Are Bottle Bills Still Relevant?" *Resource Recycling* 23, no. 9 (Sept).

Gleick, Peter H., ed. 1993. *Water in Crisis: A Guide to the World's Fresh Water Resources.* New York: Oxford Univ. Press.

Gleick, Peter H. 2002. *The World's Water: 2002–2003.* Washington, DC: Island Press.

———. 2006a. "Water and Terrorism." In *The World's Water 2006–2007: The Biennial Report on Freshwater Resources.* Washington, DC: Island Press.

———. 2006b. "Bottled Water: An Update." In *The World's Water 2006–2007: The Biennial Report on Freshwater Resources.* Washington, DC: Island Press.

———. 2009a. "China and Water." In *The World's Water 2008–2009: The Biennial Report on Freshwater Resources.* Washington, DC: Island Press.

———. 2009b. "Three Gorges Dam Project, Yangtze River, China." In *The World's Water 2008–2009: The Biennial Report on Freshwater Resources.* Washington, DC: Island Press.

———. 2009c. "Water Conflict Chronology." In *The World's Water 2008–2009: The Biennial Report on Freshwater Resources.* Washington, DC: Island Press.

Gleick, Peter H., and Heather S. Cooley. 2009. "Energy Implications of Bottled Water." *Environmental Research Letters* (Jan.–March). doi: 10.1088/1748-9326/4/1/014009.

Gleick, Peter H., Heather Cooley, and Gary Wolff. 2006. "With a Grain of Salt: An Update on Seawater Desalination." In *The World's Water 2006–2007: The Biennial Report on Freshwater Resources,* Washington, DC: Island Press.

Gleick, Peter H., Dana Haasz, and Gary Wolff. 2004. "Urban Water Conservation: A Case Study of Residential Water Use in California." In *The World's Water 2004–2005: The Biennial Report on Freshwater Resources.* Washington, DC: Island Press.

Glennon, Robert. 2002. *Water Follies: Groundwater Pumping and the Fate of America's Fresh Waters.* Washington, DC: Island Press.

Glynn, M. K. et al. 1998. "Emergence of Multidrug-Resistant *Salmonella enterica* Serotype Typhimurium DT104 Infections in the United States." *New England Journal of Medicine* 338, no. 19 (May 7): 1333–1338.

Gnaedinger, Richard H. 1993. "Lead in School Drinking Water." *Journal of Environmental Health* 55, no. 6 (April).

Goldman, Marvin. 1996. "Cancer Risk of Low-Level Exposure." *Science* 271: 1821–1822.

Goldstein, Inge F., and Martin Goldstein. 2002. *How Much Risk? A Guide to Understanding Environmental Health Hazards.* New York: Oxford Univ. Press.

Good, Brian. 2003. "A Better Vasectomy Option." *Men's Health* 18, no. 7 (Sept): 34.

Government Accountability Office (GAO). 2008. *Electronic Waste: Harmful U.S. Exports Flow Virtually Unrestricted Because of Minimal EPA Enforcement and Narrow Regulation.* GAO-08-1166T (Sept. 17).

Greczyn, Mary. 1994. "Researchers and Community Reps Call for More Bioaerosol Research." *Environmental Health Letter* 33, no. 7 (March).

Greenhouse, Linda. 1994. "Justices Decide Incinerator Ash Is Toxic Waste," *New York Times,* May 3.

Greenlee, A. R., T. E. Arbuckle, and P-H. Chou. 2003. "Risk Factors for Female Infertility in an Agricultural Region." *Epidemiology* 14: 429–436.

Gribbin, John. 1982. "Carbon Dioxide, Ammonia—and Life." *New Scientist* 94 (May 13): 413–416.

Grover, Velma I. 2007. *Water: A Source of Conflict or Cooperation?* Science Publishers.

Gustafsson, Örjan et al. 2009. "Brown Clouds Over South Asia: Biomass or Fossil Fuel Combustion?" *Science* 323, no. 5913 (Jan. 23): 495–498.

Hall, Eric J. 2000. *Radiobiology for the Radiologist.* 5th ed. Philadelphia: Lippincott.

Halweil, Brian. 2009a. "Grain Harvest Sets Record, But Supplies Still Tight." *Vital Signs 2009: The Trends That Are Shaping Our Future.* New York: Worldwatch Institute/W. W. Norton.

———. 2009b. "Meat Production Continues to Rise." *Vital Signs 2009: The Trends That Are Shaping Our Future.* New York: Worldwatch Institute/W. W. Norton.

Hamilton, John Maxwell. 1989. "Rescuing the Bounty of Rain Forests," *The Christian Science Monitor*, Jan. 26.

Hardoy, Jorge E., Diana Mitlin, and David Satterthwaite. 2001. *Environmental Problems in an Urbanizing World*. London: Earthscan Publications.

Harris, Gardiner. 2009. "Food Safety Has Reached a Plateau, U.S. Finds," *New York Times*, April 10.

Harris, John A., M.D., and Jackie W. Wynne. 1994. "Birth Defects Clusters: Evaluating Community Reports." *Health & Environment Digest* 7 (Feb).

Harris, Lilieth V., and Ishenkumba A. Kahwa. 2003. "Asbestos: Old Foe in 21st Century Developing Countries." *The Science of the Total Environment* 307, no. 1–3 (May 20): 1–9.

Hartzler, Bob, and Mike Owen. 2003. "Status and Concerns for Glyphosate Resistance." *Integrated Crop Management*. Ames: Department of Entomology, Iowa State University (March 17).

Harvell, C. Drew, Charles E. Mitchell, Jessica R. Ward, Sonia Altizer, Andrew P. Dobson, Richard S. Ostfeld, et al. 2002. "Climate Warming and Disease Risks for Terrestrial and Marine Biota." *Science* 296, no. 5576 (June 21).

Haub, Carl. 1993. "Tokyo Now Recognized as World's Largest City." *Population Today* 21, no. 3 (March).

Hawkes, Nigel, Geoffrey Lean, David Leigh, Robin McVie, P. Pringle, and A. Wilson. 1987. *Chernobyl: The End of the Nuclear Dream*. New York: Vintage Books.

Henderson, Charles W. 1999. "Thalidomide Making Comeback to Treat Cancer, AIDS." *Cancer Weekly Plus* (Jan. 25).

Henkel, John. 1993. "From Shampoo to Cereal: Seeing to the Safety of Color Additives." *FDA Consumer* (Dec).

Herring, Herbert. 1960. *A History of Latin America*. New York: Alfred A. Knopf.

Hinrichsen, Don. 2003. "A Human Thirst." *World Watch* 16, no. 1 (Jan/Feb).

Hinterthuer, Adam. 2008. "Just How Harmful Are Bisphenol-A Plastics?" *Scientific American* (Aug. 26). Accessed from http://www.scientificamerican.com/article.cfm?id=just-how-harmful-are-bisphenol-a-plastics

Hites, Ronald A., Jeffery A. Foran, David O. Carpenter, M. Coren Hamilton, Barbara A. Knuth, Steven J. Schwager. 2004. "Global Assessment of Organic Contaminants in Farmed Salmon." *Science* 303, no. 5655 (Jan. 9): 226–229.

Hoffman, Sandra. 2007. "Mending Our Food Safety Net." *Resources*, no. 166 (Summer).

Hoffman, Stephen J. 2009. *Planet Water: Investing in the World's Most Valuable Resource*. New York: John Wiley & Sons.

Holmes, Michelle D., et al. 1999. "Association of Dietary Intake of Fat and Fatty Acids with Risk of Breast Cancer." *Journal of the American Medical Association* 281, no. 10 (March 10): 914–920.

Honey, Martha. 2003. "Protecting Eden: Green Standards for the Tourism Industry." *Environment* 45, no. 6 (July/Aug).

Hoshaw, Lindsey. 2009. "Afloat in the Ocean, Expanding Islands of Trash," *New York Times*, Nov. 10, D2.

Houghton, J. T., G. J. Jenkins, and J. J. Ephraums, eds. 1990. *Climate Change: The IPCC Scientific Assessment*. Cambridge: Cambridge University Press.

Hulme, Mike, and Mick Kelly. 1993. "Exploring the Links Between Desertification and Climate Change." *Environment* 35, no. 6 (July/Aug).

Human Genome Sequencing Consortium. 2004. "Finishing the Euchromatic Sequence of the Human Genome." *Nature* 431 (Oct. 21): 931–945.

Huston, Michael, and Thomas Smith. 1987. "Plant Succession: Life History and Competition." *American Naturalist* 130: 168–198.

Hvistendahl, Mara. 2009. "Making Every Baby Girl Count." *Science* 323, no. 5918 (Feb. 27): 1164–1166.

Indermühle, A., T. F. Stocker, F. Joos, H. Fischer, H. J. Smith, M. Wahlen, et al. 1999. "Holocene Carboncycle Dynamics Based on CO_2 Trapped in Ice at Taylor Dome, Antarctica." *Nature* 398 (March 11): 121–126.

Institute of Medicine and the National Research Council (IOM and NRC). 1999. *Exposure of the American People to Iodine-131 from Nevada Nuclear-Bomb Tests*. Washington, DC: National Academy Press.

Institutes of Medicine (IOM) of the National Academies. 2000. *Clearing the Air: Asthma and Indoor Air Exposures*. Washington, DC: National Academy Press.

———. 2004. *Damp Indoor Spaces and Health*. Washington, DC: National Academy Press.

Intergovernmental Panel on Climate Change (IPCC). 2007. *Climate Change 2007: The Physical Science Basis. Contribution of Working Group I to the Fourth Assessment Report of the Intergovernmental Panel on Climate Change*. Solomon, S., D. Qin, M. Manning, Z. Chen, M. Marquis, K.B. Averyt, et al. (eds.). Cambridge, United Kingdom and New York: Cambridge University Press.

"Ionizing Radiation Exposure of the Population of the United States." 1987. National Council on Radiation Protection and Measurements, Report No. 93, Sept. 1.

Isaacson, Peter G., M.D. 1994. "Gastric Lymphoma and Helicobacter Pylori." *New England Journal of Medicine* 330, no. 18 (May 5).

Isenberg, David. 2002. *CDI Terrorism Project: Securing U.S. Water Supplies*. Centers for Defense Information.

Ising, Hartmut, Ekkehard Rebentisch, Fritz Poustka, and Immo Curio. 1990. "Annoyance and Health Risk Caused by Military Low-Altitude Flight Noise." *International Archives of Occupational and Environmental Health* 62: 357–363.

Janssen, Wallace F. 1975. "America's First Food and Drug Laws." *FDA Consumer* (June).

Jaret, Peter. 1990. "The Rock & Roll Syndrome." *In Health* (July/Aug).

Jaworowski, Zbigniew. 1999. "Radiation Risk and Ethics." *Physics Today* 52, no. 9 (Sept).

Jemal, Ahmedin et al. 2010. "Cancer Statistics, 2010." *CA, A Cancer Journal for Clinicians* (online). American Cancer Society. Accessed from http://caonline.amcancersoc.org/cgi/content/full/caac.20073v1

Jepson, P.D. et al. 2003. "Gas-Bubble Lesions in Stranded Cetaceans." *Nature* 425, no. 6958 (Oct. 9).

Jerrett, Michael et al. 2009. "Long-Term Ozone Exposure and Mortality." *New England Journal of Medicine* 360, no. 11 (March 12): 1085–1095.

Jiang, Leiwen, Malea Hoepf Young, and Karen Hardee. 2008. "Population, Urbanization, and the Environment." *WorldWatch* 21, no. 5 (Sept/Oct): 34–39.

Jones, Rachel K., Mia R.S. Zolna, Stanley K. Henshaw, and Lawrence B. Finer. 2008. "Abortion in the United States: Incidence and Access to Services, 2005." *Perspectives on Sexual and Reproductive Health,* 40 (1): 6–16.

Jorde, Lynn B., John C. Carey, Michael J. Bamshad, and Raymond L. White. 1999. *Medical Genetics.* St. Louis, MO: Mosby.

Kahn, Patricia. 1993. "A Grisly Archive of Key Cancer Data." *Science* 259 (Jan. 22).

Kanter, James. 2009. "Not So Fast, Nukes: Cost Overruns Plague a New Breed of Reactor," *New York Times,* May 29.

Kantor, Linda S., et al. 1997. "Estimating and Addressing America's Food Losses." *Food Review* 20, no. 1.

Kashefi, Kazem, and Dereck L. Lovely. 2003. "Extending the Upper Temperature for Life." *Science* 301, no. 5635 (Aug. 15).

Kasting, James F. 1993. "Earth's Early Atmosphere." *Science* 259, no. 5097 (Feb. 12).

Kaufman, Leslie, and Shaila Dewan. 2010. "Oiled Gulf May Defy Direst Predictions," *New York Times,* Sept. 14, D1, 3.

Kaufman, Scott M., Nora Goldstein, Karsten Millrath, and Nickolas J. Themelis. 2004. "The State of Garbage in America: 14th Annual Nationwide Survey of Solid Waste Management in the United States." *BioCycle* 45, no. 1 (Jan).

Kerr, J. B., and C. T. McElroy. 1993. "Evidence for Large Upward Trends of Ultraviolet-B Radiation Linked to Ozone Depletion." *Science* 262 (Nov).

Kerr, Richard A. 1998. "Acid Rain Control: Success on the Cheap." *Science* 282 (Nov. 6): 1024–1027.

———. 1999. "For Radioactive Waste from Weapons, A Home at Last." *Science* 283 (March 12): 1626–1628.

———. 2009. "Northern India's Groundwater is Going, Going, Going . . ." *Science* 325 (Aug. 14): 798.

Kevles, Bettyann Holtzmann. 1997. *Naked to the Bone.* New Brunswick, NJ: Rutgers University Press.

Kimbrough, R. D., M. L. Doemland, and M. E. LeVois. 1999. "Mortality in Male and Female Capacitor Workers Exposed to Polychlorinated Biphenyls." *Journal of Occupational and Environmental Medicine* 41, no. 3 (March 10): 161–171.

Kinley, David H. 1998. "Aerial Assault on the Tsetse Fly." *Environment* 40, no. 7 (Sept).

Kintisch, Eli. 2007. "Tougher Ozone Accord Also Addresses Global Warming." *Science* 317 (Sept. 28): 184.

———. 2009. "Projections of Climate Change Go From Bad to Worse, Scientists Report." *Science* 323 (March 20): 1546–1547.

Klein, Richard M. 1979. *The Green World: An Introduction to Plants and People.* New York: Harper & Row.

Kleinman, R. L., and P. Senanayake. 1984. *Breastfeeding, Fertility, and Contraception.* IPPF Medical Publications.

Kliewer, Erich, and Ken Smith. 1995. "Breast Cancer Mortality among Immigrants in Australia and Canada." *Journal of the National Cancer Institute* 87, no. 15 (Aug. 2): 1154–1161.

Kneale, George W., and Alice M. Stewart. 1993. "Reanalysis of Hanford Data: 1944–1986 Deaths." *American Journal of Industrial Medicine* 23 (March).

Knowlton, Kim, Gina Solomon, and Miriam Rotkin-Ellman. 2009. *Fever Pitch: Mosquito-Borne Dengue Fever Threat Spreading in the Americas.* Natural Resources Defense Council Issue Paper (July).

Knutson, Thomas R., and Robert E. Tuleya. 2004. "Impact of CO_2-Induced Warming on Simulated Hurricane Intensity and Precipitation: Sensitivity to the Choice of Climate Model and Convective Parameterization." *Journal of Climate* 17, no. 18 (Sept. 15).

Kolbert, Elizabeth. 2006. *Field Notes from a Catastrophe: Man, Nature, and Climate Change.* New York: Bloomsbury Publishing.

Koren, Herman. 1980. *Handbook of Environmental Health and Safety.* Vol. 1. Oxford: Pergamon Press.

Kramer, Andrew E. 2009. "Electricity for Americans from Russia's Dismantled Nuclear Weapons," *New York Times,* Nov. 10, B1.

Krauss, Clifford. 2009. "Ethanol, Just Recently a Savior, Is Struggling," *New York Times,* Feb. 12, A1.

LaDou, Joseph. 2004. "The Asbestos Cancer Epidemic." *Environmental Health Perspectives* 112, no. 3 (March).

Lake, James A., Ralph G. Bennett, and John F. Kotek. 2002. "Next Generation of Nuclear Power." *Scientific American* 286, no. 1 (Jan).

Landers, Peter. 1999. "Uranium Leak Feeds Antinuclear Sentiment in Japan." *Wall Street Journal,* Oct. 4.

Larsen, Kim. 2009. "The New Diseases on Our Doorstep." *On Earth* 31, no. 3 (Fall): 26–35.

Lawrence, Gregory B., and T. G. Huntington. 1999. *Soil Calcium Depletion Linked to Acid Rain and Forest Growth in the Eastern United States.* U.S. Geological Survey, WRIR 98–4267 (Feb).

Leach, F. S., et al. 1993. "Mutations of a mutS Homolog in Hereditary Nonpolyposis Colorectal Cancer." *Cell* 75, no. 6 (Dec. 17).

The Lead Education and Abatement Design Group (The LEAD Group). 2010. Accessed from http://www.lead.org

Leadership in Energy and Environmental Design (LEED). Accessed May 2009 from http://en.wikipedia.org/wiki/Leadership_in_Energy_and_Environmental_Design

League of Women Voters Education Fund. 1982. *Public Policy on Reproductive Choice.* No. 286 (July).

———. 1993. *The Garbage Primer.* New York: Lyon & Burford.

Leahy, Elizabeth, and Sean Peoples. 2008. "Population and Security: Risks from Growth, Youth, Migration, and Environmental Stress." *WorldWatch* 21, no. 5 (Sept/Oct): 40–45.

Leahy, Stephen. 2005. "Wetlands Loss Left Gulf Coast Naked to Storm." Inter Press Service News Agency. Accessed from http://ipsnews.net/print/asp?idnews=30112

Levine, Adeline G. 1982. *Love Canal: Science, Politics, and People.* Lexington Books, DC: Heath.

Levine, Arnold J. 2002. "The Origins of Cancer and the Human Genome." In *The Genomic Revolution: Unveiling the Unity of Life,* Michael Yudell and Robert DeSalle (eds.). Washington, DC: Joseph Henry Press, with the American Museum of Natural History.

Levitus, S., J. Antonov, and T. Boyer. 2005. "Warming of the World Ocean, 1955–2003." *Geophysical Research Letters* 32: L02604. doi 10.1029/2004GL021592.

"Licensing Board Rejects Obama's Attempt to Pull Yucca Mountain License." 2010. *Nuclear Waste News* 30, no. 13 (July 5): 1, 7–8.

Likens, G. E., C. T. Driscoll, and D.C. Buso. 1996. "Long-Term Effects of Acid Rain: Response and Recovery of a Forest Ecosystem." *Science* 272, no. 5259 (April 16): 244–246.

Linet, M. S., E. E. Hatch, R. A. Kleinerman, L. L. Robison, W. T. Kaune, D. K. Friedman, et al. 1997. "Residential Exposure to Magnetic Fields and Acute Lymphoblastic Leukemia in Children." *New England Journal of Medicine* 337, no. 1 (July 3): 1–7.

Lipscomb, David M. 1974. *Noise: The Unwanted Sounds.* Nelson-Hall.

Lobell, David B., and Gregory P. Asner. 2003. "Climate and Management Contributions to Recent Trends in U.S. Agricultural Yields." *Science* 299, no. 5609 (Feb. 14).

Loffredo, C. A. et al. 2001. "Association of Transposition of the Great Arteries in Infants with Maternal Exposures to Herbicides and Rodenticides." *American Journal of Epidemiology* 153 (6): 529–536.

LUMCON News. 2010. *2010 Dead Zone among Five Largest to Date.* Louisiana Universities Marine Consortium. Accessed from http://www.lumcon.edu

Macklis, Roger M. 1993. "The Great Radium Scandal." *Scientific American* (Aug).

"Mad About the Noise." 1998. *Time International* 150, no. 48 (July 27): 38.

Mahler, K. 1997. "Strong Son Preference among Nepalese Couples May Outweigh Their Desire for Smaller Families." *International Family Planning Perspectives* 23, no. 1 (March).

Makower, Joel, Ron Pernick, and Clint Wilder. 2009. "Clean Energy Trends 2009." *Clean Edge* (March).

Mallis, Arnold. 1997. *Handbook of Pest Control.* 8th ed. Mallis Handbook and Technical Training Company.

Markoff, John. 1992. "Danger of Miscarriage Found for Chip Workers," *New York Times*, Dec. 4.

Martin, Andrew, and Griff Palmer. 2007. "China Not Sole Source of Dubious Food," *New York Times*, July 12, C1, 4.

Martin, Daniel D. 2009. "Speculation on Solar Future Hits Overdrive." *Renewable Energy World Magazine* 12, no. 3 (May/June).

Martin, Philip, and Gottfried Zürcher. 2008. "Managing Migration: The Global Challenge." *Population Bulletin* 63, no. 1 (March): 3–20.

Mastny, Lisa. 2002. "Redirecting International Tourism." *State of the World 2002.* New York: The Worldwatch Institute/W.W. Norton.

Maugh, Thomas H. 1982. "New Link Between Ozone and Cancer." *Science* 216 (April 23).

Maurits la Riviere, J. W. 1989. "Threats to the World's Water." *Scientific American* (Sept).

Mayo Clinic. 2008. *Thalidomide: Research Advances in Cancer and Other Conditions.* Accessed from http://www.mayoclinic.com/health/thalidomide/HQ01507

McDonald, Alan. 1999. "Combating Acid Deposition and Climate Change: Priorities for Asia." *Environment* 41, no. 3 (April): 4–11, 34–41.

McDonald's Corporation. Press Release, June 19, 2003.

McKeown, Alice. 2009. "Genetically Modified Crops Only a Fraction of Primary Global Crop Production." In *Vital Signs 2009: The Trends That Are Shaping Our Future.* New York: Worldwatch Institute/W. W. Norton.

McKeown, Alice, and Brian Halweil. 2009. "Fish Farming Continues to Grow As World Fisheries Stagnate." In *Vital Signs 2009: The Trends That Are Shaping Our Future.* New York: Worldwatch Institute/W. W. Norton.

McLaren, Angus A. 1990. *A History of Contraception.* Oxford, England: Basil Blackwell.

McWilliams, James E. 2009. "Free-Range Trichinosis," *New York Times,* April 10.

Meister Publishing Co. 1996. *Ag Consultant Magazine* (March).

Melosi, Martin V. 1981. *Garbage in the Cities: Refuse, Reform, and the Environment, 1880–1980.* Texas A&M University Press.

Melrick, William. 1991. "Human Temporary Threshold Shift (TTS) and Damage Risk." *Journal of the Acoustical Society of America* 90, no. 1 (July).

Mernild, S. H., G. E. Liston, C. A. Hiemstra, and K. Steffen. 2009. "Record 2007 Greenland Ice Sheet Surface Melt Extent and Runoff." *EOS, Transactions of the American Geophysical Union* 90: 13–14.

Merrill, Richard A. 1997. "Food Safety Regulation: Reforming the Delaney Clause." *Annual Review of Public Health* 18: 313–340.

Micronutrient Initiative. 2009. *The Invisible Enemy: The Global Impact of Iron and Iodine Deficiencies.*

Mielke, Howard W. 1999. "Lead in the Inner Cities." *American Scientist* 87 (1) (Jan/Feb): 62.

Miller, Chaz. 2010. Personal communication. National Solid Waste Management Association.

Miller, Roger W. 1984. "How Onions and a Baked Potato Became Sources of Botulism Poisoning." *FDA Consumer* (Oct).

Ministry of Agriculture and Food (MoAF). 2007. *Sustainable Land Management 2007.* Government of Afghanistan.

Minkin, Mary Jane, and Toby Hanlon. 2003. "New: Permanent Birth Control." *Prevention* 55, no. 9 (Sept).

Mirza, M. Monirul Qader, R. A. Warrick, and N. J. Ericksen. 2003. "The Implications of Climate Change on Floods of the Ganges, Brahmaputra, and Meghna Rivers in Bangladesh." *Climatic Change* 57, no. 3 (April).

Moench, Marcus. 2004. "Groundwater: The Challenge of Monitoring and Management." In *The World's Water 2004–2005: The Biennial Report on Freshwater Resources.* Peter H. Gleick (ed.). Washington, DC: Island Press.

Montgomery, Mark. 2008. "The Urban Transformation of the Developing World." *Science* 319 (Feb. 8): 761–764.

———. 2009. "Urban Poverty and Health in Developing Countries." *Population Bulletin* 64, no. 2 (June).

Montgomery, Susan P. et al. 2009. "Trichinellosis Surveillance—United States, 2002–2007." *Morbidity & Mortality Weekly Report* 58, no. SS09 (Dec. 4): 1–7.

Moran, Susan, and J. Thomas McKinnon. 2008. "Hot Times for Solar Energy." *World Watch* 21, no. 2 (March/April): 26–31.

Mosher, W. D., and J. Jones. 2010. "Use of Contraception in the United States: 1982–2008." *Vital and Health Statistics* 23, no. 29 (Aug).

Munton, Don. 1998. "Dispelling the Myths of the Acid Rain Story." *Environment* 40, no. 6 (July/Aug): 4–7, 27–34.

Murphy, Elliott. 1989. "Townshend, Tinnitus and Rock & Roll." *Rolling Stone*, July 13–27.

Myers, Norman, Russell A. Mittermeier, Cristina G. Mittermeier, Gustavo A. B. daFonseca, and Jennifer Kent. 2000. "Biodiversity Hotspots for Conservation Priorities." *Nature* 403 (Feb. 24): 853–858.

Myers, Ransom A., and Boris Worm. 2003. "Rapid Worldwide Depletion of Predatory Fish Communities." *Nature* 423 (May 15): 280–283.

Napoli, Maryanne. 1998. "Sunscreens—Not the Protection We Thought." *Health Facts* 3, no. 6: 1–3.

Nash, Linda. 1993. "Water Quality and Health." In *Water in Crisis: A Guide to the World's Fresh Water Resources*, Peter H. Gleick (ed.). New York: Oxford Univ. Press.

National Cancer Institute (NCI). 2010. *BRCA 1 and BRCA 2: Cancer Risk and Genetic Testing*. Factsheet, U.S. National Institutes of Health. Accessed from http://www.cancer.gov/cancertopics/factsheet/risk/BRCA

National Climatic Data Center (NCDC). 2009. *Climate of 2008 Annual Report*, Jan. 14. Accessed from http://www.ncdc.noaa.gov/oa/climate/research/2008/ann/global.html

National Council on Radiation Protection and Measurements (NCRP). 1987. "Ionizing Radiation Exposure of the Population of the United States." NCRP Report No. 93. Bethesda, MD: NCRP.

———. 1998. "Radionuclide Exposure of the Embryo/Fetus." NCRP Report No. 128. Bethesda, MD: NCRP.

National Institute of Allergy and Infectious Disease (NIAID). 2001. *Workshop Summary: Scientific Evidence on Condom Effectiveness for Sexually Transmitted Disease (STD) Prevention*, July 20.

National Institute of Environmental Health Sciences (NIEHS). 2009. *Since You Asked—Bisphenol A (BPA)*. Accessed from http://www.niehs.nih.gov/news/media/questions/sya-bpa.cfm

National Institute for Occupational Safety and Health (NIOSH). 2009. *Cancer, Reproductive and Cardiovascular Diseases*. NIOSH program portfolio. Accessed from http://www.cdc.gov/niosh/programs/crcd/risks.html

National Oceanic and Atmospheric Administration. 2011. *2010 Tied For Warmest Year on Record*. Factsheet. Accessed from http://www.noaanews.noaa.gov/stories2011/20110112_globalstats.html

National Research Council (NRC). 1987. *Regulating Pesticides in Food: The Delaney Paradox*. Washington, DC: National Academy Press.

———. 1992. *Neem: A Tree for Solving World Problems*. Washington, DC: National Academy Press.

———. 1993. *Pesticides in the Diets of Infants and Children*. Washington, DC: National Academy Press.

———. 1996. *Carcinogens and Anti-Carcinogens in the Human Diet*. Washington, DC: National Academy Press.

———. 1997. *Possible Health Effects of Exposure to Residential Electric and Magnetic Fields*. Washington, DC: National Academy Press.

———. 1998. *Ensuring Safe Food from Production to Consumption*. Washington, DC: National Academy Press.

———. 1999. *Setting Priorities for Drinking Water Contaminants*. Washington, DC: National Academy Press.

———. 2000. *The Future Role of Pesticides in U.S. Agriculture*. Washington, DC: National Academy Press.

———. 2002a. *The Airliner Cabin Environment and the Health of Passengers and Crew*. Washington, DC: National Academy Press.

———. 2002b. *Biosolids Applied to Land: Advancing Standards and Practices*. Washington, DC: National Academy Press.

———. 2003. *Ocean Noise and Marine Mammals*. Washington, DC: National Academy Press.

Natural Resources Defense Council (NRDC). 1999. *Bottled Water: Pure Drink or Pure Hype?* New York (March).

———. 2004. *Efficient Appliances Save Energy—and Money: Consumers Get Lower Utility Bills, and We All Get a Cleaner Environment*. Accessed May 2009 from http://www.nrdc.org/air/energy/fappl.asp

———. 2009. "Grizzlies Laid Low by Declining Whitebark Pines." *Nature's Voice* (May/June).

Needleman, H. L., et al. 1979. "Deficits in Psychologic and Classroom Performance of Children with Elevated Dentine Lead Levels." *The New England Journal of Medicine* 300: 689–695.

———. 1990. "The Long-Term Effects of Exposure to Low Doses of Lead in Childhood." *The New England Journal of Medicine* 322: 83–88.

Nelson, Berlin. 1999. *Stachybotrys chartarum: The Toxic Indoor Mold*. American Phytopathological Society, APSnet Feature (Feb).

Nestle, Marion. 2003. *Safe Food: Bacteria, Biotechnology, and Bioterrorism*. Berkeley: Univ. of California Press.

Neuman, William. 2010a. "Testing Ignores 6 Germs in Food, A Growing Peril," *New York Times*, May 27, A1, 4.

———. 2010b. "Beef Recall Heats Up Fight to Tighten Rules," *New York Times*, Sept. 3, B1, 4.

Newbold, Retha R., et al. 1998. "Increased Tumors but Uncompromised Fertility in Female Descendents of Mice Exposed Developmentally to DES." *Carcinogenesis* 19, no. 9 (Sept): 1655–1663.

Newman, P. A., E. R. Nagh, S. R. Kawa, S. A. Montzka, and S. M. Schauffler. 2006. "When Will the Ozone Hole Recover?" *Geophysical Research Letters* 33: L12814.

Norman, Edward H. 1998. "Childhood Lead Poisoning and Vinyl Miniblind Exposure." *Journal of the American Medical Association* 279, no. 5 (Feb. 4): 342.

Normile, Dennis. 2008. "Reinventing Rice to Feed the World." *Science* 321 (July 18): 330–333.

———. 2009. "Bringing Coral Reefs Back from the Living Dead." *Science* 325: 559–561 (July 31).

North East Biosolids and Residuals Association (NEBRA). 2007. *A National Biosolids Regulation, Quality, End Use, & Disposal Survey: Final Report* (July 20).

Norwood, Christopher. 1980. *At Highest Risk*. New York: Penguin Books.

O'Neil, Marie S. et al., 2005. "Diabetes Enhances Vulnerability to Particulate Air Pollution—Associated Impairment in Vascular Reactivity and Endothelial Function." *Circulation* 111, no. 22 (June 7): 2913–2920.

O'Neill, Elizabeth. 2008. "Tigers: Worth More Dead than Alive." *WorldWatch* 21, no. 4 (July/Aug).

Odum, Eugene P. 1959. *Fundamentals of Ecology*. Philadelphia: W. B. Saunders.

OECD. 1991. *Fighting Noise in the 1990s*. Paris: OECD.

Oomman, Nandini, and Bela R. Ganatra. 2002. "Sex Selection: The Systematic Elimination of Girls." *Reproductive Health Matters* 10, no. 19: 184.

Ott, Wayne R., and John W. Roberts. 1998. "Everyday Exposure to Toxic Pollutants." *Scientific American* (Feb): 86–91.

Ottoboni, M. Alice. 1991. *The Dose Makes the Poison*. New York: Van Nostrand Reinhold.

"Ozone Takes a Nose Dive after the Eruption of Mt. Pinatubo." 1993. *Science* 260 (April 23).

Pachauri, R. K. 2009. "Forward." In *2009 State of the World: Into a Warming World*. The Worldwatch Institute. New York: W.W. Norton.

Palaniappen, Meena, and Peter H. Gleick. 2009. "Peak Water." In *The World's Water 2008–2009: The Biennial Report on Freshwater Resources*. Washington, DC: Island Press.

Pandey, Arvind et al. 1998. *Infant and Child Mortality in India*. National Family Health Survey Subject Reports, no. 11. International Institute for Population Sciences, Mumbai, India.

Panofsky, Hans A. 1978. "Earth's Endangered Ozone." *Environment* 20, no. 3 (April).

Papadopoulos, Nickolas, Nicholas C. Nicolaides, et al. 1994. "Mutation of a mutL Homolog in Hereditary Colon Cancer." *Science* 263 (March 18).

Parker, Tracey. 1994. "Recent Studies Document the Complex Ways Pesticides Affect Birds." *Journal of Pesticide Reform* 14, no. 1 (Spring).

Parkin, D. M., P. Pisani, N. Muñoz, and J. Ferlay. 1999. "The Global Health Burden of Infection Associated Cancers." *Cancer Survey* 33: *Infections and Human Cancer*. 5–33.

Parmesan, Camille, and Gary Yohe. 2003. "A Globally Coherent Fingerprint of Climate Change Impacts across Natural Systems." *Nature* 421 (Jan. 2): 37–42.

Parson, Edward A. 2003. *Protecting the Ozone Layer*. New York: Oxford University Press.

Parsonnet, Julie, M.D., et al. 1994. "Helicobacter Pylori Infection and Gastric Lymphoma." *New England Journal of Medicine* 330, no. 18 (May 5).

Patel, J. D., P. B. Bach, and M. G. Kris. 2004. "Lung Cancer in U.S. Women: A Contemporary Epidemic." *Journal of the American Medical Association* 291, no. 14 (April 14): 1763–1768.

Pauly, D., V. Christensen, J. Dalsgaard, R. Froese, and F. Torres Jr. 1998. "Fishing Down Marine Food Webs." *Science* 279: 860–863.

Pauly, Daniel, and Reg Watson. 2003. "Counting the Last Fish." *Scientific American* 289, no. 1 (July).

Pearce, Fred. 1999. "A Nightmare Revisited." *New Scientist* 161, no. 2172 (Feb. 6): 4.

———. 2006. *When the Rivers Run Dry: Water—The Defining Crisis of the Twenty-first Century*. Boston: Beacon Press.

Pellow, David Naguib. 2002. *Garbage Wars: The Struggle for Environmental Justice in Chicago*. Cambridge, MA: The MIT Press.

Pellow, David N., and Lisa Sun-Hee Park. 2002. *The Silicon Valley of Dreams: Environmental Injustice, Immigrant Workers, and the High-Tech Global Economy*. New York: NYU Press.

Peng, Shaobing, Jianliang Huang, John E. Sheehy, Rebecca C. Laza, Romeo M. Visperas, Xuhua Zhong, et al. 2004. "Rice Yields Decline with Higher Night Temperature from Global Warming." *Proceedings of the National Academy of Sciences* 101, no. 27 (July 6).

Pennisi, Elizabeth. 2009. "Calcification Rates Drop in Australian Reefs." *Science* 323 (Jan. 2): 27.

Perera, Frederica P. 1997. "Environment and Cancer: Who are Susceptible?" *Science* 278, no. 5340 (Nov. 7): 1068–1073.

Perera, Judith. 1997. "EU Offers Some Aid for Massive Eastern Europe Uranium Cleanup." *Nuclear Waste News* 17, no. 35 (Sept. 11): 335.

———. 1998. "Officials Charged with Misuse of Funds for Tomsk Cleanup." *Nuclear Waste News* 18, no. 14 (April 2): 132.

Pérez-Peña, Richard. 2003. "Powder Cure is Dangerous, Officials Say," *New York Times*, Nov. 6.

Perham, Chris. 1979. "The Sound of Silence." *EPA Journal* 5, no. 9 (Oct).

Perket, Cary. 2004. "Manufacturers Ship 7 Million Tons per Year to Commercial Hazardous Waste & Wastewater Facilities." *EI Digest*, Environmental Information Ltd. (June 21).

Perkins, John H. 1982. *Insects, Experts, and the Insecticide Crisis*. New York: Plenum Press.

Perkins, Sid. 2009. "Louisiana Sinks as Sea Level Rises." *Science News* 176, no. 2 (July 18): 15.

Peterson, Dale. 2003. *Eating Apes*. Berkeley: University of California Press.

Peterson, Peter G. 1999. "Gray Dawn: The Global Aging Crisis." *Foreign Affairs* 78, no. 1 (Jan/Feb): 42–55.

———. 2002. "The Shape of Things to Come: Global Aging in the Twenty-First Century." *Journal of International Affairs* 56, no. 1 (Fall): 189–210.

Petit, J. R, J. Jouzel, D. Raynaud, N. I. Barkov, J. M. Barnola, I. Basile, et al. 1999. "Climate and Atmospheric History of the Past 420,000 Years from the Vostok Ice Core, Antarctica." *Nature* 399 (June 3): 429–436.

Phipps, M. G., J. D. Blume, and S. M. DeMonner. 2002. "Young Maternal Age Associated with Increased Risk of Neonatal Death." *Obstetrics and Gynecology* 100(3): 481–486.

Pianka, Eric R. 1988. *Evolutionary Ecology*. 4th ed. New York: Harper & Row.

Pierson, Merle D., and Donald A. Corlett, Jr., eds. 1992. *HACCP: Principles and Applications*. New York: Chapman & Hall.

Pimentel, David, ed. 1997. *Techniques for Reducing Pesticide Use: Economic and Environmental Benefits*. New York: John Wiley & Sons.

Pimentel, David, et al. 1991. "Environmental and Economic Impacts of Reducing U.S. Agricultural Pesticide Use." *Handbook of Pest Management in Agriculture*. CRC Press.

Pitot, Henry C. 2002. *Fundamentals of Oncology*. 4th ed. New York: Marcel Dekker, Inc.

"Planned Barnwell Closure Sparks NRC Low-Level Waste Review." 2005. *The International Radioactive Exchange* 24, no. 8 (May 2): 4.

Plotkin, Steven. 2004. "Is Bigger Better? Moving Toward a Dispassionate View of SUVs." *Environment* 46, no. 9 (Nov).

Pollack, Andrew. 1997. "Japan Calls Mercury-Tainted Bay Safe Now," *New York Times*, July 30.

Pollycove, Myron. 1997. "The Rise and Fall of the Linear No-Threshold Theory of Radiation Carcinogenesis." *Nuclear Waste News* (June): 34–37.

Pope, C. A., R. T. Burnett, M. J. Thun, E. Calle, D. Krewski, K. Ito, et al. 2002. "Lung Cancer, Cardiopulmonary Mortality, and Long-Term Exposure to Fine Particulate Air Pollution." *Journal of the American Medical Association* 287, no. 9 (March 6).

Pope, C. Arden, and Douglas W. Dockery. 2006. "Health Effects of Fine Particulate Air Pollution: Lines that Connect." *Journal of Air & Waste Management Association* 56: 709–742.

Population Reference Bureau (PRB). 2002. *Family Planning Worldwide: 2002 Data Sheet*. Washington, DC: PRB.

———. 2010. *2010 World Population Data Sheet*. Washington, DC: PRB.

Postel, Sandra. 1992. *Last Oasis: Facing Water Scarcity*. New York: W. W. Norton.

———. 1996. "Dividing the Waters: Food Security, Ecosystem Health, and the New Politics of Scarcity." *Worldwatch Paper* 132 (Sept).

Potter, Andrew R. 1997. "Reducing Vitamin A Deficiency Could Save the Eyesight and Lives of Countless Children." *British Medical Journal* 314, no. 7077 (Feb. 1): 317–318.

Potts, Malcolm. 2000. "The Unmet Need for Family Planning." *Scientific American* 282, no. 1 (Jan): 88–93.

Pounds, J. Alan, Michael P. L. Fogden, and John H. Campbell. 1999. "Biological Response to Climate Change." *Nature* 398 (April 15): 611–615.

Preventing Lead Poisoning in Young Children. 1991. U.S. Dept. of Health and Human Services, Centers for Disease Control.

Rahmstorf, S., A. Cazenave, J. A. Church, J. E. Hansen, R. F. Keeling, D. E. Parker, et al. 2007. "Recent Climate Observations Compared to Projections." *Science* 316 (May 4): 709.

Rail, Chester D. 1989. *Groundwater Contamination: Sources, Control, and Preventive Measures*. Technomic Publishing.

Raloff, Janet. 2003. "Munching Along." *Science News* 164, no. 22 (Nov. 29): 344–346.

———. 2009. "Bad Breath." *Science News* 176 (2): 26–29.

Randolph, John, and Gilbert M. Masters. 2008. *Energy for Sustainability: Technology, Planning, Policy*. Washington, DC: Island Press.

Rao, Serin. 2010. Biofuels Manufacturers of Illinois (BMI). Personal communication.

Raoult, Didier, et al. 2006. "Evidence for Louse-Transmitted Diseases in Soldiers of Napoleon's Grand Army in Vilnius." *Journal of Infectious Diseases* 193, no. 1 (Jan. 1): 112–120.

Regenstein, Lewis. 1982. *The Poisoning of America*. Washington, DC: Acropolis Books.

Renner, Michael. 2004. "Moving Toward a Less Consumptive Economy." In *State of the World 2004*. New York: Worldwatch Institute/W. W. Norton.

"Reprocessing Facility Blast Leads to Review of Japan's Nuclear Plans." 1997. *Nuclear Waste News* 17, no. 12 (March 20): 115.

Revkin, Andrew. 1992. *Global Warming: Understanding the Forecast*. New York: Abbeville Press.

———. 2001. "New Pollution Tool: Toxic Avengers with Leaves," *New York Times*, March 6, D1, 7.

Rhodes, S. L., and P. Middleton. 1983. "The Complex Challenge of Controlling Acid Rain." *Environment* 22, no. 4 (May).

Riddle, John M. 1992. *Contraception and Abortion from the Ancient World to the Renaissance*. Cambridge, MA: Harvard Univ. Press.

Riley, Nancy E. 1997. "Gender, Power, and Population Change." *Population Bulletin* 52, no. 1 (May).

Riman, Tomas, Paul Pickman, Staffan Nilsson, and Nestor Correia, et al. 2002. "Risk Factors for Invasive Ovarian Cancer: Results from a Swedish Case-Control Study." *American Journal of Epidemiology* 156 (4): 363–373.

Robbins, Jim. 2008. "Spread of Bark Beetles Kills Millions of Acres of Trees in West," *New York Times,* Nov. 18, D3.

Rohe, John F. 1998. *A Bicentennial Malthusian Essay: Conservation, Population and the Indifference to Limits*. Traverse City, MI: Rhodes & Easton.

Romieu, Isabelle, and Mauricio Hernandez-Avila. 2003. "Air Pollution and Health in Developing Countries." In *Air Pollution & Health in Rapidly Developing Countries*, Gordon McGranahan and Frank Murray (eds.). London: Earthscan Publications.

Ronsmans, Carine, and Oona Campbell. 1998. "Short Birth Intervals Don't Kill Women: Evidence from Matlab, Bangladesh." *Studies in Family Planning* 29, no. 3 (Sept): 282–290.

Ropp, Kevin L. 1994. "Juice Maker Cheats Consumers of $40 Million." *FDA Consumer* (Jan/Feb).

Rose, Craig. 2009. "Here Comes the Sun." *The Nation* 288, no. 6 (Feb. 16): 26–29.

Rose, P. G. 1996. "Endometrial Carcinoma." *New England Journal of Medicine* 335: 640–649.

Rosenstreich, David L., Peyton Eggleston, Meyer Kattan, Dean Baker, Raymond G. Slavin, Peter Gergen, et al. 1997. "The Role of Cockroach Allergy and Exposure to Cockroach Allergen in Causing Morbidity Among Inner-City Children with Asthma." *New England Journal of Medicine* 336, no. 19: 1356–1363.

Rosenthal, Elisabeth, and Felicity Barringer. 2009. "Green Promise Seen in Switch to LED Lighting," *New York Times*, May 30, A1.

Ruder, Kate. 2004. "Ferns Remove Arsenic from Soil and Water." *Arsenic Crisis Group* (Aug. 6).

Russell, Armistead G., and Bert Brunekreef. 2009. "A Focus on Particulate Matter and Health." *Environmental Science & Technology* 43 (13): 4620–4625.

Sack, George H. 1999. *Medical Genetics*. New York: McGraw-Hill.

Salam, M. T., Y-F. Li, B. Langholz, and F. D. Gilliland. 2004. "Early Life Environmental Risk Factors for Asthma: Findings from the Children's Health Study." *Environmental Health Perspectives* 112, no. 6 (May): 760–765.

Sanford, Cynthia, and Joe Oosterhaut. 1991. "Protecting Groundwater: The Unseen Resource." *The National Voter* 40, no. 5 (June/July).

Santer, B. D. et al. 2003. "Contributions of Anthropogenic and Natural Forcing to Recent Tropopause Height Changes." *Science* 301: 479–483.

Sawai, Masako. 2009. "Rokkasho Reprocessing Plant: 14 Month Delay." Citizens' Nuclear Information Center, Tokyo, Japan. Accessed from http://cnic.jp/english

Sayare, Scott, and Maïa de la Baume. 2010. "Revelers See a Dimming in a Capital's Night Life," *New York Times,* Jan. 11, A8.

Schill, Susanne Retka. 2008. "Making Pennycress Pay Off." *Biodiesel Magazine* (Feb.).

———. 2009. "Mission Jatropha." *Biodiesel Magazine* (May).

Schluep, Mathias et al. 2009. *Recycling—From E-Waste to Recycling.* United Nations Environment Programme (UNEP), Sustainable Innovation and Technology Transfer.

Schneider, Keith. 1983. "Faking It." *Amicus Journal,* no. 4 (Spring).

———. 1994. "Progress, Not Victory, on Great Lakes Pollution," *New York Times,* May 7.

Schreiber, Michael M. 1986. "Exposure to Sunlight." *Comprehensive Therapy* 12, no. 5.

Scudder, B. C., L. C. Chasar, D. A. Wentz, N. J. Bauch, M. E. Brigham, P. W. Moran, et al. 2009. "Mercury in Fish, Bed Sediment, and Water from Streams across the United States, 1998–2005." *U.S. Geological Survey Scientific Investigations Report 2009-5109,* 74 p.

Searchinger, Timothy, Ralph Heimlich, R.A. Houghton, Fengxia Dong, Amani Elobeid, Jacinto Fabiosa, et al. 2008. "Use of U.S. Croplands for Biofuels Increases Greenhouse Gases through Emissions from Land-Use Change." *Science* 319, no. 5867 (Feb. 29): 1238–1240.

Semenza, Jan C., and Lisa H. Weasel. 1997. "Molecular Epidemiology in Environmental Health: The Potential of Tumor Suppressor Gene p53 as a Biomarker." *Environmental Health Perspectives* 105, suppl. 1 (Feb): 155–162.

Severance, Craig A. 2009. *Business Risks and Costs of New Nuclear Power.* Accessed from http://climateprogress.org/2009/01/05/study-cost-risks-new-nuclear-plants

Severinghaus, J. P., T. Sowers, E. J. Brooke, R. B. Alley, and M. L. Bender. 1998. "Timing of Abrupt Climate Change at the End of the Younger Dryas Interval from Thermally Fractionated Gases in Polar Ice." *Nature* 391 (Jan. 8): 141–146.

Shankman, Sabrina. 2009. "California Gives Desalination Plants a Fresh Look," *The Wall Street Journal,* July 9, A4.

Shaw, Gary, et al. 1996. "Orofacial Clefts, Parental Cigarette Smoking, and Transforming Growth Factor-Alpha Gene Variants." *American Journal of Human Genetics* 58, no. 3 (March): 551–561.

Sheehan, Molly O. 2003. "Population Growth Slows." *Vital Signs 2003.* New York: Worldwatch/W.W. Norton.

Shertzer, Richard H. 1986. "Wastewater Disinfection—Time for a Change?" *Journal of the Water Pollution Control Federation* 58, no. 3 (March).

Shindell, Drew, and Greg Faluvegi. 2009. "Climate Response to Regional Radiative Forcing During the Twentieth Century." *Nature Geoscience* 2 (April): 294–300.

Siikamaki, Juha. 2008. "Climate Change and U.S. Agriculture: Examining the Connections." *Environment* 50, no. 4 (July/Aug): 37–49.

Simon, Paul. 1998. *Tapped Out.* Welcome Rain Publishers.

Simpson, Kevin. 1997. "Train Kills Teen in B-N," *The Pantagraph,* Bloomington, IL, Oct. 18, A-1.

Smil, Vaclav. 1991. "Population Growth and Nitrogen: An Exploration of a Critical Existential Link." *Population and Development Review* 17, no. 4.

———. 2002. *The Earth's Biosphere: Evolution, Dynamics, and Change.* Cambridge, MA: The MIT Press.

Smith, Joel B., et al. 2008. "Assessing Dangerous Climate Change through an Update of the Intergovernmental Panel on Climate Change (IPCC) 'Reasons for Concern.'" *Proceedings of the National Academy of Sciences,* Dec. 9. Accessed from www.pnas.org/cgi/doi/10.1073/pnas.0812355106

Smith, K. E. et al. 1999. "Quinolone-Resistant *Campylobacter jejuni* Infections in Minnesota, 1992–1998." *New England Journal of Medicine* 340, no. 20 (May 20): 1525–1532.

Smith, Kirk R. 1988. "Air Pollution: Assessing Total Exposure in the United States." *Environment* 30, no. 8 (Oct).

Smith, Robert L. 1986. *Elements of Ecology.* 2nd ed. New York: Harper & Row.

Sohrabi, Mehdi. 1998. "The State-of-the-Art on Worldwide Studies in some Environments with Elevated Naturally Occurring Radioactive Materials (NORM)." *Applied Radiation Isotopes* 49, no. 3: 169–188.

Solomon, Susan, G. K. Plattner, R. Knutti, and P. Friedlingstein. 2009. "Irreversible Climate Change due to Carbon Dioxide Emissions." *Proceedings of the National Academy of Sciences* 106, no. 6 (Feb. 10): 1704–1709.

"Solvents Used in Making Computer Chips Linked to Workers' Miscarriages at IBM." 1992. *Environmental Health Letter,* Sept. 16.

Sontheimer, Richard D. 1992. "Photosensitivity in Lupus Erythematosus." *Lupus News* 12, no. 2.

Spencer, Robert, and Rhodes Yepsen. 2008. "Mixed Waste Composting Trends: Biocycle Nationwide Survey." *Biocycle* 48, no. 11 (Nov): 21–25.

Stauding, Kevin C., and Victor S. Roth. 1998. "Occupational Lead Poisoning." *American Family Physician* 57, no. 4 (Feb. 15): 719–728.

Stavins, Robert. 2009. "What Hath Copenhagen Wrought? A Preliminary Assessment of the Copenhagen Accord." *An Economic View of the Environment,* Belfer Center for Science and International Affairs, John F. Kennedy School of Government, Harvard University (Dec. 20). Accessed from http://belfercenter.ksg.harvard.edu/analysis/stavins/?p=464

Steenland, Kyle, Laurie Piacitelli, James Deddens, Marilyn Fingerhut, and Lih Ing Chang. 1999. "Cancer, Heart Disease, and Diabetes in Workers Exposed to 2,3,7,8–Tetrachlorodibenzo-p-dioxin." *Journal of the National Cancer Institute* 91, no. 9 (May 5): 779–786.

Steffensen, J. P., et al. 2008. "High-Resolution Greenland Ice Core Data Show Abrupt Climate Change Happens in Few Years." *Science* 321 (Aug. 1): 680–683.

Steig, E. J., D. P. Schneider, D. D. Rutherford, M. E. Mann, J. C. Comiso, and D. T. Shindell. 2009. "Warming of the Antarctic Ice-Sheet Surface Since the 1957 International Geophysical Year." *Nature* 45 (Jan. 22): 459–462.

Steingraber, Sandra. 1997. *Living Downstream: An Ecologist Looks at Cancer and the Environment.* Reading, MA: Addison-Wesley.

Steinhardt, Bernice. 1996. *Uranium Mill Tailings: Status and Future Costs of Cleanup.* United States General Accounting Office, GAO/T-RCED-96–85.

Stiling, Peter D. 1992. *Introductory Ecology.* Upper Saddle River, NJ: Prentice Hall.

Stokes, Bruce. 1980. "Men and Family Planning." *Worldwatch Paper* 41. Worldwatch Institute.

Stokstad, Erik. 2004. "Salmon Survey Stokes Debate About Farmed Fish." *Science* 303, no. 5655 (Jan. 9): 154–155.

Stone, Richard. 1992. "Can a Father's Exposure Lead to Illness in his Children?" *Science* 258 (Oct. 2).

Strahler, Arthur N., and Alan H. Strahler. 1973. *Environmental Geoscience.* Hamilton Publishing.

Streffer, Christian. 1997. "Biological Effects of Prenatal Irradiation." *Health Impacts of Large Releases of Radionuclides.* Wiley, Chichester (Ciba Foundation Symposium 203): 155–166.

"Studies Yield Conflicting Findings on Environment's Link to Cancer." 1994. *Environmental Health Letter*, April 27.

Suchanek, Thomas H., Manuel C. Lagunas-Solar, Otto G. Raabe, Roger C. Helm, Fiorella Gielow, Neal Peek, et al. 1996. "Radionuclides in Fishes and Mussels from the Farallon Islands Nuclear Waste Dump Site, California." *Health Physics* 71, no. 2 (Aug): 167–178.

"Sunscreens May Not Afford Protection." 1992. *Environmental Health Letter* (June 12).

Tannahill, Ray. 1973. *Food in History.* New York: Stein and Day.

Tarr, Phillip I., and Michael Doyle. 1996. "Food Safety: Everyone's Responsibility." *Pediatric Basics* no. 78 (Fall): 2–13.

Taub, Eric A. 2009. "Industry Looks to LED Bulbs for the Home," *New York Times*, May 11.

Thacker, Paul D. 2004. "Biological Clock Ticks for Men, Too: Genetic Defects Linked to Sperm of Older Fathers." *Journal of the American Medical Association* 291, no. 14 (April 14): 1683–1685.

Thomas, Chris D., et al. 2004. "Extinction Risk from Climate Change." *Nature* 427 (Jan. 8): 145–148.

Thurston, Floyd E., and Stanley L. Roberts. 1991. "Environmental Noise and Fetal Hearing." *Journal of the Tennessee Medical Association* 84, no. 1 (Jan).

Tobias, Michael. 1998. *World War III: Population and the Biosphere at the End of the Millennium.* New York: Continuum.

Tong, Shilu, Peter A. Baghurst, Michael G. Sawyer, Jane Burns, and Anthony J. McMichael. 1998. "Declining Blood Lead Levels and Changes in Cognitive Function During Childhood: The Port Pirie Cohort Study." *Journal of the American Medical Association* 280, no. 22 (Dec. 9): 1915.

Tong, Van T., Jaime R. Jones, Patricia M. Dietz, Denise D'Angelo, and Jennifer M. Bombard. 2009. "Trends in Smoking Before, During, and After Pregnancy, United States, 2000–2005." *Morbidity & Mortality Weekly Report,* Surveillance Summaries, May 29 (SS04): 1–29.

Tossavainen, Antti. 2004. "Global Use of Asbestos and the Incidence of Mesothelioma." *International Journal of Occupational and Environmental Health* 10, no. 1 (Jan/March): 22–25.

Tournemille, Harry. 2009. "Algae and its Role in Biofuels." *Energyboom Newsletter* (June 12).

Turiel, Isaac. 1985. *Indoor Air Quality and Human Health.* Palo Alto, CA: Stanford Univ. Press.

Tuxill, John. 1998. "Losing Strands in the Web of Life: Vertebrate Declines and the Conservation of Biological Diversity." *Worldwatch Paper* 141 (May).

U.S. Congress. 1991. *Turn It Down: Effects of Noise on Hearing Loss in Children and Youth.* Hearing before the Select House Committee on Children, Youth, and Families, July 22. Washington, DC: U.S. GPO.

U.S. Department of Agriculture (USDA). 1997. *The Conservation Reserve Program.* Farm Services Agency, PA-1603 (May).

U.S. Geological Survey (USGS). 1999. *Many Contaminants Found in Nation's Streams, But Few Drinking Water Standards Exceeded, USGS Report Shows.* News release, USGS Water Resources Division.

U. S. Global Change Research Program (USGCRP). 2009. *Synthesis and Assessment.*

Ultraguard Water Systems Corporation. 2004. *Industry Overview.* Accessed Aug. 27, 2004, from www.ultraguard.com/technology/IndustryOverview

Union of Concerned Scientists. 2001. "Greener Appliances . . . and We Don't Mean Avocado!" *Earthwise* 3, no. 3 (Summer).

United Nations (UN). 2003. *Water for People, Water for Life: The United Nations World Water Development Report.* UNESCO Publishing, Berghahn Books.

United Nations Population Fund (UNFPA). 2003a. *Missing . . . Mapping the Adverse Child Sex Ratio in India* (June).

———. 2003b. *Population Issues: Improving Reproductive Health: Campaign to End Fistula.* Accessed from http://www.unfpa.org/fistula/about.htm

———. 2009. *World Population Prospects: The 2009 Revision.* Extended Dataset, CD-ROM (New York, April 9).

United Nations Programme on HIV/AIDS (UNAIDS). 2008. *Executive Summary: 2008 Report on the Global AIDS Epidemic.* Accessed from http://www.unaids.org/en/KnowledgeCentre/HIVData/GlobalReport/2008/

Urbina, Ian. 2003. "New Jersey Health Officials Warn of Lead in Mexican Grasshopper Treats," *New York Times*, Nov. 21.

Vail, P. V., J. R. Coulson, W. C. Kauffman, and M. E. Dix. 2001. "History of Biological Control Programs in the United States Department of Agriculture." *American Entomologist* 47, no. 1 (Spring).

van Mantgem, Phillip J., et al. 2009. "Widespread Increase of Tree Mortality Rates in the Western United States." *Science* 323 (Jan. 23): 521–524.

Van Noord-Zaadstra, B. M. et al., 1991. "Delaying Childbearing: Effect of Age on Fecundity and Outcome of Pregnancy." *British Medical Journal* 302: 1361.

Viebahn, Peter, Manfred Fischedick, and Daniel Vallentin. 2009. "Carbon Capture and Storage." In *2009 State of the World: Into a Warming World*, 99–102. The Worldwatch Institute. New York: W. W. Norton.

Virta, Robert L. 2006. *Worldwide Asbestos Supply and Consumption Trends from 1900 through 2003.* U.S. Geological Survey. Accessed from http://pubs.usgs.gov/circ/2006/1298/c1298.pdf

Vitousek, Peter M., John D. Aber, Robert W. Howarth, Gene E. Likens, Pamela A. Matson, et al. 1997. "Human Alteration of the Global Nitrogen Cycle: Cases and Consequences." *Issues in Ecology*, no. 1 (Spring). Ecological Society of America.

Vogel, Gretchen. 2009. "Election Heats Up Nuclear Debate." *Science* 325, no. 5948 (Sept. 25): 1612.

Wald, Matthew L. 2009a. "What Now For Nuclear Waste?" *Scientific American* 301, no. 2 (Aug): 46–53.

———. 2009b. "U.S. Panel Shifts Focus to Reusing Nuclear Fuel," *New York Times,* Sept. 24, A26.

Waldbott, George L. 1978. *Health Effects of Environmental Pollutants.* St. Louis: C. V. Mosby.

Wallace, L. A. 1987. *Total Exposure Assessment Methodology* (TEAM Study: Summary and Analysis) 1. Washington, DC: Environmental Protection Agency.

Walsh, Bryan. 2009. "Going Green: Greening This Old House." *Time* 173, no. 17 (May 4): 45–46.

Walsh, Michael P. 2003. "Vehicle Emissions and Health in Developing Countries." In *Air Pollution & Health in Rapidly Developing Countries.* Gordon McGranahan and Frank Murray (eds.). London: Earthscan Publications.

Wang, M., and J. E. Overland. 2009. "A Sea Ice Free Summer Arctic within 30 Years?" *Geophysical Research Letters* 36: L07502. doi: 10.1029/2009GLO37820.

Wang, Wentao, Toby Primbs, Shu Tao, and Staci L. Massey Simonich. 2009. "Atmospheric Particulate Matter Pollution During the 2008 Beijing Olympics." *Environmental Science & Technology* 43 (14): 5314–5320.

Ward, Diane Raines. 2002. *Water Wars: Drought, Flood, Folly, and the Politics of Thirst.* New York: Riverhead Books.

Ware, J. H. et al., 1984. "Passive Smoking, Gas Cooking, and Respiratory Health of Children Living in Six Cities." *American Review of Respiratory Disease* 129: 366–374.

Wargo, John. 2009. *Green Intelligence.* New Haven & London: Yale University Press.

Warkany, J. 1972. "Trends in Teratologic Research." In *Pathobiology of Development.* E. Perrin and M. Finegold (eds.). Baltimore, MD: Williams and Wilkins.

Watson, R. T., H. Rohde, H. Oeschger, and U. Siegenthaler. 1990. "Greenhouse Gases and Aerosols." *Climate Change: The IPCC Scientific Assessment.* J. T. Houghton, G. J. Jenkins, and J. J. Ephraums (eds.). Cambridge: Cambridge University Press.

Watson, Reg, and Daniel Pauly. 2001. "Systematic Distortion in World Fisheries Catch Trends." *Nature* 414 (Nov. 29): 534–536.

Weed Science Society of America (WSSA). 2004. Accessed March 15, 2009, from http://www.weedscience.com/

Weinberg, Robert A. 1998. *One Renegade Cell: How Cancer Begins.* New York: Basic Books.

Weiss, Peter. 1993. "The Contraceptive Potential of Breastfeeding in Bangladesh." *Studies in Family Planning* 24, no. 2 (March/April).

Weisskopf, Michael. 1987. "Japanese Town Still Staggered by Legacy of Ecological Disaster," *The Washington Post,* April 18.

Weitzman, Michael, et al. 1993. "Lead-Contaminated Soil Abatement and Urban Children's Blood Lead Levels." *Journal of the American Medical Association* 269, no. 13 (April 7).

Weller, Phil. 1980. *Acid Rain: The Silent Crisis.* Between the Lines & the Waterloo Public Interest Research Group.

Whittaker, Robert H. 1975. *Communities and Ecosystems.* New York: Macmillan.

Whyatt, R. M., et al. 1998. "Relationship Between Ambient Air Pollution and DNA Damage in Polish Mothers and Newborns." *Environmental Health Perspectives* 106, suppl. 3 (June): 821–826.

Wiencke, John K., et al. 1999. "Early Age at Smoking Initiation and Tobacco Carcinogen DNA Damage in the Lung." *Journal of the National Cancer Institute* 91, no. 7 (April 7): 614–619.

Wiener, Jonathan B. 2009. "Engaging China in Climate Change." *Resources* 171 (Winter/Spring): 29–33.

Wilcove, David S., Margaret McMillan, and Keith C. Winston. 1993. "What Exactly Is an Endangered Species? An Analysis of the U. S. Endangered Species List, 1985–91." *Conservation Biology* 7, no. 1.

Wilford, John Noble. 1991. "The Gradual Greening of Mt. St. Helens," *New York Times,* Oct. 8, B9.

Willett, Walter C. 1994. "Diet and Health: What Should We Eat?" *Science* 264 (April 22).

Williams, Michael. 2006. *Deforesting the Earth: From Prehistory to Global Crisis.* Chicago: The University of Chicago Press.

Wilson, Edward O. 1992. *The Diversity of Life.* Cambridge, MA: Harvard Univ. Press.

Winberry, John J., and David M. Jones. n.d. "Rise and Decline of the Miracle Vine: Kudzu in the Southern Landscape." *Southern Geographer* 13: 2, 61–70.

Wines, Michael. 2009. "Smelter in China Poisons More Than 1,300 Children," *New York Times,* Aug. 21.

"With Holidays Approaching, Work on Blue-Ribbon Panel Appears Delayed." *Nuclear Waste News* 29, no. 1: 1, 7.

Wolfson, Richard. 2008. *Energy, Environment, and Climate.* New York: W.W. Norton.

Wolkomir, Richard, and Joyce Wolkomir. 2001. "Noise Busters." *Smithsonian* 31, no. 12 (March).

Woody, Todd. 2009. "Desert Vistas vs. Solar Power," *New York Times,* Dec. 22, B5.

World Health Organization (WHO). 2004. "Impact of Plague: Human Plague Cases from 1989 to 2003." *Weekly Epidemiological Record* 79: 33.

———. 2009. *Global Prevalence of Vitamin A Deficiency in Populations at Risk: 1995–2005.* Geneva, Switzerland: WHO.

World Resources Institute (WRI). 1998. *World Resources 1998–1999.* New York: Oxford Univ. Press.

———. 1992. *World Resources 1992–1993: Toward Sustainable Development.* New York: Oxford Univ. Press.

———. 1994. *World Resources 1994–1995.* New York: Oxford Univ. Press.

———. 1996. *World Resources 1996–1997.* New York: Oxford Univ. Press.

———. 1998. *World Resources 1998–1999.* New York: Oxford Univ. Press.

———. 2000. *World Resources 2000–2001: People and Ecosystems: The Fraying Web of Life.* New York: Oxford Univ. Press.

Wright, Michal, ed. 1993. *The View from Airlie: Community-Based Conservation in Perspective.* Liz Claiborne and Art Ortenberg Foundation, narrative sampling of discussions during workshop held at Airlie, Virginia, Oct. 17.

Xintaras, Charles. 1992. "Impact of Lead-Contaminated Soil on Public Health." Agency for Toxic Substances and Disease Registry, U.S. Dept. of Health and Human Services (May).

Yardley, Jim. 2003. "Rat Poison: Murder Weapon of Choice in Rural China," *New York Times,* Nov. 17.

———. 2007. "Beneath Booming Cities, China's Future is Drying Up," *New York Times,* Sept. 28.

Yin, J., M. E. Schlesinger, and R. J. Stouffer. 2009. "Model Projections of Rapid Sea-Level Rise on the Northeast Coast of the United States." *Nature Geoscience* 2, no. 4 (April): 262–266.

Yoder, Jonathan S., and Michael J. Beach. 2007. "Cryptosporidiosis Surveillance—United States, 2003–2005." *Morbidity & Mortality Weekly Report,* Surveillance Summaries 56, no. SS-7 (Sept. 7).

Zeng, Ning, Yihui Ding, Jiahua Pan, Huijun Wang, and Jay Gregg. 2008. "Climate Change—The Chinese Challenge." *Science* 319 (Feb. 8): 730–731.

Zimmerman, Peter D., and Cheryl Loeb. 2004. "Dirty Bombs: The Threat Revisited." *Defense Horizons*, no. 38. Center for Technology and National Security Policy, National Defense University.

Index